国家卫生和计划生育委员会"十三五"英文版规划教材
全国高等学校教材

供临床医学专业及来华留学生（MBBS）双语教学用

Clinical Pharmacology

临床药理学 改编教学版 Annotated Edition

Morris J. Brown, Pankaj Sharma, Fraz A. Mir, Peter N. Bennett

主　编　李　俊
Chief Editor　Jun Li

副主编　袁　洪　　何金汗　　汪逊
Vice Chief Editor　Hong Yuan　Jinhan He　Xuanbin Wang

人民卫生出版社
·北京·

图书在版编目（CIP）数据

临床药理学：英、汉／（英）莫瑞斯·布朗
（Morris J. Brown）原著；李俊主编. —北京：人民
卫生出版社，2020.12
全国高等学校临床医学专业第一轮英文版规划教材
ISBN 978-7-117-30925-7

Ⅰ．①临⋯　Ⅱ．①莫⋯②李⋯　Ⅲ．①临床医学－药
理学－医学院校－教材－英、汉　Ⅳ．①R969

中国版本图书馆 CIP 数据核字（2020）第 244187 号

人卫智网　www.ipmph.com	医学教育、学术、考试、健康，	
	购书智慧智能综合服务平台	
人卫官网　www.pmph.com	人卫官方资讯发布平台	

图字：01-2019-6954 号

临床药理学
Linchuang Yaolixue

主　　编：李　俊
出版发行：人民卫生出版社（中继线 010-59780011）
地　　址：北京市朝阳区潘家园南里 19 号
邮　　编：100021
E - mail：pmph @ pmph.com
购书热线：010-59787592　010-59787584　010-65264830
印　　刷：天津安泰印刷有限公司
经　　销：新华书店
开　　本：850×1168　1/16　印张：36
字　　数：1064 千字
版　　次：2020 年 12 月第 1 版
印　　次：2021 年 2 月第 1 次印刷
标准书号：ISBN 978-7-117-30925-7
定　　价：128.00 元

打击盗版举报电话：010-59787491　E-mail：WQ @ pmph.com
质量问题联系电话：010-59787234　E-mail：zhiliang @ pmph.com

编者（按姓氏笔画排序）

石京山
Jingshan Shi
遵义医科大学
Zunyi Medical University

吕雄文
Xiongwen Lv
安徽医科大学
Anhui Medical University

刘叔文
Shuwen Liu
南方医科大学
Southern Medical University

许建华
Jianhua Xu
福建医科大学
Fujian Medical University

孙慧君
Huijun Sun
大连医科大学
Dalian Medical University

李 俊
Jun Li
安徽医科大学
Anhui Medical University

杨 俭
Jian Yang
南京医科大学
Nanjing Medical University

何金汗
Jinhan He
四川大学
Sichuan University

汪选斌
Xuanbin Wang
湖北医药学院
Hubei University of Medicine

张 菁
Jing Zhang
复旦大学
Fudan University

陈 立
Li Chen
吉林大学
Jilin University

招明高
Minggao Zhao
空军军医大学
Air Force Medical University

周家国
Jiaguo Zhou
中山大学
Sun Yat-Sen University

姜远英
Yuanying Jiang
同济大学
Tongji University

袁 洪
Hong Yuan
中南大学
Central South University

袁恒杰
Hengjie Yuan
天津医科大学
Tianjin Medical University

徐 戎
Rong Xu
华中科技大学
Huazhong University of Science and Technology

高分飞
Fenfei Gao
汕头大学
Shantou University

郭秀丽
Xiuli Guo
山东大学
Shandong University

黄仁彬
Renbin Huang
广西医科大学
Guangxi Medical University

董 志
Zhi Dong
重庆医科大学
Chongqing Medical University

魏敏杰
Minjie Wei
中国医科大学
China Medical University

ELSEVIER

Elsevier(Singapore) Pte Ltd.
3 Killiney Road
#08-01 Winsland House I
Singapore 239519
Tel: (65) 6349-0200
Fax: (65) 6733-1817

1995 年,我国首次招收全英文授课医学留学生,到 2015 年,接收临床医学专业 MBBS（Bachelor of Medicine & Bachelor of Surgery）留学生的院校达到了 40 余家,MBBS 院校数量、规模不断扩张;同时,医学院校在临床医学专业五年制、长学制教学中陆续开展不同规模和范围的双语或全英文授课,使得对一套符合我国教学实际、成体系、高质量英文教材的需求日益增长。

为了满足教学需求,进一步落实教育部《关于加强高等学校本科教学工作提高教学质量的若干意见（教高 [2001]4 号）》和《来华留学生医学本科教育（英文授课）质量控制标准暂行规定（教外来 [2007]39 号）》等相关文件的要求,规范和提高我国高等医学院校临床医学专业五年制、长学制和来华留学生（MBBS）双语教学及全英文教学的质量,推进医学双语教学和留学生教育的健康有序发展,完善和规范临床医学专业英文版教材的体系,人民卫生出版社在充分调研的基础上,于 2015 年召开了全国高等学校临床医学专业英文版规划教材的编写论证会,经过会上及会后的反复论证,最终确定组织编写一套全国规划的、适合我国高等医学院校教学实际的临床医学专业英文版教材,并计划作为 2017 年春季和秋季教材在全国出版发行。

本套英文版教材的编写结合国家卫生和计划生育委员会、教育部的总体要求,坚持"三基、五性、三特定"的原则,组织全国各大医学院校、教学医院的专家编写,主要特点如下:

1. 教材编写应教学之需启动,在全国范围进行了广泛、深入调研和论证,借鉴国内外医学人才培养模式和教材建设经验,对主要读者对象、编写模式、编写科目、编者遴选条件等进行了科学设计。

2. 坚持"三基、五性、三特定"和"多级论证"的教材编写原则,组织全国各大医学院校及教学医院有丰富英语教学经验的专家一起编写,以保证高质量出版。

3. 为保证英语表达的准确性和规范性,大部分教材以国外英文原版教科书为蓝本,根据我国教学大纲和人民卫生出版社临床医学专业第八轮规划教材主要内容进行改编,充分体现科学性、权威性、适用性和实用性。

4. 教材内部各环节合理设置,根据读者对象的特点,在英文原版教材的基础上结合需要,增加本章小结、关键术语（英中对照）、思考题、推荐阅读等模块,促进学生自主学习。

本套临床医学专业英文版规划教材共 38 种,均为国家卫生和计划生育委员会"十三五"规划教材,计划于 2017 年全部出版发行。

In 1995, China recruited overseas medical students of full English teaching for the first time. Up to 2015, more than 40 institutions enrolled overseas MBBS (Bachelor of Medicine & Bachelor of Surgery) students. The number of MBBS institutions and overseas students are continuously increasing. At the meantime, medical colleges' application for bilingual or full English teaching in different size and range in five-year and long-term professional clinical medicine teaching results to increasingly demand for a set of practical, systematic and high-qualified English teaching material.

In order to meet the teaching needs and to implement the regulations of relevant documents issued by Ministry of Education including "Some Suggestions to Strengthen the Undergraduate Teaching and to Improve the Teaching Quality" and "Interim Provisions on Quality Control Standards of International Medical Undergraduate Education (English teaching)", as well as to standardize and improve the quality of the bilingual teaching and English teaching of the five-year, long-term and international students (MBBS) of clinical medicine in China's higher medical colleges so as to promote the healthy and orderly development of medical bilingual teaching and international students education and to improve and standardize the system of English clinical medicine textbooks, after full investigation, People's Medical Publishing House (PMPH) held the writing discussion meeting of English textbook for clinical medicine department of national colleges and universities in 2015. After the repeated demonstration in and after the meeting, PMPH ultimately determined to organize the compilation of a set of national planning English textbooks which are suitable for China's actual clinical medicine teaching of medical colleges and universities. This set will be published as spring and autumn textbooks of 2017.

This set of English textbooks meets the overall requirements of the Ministry of Education and National Health and Family Planning Commission, the editorial committee includes the experts from major medical colleges and universities as well as teaching hospitals, the main features are as follows:

1. Textbooks compilation is started to meet the teaching needs, extensive and deep research and demonstration are conducted across the country, the main target readers, the model and subject of compilation and selection conditions of authors are scientifically designed in accordance with the reference of domestic and foreign medical personnel training model and experience in teaching materials.

2. Adhere to the teaching materials compiling principles of "three foundations, five characteristics, and three specialties" and "multi-level demonstration", the organization of English teaching experts with rich experience from major medical schools and teaching hospitals ensures the high quality of publication.

3. In order to ensure the accuracy and standardization of English expression, most of the textbooks are modeled on original English textbooks, and adapted based on national syllabus and main content of the eighth round of clinical medicine textbooks which were published by PMPH, fully reflecting the scientificity, authority, applicability and practicality.

4. All aspects of teaching materials are arranged reasonably, based on original textbooks,the chapter summary, key terms (English and Chinese), review questions, and recommended readings are added to promote students' independent learning in accordance with teaching needs and the characteristics of the target readers.

This set of English textbooks for clinical medicine includes 38 species which are among "13th Five-Year" planning textbooks of National Health and Family Planning Commission, and will be all published in 2017.

全国高等学校临床医学专业第一轮英文版规划教材 · 教材目录

教材名称		主 审	主编
28 皮肤性病学	Dermatovenereology	陈洪铎	高兴华
29 肿瘤学	Oncology		石远凯
30 眼科学	Ophthalmology		杨培增 刘奕志
31 康复医学	Rehabilitation Medicine		虞乐华
32 医学心理学	Medical Psychology		赵旭东
33 耳鼻咽喉头颈外科学	Otorhinolaryngology-Head and Neck Surgery		孔维佳
34 急诊医学	Emergency Medicine		陈玉国
35 法医学	Forensic Medicine		赵 虎
36 全球健康学	Global Health		吴群红
37 中医学	Chinese Medicine		王新华
38 医学汉语	Medical Chinese		李 骢

ADAPTATION PREFACE

Clinical pharmacology is an important subject plays a major role in clinical application of medical science and clinical drug treatment. The development of clinical pharmacology is relating to a number of fields and providing the scientific basis for safe and effective drug therapy. Overall framework of the twelfth edition of clinical pharmacology is refers to the eleventh edition, clinical pharmacology is rapidly changing, we have made some adjustments according to China's clinical pharmacology textbooks.

We introduce the classification of drugs used in common clinical diseases based on novel recent studies with straightforward language, improving clinical medication and focusing on clinical evaluation of drugs. In the process of revision, we keep the pre-writing style and combine the English-language clinical pharmacology textbooks, in addition, we absorb related latest research achievements. The twelfth edition of clinical pharmacology is tailored to the requirements of safe, effective, economical and clinical medication.

All editors thank the Elsevier Press for authorizing this edition of clinical pharmacology.

I appreciate all editors in editorial board who prepared the modification of clinical pharmacology. Finally, we also thank for our students, who are careful reading and feedback of each chapter.

Jun Li

DEDICATION

And I will use regimens for the benefit of the ill in accordance with my ability and my judgement.

The Hippocratic Oath c.400 BC

But doctors are lucky: the sun shines on their successes and the earth hides their failures.

Michael de Montaigne 1533–1592

Morals do not forbid making experiments on one's neighbour or on one's self … among the experiments that may be tried on man, those that can only harm are forbidden, those that are innocent are permissible, and those that may do good are obligatory.

Claude Bernard 1813–1878

It may seem a strange principle to enunciate as the very first requirement in a Hospital that it should do the sick no harm.

Florence Nightingale 1820–1910

The ingenuity of man has ever been fond of exerting itself to varied forms and combinations of medicines.

William Withering 1741–1799

A desire to take medicine is, perhaps, the great feature which distinguishes man from other animals.

William Osler 1849–1920

All things are poisons and there is nothing that is harmless, the dose alone decides that something is no poison.

Paracelsus 1493–1541

Medical science aims at the truth and nothing but the truth.

William J Mayo 1861–1939

What we find in books is like the fire in our hearths. We fetch it from our neighbors, we kindle it at home, we communicate it to others, and it becomes the property of all.

Voltaire 1694–1778

PREFACE

For your own satisfaction and for mine, please read this preface![1]

A preface should tell the prospective reader about the subject of a book, its purpose and its plan. This book is about the scientific basis and practice of drug therapy. It addresses medical students and doctors in particular, but also anyone concerned with evidence-based drug therapy and prescribing.

The scope and rate of drug innovation increase. Doctors now face a professional lifetime of handling drugs that are new to themselves – drugs that do new things as well as drugs that do old things better – and drugs that were familiar during medical training become redundant.

We write not only for readers who, like us, have a special interest in pharmacology. We try to make pharmacology understandable for those whose primary interests lie elsewhere but who recognise that they need some knowledge of pharmacology if they are to meet their moral and legal 'duty of care' to their patients. We are aware, too, of medical curricular pressures that would reduce the time devoted to teaching clinical pharmacology and therapeutics, and such diminution is surely a misguided policy for a subject that is so integral to the successful practice of medicine. Thus, we try to tell readers what they need to know without burdening them with irrelevant information, and we try to make the subject interesting. We are very serious, but seriousness does not always demand wearying solemnity.

All who prescribe drugs would be wise to keep in mind the changing and ever more exacting expectations of patients and of society in general. Doctors who prescribe casually or ignorantly now face not only increasing criticism but also civil (or even criminal) legal charges. The ability to handle new developments depends, now more than ever, on comprehension of the principles of pharmacology. These principles are not difficult to grasp and are not so many as to defeat even the busiest doctors who take upon themselves the responsibility of introducing manufactured medicines into the bodies of their patients. The exercise of prescribing calls for the meticulous selection of medicines and so the avoidance of polypharmacy, which now seems rampant.

The principles of pharmacology and drug therapy appear in Chapters 1–11 and their application in the subsequent specialist chapters, where we draw on the knowledge and authority of a range of experts, to whom we express our gratitude. The names of those who contributed to the present and previous editions appear on subsequent pages.

We seek to offer a reasonably brief solution to the problem of combining practical clinical utility with an account of the principles on which clinical practice rests.

The quantity of practical technical detail to include is a matter of judgment. In general, where therapeutic practices are complex, potentially dangerous or commonly updated, e.g. anaphylactic shock, we provide more detail, together with websites for the latest advice; we give less or even no detail on therapy that specialists undertake, e.g. anticancer drugs. Nevertheless, especially with modern drugs

---

[1] St Francis of Sales: Preface to *Introduction to the devout life* (1609).

that are unfamiliar, prescribers should consult formularies, approved guidelines or the manufacturer's current literature, relevant to their country and region of practice.

Use of the book. Francis Bacon[2] wrote that 'Some books are to be tasted, others to be swallowed, and some few to be chewed and digested.' Perhaps elements of each activity can apply to parts of our text. Students and doctors are, or should be, concerned to understand and to develop a rational, critical attitude to drug therapy, and they should therefore chiefly address issues of how drugs act and interact in disease and how evidence of therapeutic effect is obtained and evaluated.

To this end, they should read selectively and should not impede themselves by attempts to memorise lists of alternative drugs and doses and minor differences among them, which should never be required of them in examinations. Thus, we do not encumber the text with exhaustive lists of preparations, which properly belong in a formulary, although we hope that enough has been mentioned to cover much routine prescribing, and many drugs have been included solely for identification.

The role and status of a textbook. In this computer age, a textbook still plays a coveted role. Unlike electronic search engines, a textbook allows one to browse and amble a route to the question posed, perhaps acquiring information along the way that one had never thought existed. We aspire to provide one such route.

A useful guide to drug use must offer clear conclusions and advice. If it is to be of reasonable size, it may often omit alternative acceptable courses of action. What it recommends should rest on sound evidence, where this exists, and on an assessment of the opinions of the experienced where it does not.

Increasingly, guidelines produced by specialist societies and national and international bodies have influenced the selection of drugs. We provide or refer to these as representing a consensus of best practice in particular situations. Similarly, we assume that the reader possesses a formulary, local or national, that will provide guidance on the availability, including doses, of a broad range of drugs. Yet the practice of medicinal therapeutics by properly educated and conscientious doctors working in settings complicated by intercurrent disease, metabolic differences or personality, involves challenges beyond the rigid adherence to published recommendations. The role of a textbook is to provide the satisfaction of understanding the basis for a recommended course of action and to achieve an optimal result by informed selection and use of drugs. In this our twelfth edition, we can but reassert our belief in this principle. The textbook is dead: long live the textbook.

MJB, PS, FAM, PNB

---

[2] Francis Bacon (1561–1626) *Essays* (1625) 'Of studies'. Philosopher and scientist, Bacon introduced the idea of the experimental or inductive method of reasoning for understanding nature.

CONTRIBUTORS

Mark Abrahams MB ChB DA FRCA FFPMRCA
Clinical Director,
Musculoskeletal Services,
Cambridge University Hospitals NHS Foundation
Trust,
Cambridge, UK
Chapter 18 Pain and analgesics

Graeme Alexander MB ChB, MA, MD, FRCP
UCL Professor, Institute for Liver and Digestive
Health, Royal Free Hospital Pond St, Hampstead,
London, UK.
Chapter 34 Liver and biliary tract

Sani H Aliyu MBBS FRCP FRCPath
Consultant in Microbiology and Infectious Diseases,
Cambridge University Hospitals NHS Foundation
Trust,
Cambridge, UK
Chapter 15 Viral, fungal, protozoal and helminthic
infections

John Louis-Auguste BA MB ChB MRCP
Specialist Registrar in Gastroenterology,
Charing Cross Hospital,
London, UK
Chapter 32 Oesophagus, stomach and duodenum,
Chapter 33 Intestines

Trevor Baglin MA MB Ch B PhD FRCP FRCPath
Consultant Haematologist,
Cambridge University Hospitals NHS Foundation
Trust,
Cambridge University Teaching Hospitals NHS
Trust,
Cambridge, UK
Chapter 29 Drugs and haemostasis

Devinder Singh Bansi BM DM FRCP
Consultant Gastroenterologist,
Imperial College Healthcare NHS Trust,
London, UK
Chapter 32 Oesophagus, stomach and duodenum,
Chapter 33 Intestines

Paul Bentley MA, MRCP, PhD
Clinical Senior Lecturer and Honorary Consultant in
Neurology and Stroke Medicine,
Imperial College,
London, UK
Chapter 21 Neurological disorders – epilepsy, Par-
kinson's disease and multiple sclerosis

**Blanca M. Bolea-Alamanac MD MSc (Affective
Neuroscience) PhD**
Assistant Professor,
Department of Psychiatry,
University of Toronto and Staff Psychiatrist,
Centre for Addiction and Mental Health, Toronto,
Canada
Chapter 20 Psychotropic drugs

Chrysothemis Brown MA MBBS PhD MRCPCH
Wellcome Trust Post-doctoral Clinical Research
Fellow,
Institute of Child Health,
UCL,
London, UK
Chapter 39 Vitamins, calcium, bone

Diana C. Brown MD MSc FRCP
Consultant Endocrinologist,
BUPA Cromwell Hospital,
London, UK

Chapter 35 Adrenal corticosteroids, antagonists, corticotrophin, Chapter 37 Thyroid hormones, anti-thyroid drugs

Simon Davies DM (Oxon) MBBS MRCPsych MSc (Epidemiol) MSc (Affective Neuroscience)
Associate Professor,
Department of Psychiatry,
University of Toronto and Staff Psychiatrist,
Centre for Addiction and Mental Health, Toronto,
Canada
Chapter 20 Psychotropic drugs

David A. Enoch BSc MBBS MSc MRCP FRCPath DTM&H
Consultant Medical Microbiologist,
Clinical Microbiology & Public Health Laboratory,
National Infection Service
Public Health England,
Cambridge University Hospitals NHS Foundation Trust,
Cambridge, UK
Chapter 12 Chemotherapy of infections, Chapter 13 Antibacterial drugs, Chapter 14 Chemotherapy of bacterial infections

Wendy N. Erber MBBS MD DPhil FRCPath FRCPA FAHMS
Pro Vice-Chancellor & Executive Dean and Professor of Pathology and Laboratory Medicine,
Faculty of Health and Medical Sciences,
University of Western Australia,
Perth, Australia
Chapter 30 Red blood cell disorders

Mark Evans MD FRCP
University Lecturer,
University of Cambridge;
Honorary Consultant Physician,
Wellcome Trust/MRC Institute of Metabolic Science,
Cambridge University Hospitals Foundation Trust,
Cambridge, UK
Chapter 36 Diabetes mellitus, insulin, oral antidiabetes agents, obesity

Mark Farrington MA MB BChir FRCPath
Consultant Medical Microbiologist,
National Infection Service, Public Health England,
Cambridge University Hospitals NHS Foundation Trust,
Cambridge, UK
Chapter 12 Chemotherapy of infections, Chapter 13 Antibacterial drugs, Chapter 14 Chemotherapy of bacterial infections

Andrew Grace MB PhD FRCP FACC FESC FAHA
Research Group Head,
Department of Biochemistry,
University of Cambridge;
Consultant Cardiologist,
Cambridge University Health Partners,
Cambridge, UK
Chapter 25 Cardiac arrhythmia

Thomas K. K. Ha MD FRACP FRCP
Consultant Dermatologist,
Cambridge University Hospitals NHS Foundation Trust,
Cambridge, UK
Chapter 17 Drugs and the skin

Charlotte Hateley MBBS MRes MRCP (UK) DTM&H
ST3 Gastroenterology and Hepatology Registrar,
Imperial College Healthcare NHS Trust,
London, UK
Chapter 32 Oesophagus, stomach and duodenum, Chapter 33 Intestines

Stephen Haydock PhD FRCP
Consultant Physician,
Musgrove Park Hospital,
Taunton, UK
Chapter 10 Poisoning, overdose, antidotes, Chapter 11 Drug dependence

Thomas F. Hiemstra PhD FRCPE
University Lecturer in Trials,
University of Cambridge;
Honorary Consultant Nephrologist,

Cambridge University Hospitals NHS Foundation Trust,
Cambridge, UK

Chapter 27 Kidney and genitourinary tract

Ian Hudson BSc MBBS MD DCH DipPharmMed FFPM FRCP
Chief Executive,
Medicines and Healthcare Products Regulatory Agency

Chapter 4 Evaluation of drugs in humans,Chapter 6 Regulation of medicines

Lucinda Kennard BSc MBBS MRCP (UK) AFHEA
Specialist Registrar in Clinical Pharmacology & Allergy,
Cambridge University Hospitals NHS Foundation Trust,
Cambridge, UK

Chapter 28 Respiratory system

Mike Laffan DM FRCP FRCPath
Professor of Haemostasis and Thrombosis,
Centre for Haematology,
Imperial College,
London, UK

Chapter 29 Drugs and haemostasis

Michael C. Lee MBBS FRCA PhD FFPMRCA
Consultant and University Lecturer,
Department of Medicine,
Division of Anaesthesia,
University of Cambridge,
Cambridge, UK

Chapter 18 Pain and analgesics

Keith MacDonald MSc BSc (Hons) DipRadPharmSci FRPharmS
Deputy Director, Licensing Division,
Medicines and Healthcare Products Regulatory Agency, London, UK

Chapter 6 Regulation of medicines

Justin C. Mason PhD FRCP
Professor of Vascular Rheumatology,
Imperial College,
London, UK

Chapter 16 Drugs for inflammation and joint disease

Karim Meeran MD FRCP FRCPath
Professor of Endocrinology,
Faculty of Medicine,
Imperial College,
London, UK

Chapter 38 Hypothalamic, pituitary and sex hormones

Jerry P. Nolan FRCA FRCP FFICM FRCEM (Hon)
Honorary Professor of Resuscitation Medicine,
School of Clinical Sciences,
University of Bristol;
Consultant in Anaesthesia & Intensive Care Medicine,
Royal United Hospital,
Bath, UK

Chapter 19 Anaesthesia and neuromuscular block

David Nutt DM FRCP FRCPsych FMedSci
The Edmond J Safra Chair in Neuropsychopharmacology,
Imperial College,
London, UK

Chapter 20 Psychotropic drugs

Sir Munir Pirmohamed MB ChB (Hons) PhD FRCP FRCP(E) FBPhS FMedSci
David Weatherall Chair of Medicine and NHS Chair of Pharmacogenetics,
University of Liverpool;
Associate Executive Pro-Vice Chancellor for Clinical Research,
University of Liverpool;
Director,
MRC Centre for Drug Safety Science and Wolfson Centre for Personalised Medicine,
Liverpool, UK

Chapter 8 General pharmacology

June Raine BM BCh MSc FRCP
Director,
Vigilance and Risk Management of Medicines,
Medicines and Healthcare Products, Regulatory Agency,
London, UK

Chapter 4 Evaluation of drugs in humans, Chapter 6 Regulation of medicines

Sir Michael Rawlins GBE MD FRCP FMedSci
Chair,
Medicines and Healthcare Products Regulatory
Agency (MHRA),
London, UK
Chapter 5 Health technology assessment

John P. D. Reckless DSc, MD, FRCP
Honorary Reader,
University of Bath,
Bath, UK
Chapter 26 Hyperlipidaemias

Mike Schachter MB BSc FRCP
Principal Teaching Fellow in Clinical Pharmacology,
Imperial College,
London, UK
Chapter 1 Clinical pharmacology, Chapter 2 Topics
in drug therapy, Chapter 8 General pharmacology,
Chapter 9 Unwanted effects and adverse drug reactions

Surender K. Sharma MD PhD
Chief,
Division of Pulmonary,
Critical Care and Sleep Medicine;
Head,
Department of Medicine;
All India Institute of Medical Sciences,
New Delhi, India
Chapter 14 Chemotherapy of bacterial infections

M. Hasib Sidiqi MBBS FRACP FRCPA
Advance Hematology Fellow,
Mayo Clinic Rochester, MN, USA;
Clinical Lecturer,
University of Western Australia,
Perth, Australia
Chapter 30 Red blood cell disorders

Rahat Tauni BSc MBBS (Hons) MRCP CertMedEd
Specialist Registrar,
Diabetes and Endocrinology,
Cambridge University Hospitals NHS Foundation
Trust,
Cambridge, UK
Chapter 36 Diabetes mellitus, insulin, oral antidiabetes agents, obesity

Clare Thornton PhD MRCP (Rheum)
Consultant Rheumatologist,
Homerton University Hospital,
London, UK
Chapter 16 Drugs for inflammation and joint disease

Patrick Vallance FRCP FMedSci FRS
President Research and Development,
GlaxoSmithKline,
Brentford, UK
Chapter 3 Discovery and development of drugs

Harpreet Wasan MBBS FRCP
Consultant & Reader in Medical Oncology,
Hammersmith Hospital,
Imperial College Healthcare NHS Trust,
London, UK
Chapter 31 Neoplastic disease and immunosuppression

ACKNOWLEDGEMENTS

The present work reflects our wide reuse of material by those who wrote chapters for previous editions of this book. The editors have pleasure in acknowledging their proficiency and take this opportunity of expressing to them our grateful thanks. Those who contributed to the tenth edition are:

Dr Nigel S Baber (Chapters 4, 5, 7, 8), Professor Sir Peter Rubin (Chapter 3), Dr Francis Hall (Chapter 16), Dr Charles R J Singer (Chapter 30), Dr Pippa G Corrie and Dr Charles R J Singer (Chapter 31), Dr Michael Davis (Chapters 33, 34, 35), Dr Gerard S Conway (Chapter 38).

MJB, PS, FAM, PNB

CONTENTS

Chapter | 1 |

Clinical pharmacology

Clinical pharmacology comprises all aspects of the scientific study of drugs in humans. Its objective is to optimize drug therapy and it is justified in so far as it is put to practical use.

The use of drugs to increase human happiness by elimination or suppression of diseases and symptoms and to improve the quality of life in other ways is a serious matter and involves not only technical, but also psychosocial considerations. Overall, the major benefits of modern drugs are on quality of life (measured with difficulty), and exceed those on quantity of life (measured with ease). In some situations we can attempt both objectives.

Medicines are part of our way of life from birth, when we may enter the world with the aid of drugs, to death, where drugs assist (most of) us to depart with minimal distress and perhaps even with a remnant of dignity. In between these events we regulate our fertility, often, with drugs. We tend to take such usages for granted.

But during the intervals remaining, an average family experiences illness on 1 day in 4 and between the ages of 20 and 45 years a lower-middle-class man experiences approximately one life-endangering illness, 20 disabling (temporarily) illnesses, 200 nondisabling illnesses and 1000 symptomatic episodes: the average person in the USA can expect to have about 12 years of bad health in an average lifespan, and medicines play a major role: 'At any time, 40%–50% of adults [UK] are taking a prescribed medicine.'

Over the centuries humans have sought relief from discomfort in 'remedies' concocted from parts of plants, animals and other sources; numerous formularies attest to their numbers and complexity. Gradually, a more critical view emerged, recognising the need for proper investigation of medications. In 1690, John Locke was moved to write, 'we should be able to tell beforehand that rhubarb will purge, hemlock kill, and opium make a man sleep...'.

Yet it was only in the early years of the 20th century that we began to see the use of specific chemical substances to achieve particular biological effects; that is, the exact science of drug action, which is pharmacology. Subsequently the discipline underwent a major expansion resulting from technology that allowed the understanding of molecular action and the capacity to exploit this. The potential consequences for drug therapy are enormous. All cellular mechanisms (normal and pathological), in their immense complexity, are, in principle, identifiable. What seems almost an infinite number of substances, transmitters, local hormones, cell growth factors, can be made, modified and tested to provide agonists, partial agonists, inverse agonists and antagonists. Moreover, the unravelling of the human genome opens the way for interference with disease processes in ways that were never thought possible before now.

Increasingly large numbers of substances will deserve to be investigated and used for altering physiology to the advantage of humans. With all these developments, and their potential for good, comes capacity for harm, whether inherent in the substances themselves or resulting from human mis-application. Successful use of the power conferred (by biotechnology in particular) requires understanding of the growing evidence base of the true consequences of interference. The temporary celebrity of new drugs is not a new phenomenon. Jean Nicholas Corvisart (1755—1821) reputedly expressed the issue in the dictum: 'Here is a new remedy; take it fast, as long as it still works'.

Clinical pharmacology provides the scientific basis for:

- the general aspects of rational, safe and effective drug therapy
- drug therapy of individual diseases
- the safe introduction of new medicines.

The drug and information explosion of the past six decades, combined with medical need, has called into being a new discipline, clinical pharmacology. The discipline finds recognition as both a health-care and an academic specialty; indeed, no medical school can be considered complete without a department or sub-department of clinical pharmacology.

A signal pioneer was Harry Gold (1899—1972), of Cornell University, USA, whose influential studies in the 1930s showed the qualities needed to be a clinical pharmacologist. In 1952, he wrote in a seminal article:

a special kind of investigator is required, one whose training has equipped him not only with the principles and technics of laboratory pharmacology but also with knowledge of clinical medicine...

Clinical scientists of all kinds do not differ fundamentally from other biologists; they are set apart only to the extent that there are special difficulties and limitations, ethical and practical, in seeking knowledge from man.

Willingness to learn the principles of pharmacology, and how to apply them in individual circumstances of infinite variety is vital to success without harm: to maximize benefit and minimise risk. All of these issues are the concern of clinical pharmacology and are the subject of this book.

More detailed aspects comprise:

1. Pharmacology
   - Pharmacodynamics: how drugs, alone and in combination, affect the body (young, old, well, sick).
   - Pharmacokinetics: absorption, distribution, metabolism, excretion or how the body – well or sick – affects drugs.
2. Therapeutic evaluation
   - Whether a drug is of value.
   - How it may best be used.
   - Formal therapeutic trials.
   - Surveillance studies for both efficacy and safety (adverse effects) – pharmacoepidemiology and pharmacovigilance.
3. Control
   - Rational prescribing and formularies.
   - Official regulation of medicines.
   - Social aspects of the use and misuse of medicines.
   - Pharmacoeconomics.

Clinical pharmacology finds expression in concert with other clinical specialties. Therapeutic success with drugs is becoming more and more dependent on the user having at least an outline understanding of both pharmacodynamics and pharmacokinetics. This outline is quite simple and easy to acquire. However humane and caring doctors may be, they cannot dispense with scientific skill. Knowledge of clinical pharmacology underpins decisions in therapeutics, which is concerned with the prevention, suppression or cure of disease and, from the point of view of society, is the most vital aspect of medicine.

Pharmacology is the same science whether it investigates animals or humans. The need for it grows rapidly as not only scientists, but now the whole community, can see its promise of release from distress and premature death over yet wider fields. The concomitant dangers of drugs (fetal deformities, adverse reactions, dependence) only add to the need for the systematic and ethical application of science to drug development, evaluation and use, i.e. clinical pharmacology.

IMPORTANT TERMINOLOGY

clinical pharmacology　临床药理学

pharmacoepidemiology　药物流行病学

pharmacovigilance　药物警戒

pharmacoeconomics　药物经济学

CHALLENGE YOURSELF

1. Please descript the subject of clinical pharmacology.
2. Please descript the application of clinical pharmacology.
3. Please descript that what clinical pharmacology provides the scientific basis for.

Jun Li

Chapter 2

Discovery and development of drugs

MAKING A NEW MEDICINE

Discovering and developing a new medicine requires combining the skills of biology, chemistry, clinical medicine and, of course, pharmacology. There are three key decision points along the way:

- Selecting the molecular target you want the drug to act on to produce the desired effect.
- Choosing the right chemical as the drug candidate. All the promise and all the faults become fixed at this point.
- Designing the right clinical experiment to show that the medicine will really do what you want it to do.

Medicinal therapeutics rests on the two great supporting pillars of pharmacology:

1. Selectivity – the desired effect alone is obtained.
2. Dose – The dose alone decides that something is no poison.

Once a target has been selected the process of finding the right chemical to act as an antagonist, agonist, inhibitor, activator or modulator of the protein function depends on a process of screening. For decades, the rational discovery of new medicines depended on modifications of the structures of natural chemical mediators. This may still be the route to find the drug, but more often now large libraries of compounds are screened against the target in robotic high throughput screens. However, it is worth remembering that the exact molecular basis of drug action may remain unknown, and this book contains frequent examples of old drugs whose mechanism of action remains mysterious. The evolution of molecular biology (including recombinant DNA technology) in the past 30 years has led to identification of many thousands of potential drug targets, but the function of many of these genes remains unknown. The hope was that the identification of targets identified by genetics coupled with high throughout screening would lead to a great increase in the productivity of drug discovery. This has turned out not to be the case since it is clearly important to understand both the function of the target and the nature of the interaction of the chemical drug with the target in order to make a selective and safe medicine. The skills of quantitative pharmacology are key.

The chances of discovering a truly novel medicine, i.e. one that does something valuable for patients that had previously not been possible (that does safely what could previously have been achieved only with substantial risk), are increased when the discovery and development programme is founded on precise knowledge of the biological processes it is desired to change. The commercial rewards of a successful product are potentially enormous and provide a great incentive for developers to invest and risk huge sums of money. Most projects in drug discovery and development fail. Indeed the chances of making it through from target selection to having a medicine on the market are under 1 in 100.

The huge increase in understanding of molecular signalling – both between cells and within cells – has opened many new opportunities to develop medicines that can target discrete steps in the body's elaborate pathways of chemical reactions. The challenge, of course, is to do so in a way that produces benefit without harm. The more fundamental the pathway targeted the more likely there is to be a big effect, whether beneficial, harmful or both. No benefit comes without some risk.

The industrialised and automated approach to drug discovery that followed sequencing of the genome and application of high throughput chemical approaches led to two consequences:

1. More potential drugs and therapeutic targets were identified that could be experimentally validated in animals and humans. This 'production line' approach also led to a loss of integration of the established specialities (chemistry, biochemistry, pharmacology) and to an overall lack of understanding of how physiological and pathophysiological processes contribute to the interaction of drug and disease.

2. Theoretically, new drugs could be targeted at selected groups of patients based on their genetic make-up. This concept of 'the right medicine for the right patient' is the basis of pharmacogenetics, the genetically determined variability in drug response. Pharmacogenetics has gained momentum from recent advances in molecular genetics and genome sequencing, due to:

- rapid screening for gene variants.
- knowledge of the genetic sequences of target genes such as those coding for enzymes, ion channels, and other receptor types involved in drug response.

Expectations of pharmacogenetics and its progeny, pharmacoproteomics (understanding of and drug effects on protein variants) remain high, but the applicability will not be universal. They include the following:

- The identification of subgroups of patients with a disease or syndrome based on their genotype. The most extreme of obvious examples of this are diseases caused by single gene defects. The ability accurately to subclassify based on common genetic variation is less clear.
- Targeting of specific drugs for patients with specific gene variants. This is most advanced in the field of cancer (usually targeting somatic changes in cancers) and increasingly in the field of the pharmacogenetics of safety (i.e. unwanted drug effects).

Consequences of these expectations include: smaller clinical trial programmes with well-defined patient groups (based on phenotypic and genotypic characterisation), better understanding of the pharmacokinetics and dynamics according to genetic variation, and improved monitoring of adverse events after marketing.

New drug development proceeds thus:

- Idea or hypothesis. 'This protein causes this disease/these effects which I could stop by affecting protein function.'
- Design and synthesis of substances. 'This molecule produces the wanted effect on protein function and has the physico-chemical characteristics that make it a potential medicine.'
- Studies on tissues and whole animal (preclinical studies). 'When I test it in appropriate models it does what I expect and that allows me to believe it would do the same in humans.'
- Studies in humans (clinical studies). 'Initially I want to know whether the molecule has drug-like properties in terms of its kinetics. I then want to know that it does what I need it to do in terms of the effect on disease.'
- Granting of an official licence to make therapeutic claims and to sell. 'Is my medicine better than placebo? Does it do more than existing medicines and is it well tolerated.'
- Post-licensing (marketing) studies of safety and comparisons with other medicines. 'Now many thousands of patients have taken it, am I still sure that it is safe.'

The (critical) phase of progress from the laboratory to humans is often termed translational science or experimental medicine. It was defined as 'the application of biomedical research (pre-clinical and clinical), conducted to support drug development, which aids in the identification of the appropriate patient for treatment (patient selection), the correct dose and schedule to be tested in the clinic (dosing regimen) and the best disease in which to test a potential agent'.

It will be obvious from the account that follows that drug development is an extremely arduous, highly technical and enormously expensive operation. Successful developments (1% of compounds that proceed to full test eventually become licensed medicines) must carry the cost of the failures (99%). It is also obvious that such programmes are likely to be carried to completion only when the organizations and the individuals within them are motivated overall by the challenge to succeed and to serve society, as well as to make money. A previous edition of this chapter included a quote from a paper I wrote from my time in academia and I leave it here:

Let us get one thing straight: the drug industry works within a system that demands it makes a profit to satisfy shareholders. Indeed, it has a fiduciary duty to do so. The best way to make a lot of money is to invent a drug that produces a dramatically beneficial clinical effect, is far more effective than existing options, and has few unwanted effects. Unfortunately most drugs fall short of this ideal.

TECHNIQUES OF DISCOVERY

Drug discovery sources in context. Different types of chemical compounds (top left) are tested against bioassays that are relevant to therapeutic targets, which are derived from several possible sources of information (right). The initial lead compounds discovered by the screening process are optimised by analogue synthesis and tested for appropriate pharmacokinetic properties. The candidate compounds then enter the development process involving regulatory toxicology studies and clinical trials.

Molecular modelling and structural biology aided by three-dimensional computer graphics (including virtual reality) allows the design of structures based on new and known molecules to enhance their desired, and to eliminate their undesired, properties to create highly selective targeted compounds. In principle all molecular structures capable of binding to a single high-affinity site can be modeled.

High throughput screening allows the screening of millions of compounds against a single target or a cell-based screen to determine activity against the target. Traditionally these are large robotic screens but newer technologies, including use of small molecules using coding tags, allow miniaturisation of the process. The quality of the 'hit' which is the starting point for medicinal chemistry 'lead optimisation', depends on the quality of the molecules in the compound collection and the nature of the biochemical target used for the screen.

Fragments. If the crystal structure of the protein target is known it is possible to screen small fragments of potential drugs to find those that bind and where they bind. It is then possible to construct a drug by adding fragments.

Proteins as medicines: biotechnology. The targets of most drugs are proteins (cell receptors, enzymes) and it is only lack of technology that has hitherto prevented the exploitation of proteins (and peptides) as medicines. This technology is now available and some of the most successful new medicines of the last few years have been biological – antibodies or proteins. The practical limitations are that ① they need to be injected, as they are digested when swallowed and ② they target soluble factors and targets on the cell membrane but are generally unable to target intracellular proteins. However, these limitations are offset by their high degree of specificity, their often very long halflife (for antibodies) that means that the medicine may be given by monthly injections, and the more predictable toxicity when compared to the rather unpredictable effect of classical small molecule drugs (the usual 'white pills'). Biotechnology involves the use of recombinant DNA technology/genetic engineering to clone and express human genes, for example in microbial (*Escherichia coli or yeast*) or mammalian (Chinese hamster ovary, CHO) cells so that they manufacture proteins. Such techniques can deliver hormones and autacoids in commercial amounts (such as insulin and growth hormone, erythropoietins, cell growth factors and plasminogen activators, interferons, vaccines and – probably most important – antibodies).

Transgenic animals (that breed true for the gene) are also used as models for human disease as well as for production of medicines.

Antisense approaches. Nucleic acid approaches are being developed to silence gene expression and therefore reduce the expression of culprit proteins. There are various different ways of achieving this including antisense, locked nucleic acids, small interfering RNAs, and interfering with microRNAs. The problems are ① delivery – they are injectables, ② the distribution in the body – mainly liver and kidney – and ③ the difficulty in getting the nucleic acid into cells. Nonetheless, where the treatment aim is local (intraocular injection or inhalation to the lung), or where a liver effect is desired, it is clear that this approach works and provides a potentially attractive approach to targeting those proteins or protein–protein interactions that are intractable to a small molecule, peptide or antibody approach.

Gene therapy of human genetic disorders is 'a strategy in which nucleic acid, usually in the form of DNA, is administered to modify the genetic repertoire for therapeutic purposes', e.g. in diseases caused by single gene defects. Once again significant problems remain, in particular the methods of delivery and the safety and efficiency of the vectors used to deliver the genes. So far success has been seen in the treatment of certain rare haemopoetic disorders and genetic immunodeficiency states where the gene transfer can be done ex vivo and the modified cells reinjected.

Stem cells. Stem cells are impacting drug discovery as they potentially provide a source of human cells, or even disease-specific human cells that can be used for screening and safety testing. Stem cell therapy is a reality in the form of bone marrow transplants but in other areas is still at a very early stage. However, the promise is of regenerative treatments based either on stem cell replacement or chemical stimulation of endogenous stem cells.

Immunopharmacology. Understanding of the molecular basis of immune responses has allowed the definition of mechanisms by which cellular function is altered by a legion of local hormones or autacoids in, for example, infections, cancer, autoimmune diseases, organ transplant rejection. These processes present targets for therapeutic intervention – hence the rise of immunopharmacology.

Older approaches to the discovery of new medicines that continue in use include:

- Animal models of human disease or an aspect of it of varying relevance to humans. It is always the case that the animal model is never a true model of human disease and can only model parts of the disease process. The trend in industry is to move fast to the clinic and not to rely too heavily on animal models.

- Natural products: modern technology for screening has revived interest and intensified the search. Multinational pharmaceutical companies now scour the world for leads from microorganisms (in soil or sewage or even from insects entombed in amber 40 million years ago), fungi, plants and animals. Developing countries in the tropics (with their luxuriant natural resources) are prominent targets in this search and have justly complained of exploitation ('gene robbery'). Many now require formal profit-sharing agreements to allow such searches. Natural products have been particularly successful for finding antibiotics as evolution has done over a much longer time period what medicinal chemists struggle to do. The problem with natural product drug discovery is often that identifying the precise active ingredient is hard and the molecules usually cannot easily be synthesised.

- Traditional medicine, which is being studied for possible leads to usefully active compounds. This is particularly true in China where traditional medicines are being re-evaluated for effects. The most notable example in recent years is the rediscovery of artemisinin for malaria treatment.

- Modifications of the structures of known drugs: these are obviously likely to produce more agents with similar basic properties, but may deliver worthwhile improvements. It is in this area that the 'me too' and 'me again' drugs are developed. However, such approaches are very unlikely to be commercially successful in a world that rightly demands true advances in patient care as a prerequisite for making profits and charging high costs to cover the price of innovative discovery.

- Random screening of synthesised and natural products.
- New uses for drugs already in general use as a result of intelligent observation and serendipity, or advancing knowledge of molecular mechanisms, e.g. aspirin for antithrombotic effect. Once a good drug is on the market new uses are often discovered. A recent example is rituximab, a monoclonal antibody that kills B cells. Initially developed for the treatment of B cell lymphoma it was found to be effective for suppressing B cell autoimmunity in diseases such as rheumatoid arthritis.

DRUG QUALITY

It is easy for an investigator or prescriber, interested in pharmacology, toxicology and therapeutics, to forget the fundamental importance of chemical and pharmaceutical aspects. An impure, unstable drug or formulation is useless. Pure drugs that remain pure after 3-5 years of storage in hot, damp climates are vital to therapeutics. The record of manufacturers in providing this is impressive. Much of the early work in drug discovery is spent trying to identify the right molecule with the appropriate physical and chemical properties to make it reliable as a medicine.

STUDIES IN ANIMALS

Mouse, rat, hamster, guinea-pig, rabbit, cat, dog, and sometimes monkey are used (but not all for any one drug). Non-clinical (pharmacotoxicological) studies must be carried out in conformity with the provisions of internationally agreed standards known as good laboratory practice (GLP). Certain studies in animals can be substituted by validated in vitro tests provided that the test results are of comparable qual-

ity and usefulness for the purpose of safety evaluation. The pharmacological and toxicological tests must demonstrate the potential toxicity of the product and any dangerous or undesirable toxic effects that may occur under the proposed conditions of use in human beings; these should be evaluated in relation to the pathological condition concerned. The studies must also demonstrate the pharmacological properties of the product, in both qualitative and quantitative relationship to the proposed use in human beings.

Generally, the following are undertaken:

Pharmacodynamics – to investigate the actions relating to the proposed therapeutic use. In addition, there is a need to investigate potential undesirable pharmacodynamic effects of the substance on physiological functions.

Pharmacokinetics – the study of the fate of the active substance and its metabolites within the organism (absorption, distribution, metabolism and excretion of these substances). The programme should be designed to allow comparison and extrapolation between animal and human.

Toxicology – to reveal physiological and/or histopathological changes induced by the drug, and to determine how these changes relate to dose. These involve:

- Acute toxicity: single-dose studies that allow qualitative and quantitative assessment of toxic reactions.
- Chronic and subchronic toxicity: repeat-dose studies to characterise the toxicological profile of a drug following repeated administration. This includes the identification of potential target organs and exposure–response relationships, and may include the potential for reversibility of effects.

Generally, it is desirable that tests be performed in two relevant species, based on the pharmacokinetic profile, one a rodent and one a non-rodent. The duration of the studies depends on the conditions of clinical use and is defined by Regulatory Agencies.

Genotoxicity – to reveal the changes that a drug may cause in the genetic material of individuals or cells. Mutagenic substances present a hazard to health because exposure carries the risk of inducing germline mutation (with the possibility of inherited disorders) and somatic mutations (including those leading to cancer). A standard battery of investigations includes: a test for gene mutation in bacteria (e.g. the Ames test); an in vitro test with cytogenetic evaluation of chromosomal damage with mammalian cells or an in vitro mouse lymphoma thymidine kinase (tk) assay; an in vivo test for chromosomal damage using rodent haematopoietic cells (e.g. the mouse micronucleus test).

Carcinogenicity – to reveal carcinogenic effects. These studies are performed for any medicinal product if its expected clinical use is prolonged (about 6 months), either continuously or repeatedly. These studies are also recommended if there is concern about their carcinogenic potential, e.g. from a product of the same class or similar structure, or from evidence in repeated-dose toxicity studies. Studies with unequivocally genotoxic compounds are not needed, as they are presumed to be trans-species carcinogens, implying a hazard to humans.

Reproductive and developmental toxicity – these tests study effects on adult male or female reproductive function, toxic and teratogenic effects at all stages of development from conception to sexual maturity and latent effects, when the medicinal product under investigation has been administered to the female during pregnancy. Embryo/fetal toxicity studies are normally conducted on two mammalian species, one a non-rodent. If the metabolism of a drug in particular species is known to be similar to that in humans, it is usual to include this species. Studies in juvenile animals may also be required prior to developing drugs for use in children.

Local tolerance – to ascertain whether drugs are tolerated at sites in the body at which they may come into contact in clinical use. The testing strategy is such that any mechanical effects of administration or purely physicochemical actions of the product can be distinguished from toxicological or pharmacodynamic ones.

Biotechnology-derived pharmaceuticals – present a special case and the standard regimen of toxicology studies is not appropriate. The choice of species used depends on the expression of the relevant receptor. If no suitable species exists, homologous proteins or transgenic animals expressing the human receptor may be studied and additional immunological studies are required. The study of biopharmaceutical safety provides challenges different from small molecules. Whereas the promiscuity of small molecules can lead to unexpected scaffold-related toxicity, this is usually not the case for biopharmaceuticals. But biopharmaceuticals may produce very different kinetics, binding and immunological effects in different species and therefore predictions of receptor occupancy and detailed analysis of immunological differences between species become of key importance.

ETHICS AND LEGISLATION

Controversy surrounding the use of animals in scientific research is not new. The renowned Islamic physician Avicenna (980—1037) was aware of the issues for he held that 'the experimentation must be done with the human body, for testing a drug on a lion or a horse might not prove anything about its effect on man'. Leonardo da Vinci (1452—1519) predicted that one day experimentation on animals would be judged a crime, but Descartes asserted that 'Animals do not speak, therefore they do not think, therefore they do not feel'. Later, Jeremy Bentham (1748—1832), the founding father of utilitarian philosophy, asked of animals: 'The question is not, Can they reason? nor Can they talk? but Can they suffer?'.

In our present world, billions of animals are raised to provide food and many to be used for scientific experiments. The arguments that evolve from this activity centre on the extent to which non-human animals can be respected as sentient beings of moral worth, albeit with differences between species. In recent years, a boisterous animal rights movement, asserting the moral status of animals, has challenged their use as experimental subjects. Mainstream medical and scientific opinion around the world accepts that animal research continues to be justified, subject to important protections. This position is based on the insight that research involving animals has contributed hugely to advances in biological knowledge that have in turn allowed modern therapeutics to improve human morbidity and mortality. However, each experiment must be justified and its results must be expected to deliver insight into safety or efficacy. Animal models do contribute to the understanding of human physiology and disease because we share so many biological characteristics and a medicine when introduced into the organism is exposed to a vast array of conditions that we do not fully understand and are unable to reproduce outside the living body. The study of a drug in the whole organism remains an essential step in the process of discovery and development of medicines.

Safety testing in animals is at present the only reliable way to evaluate risks before undertaking clinical trials of potentially useful medicines in humans. The investigation of reproductive effects and potential carcinogenicity would not be undertaken in humans for both ethical and practical reasons. Animal testing eliminates many unsafe test materials before clinical testing on humans, and minimises the risk of possible adverse effects when people are exposed to potential new medicines. In other words, experiments in animal models provide a critical safety check on candidate drugs; potentially hazardous or ineffective drugs can be eliminated and for those drugs that do progress to clinical trials, target organs identified in animal studies can be monitored.

Animal research has contributed to virtually every area of medical research, and almost all best known drug and surgical treatments of the past and present owe their origins in some way to evidence from animals. The antibacterial effectiveness of penicillin was proved in tests on mice. Insulin came about because of research on rabbits and dogs in the 1920s. Poliomyelitis epidemics, which until the 1950s killed and paralysed millions of children, were consigned to history by vaccines resulting from studies on a range of laboratory animals, including monkeys. Major heart surgery, such as coronary artery bypass grafts and heart transplants, was developed through research

on dogs and pigs. The BCG (Bacille Calmette–Guérin) vaccine for tuberculosis was developed through research on rats and mice. Meningitis due to Haemophilus influenzae type b, formerly common especially in children, is now almost unknown in the UK because of a vaccine developed through work on mice and rabbits. Almost all of the highly effective drug treatments we currently use were developed using animals: β-adrenoceptor blockers, angiotensin-converting enzyme inhibitors, cytotoxics, analgesics, psychotropics, and so on.

Given this evidence, there is broad public support for the position that experiments on animals are a regrettable necessity that should be limited to what is deemed essential until alternatives are developed. In the UK, for example, this reservation is expressed in progressively more stringent legislation. The Animals (Scientific Procedures) Act 1986 makes it an offence to carry out any scientific procedure on animals except under licence, the requirements of which include that:

- Animals are only used as a last resort.
- Every practical step is taken to avoid distress or suffering.
- The smallest possible number of animals is used.
- The potential benefits have to be weighed against the cost to the animals; the simplest or least sentient species is used.
- The work is realistic and achievable, and the programme designed in the way most likely to produce satisfactory results.
- The results must impact the decision-making process for discovery or development of the medicine.

Despite the continued necessity of animal studies in drug discovery and development there is now a very clear aim to move medicines into the clinic as soon as safely possible. Detailed clinical experimentation is often a better way to sort out questions related to effects on human biology and pharmacokinetics.

SAFETY PREDICTION

Knowledge of the mode of action of a potential new drug obviously greatly enhances prediction from animal studies of what will happen in humans. Whenever practicable, such knowledge should be obtained; sometimes this is quite easy, but sometimes it is impossible. Many drugs have been introduced safely without such knowledge, the later acquisition of which has not always made an important difference to their use (e.g. antimicrobials). Pharmacological studies are integrated with those of the toxicologist to build up a picture of the undesired as well as the desired drug effects.

In pharmacological testing, the investigators know what they are looking for and choose the experiments to gain their objectives.

In toxicological testing, the investigators have a less clear idea of what they are looking for; they are screening for risk, unexpected as well as predicted, and certain major routines must be done. Toxicity testing is therefore liable to become a routine to meet regulatory requirements to a greater extent than the pharmacological studies. The predictive value of special toxicology (above) is particularly controversial. All drugs are poisons if enough is given, and the task of the toxicologist is to find out whether, where and how a compound acts as a poison to animals, and to give an opinion on the significance of the data in relation to risks likely to be run by human beings. This will remain a nearly impossible task until molecular explanations of all effects can be provided.

Toxicologists are in an unenviable position. When a useful drug is safely introduced, they are considered to have done no more than their duty. When an accident occurs, they are invited to explain how this failure of prediction came about. When they predict that a chemical is unsafe in a major way for humans, this prediction is never tested. The easiest decision to make in drug discovery is to stop a project, and it is the only decision that can never be shown to be wrong. However, it is also a decision that may deny the world a new and effective medicine.

ORPHAN DRUGS AND DISEASES

In order to stimulate drug discovery and development in rare diseases, legislation in some countries has provided specific incentives to industry to develop medicines for 'orphan diseases'. Interestingly, many rare diseases are monogenic and the cause is clear. This, unlike most common diseases, means that the drug target is absolutely clear. In view of the greater certainty around cause, the smaller clinical trials and the more receptive regulatory environment, several pharmaceutical companies are beginning to work more assiduously in this area. It is also the case that some rare diseases give significant insights into common diseases and how to approach them.

SUMMARY

There are three key decision points along the way of discovering and developing a new medicine. ① Selecting the molecular target you want the drug to act on to produce the desired effect. ② Choosing the right chemical as the drug candidate. All the promise and all the faults become fixed at this point. ③ Designing the right clinical experiment to show that the medicine will really do what you want it to do. Several approaches, including using synthetic small molecules, natural products, traditional medicines, large proteins and nucleic-based approaches, broaden what we think of as a medicine. Studies in animals are required by regulation (for safety), or by giving insight into the effect of the drug in the whole body, but none replaces the need for clinical testing. Getting the medicine into the clinic to test its properties and its effects on biological systems of human being is a key step. A drug may be abandoned at any stage, including after marketing. New drug development is a colossally expensive and commercially driven activity.

IMPORTANT TERMINOLOGY

molecular target　分子靶标

drug candidate　候选药物

clinical experiment　临床试验

high throughput screening　高通量筛选

proteins as medicines　蛋白质药物

gene therapy　基因治疗

stem cells　干细胞
natural products　天然产物
traditional medicines　传统药物
pharmacodynamics　药效学
pharmacokinetics　药动学
toxicology　毒理学
orphan drugs　孤儿药物

CHALLENGE YOURSELF

1. What are the three key decision points along the way of discovering and developing a new medicine?
2. Write down the important techniques of drug discovery and development.
3. What are the purposes of studies in animals in the process of discovering and developing a new drug?

Yuanying Jiang

Chapter 3

Clinical Research of Drugs

EXPERIMENTAL THERAPEUTICS

After preclinical evidence of efficacy and safety have been obtained in animals, potential medicines are tested in healthy volunteers and volunteer patients. Studies in healthy normal volunteers can help to determine the safety, tolerability, pharmacokinetics and, for some drugs (e.g. anticoagulants and anaesthetic agents), their dynamic effect and likely dose range. For many drugs, the dynamic effect and hence therapeutic potential can be investigated only in patients, e.g. drugs for parkinsonism and antimicrobials will have no measurable efficacy in subjects without movement disorder or infection, respectively.

Modern medicine is sometimes accused of callous application of science to human problems and of subordinating the interest of the individual to those of the group (society). Now, the guidance to researchers in this matter is clear. The World Medical Association Declaration of Helsinki (Edinburgh revision 2000) states that 'considerations related to the well-being of the human subject should take precedence over the interests of science and society'. The General Assembly of the United Nations adopted in 1966 the International Covenant on Civil and Political Rights, of which Article 7 states, 'In particular, no one shall be subjected without his free consent to medical or scientific experimentation'. This means that subjects are entitled to know that they are being entered into research even though the research be thought 'harmless'. But there are people who cannot give (informed) consent, e.g. the demented. The need for special procedures for such is now recognised, for there is a consensus that, without research, they and the diseases from which they suffer will become therapeutic 'orphans'. Official regulatory bodies rightly require scientific evaluation of drugs. Drug developers need to satisfy the official regulators and they also seek to persuade the medical profession to prescribe their products. Patients, too, are more aware of the comparative advantages and limitations of their medicines than they used to be. To some extent, this helps encourage patients to participate in trials so that future patients can benefit, as they do now, from the knowledge gained from such trials. An ethical framework is required to ensure that the interests of the individual participant take precedence over those of society (and, more obviously, those of an individual or corporate investigator).

ETHICS OF RESEARCH

Principle 1 of the Nuremberg Code states:

The voluntary consent of the human subject is absolutely essential. This means that the person involved should have legal capacity to give consent; should be so situated as to be able to exercise free power of choice, without the intervention of any element of force, fraud, deceit, duress, overreaching, or other ulterior form of constraint or coercion; and should have sufficient knowledge and comprehension of the elements of the subject matter involved as to enable him to make an understanding and enlightened decision.

The issue of (adequately informed) consent is a principal concern for Research Ethics Committees (also called Institutional Review Boards). People have the right to choose for themselves whether or not they will participate in research, i.e. they have the right to self-determination (the ethical principle of autonomy). They should be given whatever information is necessary for making an adequately informed choice (consent) with the right to withdraw at any stage. Consent procedures, especially information on risks, loom larger in research than they do in medical practice. This is appropriate given that in research, patients may be submitting themselves to extra risks, or simply to extra inconvenience (e.g. more or longer visits). It is a moot point whether more consent in routine practice might not go amiss. It is also likely that patients participating in well-conducted trials receive more, and sometimes better, care and attention than might otherwise be available. Sometimes the unintended consequences of ethical procedures include causing unnecessary apprehension to patients with long, legalistic documents, and creating a false impression of clinical researchers as people from whom patients need protection.

RATIONAL INTRODUCTION OF A NEW DRUG TO HUMANS

When studies in animals predict that a new molecule may be a useful medicine, i.e. effective and safe in relation to its benefits, then the time has come to put it to the test in humans. Most doctors will be involved in clinical trials at some stage of their career and need to understand the principles of drug development. When a new chemical entity offers a possibility of doing something that has not been done before or of doing something familiar in a different or better way, it can be seen to be worth testing. But where it is a new member of a familiar class of drug, potential advantage may be harder to detect. Yet these 'me too' drugs are often worth testing. Predic-

tion from animal studies of modest but useful clinical advantage is particularly uncertain and, therefore, if the new drug seems reasonably effective and safe in animals it is rational to test it in humans.

Phases of clinical development

Human experiments progress in a commonsense manner that is conventionally divided into four phases (Fig. 3.1). These phases are divisions of convenience in what is a continuous expanding process. It begins with a small number of subjects (healthy subjects and volunteer patients) closely observed in laboratory settings, and proceeds through hundreds of patients, to thousands before the drug is agreed to be a medicine by a national or international regulatory authority. It is then licensed for general prescribing (though this is by no means the end of the evaluation). The process may be abandoned at any stage for a variety of reasons, including poor tolerability or safety, inadequate efficacy and commercial pressures. The phases are:

Phase 1   Human pharmacology (20–50 subjects):
- healthy volunteers or volunteer patients, according to the class of drug and its safety
- pharmacokinetics (absorption, distribution, metabolism, excretion)
- pharmacodynamics (biological effects) where practicable, tolerability, safety, efficacy

Phase 2   Therapeutic exploration (50–300 subjects):
- patients
- pharmacokinetics and pharmacodynamic dose ranging, in carefully controlled studies for efficacy and safety (Moderate to severe adverse events have occurred in about 0.5% of healthy subjects), which may involve comparison with placebo

Phase 3   Therapeutic confirmation (randomized controlled trials; 250–1 000+ subjects):
- patients
- efficacy on a substantial scale; safety; comparison with existing drugs

Phase 4   Therapeutic use (pharmacovigilance, post-licensing studies) (2 000–10 000+ subjects):
- surveillance for safety and efficacy: further formal therapeutic trials, especially comparisons with

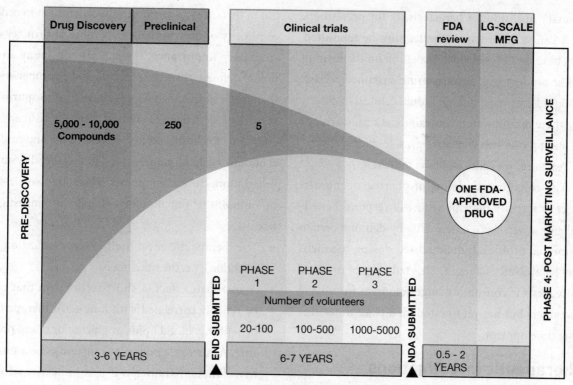

Fig. 3.1 The phases of drug discovery and development

other drugs, marketing studies and pharmaco-economic studies

As indicated in above, Phase 1 studies aim to investigate the metabolism of a drug and its pharmacodynamics and pharmacokinetics. Phase 2 trials aim to set the scene for subsequent confirmatory Phase 3 trials. Typically, although exceptions may occur, these will be the first 'trials' in patients. Phase 3 is designed to assess the effectiveness of the new intervention and, thereby, its value in clinical practice. Phase3 studies are randomized controlled multicenter trials on large patient groups and are aimed at being the definitive assessment of how effective the drug is, in comparison with current 'gold standard' treatment. Phase 4 trials are generally considered as 'post-registration' trials: that is, a marketing authorization was already possed by trials of products.

Official regulatory guidelines and requirements

For studies in humans these ordinarily include:

- Studies of pharmacokinetics and bioavailability and, in the case of generics, bioequivalence (equal bioavailability) with respect to the reference product.

- Therapeutic trials (reported in detail) that substantiate the safety and efficacy of the drug under likely conditions of use, e.g. a drug for long-term use in a common condition will require a total of at least 1 000 patients (preferably more), depending on the therapeutic class, of which (for chronic diseases) at least 100 have been treated continuously for about 1 year.

- Special groups. If the drug will be used in, for example, the elderly or children, then these populations should be studied. New drugs are not normally studied in pregnant women. Studies in patients having disease that affects drug metabolism and elimination may be needed, such as patients with impaired liver or kidney function.

- Fixed-dose combination products will require explicit justification for each component.

- Interaction studies with other drugs likely to be taken simultaneously. Plainly, all possible combinations cannot be evaluated; a rational choice, based on knowledge of pharmacodynamics and pharmacokinetics, is made.

- The application for a licence for general use (marketing application) should include a draft Summary of Product Characteristics for prescribers. A Patient Information Leaflet must be submitted. These should include information on the form of the product (e.g. tablet, capsule, sustained-release, liquid), its uses, dosage (adults, children, elderly where appropriate), contraindications, warnings and precautions (less strong), side-effects/adverse reactions, overdose and how to treat it.

The emerging discipline of pharmacogenomics seeks to identify patients who will respond beneficially or adversely to a new drug by defining certain genotypic profiles. Individualized dosing regimens may be evolved as a result. This tailoring of drugs to individuals is consuming huge resources from drug developers but has yet to establish a place in routine drug development.

Therapeutic investigations

There are three key questions to be answered during drug development: Does it work? Is it safe? What is the dose?

With few exceptions, none of these is easy to answer definitively within the confines of a pre-registration clinical trials program. Effectiveness and safety have to be balanced against each other. What may be regarded as 'safe' for a new oncology drug in advanced lung cancer would not be so regarded in the treatment of childhood eczema. The use of the term 'dose', without explanation, is irrational as it implies a single dose for all patients. Pharmaceutical companies cannot be expected to produce a large array of different doses for each medicine, but the maxim to use the smallest effective dose that results in the desired effect holds true. Some drugs require titration, others have a wide safety margin so that one 'high' dose may achieve optimal effectiveness with acceptable safety.

It is crucial that these endpoints are unambiguously defined so that they can be determined for each patient recruited to the trial. It is fine practice to define which endpoint is the major endpoint of the trial as this will be used to determine trial size and be the main focus for the efficacy evaluation. In many situations, there may be several endpoints of interest,

but in this case it is significant to order them in order of priority or at least to identify those of primary or secondary importance. If there are too many endpoints defined, then the multiplicity of comparisons then made at the analysis stage may lead to spurious statistical significance. This is a major concern if endpoints for health-related quality of life and health economic evaluations are added to the already established more clinical endpoints. There are two classes of endpoint or outcome of a therapeutic investigation:

- The therapeutic effect itself (sleep, eradication of infection), i.e. the outcome.
- A surrogate effect, a short-term effect that can be reliably correlated with long-term therapeutic benefit, e.g. blood lipids or glucose or blood pressure. A surrogate endpoint might also be a pharmacokinetic parameter, if it is indicative of the therapeutic effect, e.g. plasma concentration of an antiepileptic drug.

Use of surrogate effects presupposes that the disease process is fully understood. They are best justified in diseases for which the true therapeutic effect can be measured only by studying large numbers of patients over many years. Such long-term outcome studies are indeed always prefer-able but may be impracticable on organizational, financial and sometimes ethical grounds prior to releasing new drugs for general prescription. It is in areas such as these that the techniques of large-scale surveillance for efficacy, as well as for safety, under conditions of ordinary use (below), would be needed to supplement the necessarily smaller and shorter formal therapeutic trials employing surrogate effects. Surrogate endpoints are of particular value in early drug development to select candidate drugs from a range of agents.

Therapeutic evaluation

The aims of therapeutic evaluation are three-fold:

1. To assess the efficacy, safety and quality of new drugs to meet unmet clinical needs.
2. To expand the indications for the use of current drugs (generic drug, A drug for which the original patent has expired, so that any pharmaceuti-

cal company may market it in competition with the inventor) in clinical and marketing terms.

3. To protect public health over the lifetime of a given drug.

The process of therapeutic evaluation may be divided into pre- and post-registration phases, the purposes of which are set out below.

When a new drug is being developed, the first therapeutic trials are devised to find out the best that the drug can do under conditions ideal for showing efficacy, e.g. uncomplicated disease of mild to moderate severity in patients taking no other drugs, with carefully supervised administration by specialist doctors. Interest lies particularly in patients who complete a full course of treatment. If the drug is ineffective in these circumstances there is no point in proceeding with an expensive development program. Such studies are sometimes called explanatory trials as they attempt to 'explain' why a drug works (fails to work) in ideal conditions.

If the drug is found useful in these trials, it becomes desirable next to find out how closely the ideal may be approached in the rough and tumble of routine medical practice: in patients of all ages, at all stages of disease, with complications, taking other drugs and relatively unsupervised. Interest continues in all patients from the moment they are entered into the trial and it is maintained if they fail to complete, or even to start, the treatment; the need is to know the outcome in all patients deemed suitable for therapy, not only in those who successfully complete therapy.

The methods used to test the therapeutic value depend on the stage of development, who is conducting the study (a pharmaceutical company, or an academic body or health service at the behest of a regulatory authority), and the primary endpoint or outcome of the trial. The methods include:

- Formal therapeutic trials.
- Equivalence and non-inferiority trials.

Safety surveillance methods. Formal therapeutic trials are conducted during Phase 2 and Phase 3 of pre-registration development, and in the post-registration phase to test the drug in new indications. Equivalence trials aim to show the therapeutic equivalence of two treatments, usually the new drug under development and an existing drug used as a standard active comparator. Equivalence trials may be conducted before or after registration for the first therapeutic indication of the new drug. Safety surveillance methods use the principles of pharmacoepidemiology and are concerned mainly with evaluating adverse events and especially rare events, which formal therapeutic trials are unlikely to detect.

Economic evaluation

Most trials are intended primarily to address questions of efficacy and safety. Health economics is becoming increasingly important, And we often now evaluate it as part of a randomized controlled trial.

There are four main types of cost analyses that are usually considered:

- *cost minimization*, simply to determine the best therapy to minimize the total cost of treating the disease
- *cost effectiveness*, a trade-off between the cost of caring for a patient and the level of efficacy offered by a remedy
- *cost benefit*, a trade-off between the cost of caring for a patient and the overall benefit (not restricted to efficacy)
- *cost utility*, the trade-off between costs and all measures of 'utility'. This may include efficacy, quality of life, greater life expectancy or increased productivity

Determining what indirect costs should be considered is one of the big difficulties in pharmacoeconomic evaluations. *Direct costs* are usually easier: costs of medication, costs of those giving the care (doctors, nurses, health visitors) and the basic costs of occupation of a hospital bed. Indirect costs include loss of earnings and productivity, loss of earnings and productivity of spouses or other family members. These family members may care for a sick relative and contribution to hospital/pharmacy overhead costs. Due to the ambiguity associated with these indirect costs, most pharmacoeconomic evaluations performed as part of a clinical trial incline to focus solely on direct costs.

NEED FOR STATISTIC

In order truly to know whether patients treated in one way are benefited more than those treated in another, it is essential to use numbers. Statistics has been defined as 'a body of methods for making wise decisions in the face of uncertainty'. Used properly, they are tools of great value for promoting efficient therapy.

Hypothesis of no difference

When it is suspected that treatment A may be superior to treatment B, and the truth is sought, it is convenient to start with the proposition that the treatments are equally effective-the 'no difference' hypothesis (null hypothesis). After two groups of patients have been treated and it has been found that improvement has occurred more often with one treatment than with the other, it is necessary to decide how likely it is that this difference is due to a real superiority of one treatment over the other. To make this decision we need to understand two major concepts, *statistical significance* and *confidence intervals*.

A statistical significance test such as the Student's *t*-test or the chi-squared (χ^2) test will tell how often an observed difference would occur due to chance (random influences) if there is, in reality, no difference between the treatments. Where the statistical significance test shows that an observed difference would occur only five times if the experiment were repeated 100 times, this is often taken as sufficient evidence that the null hypothesis is unlikely to be true. Therefore, the conclusion is that there is (probably) a real difference between the treatments. This level of probability is generally expressed in thera-

peutic trials as: 'the difference was statistically significant', or 'significant at the 5% level' or 'P=0.05' (P is the probability based on chance alone). Statistical significance simply means that the result is unlikely to have occurred if there was no genuine treatment difference, i.e. there probably is a difference.

If the analysis reveals that the observed difference, or greater, would occur only once if the experiment were repeated 100 times, the results are generally said to be 'statistically highly significant', or 'significant at the 1% level' or 'P =0.01'.

Confidence intervals. The problem with the P value is that it conveys no information on the amount of the differences observed or on the range of possible differences between treatments. A result that a drug produces a uniform 2% reduction in heart rate may well be statistically significant but it is clinically meaningless. What doctors are interested to know is the size of the difference, and what degree of assurance (confidence) they may have in the precision (reproducibility) of this estimate. To obtain this it is necessary to calculate a confidence interval (see Figs 3.2 and 3.3).

The treatment differences a, b, care all in favour of 'New treatment', but superiority is shown only in A and B. In C, superiority has not been shown. This may be because the effect is small and not detected. The result, nevertheless, is compatible with equivalence or non-inferiority. Adequate precision and power are assumed for all the trials.

In practice, the actual number would be calculated from standard equations. In this example the curves are constructed for 16, 40, 100 and 250 subjects per group in a two-limb comparative trial. The graphs can provide three pieces of information: ① the

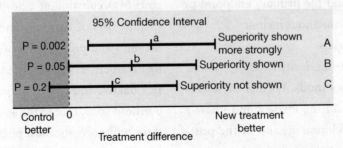

Fig. 3.2 Relationship between significance tests and confidence intervals for the comparisons between a new treatment and control.

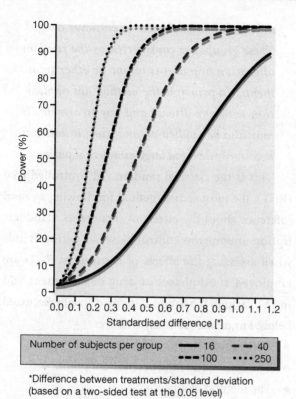

*Difference between treatments/standard deviation
(based on a two-sided test at the 0.05 level)

Fig. 3.3 Power curves - an illustrative method of defining the number of subjects required in a given study.

number of subjects that need to be studied, given the power of the trial and the difference expected between the two treatments; ② the power of a trial, given the number of subjects included and the difference expected; and ③ the difference that can be detected between two groups of subjects of given number, with varying degrees of power.

A confidence interval expresses a range of values that contains the true value with 95% (other chosen percent- age) certainty. The range may be broad, indicating uncertainty, or narrow, indicating (relative) certainty. A wide confidence interval occurs when numbers are small or differences observed are variable and points to a lack of information, whether the difference is statistically significant or not; it is a warning against placing much weight on (confidence in) the results of small or variable studies. Confidence intervals are extremely helpful in interpretation, particularly of small studies, as they show the degree of uncertainty related to a result. Their use in conjunction with non-significant results may be especially enlightening.

A finding of 'not statistically significant' can be interpreted as meaning there is no clinically useful difference only if the confidence intervals for the results are also stated in the report and are narrow. If the confidence intervals are wide, a real difference may be missed in a trial with a small number of subjects, i.e. the absence of evidence that there is a difference is not the same as showing that there is no difference. Small numbers of patients inevitably give low precision and low power to detect differences.

Types of error

The above discussion provides us with information on the likelihood of falling into one of the two principal kinds of error in therapeutic experiments, for the hypothesis that there is no difference between treatments may either be accepted incorrectly or rejected incorrectly.

Type I error (α) is the finding of a difference between treatments when in reality they do not differ, i.e. rejecting the null hypothesis incorrectly. Investigators decide the degree of this error which they are prepared to tolerate on a scale in which 0 indicates complete rejection of the null hypothesis and 1 indicates its complete acceptance; clearly the level for α must be set near to 0. This is the same as the significance level of the statistical test used to detect a difference between treatments. Thus α (P=0.05) indicates that the investigators will accept a 5% chance that an observed difference is not a real difference.

Type II error (β) is the finding of no difference between treatments when in reality they do differ, i.e. accepting the null hypothesis incorrectly. The probability of detecting this error is often given wider limits, e.g. β=0.1–0.2, which indicates that the investigators are willing to accept a 10%–20% chance of missing a real effect. Conversely, the power of the study (1–β) is the probability of avoiding this error and detecting a real difference, in this case 80%–90%.

It is up to the investigators to decide the target difference and what probability level (for either type of error) they will accept if they are to use the result as a guide to action.

Plainly, trials should be devised to have adequate

precision and power, both of which are consequences of the size of study. It is also necessary to make an estimate of the likely size of the difference between treatments, i.e. the target difference. Adequate power is often defined as giving an 80%–90% chance of detecting (at 1%–5% statistical significance, P=0.01–0.05) the defined useful target difference (say 15%). It is rarely worth starting a trial that has less than a 50% chance of achieving the set objective, because the power of the trial is too low.

Statistics of reporting clinical trials

The first rule after completing a clinical trial is to report the results - whether they are positive, negative or equivocal. A distorted view of the true situation is presented by the selective reporting whereby results of positive studies tend to be published and negative studies tend not to be published. This approach to reporting is particularly important for clinical trial overviews and meta-analysis. In these studies, it is clearly important to be able to include all relevant studies (not just the published ones) in the overall synthesis.

The second aspect of reporting is the standard of reporting, particularly the amount of necessary detail which is given in any trial report. The most basic feature that has repeatedly been emphasised is to give estimates (with confidence intervals) of treatment effects and not just P-values. Guidelines for referees (useful also for authors) have been published in several journals including the *British Medical Journal*. The Consolidation of the Standards of Reporting Trials (CONSORT) statement is an international recommendation and it is adopted by many leading medical journals.

TYPES OF THERAPEUTIC TRIAL

A therapeutic trial is:

a carefully, and ethically, designed experiment with the aim of answering some precisely framed question. In its most rigorous form it demands equivalent groups of patients concurrently treated in different ways or in ran-domized sequential order in crossover designs. These groups are constructed by the random allocation of patients to one or other treatment... In principle the method has application with any disease and any treatment. It may also be applied on any scale; it does not necessarily demand large numbers of patients.

This is the classical randomized controlled trial (RCT), the most secure method for drawing a causal inference about the effects of treatments. Randomization attempts to control biases of various kinds when assessing the effects of treatments. RCTs are employed at all phases of drug development and in the various types and designs of trials discussed below. Fundamental to any trial are:

- A hypothesis.
- The definition of the primary endpoint.
- The method of analysis.
- A protocol.

Other factors to consider when designing or critically appraising a trial are:

- The characteristics of the patients.
- The general applicability of the results.
- The size of the trial.
- The method of monitoring.
- The use of interim analyses.
- The interpretation of subgroup comparisons.

The aims of a therapeutic trial, not all of which can be attempted at any one occasion, are to decide:

- Whether a treatment is effective.
- The magnitude of that effect (compared with other remedies – or doses, or placebo).
- The types of patients in whom it is effective.
- The best method of applying the treatment (how often, and in what dosage if it is a drug).
- The disadvantages and dangers of the treatment.

Dose–response trials. Response in relation to the dose of a new investigational drug may be explored in all phases of drug development. Dose–response trials serve a number of objectives, of which the following are of particular importance:

- Confirmation of efficacy (hence a therapeutic trial).
- Investigation of the shape and location of the dose–response curve.

- The estimation of an appropriate starting dose.
- The identification of optimal strategies for individual dose adjustments.
- The determination of a maximal dose beyond which additional benefit is unlikely to occur.

Superiority, equivalence and non-inferiority in clinical trials. The therapeutic efficacy of a novel drug is most convincingly established by demonstrating superiority to placebo, or to an active control treatment, or by demonstrating a dose–response relationship (as above). In some cases the purpose of a comparison is to show not necessarily superiority, but either equivalence or non-inferiority. Such trials avoid the use of placebo, explore possible advantages of safety, dosing convenience and cost, and present an alternative or 'second-line' therapy. Examples of a possible outcome in a 'head to head' comparison of two active treatments appear in Figure 3.2. There are in general, two types of equivalence trials in clinical development: bio-equivalence and clinical equivalence. In the former, certain pharmacokinetic variables of a new formulation have to fall within specified (and regulated) margins of the standard formulation of the same active entity. The advantage of this type of trial is that, if bioequivalence is 'proven', then proof of clinical equivalence is not required.

Methods to avoid bias

The two most important techniques to avoid bias are randomization and blinding.

Randomization. The use of randomization was a contribution by the statistician R.A. Fisher in agriculture. Fisher randomized plots of crops to receive different administrations and in clinical trials there were early schemes to use 'group randomization': patients were divided into two groups and then the treatment for each group was randomly selected. Introduces a deliberate element of chance into the assignment of treatments to the subjects in a clinical trial. It provides a sound statistical basis for the evaluation of the evidence relating to treatment effects, and tends to produce treatment groups that have a balanced distribution of prognostic factors, both known and unknown. Together with blinding,

it helps to avoid possible bias in the selection and allocation of subjects.

Randomization may be accomplished in simple or more complex ways, such as:

- Sequential assignments of treatments (sequences in crossover trials).
- Randomizing subjects in blocks. This helps to increase comparability of the treatment groups when subject characteristics change over time or there is a change in recruitment policy. It also gives a better guarantee that the treatment groups will be of nearly equal size.
- By dynamic allocation, in which treatment allocation is influenced by the current balance of allocated treatments. (Note also patient preference trials. Conventionally, patients are invited to participate in a clinical trial, give consent and are then randomized to a particular treatment group. In special circumstances, randomization takes place first, the patients are informed of the treatment to be offered and are allowed to opt for this or another treatment. This is called pre-consent randomization or 'pre-randomization'. In a trial of simple mastectomy versus lumpectomy with or without radiotherapy for early breast cancer, recruitment was slow because of the disfiguring nature of the mastectomy option. A policy of pre-randomization was then adopted, letting women know the group to which they would be allocated should they consent. Recruitment increased six-fold and the trial was completed, providing sound evidence that survival was as long with the less disfiguring option).

Blinding. The fact that both doctors and patients are subject to bias due to their beliefs and feelings has led to the invention of the double-blind technique, which is a control device to prevent bias from influencing results. On the one hand, it rules out the effects of hopes and anxieties of the patient by giving both the drug under investigation and a placebo (dummy) of identical appearance in such a way that the subject (the first 'blind' person) does not know which he or she is receiving. On the other hand, it also rules out the influence of preconceived hopes of, and unconscious communication by, the investigator or observer by keeping him or her (the second 'blind' person) ignorant of whether he or she is prescribing a placebo or an active drug. At the same time, the technique provides another control, a means of comparison with the magnitude of placebo effects. The device is both philosophically and practically sound.

A non-blind trial is called an open trial.

The double-blind technique should be used wherever possible, and especially for occasions when it might at first sight seem that criteria of clinical improvement are objective when in fact they are not. For example, the range of voluntary joint movement in rheumatoid arthritis has been shown to be influenced greatly by psychological factors, and a moment's thought shows why, for the amount of pain patients will put up with is influenced by their mental state.

Blinding should go beyond the observer and the observed. None of the investigators should be aware of treatment allocation, including those who evaluate endpoints, assess compliance with the protocol and monitor adverse events. Breaking the blind (for a single subject) should be considered only when the subject's physician deems knowledge of the treatment assignment essential in the subject's best interests.

Sometimes the double-blind technique is not possible, because, for example, side effects of an active drug reveal which patients are taking it or tablets look or taste different; but it never carries a disadvantage ('only protection against biased data'). It is not, of course, used with new chemical entities fresh from the animal laboratory, whose dose and effects in humans are unknown, although the subject may legitimately be kept in ignorance (single blind) of the time of administration. Single-blind techniques have a place in therapeutics research, but only when the double- blind procedure is impracticable or unethical.

Ophthalmologists are understandably disinclined to refer to the 'double-blind' technique; they call it double-masked.

Some common design configurations

Parallel group design. This is the most common clinical trial design for confirmatory therapeutic (Phase 3) trials. Subjects are randomized to one of two or more treatment 'arms'. These treatments will include the investigational drug at one or more doses, and one or more control treatments such as placebo and/or an active comparator. Parallel group designs are particularly useful in conditions that fluctuate over a short term, e.g. migraine or irritable bowel syndrome, but are also used for chronic stable diseases such as Parkinson's disease and some types of cancer. The particular advantages of the parallel group design are simplicity, the ability to approximate more closely the likely conditions of use, and the avoidance of 'carry-over effects'.

Crossover design. In this design, each subject is randomized to a sequence of two or more treatments, and hence acts as his or her own control for treatment comparisons. The advantage of this design is that subject-to-subject variation is eliminated from treatment comparison so that the number of subjects is reduced.

In the basic crossover design each subject receives each of the two treatments in a randomized order. There are variations to this in which each subject receives a subset of treatments or ones in which treatments are repeated within the same subject.

Factorial designs. In the factorial design, two or more treatments are evaluated simultaneously through the use of varying combinations of the treatments. The simplest example is the 2×2 factorial design in which subjects are randomly allocated to one of four possible combinations of two treatments A and B. These are: A alone, B alone, A+B, neither A nor B (placebo). The main uses of the factorial design are to:

- Make efficient use of clinical trial subjects by evaluating two treatments with the same number of individuals.
- Examine the interaction of A with B.
- Establish dose–response characteristics of the combination of A and B when the efficacy of each has been previously established.

Multicentre trials. Multicentre trials are carried out for two main reasons. First, they are an efficient way of evaluating a new medication, by accruing sufficient subjects in a reasonable time to satisfy trial objectives. Second, multicentre trials may be designed to provide a better basis for the subsequent generalization of their findings. Thus they provide the possibility of recruiting subjects from a wide population and of administering the medication in a broad range of clinical settings. Multicentre trials can be used at any phase in clinical development, but are especially valuable when used to confirm therapeutic value in Phase 3. Large-scale multicentre trials using minimised data collection techniques and simple endpoints have been of immense value in establishing modest but real treatment effects that apply to a large number of patients, e.g. drugs that improve survival after myocardial infarction.

N-of-1 trials. Patients give varied treatment responses and the average effect derived from a population sample may not be helpful in expressing the size of benefit or harm for an individual. In the future, pharmacogenomics may provide an answer, but in the meantime the best way to settle doubt as to whether a test drug is effective for an individual patient is the N-of-1 trial. This is a crossover design in which each patient receives two or more administrations of drug or placebo in random manner; the results from individuals can then be displayed. Two conditions apply. First, the disease in which the drug is being tested must be chronic and stable. Second, the treatment effect must wear off rapidly. N-of-1 trials are not used routinely in drug development and, if so, only at the Phase 3 stage.

Historical controls. Any temptation simply to give a new treatment to all patients and to compare the results with the past (historical controls) is almost always unacceptable, even with a disease such as leukaemia. The reasons are that standards of diagnosis and treatment change with time, and the severity of some diseases (infections) fluctuates. The general provision stands that controls must be concurrent and concomitant. An exception to this rule is the case–control study.

Size of trials

Anticipated effect size. A major factor in determining the size of a RCT is the anticipated effect size or clinically worthwhile difference. In broad terms if this is not large then it should be of sufficient clinical, scientific or public health importance to warrant the consequentially large trial that will be required to answer the question posed. If the anticipated effect is large, the RCT will be relatively small in which case the investigators may need to question their own 'optimistic' view of the potential benefit. In either case, a realistic view of the possible effect size is important. In practice, it is usually important to calculate sample size for a range of values of the effect size. In this way the sensitivity of the resulting sample sizes to this range of values will provide options for the investigating team.

Estimates of the anticipated effect size may be obtained from the available literature, formal meta-analyses of related trials or may be elicited from clinical opinion. In circumstances where there is little prior information available, Cohen has proposed a standardized effect size, Δ. In the case when the difference between two treatments A and B is expressed by the difference between their means ($\mu_A - \mu_B$) and σ is the standard deviation (SD) of the endpoint variable which is assumed to be a continuous measure, then $\Delta = (\mu_A - \mu_B)/\sigma$. A value of $\Delta \leq 0.1$ is considered a small standardized effect, $\Delta \approx 0.5$ as moderate and $\Delta \geq 1$ as large. Experience has suggested that in many clinical areas these can be taken as a good practical guide for design purposes. However, for large simple trials, the equivalent of effects sizes as small as $\Delta = 0.05$ or less may be clinically important.

Calculation of sample size. Before the start of any controlled trial it is necessary to decide the number of patients that will be needed to deliver an answer, for ethical as well as practical reasons. This is determined by four factors:

- The magnitude of the difference sought or expected on the primary efficacy endpoint (the target difference). For between-group studies, the focus of interest is the mean difference that constitutes a clinically significant effect.
- The variability of the measurement of the primary endpoint as reflected by the standard devia-

tion of this primary outcome measure. The magnitude of the expected difference (above) divided by the standard deviation of the difference gives the standardized difference (Fig. 3.3).

- The defined significance level, i.e. the level of chance for accepting a Type I (α) error. Levels of 0.05 (5%) and 0.01 (1%) are common targets.

- The power or desired probability of detecting the required mean treatment difference, i.e. the level of chance for accepting a Type II (β) error. For most controlled trials, a power of 80%–90% (0.8–0.9) is frequently chosen as adequate, although higher power is chosen for some studies.

It will be intuitively obvious that a small difference in the effect that can be detected between two treatment groups, or a large variability in the measurement of the primary endpoint, or a high significance level (low P value) or a large power requirement, all act to increase the required sample size. Figure 3.3 gives a graphical representation of how the power of a clinical trial relates to values of clinically relevant standardized difference for varying numbers of trial subjects (shown by the individual curves). It is clear that the larger the number of subjects in a trial, the smaller is the difference that can be detected for any given power value.

A good clinical trial design is that which will answer the question posed with the minimum number of subjects possible. An excessively large trial not only incurs higher costs but is also unethical. Too small a trial size leads to inconclusive results, since there is a greater chance of missing the clinically important difference, resulting in a waste of resources.

Fixed sample size and sequential designs. Defining when a clinical trial should end is not as simple as it first appears. In the standard clinical trial the end is defined by the passage of all of the recruited subjects through the complete design. However, it is results and decisions based on the results that matter, not the number of subjects. The result of the trial may be that one treatment is superior to another or that there is no difference. These trials are of fixed sample size.

The results of this type of trial may be disappointing if they miss the agreed and accepted level of significance.

An alternative (addition) to repeating the fixed sample size trial is to use a sequential design in which the trial is run until a useful result is reached. These adaptive designs, in which decisions are taken on the basis of results to date, can assess results on a continuous basis as data for each subject become available or, more commonly, on groups of subjects (group sequential design).

Such sequential designs recognise the reality of medical practice and provide a reasonable balance between statistical, medical and ethical needs. Interim analyses, however, reduce the power of statistical significance tests each time that they are performed, and carry a risk of false positive result if chance differences between groups are encountered before the scheduled end of a trial.

Sensitivity of trials

Definitive therapeutic trials are expensive and on occasion may be so prolonged that aspects of treatment have been superseded by the time a result is obtained. A single trial, however well designed, executed and analyzed, can answer only the question addressed. The regulatory authorities give guidance as to the number and design of trials that, if successful, would lead to a therapeutic claim. But changing clinical practice in the longer term depends on many other factors, of which confirmatory trials in other centres by different investigators under different conditions are an important part.

META-ANALYSIS

Introduction to meta-analysis

The two main outcomes for therapeutic trials are to influence clinical practice and, where appropriate, to make a successful claim for a drug with the regulatory authorities. Investigators are eternally optimistic and frequently plan their trials to look for large effects. Reality is different. The results of a planned (unplanned) series of clinical trials may vary considerably for several reasons, but most significantly because the studies are too small to detect a treatment effect. In common but serious diseases such as cancer or heart disease, however, even small treatment effects can be important in terms of their total impact on public health. It may be unreasonable to expect dramatic advances in these diseases; we should be looking for small effects. Drug developers, too, should be interested not only in whether a treatment works, but also how well, and for whom.

The collecting together of a number of trials with the same objective in a systematic review and analysing the accumulated results using appropriate statistical methods is termed meta-analysis. The principles of a meta-analysis are that:

- It should be comprehensive, i.e. include data from all trials, published and unpublished.
- Only randomised controlled trials should be analysed, with patients entered on the basis of 'intention to treat'.
- The results should be determined using clearly

defined, disease-specific endpoints (this may involve a re-analysis of original trials).

Meta-analysis aims in using statistics approaches to derive a pooled estimate closest to the unknown common truth based on how this error is perceived. In essence, all existing methods yield a weighted average from the results of the individual studies and what differs is the manner in which these weights are allocated and also the manner in which the uncertainty is computed around the point estimate thus generated.

In clinical practice, and in the era of cost-effectiveness, the use of meta-analysis as a tool to aid medical decision-making and underpinning 'evidence-based medicine' is here to stay.

Figure 3.4 shows detailed results from 11 trials in which antiplatelet therapy after myocardial infarction was com- pared with a control group. The number of vascular events per treatment group is shown in the second and third columns, and the odds ratios with the point estimates (the value most likely to have resulted from the study) are represented by

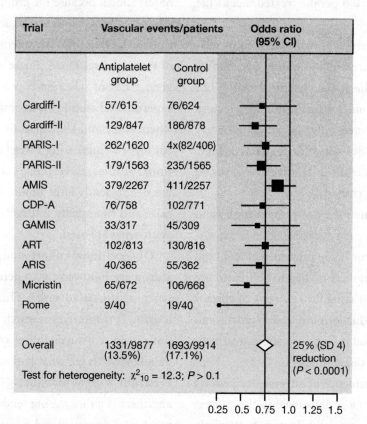

Fig. 3.4 A clear demonstration of benefits from meta-analysis of available trial data, when individual trials failed to provide convincing evidence.

black squares and their 95% confidence intervals (*CI*) in the fourth column.

The size of the square is proportional to the number of events. The diamond gives the point estimate and *CI* for overall effect.

RESULTS: IMPLEMENTATION

The way in which data from therapeutic trials are presented can influence doctors' perceptions of the advisability of adopting a treatment in their routine practice. To make clinical decisions, how many patients must be treated (and for how long) to obtain one desired result (number needed to treat) need to be known by researchers of therapeutic studies. This is the inverse (reciprocal) of absolute risk reduction.

Relative and absolute risk. The results of therapeutic trials are commonly expressed as the percentage reduction of an unfavourable (percentage increase in a favourable) outcome, i.e. as the relative risk, and this can be very impressive indeed until the figures are presented as the number of individuals actually affected per 100 people treated, i.e. as the absolute risk.

Where a baseline risk is low, a statement of relative risk alone is particularly misleading as it implies large benefit where the actual benefit is small. Thus a reduction of risk from 2% to 1% is a 50% relative risk reduction, but it saves only one patient for every 100 patients treated. But where the baseline is high, say 40%, a 50% reduction in relative risk saves 20 patients for every 100 treated.

Relative risk reductions can remain high (and thus make treatments seem attractive) even when susceptibility to the events being prevented is low (and the corresponding numbers needed to be treated are large). As a result, restricting the reporting of efficacy to just relative risk reductions can lead to great – and at times excessive – zeal in decisions about treatment for patients with low susceptibilities.

Whether a low incidence of adverse drug effects is acceptable becomes a serious issue in the context of absolute risk. Non- specialist doctors, particularly those in primary care, need and deserve clear and informative presentation of therapeutic trial results that measure the overall impact of a treatment on the patient's life, i.e. on clinically important outcomes such as morbidity, mortality, quality of life, working capacity, fewer days in hospital. Without it, they cannot adequately advise patients, who may themselves be misled by inappropriate use of statistical data in advertisements or on internet sites.

PHARMACOEPIDEMILOGY

Introduction to pharmacoepidemiology

Pharmacoepidemiology is the study of the use and effects of drugs in large numbers of people. Some of the principles of pharmacoepidemiology are used to gain further insight into the efficacy, and especially the safety, of new drugs once they have passed from limited exposure in controlled therapeutic pre-registration trials to the looser conditions of their use in the community. Trials in this setting are described as observational because the groups to be compared are assembled from subjects who are, or who are not (the controls), taking the treatment in the ordinary way of medical care. These (Phase 4) trials are subject to greater risk of selection bias and confounding than experimental studies (randomized controlled trials) where entry and allocation of treatment are strictly controlled (increasing internal validity). Observational studies, nevertheless, come into their own when sufficiently large randomized trials are logistically and financially impracticable. The following approaches are used.

Observational cohort studies. Patients receiving a drug are followed up to determine the outcomes (therapeutic or adverse). This is usually forward-looking (prospective) research. A cohort study does not re- quire a suspicion of causality; subjects can be followed 'to see what happens' (event recording). Prescription event monitoring (below) is an example, and there is an increasing tendency to recognise that most new drugs should be monitored in this way when prescribing becomes general. Major difficulties include the selection of an appropriate control group, and the need for large numbers of subjects and for prolonged surveillance. This sort of study is scientifically inferior to the experimental cohort study (the randomized controlled trial) and is cumbersome for research on drugs.

Investigation of the question of thromboembolism and the combined oestrogen - progestogen contraceptive pill by means of an observational cohort study required enormous numbers of subjects (the adverse effect is, fortunately, uncommon) followed over years. An investigation into cancer and the contraceptive pill by an observational cohort would require follow-up for 10–15 years. Happily, epidemiologists have devised a partial alternative: the case–control study.

Case–control studies. This reverses the direction of scientific logic from a forward- looking, 'what happens next' (prospective) to a backward - looking, 'what has happened in the past' (retrospective) investigation. The case–control study requires a definite hypothesis or suspicion of causality, such as an adverse reaction to a drug. The investigator assembles a group of patients who have the condition. A control group of people who have not had the reaction is then assembled (matched, e.g. for sex, age, smoking habits) from hospital admissions for other reasons, primary care records or electoral rolls. A complete drug history is taken from each group, i.e. the two groups are 'followed up' backwards to determine the proportion in each group that has taken the suspect agent. Case–control studies do not prove causation. They reveal associations and it is up to investigators and critical readers to decide the most plausible explanation.

A case–control study has the advantage that it requires a much smaller number of cases (hundreds) of disease and can thus be done quickly and cheaply. It has the disadvantage that it follows up subjects backwards and there is al- ways suspicion of the intrusion of unknown and so unavoidable biases in the selection of both patients and controls. Here again, independent repetition of the studies, if the results are the same, greatly enhances confidence in the outcome.

Surveillance systems: pharmaco-vigilance

Pharmacoepidemiology benefits from the methodology developed in general epidemiology and may further develop them for applications of methodology unique to needs of pharmacoepidemiology. There are also some areas that are altogether unique to pharmacoepidemiology, e.g, pharmacovigilance. Pharmacovigilance is a type of continual monitoring of unwanted effects and other safety-related aspects of drugs that are already placed in current growing integrating markets. In practice, Pharmacovigilance refers to spontaneous reporting systems which allow health care professionals and others to report adverse drug reactions to the central agency. The central agency combines reports from many sources to produce a more informative profile for drug products than could be done based on reports from fewer health care professionals.

Four kinds of logic can be applied to drug safety monitoring:

- To gain experience from regular reporting of suspected adverse drug reactions from health professionals during the regular clinical use of the drug.
- To attempt to follow a complete cohort of (new) drug users for as long as it is deemed necessary to have adequate information.
- To perform special studies in areas which may be predicted to give useful information.
- To examine disease trends for drug-related causality.

Drug safety surveillance relies heavily on the techniques of pharmacoepidemiology, which include the following:

Voluntary reporting. Doctors, nurses, pharmacists and patients may report suspected adverse reaction to drugs. In the UK, this is called the 'Yellow Card' system and the Commission for Human Medicines advises the Medicines and Healthcare products Regulatory Agency of the government on trends and signals. It is recommended that for:

- newer drugs: all suspected reactions should be reported, i.e. any adverse or any unexpected event, however minor, that could conceivably be attributed to the drug

- established drugs: all serious suspected reactions should be reported, even if the effect is well recognized.

Inevitably the system depends on the intuitions and willingness of those called on to respond. Surveys suggest that no more than 10% of serious reactions are reported. Voluntary reporting is effective for identifying reactions that develop shortly after starting therapy, i.e. at providing early warnings of drug toxicity, particularly rare adverse reactions. Thus, it is the first line in post-marketing surveillance. Reporting is particularly low, however, for reactions with long latency, such as tardive dyskinesia from chronic neuroleptic use. As the system has no limit of quantitative sensitivity, it may detect the rarest events, e.g. those with an incidence of 1:5 000 to 1:10 000. Voluntary systems are, however, unreliable for estimating the incidence of adverse reactions as this requires both a high rate of reporting (the numerator) and a knowledge of the rate of drug usage (the denominator).

Prescription event monitoring. This is a form of observational cohort study. Prescriptions for a drug (say, 20 000) are collected (in the UK this is made practicable by the existence of a National Health Service in which prescriptions are sent to a single central authority for pricing and payment of the pharmacist). The prescriber is sent a questionnaire and asked to report all events that have occurred (not only suspected adverse reactions) with no judgement regarding causality. Thus 'a broken leg is an event. If more fractures were associated with this drug they could have been due to hypotension, CNS effects or metabolic disease'. By linking general practice and hospital records and death certificates, both prospective and retrospective studies can be done and unsuspected effects detected. Prescription event monitoring can be used routinely on newly licensed drugs, especially those likely to be widely prescribed in general practice, and it can also be implemented quickly in response to a suspicion raised, e.g. by spontaneous reports.

Medical record linkage allows computer correlation in a population of life and health events (birth, marriage, death, hospital admission) with history of drug use. It is being developed as far as resources permit. It includes prescription event monitoring (above). The largest UK medical record linkage is the General Practice Research Database (GPRD) at the Medicines and Healthcare products Regulatory Agency.

Population statistics e.g. birth defect registers and cancer registers. These are insensitive unless a drug-induced event is highly remarkable or very frequent. If suspicions are aroused then case–control and observational cohort studies will be initiated.

STRENGTH OF EVIDENCE

A number of types of clinical investigation are described in this chapter, and elsewhere in the book. When making clinical decisions about a course of therapeutic action, it is obviously relevant to judge the strength of evidence generated by different types of study. This has been summarized as follows, in rank order:

1. Systematic reviews and meta-analyses.
2. Randomized controlled trials with definitive results (confidence intervals that do not overlap the threshold of the clinically significant effect).
3. Randomized controlled trials with non-definitive results (a difference that suggests a clinically significant effect but with confidence intervals overlapping the threshold of this effect).
4. Cohort studies.
5. Case–control studies.
6. Cross-sectional surveys.
7. Case reports.

IMPORTANT TERMINOLOGY

experimental therapeutics　实验治疗学
clinical trials　临床实验
informed consent form　知情同意书
pharmacokinetics　药物动力学
pharmacodynamics　药效学
hypothesis testing　假设检验

confidence intervals 置信区间
type I error I型错误
type II error II型错误
superiority trials 优效性试验
equivalence trials 等效性试验
non-inferiority trials 非劣效性试验
randomization 随机
parallel group design 平行组设计
crossover design 交叉设计
factorial designs 析因设计
multicentre trials 多中心试验
meta-analysis 荟萃分析

pharmacoepidemiology 药物流行病学

CHALLENGE YOURSELF

1. Please briefly introduce the four phases of clinical trials.
2. Please descript two methods to avoid bias in drug clinical trials.
3. Please descript common design of clinical trials and its application.
4. Please describe the basic principles of a meta-analysis.
5. Please briefly descript the types of surveillance system.

Hong Yuan

Chapter | 4 |

Classification and Regulatory System of drugs

Part 1. Classification and naming of drugs

CLASSIFICATION

It is evident from the way this book is organised that there is no homogeneous system for classifying drugs that suits the purpose of every user. Drugs are commonly categorized according to the convenience of whoever is discussing them: clinicians, pharmacologists or medicinal chemists.

Drugs may be classified by:

- *Body system*, e.g. alimentary, cardiovascular.
- *Therapeutic use*, e.g. receptor blockers, enzyme inhibitors, carrier molecules, ion channels.
- *Mode or site of action*:
  - *molecular interaction*, e.g. glucoside, alkaloid, steroid
  - *cellular site*, e.g. loop diuretic, catecholamine uptake inhibitor (imipramine)
- Molecular structure, e.g. glycoside, alkaloid, steroid.

In order to ensure the safe and effective clinical application of drugs, through the implementation of legislation on the classification of drugs management, which the drugs can also divided into prescription drugs and non-prescription drugs according to the pharmacological properties of drugs, clinical application and safety features.

Prescription drug means a drug that must be dispensed, purchased and used in a regular pharmacy or pharmacy by a prescribing physician.

Non-prescription drug refers to the approval of the National Medical Products Administration, does not need prescription of the practicing physician and consumers can judge, purchase and use drugs by themselves.

The significance of classification

Standardize the behavior of clinical medication to ensure safe use of drugs.

In the absence of drug classification management, people in the drugstore can buy any drugs, which can lead to many adverse consequences. Such the unreasonable use of antimicrobial agents can result in the rapid development of drug resistance and a variety of antimicrobial adverse drug reactions. And adults self-purchase **anxiety tablets and other anti-anxiety drugs, resulting in drug addiction**, and even lead to acute poisoning. Various drugs, which have strong pharmacological effects for the treatment of serious illness and prone to adverse reactions, will be limited to prescription drugs. Such as antibiotics for the treatment of bacterial infectious diseases, drugs for the treatment of nervous system diseases, the main drugs for the treatment of cardiovascular disease, hormones, biological agents and a variety of drugs through injection routes are classified in prescription drugs range. Physician to confirm the prescription for the premise of the issuance of the first dose of medication, the total amount of a prescription drug should be calculated according to the condition, so as to effectively avoid drug misuse and abuse. The specialties of prescription drugs including psychotropic substances, narcotic drugs, toxic drugs for medical use and radiopharmaceuticals should have more stringent restrictions on the sale of prescription drugs.

Provide a basis for self-medication

In 1978, World Health Organization (WHO) proposed the goal of health care for everybody in 2000 in Alma-Ata Declaration, noting that health is self-responsibility and advocates self-care and self-medication to achieve basic health care. The state drug regulatory department determined the type, dosage forms and specifications of non-prescription drugs according to the recognized non-prescription selection criteria, providing a security guarantee for people self-purchased drugs in community pharmacy and hospital pharmacy to achieve self-medication. Based on the situation of the community, the drug business enterprise shall equip the non-prescription drugstore and the medicine business network with the practicing pharmacist for the consultation service, contributing to a good social environment to develop the self-care and self-medication.

Conducive to the implementation of medical expenses for nation, group and individual sharing principles

In China, The Social Basic Medical Insurance System was gradual established for providing the community part compensation of the medical expenses, which is mainly used for treatment of patients with severe diseases in the hospital, and general minor ailments (such as headache, indigestion, etc) can rely on self-medication and bear their own drug costs. The principle of sharing the medical expenses according to the nature of the disease is conducive to consolidating the basic medical insurance system and curbing the rising medical expenditure to save the limited medical and health resources.

Conducive to improving the overall quality of medical care, and promote the development of Chinese medicine

With the implementation of drug classification management, patients can buy OTC drugs for their own common symptoms rather than to the hospital, which will not only save time and reduce expenses for patients, but also avoid the difficulties of hospital staff, so as to ensure that medical personnel have more time and energy to solve clinical problems and improve the overall quality of medical services. Hospital pharmacists can also be freed from the complexity of the general pharmacy work, and further strengthen the clinical pharmacy care for consulting rational use of drugs.

With the increasing application of non-prescription drugs and market demand, China's pharmaceutical companies put forward new requirements. Pharmaceutical companies can develop old drugs, which have been long-term clinical practice proved safe and effective, into convenient, economical and practical non-prescription drug of new formulations to meet the needs of the people self-medication through the reform of pharmaceutical formulations, which contributes to the development of the pharmaceutical industry and opens up a broader field.

NOMENCLATURE (NAMES)

Any drug may have names in all three of the following classes:

1. The full chemical name.
2. A non-proprietary (official, approved, generic) name used in pharmacopoeias and chosen by official bodies; the World Health Organization (WHO) chooses recommended International Nonproprietary Names (rINNs). The harmonisation of names began 50 years ago, and most countries have used rINNs for many years. The USA is an exception, but even here most US National Names are the same as their rINN counterparts. In the UK, there are two exceptions to the policy: adrenaline (rINN epinephrine) and noradrenaline (rINN norepinephrine). Manufacturers are advised to use both names on the product packaging and information literature.

In general we use rINNs in this book and aim to minimise some unavoidable differences with, where appropriate, alternative names in the text and index (in brackets).

3. A proprietary (brand) name that is the commercial property of a pharmaceutical company or companies. In this book proprietary names are distinguished by an initial capital letter.

The full chemical name describes the compound for chemists. It is obviously unsuitable for prescribing.

A *non-proprietary* (generic, approved) *name* is given by an official (pharmacopoeia) agency, e.g. WHO.

Three principles remain supreme and unchallenged in importance: the need for distinction in sound and spelling, especially when the name is handwritten; the need for freedom from confusion with existing names, both non proprietary and proprietary, and the desirability of indicating relationships between similar substances.

The generic names *diazepam, nitrazepam* and *flurazepam* are all of benzodiazepines. Their proprietary names are Valium, Mogadon and Dalmane respectively. Names ending in -*olol* are adrenoceptor blockers; those ending in –*pril* are angiotensin-converting enzyme (ACE) inhibitors; and those in -*floxacin* are quinolone antimicrobials. Any pharmaceutical company may manufacture a drug that has a well-established use and is no longer under patent restriction, in accordance with official pharmacopoeial quality criteria, and may apply to the regulatory authority for a licence to market. The task of authority is to ensure that these *generic* or *multi-source pharmaceuticals* are interchangeable, i.e. they are pharmaceutically and biologically equivalent, so that a formulation from one source will be absorbed and give the same blood concentrations and have the same therapeutic efficacy as that from another. (Further formal therapeutic trials are not demanded for these well-established drugs.) A prescription for a generic drug formulation may be written for any officially licensed product that the dispensing pharmacy has chosen to purchase.

The proprietary name is a trademark applied to particular formulation(s) of a particular substance by a particular manufacturer. Manufacture is confined to the owner of the trademark or to others licensed by the owner. It is designed to maximise the difference between the names of similar drugs marketed by rivals for obvious commercial reasons. To add confusion, some companies give their proprietary products the same names as their generic products in an attempt to capture the prescription market, both proprietary and generic, and some market lower-priced generics of their own proprietaries. When a prescription is written for a proprietary product, pharmacists under UK law must dispense that product only. But, by agreement with the prescribing doctor, they may substitute an approved generic product (generic substitution). What is not permitted is the substitution of a different molecular structure deemed to be pharmacologically and therapeutically equivalent (therapeutic substitution).

Non-proprietary names

The principal reasons for advocating the habitual use of non-proprietary (generic) names in prescribing are described below.

Clarity. Non-proprietary names give information on the class of drug; for example, nortriptyline and amitriptyline are plainly related, but their proprietary names, allegron and triptafen, are not. It is not unknown for prescribers, when one drug has failed, unwittingly to add or substitute another drug of the same group (even the same drug), thinking that different proprietary names must mean different classes of drugs. Such occurrences underline the wisdom of prescribing generically, so that group similarities are immediately apparent, but highlight the requirement for brand names to be as distinct from one another as possible. Relationships cannot, and should not, be shown by brand names.

Economy. Drugs sold under non-proprietary names are usually, but not always, cheaper than those sold under proprietary names.

Convenience. Pharmacists may supply whatever version they stock, whereas if a proprietary name is used they are obliged to supply that preparation alone. They may have to buy in the preparation named even though they have an equivalent in stock. Mixtures of drugs are sometimes given non-proprietary names, having the prefix *co-* to indicate more than one active ingredient, e.g. coamoxiclav for Augmentin. No prescriber can be expected to write out the ingredients, so proprietary names are used in many cases, there being no alternative. International travellers with chronic illnesses will be grateful for rINNs, as proprietary names often differ from country to country. The reasons are linguistic as well as commercial.

Proprietary names

The principal non-commercial reason for advocating the use of proprietary names in prescribing is consistency of the product, so that problems of quality, especially of bioavailability, are reduced. There is substance in this argument, though it is often exaggerated.

It is reasonable to use proprietary names when dosage, and therefore pharmaceutical bioavailability, is critical, so that small variations in the amount of drug available for absorption may have a big effect on the patient, e.g. drugs with a low therapeutic ratio, digoxin, hormone replacement therapy, adrenocortical steroids (oral), antiepileptics, cardiac antiarrhythmics, warfarin. In addition, with the introduction of complex formulations, e.g. sustained release, it is important clearly to identify these, and the use of proprietary names has a role.

The prescription and provision of proprietary drugs increases profits for the company who first invented the drug, and costs for the purchaser – variably the patient, insurer or national health-care system. There are no absolute rights or wrongs in this. Society rewards the inventer, because it requires inventions, but wishes a healthy generic market in order to restrain costs. The now widespread use of computer programmes for prescribing, which prompt the doctor to use non-proprietary names, has tilted the balance in favour of generics.

Generic names are intentionally longer than trade names to minimise the risk of confusion, but the use of accepted prefixes and stems for generic names works well and the average name length is four syllables, which is manageable. The search for proprietary names is a 'major problem' for pharmaceutical companies, increasing, as they are, their output of new preparations. A company may average 30 new preparations (not new chemical entities) a year, another warning of the urgent necessity for the doctor to cultivate a sceptical habit of mind. Names that 'look and sound medically seductive' are being picked out. 'Words that survive scrutiny will go into a stockpile and await inexorable proliferation of new drugs'. One firm (in the USA) commissioned a computer to produce a dictionary of 42 000 nonsense words of an appropriately scientific look and sound.

A more recent cause for confusion for patients (consumers) in purchasing proprietary medicines is the use by manufacturers of a well-established 'brand' name that is associated in the mind of the purchaser with a particular therapeutic effect, e.g. analgesia, when in fact the product may contain a quite different pharmacological entity. By a subtle change or addition to the brand name of the original medicine, the manufacturer aims to establish 'brand loyalty'. This unsavoury practice is called 'umbrella branding'. It is also important to doctors to be aware of what over-the-counter (OTC) medicines their patients are taking, as proprietary products that were at one time familiar to them may contain other ingredients, with the increased risk of adverse events and drug interactions.

For the practising doctor (in the UK) the *British National Formulary* provides a regularly updated and comprehensive list of drugs in their non-proprietary (generic) and proprietary names. 'The range of drugs prescribed by any individual is remarkably narrow, and once the decision is taken to "think generic" surely the effort required is small'. And, we would add, worthwhile.

Confusing names. The need for both clear thought and clear handwriting is shown by medicines of totally different class that have similar names. Serious events have occurred as a result of the confusion of names and dispensing the wrong drug, e.g. Lasix (furosemide) for Losec (omeprazole) (death); AZT (intending zidovudine) was misinterpreted in the pharmacy and azathioprine was dispensed (do not use abbreviations for drug names); Daonil (glibenclamide) for De-nol (bismuth chelate) and for Danol (danazol). It will be noted that non-proprietary names are less likely to be confused with other classes of drugs.

SUMMARY

In any science there are two basic requirements, classification and nomenclature (names):

- Classification – drugs cannot be classified and named according to a single rational system because the requirements of chemists, pharmacologists and doctors differ.
- Nomenclature – nor is it practicable always to present each drug under a single name because the formulations in which they are presented as prescribable medicines may vary widely and be influenced by commercial considerations.

Generic (non-proprietary) names should be used as far as possible when prescribing except where pharmaceutical bioavailability differences have overriding importance.

The wider availability of proprietary medicines through pharmacy sale and direct to the public has the potential for greater confusion to consumers (patients) and doctors.

Part 2. Official regulation of medicines

BASIS FOR REGULATION

Neither patients nor doctors are in a position to decide for themselves, across the range of medicines that they use, which ones are *pure* and *stable*, and *effective* and *safe*. They need assurance that the medicines they are offered fulfil these requirements and are supported by information that permits optimal use. The information about, and the usage of, medicines becomes out of date, and there is an obligation on licence holders continually to review their

licence with particular regard to safety. Marketing Authorisation Holders (MAHs), i.e. pharmaceutical companies, can also change the efficacy claims to their licence (e.g. new indications, extension of age groups) or change the safety information (e.g. add new warnings, or contraindications). The quality aspects may also need to be revised as manufacturing practices change. MAHs operate in a market economy and have strong profit motives for making claims about their drugs. Only governments can provide the assurance about all those aspects in the life of a medicine (in so far as it can be provided).

The *principles of official (statutory) medicines* regulation are that:

- No medicines will be marketed without prior licensing by the government.
- A licence will be granted on the basis of scientific evaluation of:
  1. *Safety*, in relation to its use: evaluation at the point of marketing is provisional in the sense that it is followed in the community by a pharmacovigilance programme.
  2. *Efficacy* (now often including quality of life).
  3. *Quality*, i.e. purity, stability (shelf-life).
  4. *Supply*, i.e. whether the drug is suitable to be unrestrictedly available to the public or whether it should be confined to sales through pharmacies or on doctors' prescriptions; and what printed information should accompany its sale (labelling, leaflets).
- A licence shall specify the clinical indications that may be promoted and shall be for a limited period (5 years), which is renewable on application. A regulatory authority may review the risk: benefit balance or safety of a drug at any time and restrict the licensing, or remove the drug from the market for good cause.
- A licence may be varied (altered) by an application from the pharmaceutical company to update efficacy, safety and quality sections; safety and (less commonly) efficacy variations may be initiated by the regulatory authority.

Plainly manufacturers and developers are entitled to be told what substances are regulated and what are not, and what kinds and amounts of data are likely to persuade a regulatory authority to grant a marketing application (licence) and for what medical purpose. In summary, medicines regulation aims to provide an objective, rigorous and transparent assessment of efficacy, safety and quality in order to protect and promote public health but not to impede the pharmaceutical industry. Inevitably, an interesting tension exists between regulators and regulated.

Historical background

The beginning of substantial government intervention in the field of medicines paralleled the proliferation of synthetic drugs in the early 20th century when the traditional and familiar pharmacopoeia expanded slowly and then, in mid-century, with enormous rapidity. The first comprehensive regulatory law that required pre-marketing testing was passed in the USA in 1938, following the death of about 107 people due to the use of diethylene glycol (a constituent of antifreeze) as a solvent for a stable liquid formulation of sulphanilamide for treating common infections.

Other countries did not take on board the lesson provided by the USA and it took *the thalidomide disaster* to make governments all over the world initiate comprehensive control over all aspects of drug introduction, therapeutic claims and supply. In 1960—1961 in (West) Germany, the incidence of phocomelia in newborns was noted. The term means 'seal extremities' and is a deformity in which the long bones of the limbs are defective and substantially normal or rudimentary hands and feet arise on, or nearly on, the trunk, like the flippers of a seal; other abnormalities may occur. Phocomelia is ordinarily exceedingly rare. Case–control and prospective observational cohort studies in antenatal clinics where women had yet to give birth provided evidence incriminating a sedative and hypnotic called thalidomide; it was recommended for use in pregnant women, although it had not been tested on pregnant animals. The worst had happened: a trivial new drug was the cause of the most grisly disaster in the short history of modern scientific drug therapy.

Many thalidomide babies died, but many live on with deformed limbs, eyes, ears, heart and alimentary and urinary tracts. The world total of survivors was probably about 10 000.

In the UK, two direct consequences were the development of a spontaneous adverse drug reaction reporting scheme (the Yellow Card system) and legislation to provide regulatory control on the safety, quality and efficacy of medicines through the systems of standards, authorisation, pharmacovigilance and inspection (Medicines Act 1968). A further landmark was the establishment of the Committee on Safety of Medicines in 1971 (from 2006 renamed the Commission on Human Medicines) to advise the Licensing Authority in the UK. In 1995, the new European regulatory system was introduced.

Despite these protective systems, other drug disasters occurred. In 1974 the β-blocking agent *practolol* was withdrawn because of a rare but severe syndrome affecting the eyes and other mucocutaneous regions in the body (not detected by animal tests), and in 1982 benoxaprofen, a non-steroidal anti-inflammatory drug, was found to cause serious adverse effects including onycholysis and photosensitivity in elderly patients. More recent examples that have gained wide public notice include the association of serotonin-specific reuptake inhibitors with increased risk of suicide behaviour and that of cyclo-oxygenase I and II inhibitors with cardiovascular disease.

CURRENT MEDICINES REGULATORY SYSTEMS

All countries where medicines are licensed for use have a regulatory system. When a pharmaceutical company seeks worldwide marketing rights, its programmes must satisfy each of the following: the Food and Drug Administration (FDA) of the USA; the European regulations and guidance issued by the Commission and overseen by the European Medicines Agency (EMA); and the Japanese Pharmaceutical Affairs Bureau. The national regulatory bodies of the individual European Union members remain in place but work with the EMA, which acts as a single source of authority. National licences can still be granted through individual member states, which maintain particular responsibility for their own public health issues. Significant harmonisation of practices and procedures at a global level was also achieved through the International Conferences on Harmonisation (ICH) involving Europe, Japan and the USA.

In the European Union drugs can be licensed in three ways:

1. *The centralised procedure* allows applications to be made directly to the EMA; applications are allocated for assessment to one member state (the rapporteur) assisted by a second member state (co-rapporteur). Approval of the licence is then binding on all member states. This approach is mandatory for biotechnology products and for certain new medicinal products.

2. *The mutual recognition (decentralised) procedure* allows applicants to nominate one member state (known as a reference member state), which assesses the application and seeks opinion from the other (concerned) member states. Granting the licence will ensure simultaneous mutual recognition in these other states, provided agreement is reached among them. There is an arbitration procedure to resolve disputes.

3. A product to be marketed in a single country can have its licence applied for through the *national route*.

The European systems are conducted according to strict timelines and written procedures. Once a medicine has been licensed for sale by one of the above procedures, its future regulatory life remains within that procedure. Safety updates have to be reviewed every 6 months for the first 2 years, then annually until 5 years. Thereafter, there may be a second renewal at 10 years, if safety issues demand. The renewal of a licence is primarily the responsibility of the pharmaceutical company, but requires approval from the regulatory authority. This provides the opportunity for companies to review, in particular, the safety aspects to keep the licence in line with cur-

rent clinical practice. Any major changes to licences must be made by variation of the original licence and supported by data, which for a major indication can be substantial.

In China, essential medicines policy is the heart of the national drug policy. WHO stressed that protection of the people's basic medical and health needs should be agreed by their governments to develop a number of supporting policies and regulations that the national drug policy, to guide drug development, production, circulation, application and supervision and management. The national drug policy is made up of a series of policy objectives and policy measures, including legislation and regulation of pharmaceuticals, drug selection, drug supplication, rational drug use, pharmacoeconomic strategies, drug monitoring and evaluation, drug research and development and international technical cooperation. In countries with relatively short medical resources, the key to the implementation of national drug policy is to ensure that the limited resources of the society are used rationally.

Since the 1980s, WHO has emphasized the need to develop and promote standard treatment guidelines and prescription sets in order to achieve the goal of safe, effective, convenient and economical application of clinical medication in the promotion of essential medicines. At the same time, the development and implementation of sound standard-setting guidelines is also known as the basis for the selection of essential medicines. The basic common points of any national drug policy:

- Ensure the supply and availability of essential drugs.
- Ensure to provide the public safe, effective, quality qualified drugs.
- Improve the clinical prescription and drug allocation for improving the level of rational drug use.

The Selection Principles of Essential Medicines in China as follows:

1. *Clinical necessity*: To meet the needs of the vast majority of population health care, at all times should ensure that sufficient quantities of essential drugs and appropriate dosage forms of sup-

ply, and should be dominated by national drugs.

2. *Safety and efficiency*: The available information and clinical experience can confirm the efficacy of selected drugs, less adverse reactions, quality and stability. The results of clinical evaluation were used as the main basis for the selection, if necessary, the laboratory evaluation and clinical trial reassessment of the pharmacy quality were carried out, and the evaluation conclusion was used as the basis.

3. *Reasonable prices*: Combined with the unit price of drugs and the total cost of treatment. Reasonable price is an important indicator of drug selection.

4. *Convenience*: Drug dosage forms and packaging should be suitable for different medical units in the convenience of both doctors and patients, but also conducive to the transport and storage of drugs.

5. *Preferred selection*: Choosing the best selection is based on the effectiveness, safety, quality stability, standard perfectness, price rationality and availability and other aspects of comprehensive comparison.

6. Same importance between Chinese and Western medicine: Emphasizing the equal importance of traditional Chinese medicine and western medicine in order to facilitate common development

7. *Selection of Traditional Chinese Medicine*: Base on the rectification of proprietary Chinese medicines and pay attention to gradually improve the quality standards of the varieties In the process of reviewing the process and standards of pharmaceuticals.

REQUIREMENTS

Authorisation for clinical trials in the UK

The EU Clinical Trial Directive 2001/20/EC harmonized the laws and administrative procedures relating to the regulation of clinical trials across Europe and replaced the previous legislation in each of the separate member states. It is implemented in the UK through the Medicines for Human Use (Clinical Trials) Regulations. All interventional clinical trials of an investigational medical product (so called CTIMPs), including human volunteer trials, require regulatory approval through a Clinical Trial Authorisation (CTA) application that must include summaries of preclinical, clinical and pharmaceutical data. For most trials a response must be provided by the regulatory authority within 30 days, with a maximum of up to 60 days. There is a complementary process to allow for amendments to the original application, and there is a requirement to notify each involved regulatory agency when the trial is completed.

Regulatory review of a new drug application

A drug regulatory authority requires the following:

- *Quality checks*. Full information on manufacturing process including purity, stability, formulation.
- *Preclinical tests*: tests carried out in animals to allow some prediction of potential efficacy and safety in humans.
- Clinical (human) tests.
- Knowledge of the environmental impact of pharmaceuticals. Regulatory authorities expect manufacturers to address this concern in their application to market new chemical entities. Aspects include manufacture (chemical pollution), packaging (waste disposal), pollution in immediate use, e.g. antimicrobials and, more remotely, drugs or metabolites entering the food chain or water where use may be massive, e.g. hormones.

The full process of regulatory review of a truly novel drug (new chemical entity) may take months.

In China, *application for new drugs* should submitted the development method, quality indicators, pharmacological and toxicological test results and other relevant information and samples to the state supervision and administration department or the drug regulatory department of the province, autonomous region or municipality directly under the Central Government, approved by the clinical trials before. New drugs, which have completed the clinical trials and production approval, will be issued a 'new drug certificate' by the State Drug Administration Department. Production of new drugs, will need 'approval number' approved by State Drug Administration Department. The State Drug Administration shall ensure the quality of new drug development and the conditions necessary for the clinical trial of new drug by grasping the two main links of clinical examination and approval and production approval of new drug in the process of drug research and development, so as to further ensure the quality controllability, safety and effectiveness of new drugs production market.

Generic drugs refer to the drugs prepared by the national standard of the original drug that has passed the patent protection period. Generic drugs should have the same active ingredients, routes of administration, dosage forms, specifications, and the same therapeutic effect as the generic. The development and production of generic drugs is beneficial to reduce the medical expenses, and it is of great significance to protect the people's access to basic medical services.

Drugs applied for import shall get the marketing approval in the country or region where the overseas enterprise is located, and its production should meet pharmaceutical production quality management practices of the country or region and the Chinese "pharmaceutical production quality management practices" requirements. The State Drug Administration shall be responsible for the formal examination of the declared materials. China Pharmaceutical and Biological Products Testing Institute is responsible for organizing registration test of the production and samples; and organizing on-site inspections of the development and production and taking samples. The State Food and Drug Administration Drug Evaluation Center is responsible for the review of the submitted information to form a comprehensive opinion so that The State Food and Drug Administration make the decision to approve. The drug for declaration, in compliance with the provisions,

is issued to "drug clinical trial documents". After completed with drug clinical trials and identified as qualified, the drug can be followed by production reporting and approval.

Regulatory review

Using one of the regulatory systems described above, an authority normally conducts a review in two stages:

1. Examination of preclinical data to determine whether the drug is safe enough to be tested for (predicted) human therapeutic efficacy.

2. Examination of the clinical studies to determine whether the drug has been shown to be therapeutically effective with safety appropriate to its use. If the decision is favourable, the drug is granted a marketing authorisation (for 5 years: renewable), which allows it to be marketed for *specified therapeutic uses*. The authority must satisfy itself of the adequacy of the information to be provided to prescribers in a Summary of Product Characteristics (SPC) and also a Patient Information Leaflet (PIL).

The PIL must also be approved by the licensing authority, be deemed fairly to represent the SPC, and be comprehensive and understandable to patients and carers. Where a drug has special advantage, but also has special risk, restrictions on its promotion and use can be imposed, e.g. isotretinoin and clozapine.

Central to the decision to grant a marketing authorisation is the assessment procedure undertaken by professional medical, scientific, statistical and pharmaceutical staff at one of the national agencies. In the UK these are employed as civil servants within the Medicines and Healthcare products Regulatory Agency (MHRA) and are advised by various independent expert committees.

When a novel drug is granted a marketing authorization it is recognised as a medicine and there is rejoicing among those who have spent many years developing it. But the testing is not over: the most stringent test of all is about to begin. It will be used in all sorts of people of all ages and sizes, and having all sorts of other conditions. Its use can no longer be supervised so closely as hitherto. Doctors will prescribe it and patients will use it correctly and incorrectly. It will have effects that have not been anticipated. It will be taken in overdose. It has to find its place in therapeutics, through extended comparisons with other drugs available for the same diseases.

Drugs used to prevent a long-term morbidity, e.g. stroke in hypertensive patients, can be proven effective only in *outcome* trials that are usually considered too expensive even to start until marketing of the drug is guaranteed. The effect of a drug at preventing rare occurrences requires many thousands of patients, more than are usually studied during development. Similarly rare adverse events cannot be detected prior to marketing, and it would be unethical to expose large numbers of trial patients to a novel drug for purely safety reasons.

Post-licensing responsibilities

The pharmaceutical company is predominantly interested in gaining as widespread a usage as fast as possible, based on the efficacy of the drug demonstrated in pre-registration trials. The regulatory authorities are more concerned with the safety profile of the drug and protection of public health. The most important source of safety data once the drug is in clinical use is spontaneous reporting of adverse events, which will generate 'signals' and raise suspicion of infrequent but potentially serious adverse events caused by the drug. Proving the causal link from sporadic signals can be extremely difficult, and is entirely dependent on the number and quality of these spontaneous reports. In the UK, these reports are captured through the Yellow Card system, which may be completed by doctors, nurses or pharmacists and, most recently, by patients. Other countries have their own systems. The importance of encouraging accurate spontaneous reporting of adverse events cannot be overemphasised.

Since 2005, companies are required to submit at the time of licence application the details of subsequent review and management systems. This may include a postauthorisation surveillance study (PASS). Other studies investigating the safety of a medicine that are not directly sponsored by the manufacturer may be identified from various organisations. These include the Drug Safety Research Unit (Southampton, UK) using Prescription Event Monitoring (PEM), the Medicines Monitoring Unit (MEMO) (Tayside, UK), and the use of computerised record linkage schemes (in place in the USA for many years) such as the UK General Practice Research Database (GPRD) at the MHRA. All these systems have the important capacity to obtain information on very large numbers of patients (10 000–20 000) in observational cohort studies and case– control studies, complementing the spontaneous reporting system.

In the UK, many new drugs are highlighted as being under special consideration by the regulatory authorities, by marking the drug with a symbol, the inverted black triangle (▼), in formularies. The regulatory authority communicates emerging data on safety of drugs to doctors through letters or papers in journals, through specialist journals, e.g. Current Problems in Pharmacovigilance, in the UK, and for very significant issues by direct ('Dear Doctor') letters and fax messages.

Two other important regulatory activities that affect marketed drugs are:

- Variations to licences.
- Reclassifications.

Variations are substantial changes instigated usually by pharmaceutical companies, but sometimes by the regulatory authority, to the efficacy, safety or quality aspects of the medicine. Most significant variations involve additions to indications or dosing regimens, or to the warnings and contraindication sections of the SPC. They need to be supported by evidence and undergo formal assessment.

Reclassification means change in the legal status of a medicine and is the process by which a prescription-only medicine can be converted to one that is available directly to the public through pharmacies and shops. It follows a rigorous assessment process with a particular stress on safety aspects of the medicine; it involves advice from the Commission on Human Medicines and public consultation. The purpose of reclassification is to allow easier access of the general public to effective and safe medicines for self-medication. In the UK, emergency contraception ('morning after' pill), simvastatin and omeprazole have been reclassified to be available from pharmacies without prescription, under supervision of a pharmacist.

DISCUSSION

Common sense would seem to dictate that safety and efficacy of a drug should be fully defined before it is granted marketing authorisation. For practical and ethical reasons, pre-licensing trials with very close supervision are limited to hundreds, sometimes thousands, of patients and are powered to detect efficacy. Post-licensing studies are increasingly regarded as essential to complete the evaluation of drugs under conditions of ordinary use on a large scale, these programmes being preferable to attempts to enlarge and prolong formal therapeutic trials.

It would also seem sensible to require developers to prove that a new drug is not only effective but is actually needed in medicine before it is licensed. Strong voices are now arguing that a *risk: benefit* assessment of new (candidate) medicines against old medicines should be part of a regulatory application. It is argued that a novel drug finds its place only after several, sometimes many, years, and to delay licensing is simply impracticable on financial grounds. Thus a 'need clause' in licensing is not generally practicable if drug developers are to stay in that business. This is why *comparative* therapeutic studies of a new drug with existing drugs are not required for licensing in countries having a research-based pharmaceutical industry. A 'need clause' is, however, appropriate for economically deprived countries; indeed, such countries have no alternative.

The licensing authority in the UK is not concerned with the pricing of drugs or their cost-effectiveness. The cost of medicines does, however, concern all governments, as part of the rising costs of national health services. A serious attempt to control costs on drug usage by the introduction of national guidelines on disease management (including the

use of individual drugs) and the appraisal of new and established medicines for cost-effectiveness now operate through a government-funded body called the National Institute for Health and Clinical Excellence (NICE). The present text includes a section on what is called health technology assessment by the Chairman of NICE. In addition, elements of guidance notes issued by NICE appear throughout the book.

Licensed medicines for unlicensed indications

Doctors may generally prescribe any medicine for any legitimate medical purpose, when they judge it to be in the best interest of the patient. But if they use a drug for an indication that is not formally included in the product licence ('off-label' use) they would be wise to think carefully and to keep particularly good records, for, if a patient is dissatisfied, prescribers may find themselves having to justify the use in a court of law. (Written records made at the time of a decision carry substantial weight, but records made later, when trouble is already brewing, lose much of their power to convince, and records that have been altered later are quite fatal to any defence.) Manufacturers are not always willing to go to the trouble and expense of the rigorous clinical studies required to extend their licence unless a new use is likely to generate significant profits. They are prohibited by law from promoting an unlicensed use. Much prescribing for children is in fact 'off licence' because clinical trials are usually conducted in adults and information sufficient for regulatory purposes in children does not exist. Paediatricians have to use adult data, scaled by body-weight or surface area, together with their clinical experience. To address this issue, companies are now required to conduct trials in children.

Unlicensed medicines and accelerated licensing

Regulatory systems make provision for the supply of an unlicensed medicine, e.g. one that has not yet completed its full programme of clinical trials, for patients who, on the judgement of their doctors, have no alternative among licensed drugs. The doctor must apply to the manufacturer, who may supply the drug for that particular patient and at the doctor's own responsibility. Various terms are used, e.g. supply on a 'named patient' basis (UK); 'compassionate' drug use (USA). It is illegal to exploit this sensible loophole in supply laws to conduct research. Precise record-keeping of such use is essential. But there can be desperate needs involving large numbers of patients, e.g. AIDS, and regulatory authorities may respond by licensing a drug before completion of the usual range of studies (making it clear that patients must understand the risks they are taking). Unfortunately such well-intentioned practice discourages patients from entering formal trials and may, in the long run, actually delay the definition of life-saving therapies.

Decision-taking

The responsibility to protect public health on the one hand, yet to allow timely access to novel medicines on the other, is one shared by drug regulators, expert advisory bodies and developers. It is complicated by an ever-increasing awareness of the risks and benefits (real or perceived) of medicines by the general public. Some new medicines are registered with the high expectation of effectiveness and with very little safety information; rare and unpredictable adverse events may take years to appear with sufficient conviction that causality is accepted. In taking decisions about drug regulation, it has been pointed out that there is uncertainty in three areas:

- Facts.
- Public reaction to the facts.
- Future consequences of decisions.

Regulators are influenced not only to avoid risk but also to avoid regret later (regret avoidance), and this consideration has a profound effect whether or not the decision-taker is conscious of it; it promotes defensive regulation. Regulatory authorities are frequently accused of being too cautious, and responsible, at least in part, for the stagnation in new drug development.

It is self-evident that it is much harder to detect and quantify a good that is not done than it is to detect and quantify a harm that is done. Therefore, although it is part of the decision-taker's job to facilitate the doing of good, the avoidance of harm looms larger. Attempts to blame regulators for failing to do good due to regulatory procrastination, the 'drug lag', do not induce the same feelings of horror in regulators and their advisory committees as are induced by the prospect of finding they have approved a drug that has, or may have, caused serious injury and that the victims are about to appear on television. The bitterness of people injured by drugs, whether or not there is fault, could be much reduced by the institution of simple non-adversarial arrangements for compensation.

Counterfeit drugs

Fraudulent medicines make up as much as 6% of pharmaceutical sales worldwide. They present a serious health (and economic) problem in countries with weak regulatory authorities and lacking money to police drug quality. In these countries counterfeit medicines may make up 20%–50% of available products. The trade may involve: false labelling of legally manufactured products, in order to play one national market against another; also, low-quality manufacture of correct ingredients; wrong ingredients, including added ingredients (such as corticosteroids added to herbal medicine for arthritis); no active ingredient; false packaging. The trail from raw material to appearance on a pharmacy shelf may involve as many as four countries, with the final stages (importer, wholesaler) quite innocent, so well has the process been obscured. Developed countries have inspection and enforcement procedures to detect and take appropriate action on illegal activities.

The public has a role to play. A patient with obsessive–compulsive disorder was receiving treatment with olanzapine. His custom was rigorously to polish the tablets each day before consumption. After one of his repeat prescriptions, his polishing became ever more thorough until the blue colour started to wear off the tablets. He rang the company to complain. Instead of being dismissed as a touch eccentric, the company investigated and found the tablets to be – well, not true blue.

Complementary and alternative medicine

The broad term complementary and alternative medicine (CAM) covers a range of widely varied diagnostic and therapeutic practices; it includes herbal and traditional (mainly Chinese) medicines, homoeopathic remedies and dietary supplements. The public demand for these substances is substantial and the financial interests are huge: annual global sales of complementary medicines have reached an estimated US$83 billion. The efficacy, safety and quality of herbal and homoeopathic preparations have been critically reviewed. Physicians need to be aware that their patients may be taking CAM preparations, not least because of the risk of adverse reactions and drug–drug interactions, e.g. enzyme induction with St John's wort (*Hypericum perforatum*).

In the UK, largely for historical reasons, the regulation of CAM is problematic and rife with inconsistencies. Some herbal medicines are licensed as such; some are exempt from licensing; some are sold as food supplements; and some products are available in all three categories. Herbal products were granted a Product Licence of Right (PLR) when the licensing system was introduced in the 1970s. Proof of efficacy, safety and quality (mandatory for 'regular' chemical and biologically developed medicinal products) is usually absent. From 2011, European legislation requires registration of CAM based on quality, safety and traditional use. Manufacturers are obliged to report adverse reactions.

Medicines regulation: the future

In the UK, the principal responsibilities of medicine regulation, i.e. for safe and effective medicines of high quality, will remain the same but the following themes will provide special attention:

- The promotion and protection of public health: the obligations to ministers, the public and industry are unchanged but regulators will operate in an environment in which the public increasingly expects more effective medicines without sacrifice of safety. Some results of this are already apparent.

- A wider and more rapid international pharmacovigilance.
- Greater transparency in regulatory decision-making.
- More biological, especially therapeutic, antibodies.
- Pharmacogenetics.
- The results of assessed applications for new medicines will see a shift from complex technical to patientoriented documents with clear expressions of risk and benefit.
- A widening of the availability of medicines for chronic disorders through pharmacies, by nurses and other nonmedical professionals, and directly to the public.
- Attention to the regulation of medicines for special populations, e.g. the licensing of old and new medicines for children.
- Benefit–risk management throughout product lifecycle.

SUMMARY

This part mainly describes the background why it's necessary to regulate the use and supply of drugs, and the ways in which these processes are managed. The basis for regulation is safety, efficacy, quality and supply. All countries where medicines are licensed for use have a regulatory system including the Food and Drug Administration (FDA) of the USA, the European Medicines Agency (EMA) and the Japanese Pharmaceutical Affairs Bureau.

Part 3. Health technology assessment

Before embarking on the health technology assessment of a product the scope of the enquiry needs to be carefully defined:

1. Obviously the product, or group of products, under investigation needs to be characterised.
2. The nature of the comparator health technology (technologies) also requires definition. Depending on the circumstances, the comparator might be another pharmaceutical product indicated for

the samecondition; it might be a device or procedure used for the same or similar purposes; or it might be 'best supportive care'. In any event, the comparator should reflect current clinical practice.

Difficulties arise when a potential comparator is not licensed for a particular indication but is, nevertheless, used in clinical practice. This is a particular problem in the heath technology assessment of products for use in children and for whom potential comparators reflect 'custom and practice' even though unlicensed. The wise course of action, in such circumstances, is to include comparators that reflect current clinical practice.

3. At the start of any health technology assessment, the clinical outcome(s) of interest should be decided. The most desirable, of course, is the 'ultimate outcome', such as dead versus alive or recovered versus not recovered. There are circumstances, however, when an assessment is focused on an 'intermediate' (surrogate) outcome where there is confidence that this reflects the ultimate outcome. For example, in the assessment of statins for the treatment of hypercholesterolaemia, a decision would need to be taken as to whether the long-term 'ultimate' outcome (i.e. reduction in coronary artery disease) should be used; or whether the assessment should be concerned with an 'intermediate' outcome (i.e. a reduction in LDL cholesterol).

4. The type of evidence required to demonstrate the effectiveness of a product must also be determined. In many instances this may be restricted to the results of randomised controlled trials. There may be circumstances where other study designs are more appropriate. In the assessment of a vaccine, for example, evidence from randomised controlled trials may usefully be supplemented by the results of observational studies that have examined its efficacy under circumstances that more closely reflect its performance in the 'real world'.

5. Decisions must also be made about the form any economic evaluation should take. These include the economic perspective and the type of analysis that is most appropriate. These issues are discussed later.

CLINICAL EFFECTIVENESS

An assessment of the clinical effectiveness of a product requires a full 'systematic review' of the available evidence. A systematic review involves four steps:

Developing the protocol

The development of a protocol for a systematic review is just as important in secondary research as it is for primary research. The objectives of the review will usually have been defined by the scope (as above). The protocol will, in addition, include the relevant:

- pharmacological product or therapeutic class
- comparator(s) which may include a nonpharmacological procedure
- study designs for assessing the effectiveness of the product
- clinical endpoints used in the studies that are to be included in the review.

Defining the methods

The literature search will, at a minimum, involve a comprehensive search of the three major electronic databases (MEDLINE, EMBASE and CENTRAL). Although there is some overlap between each database, one alone is inadequate. The usual approach is to start the search in a broad manner by looking at the abstracts of all the studies that appear to be relevant and then only include those that match the criteria that have been established for the review. In a review of the clinical effectiveness of statins, for example, the review criteria may have required the assessment to be restricted to randomised controlled trials where the outcome is the secondary prevention of vascular death or disability. All other study designs, involving different patient populations or surrogate outcomes, would be excluded. The search will also include any relevant references gleaned from scrutiny of the list of publications in the included studies.

43

One of the major problems in identifying appropriate studies in any systematic review is so-called 'publication bias'. There is a tendency for negative studies, or those demonstrating only very modest benefits, to either remain unpublished or to be published in a non-English language journal. The inclusion of such studies is extremely important if a reliable indication of the product's 'effect size' is to be made. Common techniques to avoid publication bias include enquiry of both the particular manufacturer as well as of known experts in the particular field. The assessment team must also decide whether to attempt to identify articles in non-English language journals and get them translated. This step substantially increases the cost of the review and is not invariably undertaken.

Analysing the data

After extracting the relevant data from each of the studies that meet the review inclusion criteria an 'evidence table' is constructed. In such a table the relevant data for each study are summarised and usually include:

- The study's bibliographic reference.
- The type of study (e.g. randomised controlled trial case–control study).
- Number of patients in each arm.
- Patient characteristics (e.g. age, gender).
- Study setting (e.g. hospital inpatients, GPs' surgeries).
- Intervention(s) including dose(s) and route(s) of administration.
- Comparator interventions (e.g. placebo, active comparator).
- Length of follow-up.
- Outcome measure(s) and effect size(s).
- Additional comments.

The evidence table may also include some attempt to assess the quality of each study. There is no generally accepted approach to doing this but one of the more common methods is to use the Jadad score. This itemises those elements in the design and conduct of a study (i.e. randomisation and blinding) that contribute most to a study's internal validity. A

score of 5 would indicate that the particular study appeared to avoid both selection and ascertainment biases. A score of 0 would cast considerable doubt on a study's internal validity.

Qualitative synthesis

Almost all systematic reviews include an element of narrative or 'qualitative' synthesis outlining, or expanding on, aspects of the included studies. Narrative syntheses become a more significant component in systematic reviews of complex interventions (such as a comparison between an antidepressant and cognitive behavioural therapy in the treatment of mild depression). The defining characteristic of a formal narrative synthesis is the use of a textual approach that provides an analysis of the relationships within and between studies, and an overall assessment of the robustness of the evidence. It is a more subjective process than meta-analysis and, when used, needs to be rigorous and transparent to reduce the potential for bias.

Quantitative synthesis (meta-analysis)

A qualitative synthesis of the results in a systematic review may itself be sufficient. It is very common, however, to attempt a quantitative synthesis – or meta-analysis – of the individual outcomes from each study so as to provide the most reliable estimate of the overall size of a product's effects.

A meta-analysis, at its most simple level, involves extracting the summary statistical data for each study. The relevant data are the mean differences in outcomes at the end of the study with their 95% confidence intervals. Estimates of the effect size for of the included studies, and the pooled estimate from all the studies, are often depicted as a 'forest plot'; an example is shown in Figure 4.1.

This forest plot summarises the results of each of five placebo-controlled trials, designed to assess the effect of anticoagulation with warfarin on the frequency of ischaemic stroke in patients with non-valvular atrial fibrillation. In a typical forest plot, there is an abbreviated reference to each trial on the left. The point estimate (mean) of the results of each study is represented as a square; and the horizontal line running through the square is its 95% confidence interval. The size of each square is proportional to the size of the study compared to the others. The column at the right shows the individual odds ratios (the expression of benefit used in this meta-analysis), and their 95% confidence intervals, for each study. By convention, improvement (a decrease in the frequency of ischaemic stroke) is shown to the left of the vertical 'no effect' line; a worsening (an increase in the frequency of ischaemic stroke) is shown to the right. In the forest plot in Figure 4.1 the outcome is expressed as odds ratios. In each of five studies, the frequency of ischaemic stroke is reduced by treatment with warfarin and all five 'squares' are to the left of the 'no effect' (odds ratio=1) vertical line. In three of the studies the 95% confidence interval does not cross the 'no effect' line and the results would be statistically significant with P values of less than 0.05. In the other two studies, the upper boundaries of the 95% confidence interval cross the 'no effect' line and would not reach conventional levels of statistical significance (i.e. the P value is more

than 0.05). The overall pooled mean effect size, taking account of the results of all five studies, is shown as a diamond in Figure 4.1; and the horizontal line again represents its 95% confidence interval.

The value of a forest plot is that the results can be seen and interpreted almost at a glance. Although not all the studies were statistically significant the mean effects of each study showed benefit; and those that failed to meet statistical significance were the smaller studies (as evidenced by their smaller squares).

Drawing conclusions

The final step in a systematic review is to discuss it strengths and weaknesses, and to draw conclusions. Both strengths and weaknesses will depend in large part on the range and quality of the included studies. The veracity of any conclusions will also depend on the extent to which there might have been publication bias so that important trials with negative results were never published. There are statistical techniques that can sometimes be helpful in establishing probable publication bias. Scrutiny of Figure 4.1 suggests that it would be reasonable, by any stan-

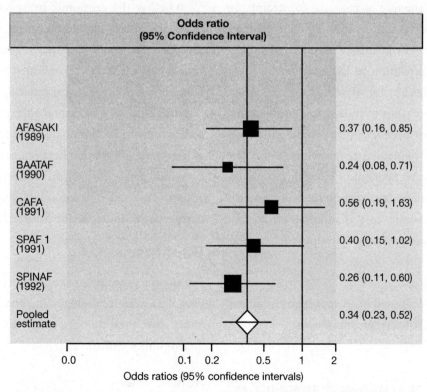

Fig. 4.1 Forest plot of five placebo-controlled trials of warfarin's efficacy in preventing ischaemic stroke in patients with non-valvularatrial fibrillation (Odds ratios with 95% confidence intervals.).

dards, to regard warfarin as effective in the prevention of ischaemic stroke in patients with nonvalvular atrial fibrillation. Moreover, the authors were able to estimate that about 25 strokes and about 12 disabling or fatal strokes would be prevented yearly for every 1 000 patients with atrial fibrillation treated with warfarin.

COST-EFFECTIVENESS

No health-care system is able to meet all the demands of its patients. The resources used to provide health care, in any individual country, are directly proportional to its wealth, so that wealthier nations with higher gross domestic products are able to devote more resources to health care than poorer ones. The manner in which health-care priorities are decided varies between countries, but rationing decisions are necessary – explicitly or implicitly – in all countries because resources are finite and demand is (almost) infinite.

A cost–effectiveness analysis attempts to provide a health-care system with a rational basis for decision making in the face of resource constraints. In pharmacoeconomics this involves trying to estimate the extra cost to the health-care system of adopting a product in relation to the additional benefit the product might bring. If a health-care system devotes very large sums of money to a product that gives only modest benefits, other people, with other conditions, will be denied cost effective care. The cost-effectiveness component of a health technology assessment thus attempts to provide some indication of the 'opportunity cost' of adopting a particular technology. In doing so, the assessment has to take account of:

- The relevant costs.
- The benefits expressed in an appropriate manner.
- The type of analysis that will be used.

The costs

The costs of using a particular pharmaceutical will include the acquisition costs of the product, as well as the costs associated with its use (such as any spe-

cial monitoring requirements, additional visits to hospital). In using warfarin for the prevention of ischaemic stroke, the costs will therefore have to include the costs of the warfarin itself, the costs of attending a hospital anticoagulant clinic and the laboratory monitoring costs.

The costs will also have to include the consequences of any adverse effects which, in the case of warfarin, would need to encompass the costs associated with warfarin-induced bleeding. The costs will also have to take account of any savings from which a health-care system would benefit. These are often known as 'cost offsets' which, in the case of warfarin to prevent ischaemic stroke, would include the savings made by the reduction in strokes among treated patients.

The costs might also include the wider costs and savings to society as a whole. In this case the costs (and cost offsets) would be extended to include any reduction in time off work; or, continuing the warfarin example, the savings resulting from fewer strokes that would reduce the costs associated with unemployment or disability.

Whether the economic perspective (as economists describe it) should be based on the costs and savings to the health-care system alone, or whether it should be societal, is a complicated and controversial issue. It is a political, fiscal (relating to government revenue, especially taxes) and governmental problem rather than an economic one. For this reason there is considerable variation between countries as to the economic perspective taken. A societal perspective is adopted in Sweden, for example, but in the UK the perspective is limited to the National Health Service.

Benefits

For the purposes of an economic analysis, the benefits of a health technology can, broadly, be expressed either in 'natural units' (e.g. life years gained), or as 'health utility' gained.

Natural units

The number of life years saved as a result of using a product is a commonly used natural unit for products that extend life. Other natural units might include the number of additional centimetres of height gained from the use of human growth hormone in the treatment of children with congenital growth hormone deficiency; or, again using the warfarin example, the number of strokes prevented.

The use of natural units is relatively simple and they can be used effectively in comparing the costs and benefits of products that are used to treat the same condition. The disadvantage is that it is impossible to use natural units for comparing the costs and benefits of treatments for different conditions. It is for this reason that most economic analyses prefer to use health 'utilities' as the measure of benefit.

Health utilities

Utilities are numbers assigned to preferences according to a rule. There are a number of ways by which health utilities can be captured and all are based on an assessment, by each person, of the improvement in their quality of life. These are then aggregated across the patients using the product of interest as well as those using the comparator(s). If the study itself did not collect health-related quality of life data, there are techniques that allow it to be imputed.

The most widely used technique for capturing health related quality-of-life data is the so-called EuroQol EQ-5D questionnaire. It is not disease-specific and captures patients' preferences for particular health states.

The health utility measure provided by the EQ-5D ranges from 0 (dead) to 1 (perfect health). When patients benefit from a particular treatment their health state might move from (say) 0.5 to 0.8 with a corresponding utility gain of 0.3. This is multiplied by the number of years for which it is enjoyed to yield the 'quality-adjusted life years' (QALY). If patients could on average expect to enjoy a utility gain of 0.3 for 10 years, the quality-adjusted life years gained would be 3.0 (0.3 times 10).

Type of analysis

Two types of analysis are possible depending on whether the benefits are expressed in natural units or as utilities. Both require calculating an 'incremental cost-effectiveness ratio' (ICER) by dividing the incremental costs by the incremental benefits. Treatment pathways, however, can be extraordinarily complicated; and in arriving at an ICER health economists must of necessity construct an economic model. There is a great variety of these, and they vary in their complexity. No attempt is made to discuss them further here, and their interpretation requires considerable expertise.

Cost-effectiveness analysis

In a cost–effectiveness analysis the ICER is expressed as the incremental cost (£) per incremental gain in some natural unit. In the case of a product that, in advanced cancer, results in (say) a 6-month extension of life at a total cost of (say) £10 000, the ICER would be £20 000 per life year gained.

Cost-utility analysis

In this form of analysis the ICER is expressed as the ratio of the incremental costs to the incremental utility gain. The most common expression of this form of ICER is as cost (£) per incremental gain in the quality adjusted life years (£ per QALY).

A health technology assessment may also include economic evaluations in subgroups of patients, such as those aged over 65 years, or those with other identifiable prognostic characteristics. This is usually undertaken when the overall ICER for the product is likely to represent poor value for money, but when there may be subgroups who might gain greater benefit.

IN CONCLUSION

A health technology assessment is concerned with analysing the totality of the available clinical and economic evidence. Bodies undertaking health technology assessments are not, however, decision-makers. Health technology assessments should provide decision-makers with a sophisticated analysis of the available data, together with a critical evaluation of the strengths and weaknesses of the assessment as well as the limitations in the economic analyses.

One of the most critical issues, in the assessment of the clinical data, is the extent to which the benefits in trials can be extrapolated beyond the data. In the trials depicted in Figure 4.1, the average duration of follow-up was 1.5 years. Does this mean that treatment should be stopped after this? The mean age of participants was 69 years and with very few under the age of 50 years or over the age of 80 years. Does this mean that treatment should be denied to younger people? Or to the very elderly?

These are the decisions that decision-makers themselves must make. A reasonable decision-maker could reasonably conclude that to stop warfarin treatment after 1.5 years would be wrong, and that denying the very likely benefits to those younger and older than those in the trials would be equally wrong. These decisions are ones that require judgements to be made rather than strict adherence to the tenets of health technology assessment. Health technology assessment plays a crucial role in underpinning evidence-based clinical practice but it does not supplant the place of judgement.

SUMMMARY

Health technology assessments bridge the gap between licensing and everyday clinical practice and may be used by a variety of agencies. It may inform the decisions of individual practitioners in the treatment of their own patients or it may be used by a hospital to develop their treatment policies. Health technology assessments are critical for those developing clinical guidelines for the management of specific conditions; and they may be used by policy makers for an entire health-care system.

There are three stages in the health technology assessment of a product: definition of the scope of the assessment, assessment of its clinical effectiveness, and assessment of its cost-effectiveness.

IMPORTANT TERMINOLOGY

International Nonproprietary Names (INN) 国际非专利药名

proprietary name 专利名

generic names 通用名

over-the-counter (OTC) medicines 非处方药物

new drug application 新药申请

clinical effectiveness 临床疗效

qualitative synthesis 定性分析

quantitative synthesis (meta-analysis) 定量分析（荟萃分析）

cost–effectiveness analysis 成本 - 效果分析

CHALLENGE YOURSELF

1. Please descript the classification of drugs.
2. Please descript the regulatory System of drugs in different countries.
3. Please descript the main content of clinical effectiveness.

Xiongwen Lv

Chapter | 5 |

Pharmacodynamics and Pharmacokinetics

QUALITATIVE ASPECTS

The starting point is to consider what drugs do and how they do it, i.e. the nature of drug action. The body functions through control systems that involve chemotransmitters or local hormones, receptors, enzymes, carrier molecules and other specialised macromolecules such as DNA.

Most medicinal drugs act by altering the body's control systems and, in general, they do so by binding to some specialised constituent of the cell, selectively to alter its function and consequently that of the physiological or pathological system to which it contributes. Such drugs are structurally specific in that small modifications to their chemical structure may profoundly alter their effect.

Mechanisms

An overview of the mechanisms of drug action shows that drugs act on *specific receptors* in the cell membrane and interior by:

- *Ligand-gated ion channels*, i.e. receptors coupled directly to membrane ion channels; neurotransmitters act on such receptors in the postsynaptic membrane of a nerve or muscle cell and give a response within milliseconds.
- *G-protein-coupled receptor systems*, i.e. receptors bound to the cell membrane and coupled to intracellular effector systems by a *G-protein*. For

instance, catecholamines (*the first messenger*) activate β-adrenoceptors through a coupled G-protein system. This increases the activity of intracellular adenylyl cyclase, increasing the rate of formation of cyclic AMP (*the second messenger*), a modulator of the activity of several enzyme systems that cause the cell to act. The process takes seconds.

- *Protein kinase receptors*, so called because the structure incorporates a protein kinase, are targets for peptide hormones involved in the control of cell growth and differentiation, and the release of inflammatory mediators over a course of hours.
- *Cytosolic (nuclear) receptors*, i.e. within the cell itself, regulate DNA transcription and, thereby, protein synthesis, e.g. by steroid and thyroid hormones, a process that takes hours or days.

Drugs also act on processes within or near the cell by:

- *Enzyme inhibition*, e.g. platelet cyclo-oxygenase by aspirin, cholinesterase by pyridostigmine, xanthine oxidase by allopurinol.
- Inhibition or induction of *transporter processes* that carry substances into, across and out of cells, e.g. blockade of anion transport in the renal tubule cell by probenecid is used to protect against the nephrotoxic effects of cidofovir (used for cytomegalovirus retinitis).
- *Incorporation into larger molecules*, e.g. 5-fluorouracil, an anticancer drug, is incorporated into messenger RNA in place of uracil.

- In the case of successful antimicrobial agents, *altering metabolic processes* unique to microorganisms, e.g. penicillin interferes with formation of the bacterial cell wall; or by showing enormous quantitative differences in affecting a process common to both humans and microbes, e.g. inhibition of folic acid synthesis by trimethoprim. Outside the cell drugs act by:

- Direct *chemical interaction*, e.g. chelating agents, antacids.

- *Osmosis*, as with purgatives, e.g. magnesium sulphate, and diuretics, e.g. mannitol, which are active because neither they nor the water in which they are dissolved is absorbed by the cells lining the gut and kidney tubules respectively.

Receptors

Most receptors are protein macromolecules. When the agonist binds to the receptor, the proteins undergo an alteration in conformation, which induces changes in systems within the cell that in turn bring about the response to the drug over differing time courses. Many kinds of effector response exist, but those indicated above are the four basic types.

Radioligand binding studies have shown that the receptor numbers do not remain constant but change according to circumstances. When tissues are continuously exposed to an agonist, the number of receptors decreases (*down-regulation*) and this may be a cause of *tachyphylaxis* (loss of efficacy with frequently repeated doses), e.g. in asthmatics who use adrenoceptor agonist bronchodilators excessively. Prolonged contact with an antagonist leads to formation of new receptors (*up-regulation*). Indeed, one explanation for the worsening of angina pectoris or cardiac ventricular arrhythmia in some patients following abrupt withdrawal of a β-adrenoceptor blocker is that normal concentrations of circulating catecholamines now have access to an increased (up-regulated) population of β-adrenoceptors.

Agonists. Drugs that activate receptors do so because they resemble the natural transmitter or hormone, but their value in clinical practice often rests on their greater capacity to resist degradation and so to act for longer than the natural substances (endogenous ligands) they mimic; for this reason, bronchodilatation produced by salbutamol lasts longer than that induced by adrenaline/epinephrine.

Antagonists (blockers) of receptors are sufficiently similar to the natural agonist to be 'recognised' by the receptor and to occupy it without activating a response, thereby preventing (blocking) the natural agonist from exerting its effect. Drugs that have no activating effect whatever on the receptor are termed pure antagonists. A receptor occupied by a low-efficacy agonist is inaccessible to a subsequent dose of a high-efficacy agonist, so that, in this specific situation, a low-efficacy agonist acts as an antagonist. This can happen with opioids.

Partial agonists. Some drugs, in addition to blocking access of the natural agonist to the receptor, are capable of a low degree of activation, i.e. they have both antagonist and agonist action. Such substances show partial agonist activity (PAA). The β-adrenoceptor antagonists pindolol and oxprenolol have partial agonist activity (in their case it is often called intrinsic sympathomimetic activity, ISA), while propranolol is devoid of agonist activity, i.e. it is a pure antagonist.

A patient may be as extensively 'β-blocked' by propranolol as by pindolol, i.e. with eradication of exercise tachycardia, but the resting heart rate is lower on propranolol; such differences can have clinical importance.

Inverse agonists. Some substances produce effects that are specifically opposed to those of the agonist. The agonist action of benzodiazepines on the benzodiazepine receptor in the central nervous system produces sedation, anxiolysis, muscle relaxation and controls convulsions; substances called β-carbolines, which also bind to this receptor, cause stimulation, anxiety, increased muscle tone and convulsions; they are *inverse agonists*. Both types of drug act by modulating the effects of the neurotransmitter γ-aminobutyric acid (GABA).

Receptor binding (and vice versa). If the forces that bind drug to receptor are weak (hydrogen bonds, van der Waals bonds, electrostatic bonds), the binding will be easily and rapidly reversible; if the forces involved are strong (covalent bonds), then binding will be effectively irreversible.

Physiological (functional) antagonism

An action on the same receptor is not the only mechanism by which one drug may oppose the effect of another. Extreme bradycardia following overdose of a β-adrenoceptor blocker can be relieved by atropine, which accelerates the heart by blockade of the parasympathetic branch of the autonomic nervous system, the cholinergic tone of which (vagal tone) operates continuously to slow it.

Adrenaline/epinephrine and theophylline counteract bronchoconstriction produced by histamine released from mast cells in anaphylactic shock by relaxing bronchial smooth muscle (β₂-adrenoceptor effect). In both cases, a second drug overcomes the pharmacological effect, by a different physiological mechanism, i.e. there is *physiological* or *functional* antagonism.

Enzymes

Interaction between drug and enzyme is in many respects similar to that between drug and receptor. Drugs may alter enzyme activity because they resemble a natural substrate and hence compete with it for the enzyme. For example, enalapril is effective in hypertension because it is structurally similar to the part of angiotensin I that is attacked by angiotensin-converting enzyme (ACE); enalapril prevents formation of the pressor angiotensin II by occupying the active site of the enzyme and so inhibiting its action.

Irreversible inhibition occurs with organophosphorus insecticides and chemical warfare agents, which combine covalently with the active site of acetylcholinesterase; recovery of cholinesterase activity depends on the formation of new enzyme. Covalent binding of aspirin to cyclo-oxygenase (COX) inhibits the enzyme in platelets for their entire lifespan because platelets have no system for synthesising new protein; this is why low doses of aspirin are sufficient for antiplatelet action.

Selectivity

The pharmacologist who produces a new drug and the doctor who gives it to a patient share the desire that it should possess a selective action so that additional and unwanted (adverse) effects do not complicate the management of the patient. Approaches to obtaining selectivity of drug action include the following.

Modification of drug structure. Many drugs have in their design a structural similarity to some natural constituent of the body, e.g. a neurotransmitter, a hormone, a substrate for an enzyme; replacing or competing with that natural constituent achieves selectivity of action. Enormous scientific effort and expertise go into the synthesis and testing of analogues of natural substances in order to create drugs capable of obtaining a specified effect, and that alone. The approach is the basis of modern drug design and it has led to the production of adrenoceptor antagonists, histamine receptor antagonists and many other important medicines.

Selective delivery (drug targeting). Simple topical application, e.g. skin and eye, and special drug delivery systems, e.g. intrabronchial administration of β₂-adrenoceptor agonist or corticosteroid (inhaled, pressurised, metered aerosol for asthma) can achieve the objective of target tissue selectivity. Selective targeting of drugs to less accessible sites of disease offers considerable scope for therapy as technology develops, e.g. attaching drugs to antibodies selective for cancer cells.

Stereoselectivity. Drug molecules are three-dimensional and many drugs contain one or more *asymmetrical* or *chiral* centres in their structures, i.e. a single drug can be, in effect, a mixture of two non-identical mirror images (like a mixture of left- and right-handed gloves). The two forms, which are known as *enantiomorphs*, can exhibit very different pharmacodynamic, pharmacokinetic and toxicological properties.

For example, ① the S form of warfarin is four times more active than the R form, ② the peak plasma concentration of S fenoprofen is four times that of

R fenoprofen after oral administration of RS fenoprofen, and ③ the S, but not the R, enantiomorph of thalidomide is metabolised to primary toxins.

QUANTITATIVE ASPECTS

That a drug has a desired qualitative action is obviously all important, but is not by itself enough. There are also quantitative aspects, i.e. the right amount of action is required, and with some drugs the dose has to be adjusted very precisely to deliver this, neither too little nor too much, to escape both inefficacy and toxicity, e.g. digoxin, lithium, gentamicin. While the general correlation between dose and response may evoke no surprise, certain characteristics of the relation are fundamental to the way drugs are used, as described below.

Dose–response relationships

Conventionally, the horizontal axis shows the dose and the response appears on the vertical axis. The slope of the dose–response curve defines the extent to which a desired response alters as the dose is changed. A steeply rising and prolonged curve indicates that a small change in dose produces a large change in drug effect over a wide dose range, e.g. with the loop diuretic furosemide (used in doses from 20 mg to over 250 mg/day). By contrast, the dose–response curve for thiazide diuretics soon reaches a plateau, and the clinically useful dose range for bendroflumethiazide, for example, extends from 5 to 10 mg; increasing the dose beyond this produces no added diuretic effect, although it adds to toxicity.

Dose–response curves for wanted and unwanted effects can illustrate and quantify selective and non-selective drug action (Fig. 5.1).

Potency and efficacy

A clear distinction between potency and efficacy is pertinent, particularly in relation to claims made for usefulness in therapeutics.

Potency is the amount (weight) of drug in relation to its effect, e.g. if weight-for-weight drug A has a greater effect than drug B, then drug A is more

Fig. 5.1 Dose–response curves for two hypothetical drugs. For drug A, the dose that brings about the maximum wanted effect is less than the lowest dose that produces the unwanted effect. The ratio ED_{50} (unwanted effect)/ED_{50} (wanted effect) indicates that drug A has a large therapeutic index; it is thus highly *selective* in its wanted action. Drug B causes unwanted effects at doses well below producing its maximum benefit. The ratio ED_{50} (unwanted effect)/ED_{50} (wanted effect) indicates that the drug has a small therapeutic index: it is thus *non-selective*.

potent than drug B, although the maximum therapeutic effect obtainable may be similar with both drugs.

The diuretic effect of bumetanide 1 mg is equivalent to that of furosemide 50 mg; thus bumetanide is more potent than furosemide but both drugs achieve about the same maximum effect. The difference in weight of drug administered is of no clinical significance unless it is great.

Pharmacological efficacy refers to the strength of response induced by occupancy of a receptor by an agonist (intrinsic activity); it is a specialised pharmacological concept. But clinicians are concerned with therapeutic efficacy, as follows.

Therapeutic efficacy or effectiveness, is the capacity of a drug to produce an effect and refers to the maximum such effect. For example, if drug A can produce a therapeutic effect that cannot be obtained with drug B, however much of drug B is given, then drug A has the higher therapeutic efficacy. Differences in therapeutic efficacy are of great clinical importance, usually more than potency.

Amiloride (*low* efficacy) can at best effect excretion of no more than 5% of the sodium load filtered by the glomeruli; there is no point in increasing the dose beyond that which achieves this, as this is its maximum diuretic effect. Bendroflumethiazide (*moderate* efficacy) can effect excretion of no more than 10% of the filtered sodium load no matter how large the dose. Furosemide can effect excretion of 25% and more of filtered sodium; it is a *high*-efficacy diuretic.

Therapeutic index. With progressive increases in dose, the desired response in the patient usually rises to a maximum beyond which further increases elicit no greater benefit but induce unwanted effects. This is because most drugs do not have a single dose–response curve, but a different curve for each action, wanted as well as unwanted. Increases in dose beyond that which gives the maximum wanted response recruit only new and unwanted actions.

A sympathomimetic bronchodilator might exhibit one dose–response relation for decreasing airway resistance (wanted) and another for increase in heart rate (unwanted). Clearly, the usefulness of any drug relates closely to the extent to which such dose–response relations overlap.

Ehrlich introduced the concept of the *therapeutic index* or ratio as the maximum tolerated dose divided by the minimum curative dose, but the index is never calculated thus as such single doses cannot be determined accurately in humans. More realistically, a dose that has some unwanted effect in 50% of humans, e.g. in the case of an adrenoceptor agonist bronchodilator a specified increase in heart rate, is compared with that which is therapeutic in 50% (ED_{50}), e.g. a specified decrease in airways resistance.

In practice, such information is not available for many drugs but the therapeutic index does embody a concept that is fundamental in comparing the usefulness of one drug with another, namely, *safety in relation to efficacy*. Figure 5.1 expresses the concept diagrammatically.

Tolerance

Continuous or repeated administration of a drug is often accompanied by a gradual diminution of the effect it produces. A state of *tolerance* exists when it becomes necessary to increase the dose of a drug to get an effect previously obtained with a smaller dose, i.e. reduced sensitivity. By contrast, the term *tachyphylaxis* describes the phenomenon of progressive lessening of effect (refractoriness) in response to frequently administered doses; it tends to develop more rapidly than tolerance.

The use of opioids readily illustrates tolerance, as witnessed by the huge doses of morphine that may be necessary to maintain pain relief in terminal care; the effect is due to reduced pharmacological efficacy at receptor sites or to down-regulation of receptors. Tolerance is acquired rapidly with nitrates used to prevent angina, possibly mediated by the generation of oxygen free radicals from nitric oxide; it can be avoided by removing transdermal nitrate patches for 4–8 h, e.g. at night, to allow the plasma concentration to fall.

Accelerated metabolism by enzyme induction also leads to tolerance, as experience shows with alcohol, taken regularly as opposed to sporadically. There is commonly cross-tolerance between drugs of similar structure.

Failure of certain individuals to respond to normal doses of a drug, e.g. resistance to warfarin, vitamin D, constitutes a form of natural tolerance.

Bioassay and standardisation

Biological assay (bioassay) is the process by which the activity of a substance (identified or unidentified) is measured on living material: e.g. contraction of bronchial, uterine or vascular muscle. It is used only when chemical or physical methods are not practicable as in the case of a mixture of active substances, or of an incompletely purified preparation, or where no chemical method has been developed. The activity of a preparation is expressed relative to that of a standard preparation of the same substance.

Biological standardisation is a specialised form of bioassay. It involves matching of material of unknown potency with an international or national standard with the objective of providing a preparation for use in therapeutics and research. The results are expressed as *units* of a substance rather than its weight, e.g. insulin, vaccines.

Part 2. Pharmacokinetics

Dosage regimens of long-established drugs grew from trial and error. Doctors learned by experience the dose, the frequency of dosing and the route of administration that was most likely to benefit and least likely to harm. But this empirical ('suck it and see') approach is no longer tenable. We now have an understanding of how drugs cross membranes to enter the body, how they are distributed round it in the blood and other body fluids, how they are bound to plasma proteins and tissues (which act as stores), and how they are eliminated from the body. Quantification of these processes paves the way for efficient development of dosing regimens.

> **Pharmacokinetics** is concerned with the rate at which drug molecules cross cell membranes to enter the body, to distribute within it and to leave the body, as well as with the structural changes (metabolism) to which they are subject within it.

The discussion covers the following topics:

- Drug passage across cell membranes.
- Order of reaction or process (first and zero order).
- Time course of drug concentration and effect:
  - plasma half-life and steady-state concentration
  - therapeutic monitoring
- The individual processes: absorption, distribution, metabolism (biotransformation), elimination.

DRUG PASSAGE ACROSS CELL MEMBRANES

Certain concepts are fundamental to understanding how drug molecules make their way around the body to achieve their effect. The first concerns the modes by which drugs cross cell membranes and cells.

Cell membranes are essentially bilayers of lipid molecules with 'islands' of protein, and they preserve and regulate the internal environment. *Lipid-soluble* substances diffuse readily into cells and therefore throughout body tissues. Adjacent epithelial or endothelial cells are linked by tight junctions, some of which are traversed by water-filled channels that allow the passage of water-soluble substances of small molecular size.

The jejunum and proximal renal tubule contain many such channels and are *leaky epithelia*, whereas the tight junctions in the stomach and urinary bladder do not have these channels and water cannot pass; they are termed *tight epithelia*. Special protein molecules within the lipid bilayer allow specific substances to enter or leave the cell preferentially, i.e. *energy-utilising transporter processes*, described later. The natural processes of passive diffusion, filtration and carrier-mediated transport determine the passage of drugs across membranes and cells, and their distribution round the body.

Passive diffusion

This is the most important means by which a drug enters the tissues and distributes through them. It refers simply to the natural tendency of any substance to move passively from an area of high concentration to one of low concentration. In the context of an individual cell, the drug moves at a rate proportional to the concentration difference across the cell membrane, i.e. it shows first-order kinetics; cellular energy is not required, which means that the process does not become saturated and is not inhibited by other substances.

The extent to which drugs are soluble in *water* or *lipid* is central to their capacity to cross cell membranes and depends on environmental pH and the structural properties of the molecule.

> Lipid solubility is promoted by the presence of a benzene ring, a hydrocarbon chain, a steroid nucleus or halogen (-Br, -Cl, -F) groups. Water solubility is promoted by the presence of alcoholic (-OH), amide ($-CO \cdot NH_2$) or carboxylic (-COOH) groups, or the formation of glucuronide and sulphate conjugates.

Drugs that ionise according to environmental pH

Many drugs are *weak electrolytes*, i.e. their structural

groups ionise to a greater or lesser extent, according to environmental pH. Most such molecules are present partly in the ionised and partly in the un-ionised state. The degree of ionisation influences lipid solubility (and hence diffusibility) and so affects absorption, distribution and elimination.

Ionisable groups in a drug molecule tend either to lose a hydrogen ion (acidic groups) or to add a hydrogen ion (basic groups). The extent to which a molecule has this tendency to ionise is given by the dissociation (ionisation) constant (K_a), expressed as the pK_a, i.e. the negative logarithm of the K_a (just as pH is the negative logarithm of the hydrogen ion concentration). In an acidic environment, i.e. one already containing many free hydrogen ions, an acidic group tends to retain a hydrogen ion and remains un-ionised; a relative deficit of free hydrogen ions, i.e. a basic environment, favours loss of the hydrogen ion from an acidic group, which thus becomes ionised. The opposite is the case for a base.

This in turn influences *diffusibility* because:

- Un-ionised drug is lipid soluble and diffusible.
- Ionised drug is lipid insoluble and non-diffusible.

pH variation and drug kinetics. The *pH partition hypothesis* expresses the separation of a drug across a lipid membrane according to differences in environmental pH. There is a wide range of pH in the gut (pH 1.5 in the stomach, 6.8 in the upper and 7.6 in the lower intestine). But the pH inside the body is maintained within a limited range (pH 7.46 ± 0.04), so that only drugs that are substantially un-ionised at this pH will be lipid soluble, diffuse across tissue boundaries and so be widely distributed, e.g. into the central nervous system (CNS). Urine pH varies between the extremes of 4.6 and 8.2, and the prevailing pH affects the amount of drug reabsorbed from the renal tubular lumen by passive diffusion.

In the stomach, aspirin (acetylsalicylic acid, pK_a 3.5) is un-ionised and thus lipid soluble and diffusible. When aspirin enters the gastric epithelial cells (pH 7.4) it will ionise, become less diffusible and so will localise there. This *ion trapping* is one mechanism whereby aspirin is concentrated in, and so harms, the gastric mucosa. In the body aspirin is

metabolised to salicylic acid (pK_a 3.0), which at pH 7.4 is highly ionised and thus remains in the extracellular fluid. Eventually the molecules of salicylic acid in the plasma are filtered by the glomeruli and pass into the tubular fluid, which is generally more acidic than plasma and causes a proportion of salicylic acid to become un-ionised and lipid soluble so that it diffuses back into the tubular cells. Alkalinising the urine with an intravenous infusion of sodium bicarbonate causes more salicylic acid to become ionised and lipid insoluble so that it remains in the tubular fluid, and passes into the urine. Treatment for salicylate (aspirin) overdose utilises this effect.

Conversely, acidifying the urine increases the elimination of the base amfetamine (pK_a 9.9).

Drugs that are incapable of becoming ionised

These include digoxin and steroid hormones such as prednisolone. Effectively lacking any ionisable groups, they are unaffected by environmental pH, are lipid soluble and so diffuse readily across tissue boundaries. These drugs are also referred to as *non-polar*.

Permanently ionised drugs

Drugs that are permanently ionised contain groups that dissociate so strongly that they remain ionised over the range of the body pH. Such compounds are termed *polar*, for their groups are either negatively charged (acidic, e.g. heparin) or positively charged (basic, e.g. ipratropium, tubocurarine, suxamethonium) and all have a very limited capacity to cross cell membranes. This is a disadvantage with heparin, which the gut does not absorb, so that it is given parenterally. Conversely, heparin is a useful anticoagulant in pregnancy because it does not cross the placenta (which the orally effective warfarin does and is liable to cause fetal haemorrhage as well as being teratogenic).

The following are particular examples of the relevance of drug passage across membranes.

Brain and cerebrospinal fluid (CSF). The capillaries of the cerebral circulation differ from those in most other parts of the body in that they lack the filtration channels between endothelial cells through which substances in the blood normally gain access to the extracellular fluid. Tight junctions between adjacent capillary endothelial cells, together with their basement membrane and a thin covering from the processes of astrocytes, separate the blood from the brain tissue, forming the *blood–brain barrier*. Compounds that are *lipid insoluble* do not cross it readily. Therapy with methotrexate (lipid insoluble) may fail to eliminate leukaemic deposits in the CNS. Conversely *lipid-soluble* substances enter brain tissue with ease; thus diazepam (lipid soluble) given intravenously is effective within 1 min for status epilepticus.

Placenta. Maternal blood bathes the chorionic villi, which consist of a layer of trophoblastic cells that enclose fetal capillaries. Their large surface area and the high placental blood flow (500 mL/min) are essential for gas exchange, uptake of nutrients and elimination of waste products. Thus a lipid barrier separates the fetal and maternal bloodstreams, allowing the passage of lipid-soluble substances but excluding water-soluble compounds, especially those with a molecular weight exceeding 600.

This exclusion is of particular importance with short-term use, e.g. tubocurarine (mol. wt. 772) (lipid insoluble) or gallamine (mol. wt. 891) used as a muscle relaxant during caesarean section do not affect the infant; with prolonged use, however, all compounds will eventually enter the fetus to some extent.

Filtration

Aqueous channels in the tight junctions between adjacent epithelial cells allow the passage of some water-soluble substances. Neutral or uncharged, i.e. non-polar, molecules pass most readily because the pores are electrically charged. Within the alimentary tract, channels are largest and most numerous in jejunal epithelium, and filtration allows for rapid equilibration of concentrations and consequently of osmotic pressures across the mucosa. Ions such as sodium enter the body through the aqueous chan-

nels, the size of which probably limits passage to substances of low molecular weight, e.g. ethanol (mol. wt. 46). Filtration seems to play at most a minor role in drug transfer within the body except for glomerular filtration, which is an important mechanism of drug excretion.

Carrier-mediated transport

The membranes of many cells incorporate carrier-mediated transporter processes that control the entry and exit of endogenous molecules, and show a high degree of specificity for particular compounds because they have evolved from biological needs for the uptake of essential nutrients or elimination of metabolic products. Drugs that bear some structural resemblance to natural constituents of the body are likely to utilise these mechanisms.

Some carrier-mediated transport processes operate passively, i.e. do not require cellular energy, and this is *facilitated diffusion*, e.g. vitamin B_{12} absorption. Other, energy-requiring processes move substrates into or out of cells against a concentration gradient very effectively, i.e. by *active transport*; they are subject to saturation, inhibition and induction.

THE ORDER OF REACTION OR PROCESS

In the body, drug molecules reach their sites of action after crossing cell membranes and cells, and many are metabolised in the process. The rate at which these movements or changes take place is subject to important influences called the *order of reaction* or process. In biology generally, two orders of such reactions are recognised as first-order processes and zero-order processes.

First-order (exponential) processes

First-order processes by which a constant fraction of drug is transported/metabolised in unit time. In the majority of instances, the rates at which absorption, distribution, metabolism and excretion of a drug occur are directly proportional to its concentration in the body. In other words, transfer of drug across a cell membrane or formation of a metabolite is high at high concentrations and falls in direct proportion to be low at low concentrations (an exponential relationship). Processes for which the rate of reaction is proportional to the concentration of participating molecules are *first-order processes*.

In doses used clinically, most drugs are subject to first-order processes of absorption, distribution, metabolism and elimination, and this knowledge is useful. The current chapter later describes how the rate of elimination of a drug from the plasma falls as the concentration in plasma falls, and the time for any plasma concentration to fall by 50% ($t_{1/2}$, the plasma half-life) is always the same. Thus, it becomes possible to quote a constant value for the $t_{1/2}$ of the drug. This occurs because rate and concentration are in proportion, i.e. the process obeys first-order kinetics.

Knowing that first-order conditions apply to a drug allows accurate calculations that depend on its $t_{1/2}$, i.e. time to achieve steady-state plasma concentration, time to elimination, and the construction of dosing schedules.

Zero-order processes (saturation kinetics)

Zero-order processes by which a constant amount of drug is transported/metabolised in unit time. As the amount of drug in the body rises, metabolic reactions or processes that have limited capacity become saturated. In other words, the rate of the process reaches a maximum amount at which it stays constant, e.g. due to limited activity of an enzyme, and any further increase in rate is impossible despite an increase in the dose of drug. In these circumstances, the rate of reaction is no longer proportional to dose, and exhibits *rate-limited* or *dose-dependent* or *zero-order* or *saturation* kinetics. In practice, enzyme-mediated metabolic reactions are the most likely to show rate limitation because the amount of enzyme present is finite and can become saturated. Passive diffusion does not become saturated. There are some important consequences of zero-order kinetics.

Order of reaction and $t_{1/2}$. When a drug is subject to first-order kinetics, the $t_{1/2}$ is a constant characteristic, i.e. a constant value can be quoted throughout the plasma concentration range (accepting that there will be variation in $t_{1/2}$ between individuals), and this is convenient. But if the rate of a process is not directly proportional to plasma concentration, then the $t_{1/2}$ cannot be constant. Consequently, no single value for $t_{1/2}$ describes overall elimination when a drug exhibits zero-order kinetics. In fact, $t_{1/2}$ decreases as plasma concentration falls and the calculations on elimination and dosing that are so easy with first-order elimination become more complicated.

Zero-order absorption processes apply to iron, to depot intramuscular formulations and to drug implants, e.g. antipsychotics and sex hormones.

TIME COURSE OF DRUG CONCENTRATION AND EFFECT

Plasma half-life and steady-state concentration

The manner in which plasma drug concentration rises or falls when dosing begins, alters or ceases follows certain simple rules, which provide a means for rational control of drug effect. Central to understanding these is the concept of *half-life* ($t_{1/2}$) or half-time.

Decrease in plasma concentration after an intravenous bolus injection

Following an intravenous bolus injection (a single dose injected in a period of seconds as distinct from a continuous infusion), plasma concentration rises quickly as drug enters the blood to reach a peak. There is then a sharp drop as the drug distributes round the body (distribution phase), followed by a steady decline as drug is removed from the blood by the liver or kidneys (elimination phase). If the elimination processes are first order, the time taken for any concentration point in the elimination phase to fall to half its value (the $t_{1/2}$) is always the same; see Figure 5.2. Note that the drug is virtually eliminated from the plasma in five $t_{1/2}$ periods.

Fig. 5.2 Changes in plasma concentration following an intravenous bolus injection of a drug in the elimination phase (the distribution phase, see text, is not shown). As elimination is a first-order process, the time for any concentration point to fall by 50% ($t_{1/2}$) is always the same.

> The $t_{1/2}$ is the one pharmacokinetic value of a drug that it is most useful to know.

Increase in plasma concentration with constant dosing

With a constant rate infusion, the amount of drug in the body and with it the plasma concentration rise until a state is reached at which the rate of administration to the body is exactly equal to the rate of elimination from it: this is called the *steady state*. The plasma concentration is then on a plateau, and the drug effect is stable. Figure 5.3 depicts the smooth changes in plasma concentration that result from a constant intravenous infusion. Clearly, giving a drug by regularly spaced oral or intravenous doses will result in plasma concentrations that fluctuate between peaks and troughs, but in time all of the peaks will be of equal height and all of the troughs will be of equal depth; this is also called a steady-state concentration, as the mean concentration is constant.

Time to reach steady state

It is important to know *when* a drug administered at a constant rate achieves a steady-state plasma concentration, for maintaining the same dosing schedule then ensures a constant amount of drug in the body and the patient will experience neither acute toxicity nor decline of effect. The $t_{1/2}$ provides the answer. Taking *ultimate* steady state attained as 100%: in $1 \times t_{1/2}$ the concentration will be (100/2) 50%

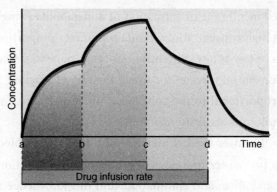

Fig. 5.3 Changes in plasma concentration during the course of a constant-rate intravenous infusion. (a) The infusion commences and plasma concentration rises to reach a steady state (plateau) in about $5 \times t_{1/2}$ periods. (b) The infusion rate is increased by 50% and the plasma concentration rises further to reach a new steady state that is 50% higher than the original steady state; the process takes another $5 \times t_{1/2}$ periods. (c) The infusion is decreased to the original rate and the plasma concentration returns to the original steady state in $5 \times t_{1/2}$ periods. (d) The infusion is discontinued and the plasma concentration falls to virtually zero in $5 \times t_{1/2}$ periods.

in $2 \times t_{1/2}$ (50 + 50/2) 75%

in $3 \times t_{1/2}$ (75 + 25/2) 87.5%

in $4 \times t_{1/2}$ (87.5 + 2.5/2) 93.75%

in $5 \times t_{1/2}$ (93.75 + 6.25/2) 96.875%

of the ultimate steady state.

> When a drug is given at a constant rate (continuous or repeated administration), the time to reach steady state depends *only* on the $t_{1/2}$ and, for all practical purposes, after $5 \times t_{1/2}$ periods the amount of drug in the body is constant and the plasma concentration is at a plateau (a–b in Fig. 5.3).

Change in plasma concentration with change or cessation of dosing

The same principle holds for *change* from any steady-state plasma concentration to a *new* steady state brought about by increase or decrease in the rate of drug administration. Provided the kinetics remain first order, increasing or decreasing the rate of drug administration (b and c in Fig. 5.3 gives rise to a new steady-state concentration in a time equal to $5 \times t_{1/2}$ periods.

Similarly, starting at any steady-state plasma concentration (100%), discontinuing the dose (d in

Fig. 5.3) will cause the plasma concentration to fall to virtually zero in $5 \times t_{1/2}$ periods, as described in Fig. 5.2.

Note that the difference between the rate of drug administration (input) and the rate of elimination (output) determines the actual *level* of any steady-state plasma concentration (as opposed to the *time taken* to reach it). If drug elimination remains constant and administration increases by 50%, in time the plasma concentration will reach a new steady-state concentration, which will be 50% greater than the original.

The relation between $t_{1/2}$ and time to reach steady-state plasma concentration applies to all drugs that obey first-order kinetics.

Therapeutic drug monitoring

Patients differ greatly in the dose of drug required to achieve the same response. The dose of warfarin that maintains a therapeutic concentration may vary as much as five-fold between individuals. This is a consequence of variation in rates of drug metabolism, disposition and tissue responsiveness, and it raises the question of how optimal drug effect can be achieved quickly for the individual patient.

In principle, drug effect relates to free (unbound) concentration at the tissue receptor site, which in turn reflects (but is not necessarily the same as) the concentration in the plasma. For many drugs, correlation between plasma concentration and effect is indeed better than that between dose and effect. Yet monitoring therapy by measuring drug in plasma is of practical use only in selected instances.

Interpreting plasma concentration measurements. Recommended plasma concentrations for drugs appear throughout this book where these are relevant but the following points ought to be kept in mind:

- The target therapeutic concentration range for a drug is a guide to optimise dosing together with other clinical indicators of progress.
- Take account of the time needed to reach steady-state dosing conditions. Additionally, some drugs alter their own rates of metabolism by enzyme induction, e.g. carbamazepine and phenytoin, and it is best to allow 2–4 weeks between change

in dose and meaningful plasma concentration measurement.

- As a general rule, when a drug has a short $t_{1/2}$ it is desirable to know both peak (15 min after an intravenous dose) and trough (just before the next dose) concentrations to provide efficacy without toxicity, as with gentamicin ($t_{1/2}$ 2.5 h). For a drug with a long $t_{1/2}$, it is usually best to sample just before a dose is due; effective immunosuppression with ciclosporin ($t_{1/2}$ 27 h) is obtained with trough concentrations of 50–200 micrograms/L when the drug is given by mouth.

Part 3. Individual pharmacokinetic processes

Drug absorption into, distribution around, metabolism by and elimination from the body are reviewed.

ABSORPTION

Commonsense considerations of anatomy, physiology, pathology, pharmacology, therapeutics and convenience determine the routes by which drugs are administered. Usually these are:

- *Enteral*: by mouth (swallowed) or by sublingual or buccal absorption; by rectum.
- *Parenteral*: by intravenous injection or infusion, intramuscular injection, subcutaneous injection or infusion, inhalation, topical application for local (skin, eye, lung) or for systemic (transdermal) effect.
- *Other routes*, e.g. intrathecal, intradermal, intranasal, intratracheal, intrapleural, are used when appropriate.

The features of the various routes, their advantages and disadvantages are relevant.

Absorption from the gastrointestinal tract

The *small intestine* is the principal site for absorption of nutrients and it is also where most orally administered drugs enter the body. This part of the gut has an enormous surface area due to the intestinal villi, and an epithelium through which fluid readily filters in response to osmotic differences caused by the presence of food. Disturbed alimentary motility can reduce drug absorption, i.e. if food slows gastric emptying, or gut infection accelerates intestinal transit. Additionally, it is becoming apparent that uptake and efflux transporters in enterocytes play a substantial role in controlling the absorption of certain drugs, e.g. digoxin, ciclosporin. Many sustained-release formulations probably depend on absorption from the colon.

Absorption of ionisable drugs from the *buccal mucosa* responds to the prevailing pH, which is 6.2–7.2. Lipid-soluble drugs are rapidly effective by this route because blood flow through the mucosa is abundant; these drugs enter directly into the systemic circulation, avoiding the possibility of first-pass (presystemic) inactivation by the liver and gut.

The *stomach* does not play a major role in absorbing drugs, even those that are acidic and thus un-ionised and lipid soluble at gastric pH, because its surface area is much smaller than that of the small intestine and gastric emptying is speedy ($t_{1/2}$ 30 min).

Enterohepatic circulation

This system is illustrated by the bile salts which are formed in the liver, then conserved by circulating round liver, intestine and portal blood about eight times a day. Several drugs form conjugates with glucuronic acid in the liver and enter the bile. Too polar (ionised) to be reabsorbed, the glucuronides remain in the gut, are hydrolysed by intestinal enzymes and bacteria, and the parent drug, thus released, is reabsorbed and reconjugated in the liver. Enterohepatic recycling appears to help sustain the plasma concentration and so the effect of sulindac, pentaerithrityl tetranitrate and ethinylestradiol (in many oral contraceptives).

Systemic availability and bioavailability

A drug injected intravenously enters the systemic circulation and thence gains access to the tissues and to receptors, i.e. 100% is available to exert its therapeutic effect. If the same quantity of the drug is swallowed, it does not follow that the entire amount will reach first the portal blood and then the systemic blood, i.e. its availability for therapeutic effect via the systemic circulation may be less than 100%. The anticipated response to a drug must take account of its availability to the systemic circulation.

While considerations of reduced availability attach to any drug given by any route other than intravenously, and intended for systemic effect, in practice the issue concerns enteral administration. The extent of systemic availability is usually calculated by relating the area under the plasma concentration–time curve (AUC) after a single oral dose to that obtained after intravenous administration of the same amount (by which route a drug is 100% systemically available). Calculation of AUCs after oral doses also allows a comparison of the bioavailability of different pharmaceutical formulations of the same drug. Factors influencing systemic availability present in three main ways, as described below.

Pharmaceutical factors

The amount of drug released from a dose form (and so becoming available for absorption) is referred to as its *bioavailability*. This is highly dependent on its pharmaceutical formulation. With tablets, for example, particle size (surface area exposed to solution), diluting substances, tablet size and pressure used in the tabletting process can affect disintegration and dissolution and so the bioavailability of the drug. Manufacturers must test their products to ensure that their formulations release the same amount of drug at the same speed from whatever manufactured batch or brand the patient may be taking.

Biological factors

Biological factors related to the gut include limitation of drug absorption by drug transporter systems, destruction of drug by gastric acid, e.g. benzylpenicillin, and impaired absorption due to rapid intestinal transit, which is important for all drugs that are absorbed slowly. Drugs may also bind to food constituents, e.g. tetracyclines to calcium (in milk), and to iron, or to other drugs (e.g. acidic drugs to colestyramine), and the resulting complex is not absorbed.

Presystemic (first-pass) elimination

Some drugs readily enter gut mucosal cells, but appear in low concentration in the systemic circulation. The reason lies in the considerable extent to which such drugs are metabolised in a single passage through the gut mucosa and (principally) the liver. As little as 10%–20% of the parent drug may reach the systemic circulation unchanged. By contrast, after intravenous administration, 100% becomes systemically available and the patient experiences higher concentrations with greater, but more predictable, effect. Dosing, particularly *initial* doses, must take account of discrepancy in anticipated plasma concentrations between the intravenous and oral routes. The difference is usually less if a drug produces active metabolites.

Once a drug is in the systemic circulation, irrespective of which route is used, about 20% is subject to the hepatic metabolic processes in each circulation time because that proportion of cardiac output passes to the liver.

As the degree of presystemic elimination differs much between drugs and individuals, the phenomenon of first-pass elimination adds to variation in systemic plasma concentrations, and thus particularly in initial response to the drugs that are subject to this process. In drug overdose, decreased presystemic elimination with increased bioavailability may account for the rapid onset of toxicity with antipsychotic drugs.

Drugs for which *presystemic elimination* is significant include: analgesics (morphine), adrenoceptor blockers (labetalol, propranolol and metoprolol), chlorpromazine, isosorbide dinitrate, nortriptyline and so on.

In severe hepatic cirrhosis with both impaired liver cell function and well-developed vessels shunting blood into the systemic circulation without passing through the liver, first-pass elimination reduces and systemic availability is increased. The result of these changes is an increased likelihood of exaggerated response to normal doses of drugs having high hepatic clearance and, on occasion, frank toxicity.

Drugs that exhibit the hepatic first-pass phenomenon do so because of the rapidity with which they are metabolised. The rate of delivery to the liver, i.e. blood flow, is then the main determinant of its rate of metabolism. Many other drugs are completely metabolised by the liver but at a slower rate and consequently loss in the first pass through the liver is unimportant. Dose adjustment to account for presystemic elimination is unnecessary, e.g. for diazepam, phenytoin, theophylline, warfarin.

DISTRIBUTION

If a drug is required to act throughout the body or to reach an organ inaccessible to topical administration, it must get into the blood and other body compartments. Most drugs distribute widely, in part dissolved in body water, in part bound to plasma proteins, in part to tissues. Distribution is often uneven, for drugs may bind selectively to plasma or tissue proteins or be localised within particular organs. Clearly, the site of localisation of a drug is likely to influence its action, e.g. whether it crosses the blood–brain barrier to enter the brain; the extent (amount) and strength (tenacity) of protein or tissue binding (stored drug) will affect the time it spends in the body and thereby its duration of action.

Distribution volume

The pattern of distribution from plasma to other body fluids and tissues is a characteristic of each drug that enters the circulation, and it varies between drugs. Precise information on the concentration of drug attained in various tissues and fluids is usually not available for humans. But *blood plasma* is sampled readily in humans, the drug concentration in which, taking account of the dose given, is a measure of whether a drug tends to remain in the circulation or to distribute from the plasma into the tissues.

Such information can be useful. In drug overdose, if a major proportion of the total body load is known to be in the plasma, i.e. the distribution volume is small, then haemodialysis/filtration is likely to be a useful option (as is the case with severe salicylate poisoning), but it is an inappropriate treatment for overdose with dosulepin. Selective distribution within the body occurs because of special affinity between particular drugs and particular body constituents. Many drugs bind to proteins in the plasma; phenothiazines and chloroquine bind to melanin-containing tissues, including the retina, which may explain the occurrence of retinopathy. Drugs may also concentrate selectively in a particular tissue because of specialised transport mechanisms, e.g. iodine in the thyroid.

Plasma protein and tissue binding

Many natural substances circulate around the body partly free in plasma water and partly bound to plasma proteins; these include cortisol, thyroxine, iron, copper and, in hepatic or renal failure, by-products of physiological intermediary metabolism.

Drugs, too, circulate in the protein-bound and free states, and the significance is that the free fraction is pharmacologically active whereas the protein-bound component is a reservoir of drug that is inactive because of this binding. Free and bound fractions are in equilibrium, and free drug removed from the plasma by metabolism, renal function or dialysis is replaced by drug released from the bound fraction.

Albumin is the main binding protein for many natural substances and drugs. Its complex structure has a net negative charge at blood pH and a high *capacity* but low (weak) *affinity* for many basic drugs, i.e. a lot is bound but it is readily released. Two particular sites on the albumin molecule bind acidic drugs with high affinity (strongly), but these sites have low capacity. Saturation of binding sites on plasma proteins in general is unlikely in the doses in which most drugs are used.

In *chronic renal failure*, hypoalbuminaemia and retention of products of metabolism that compete for binding sites on protein are both responsible for the decrease in protein binding of drugs. Most affected are acidic drugs that are highly protein bound, e.g. phenytoin, and initiating or modifying the dose of such drugs for patients with renal failure requires special attention.

Chronic liver disease also leads to hypoalbuminaemia and an increase of endogenous substances such as bilirubin that may compete for binding sites on protein. Drugs that are normally extensively protein bound should be used with special caution, for increased free concentration of diazepam, tolbutamide and phenytoin have been demonstrated in patients with this condition.

Tissue binding. Some drugs distribute readily to regions of the body other than plasma. These include many lipid-soluble drugs, which may enter fat stores, e.g. most benzodiazepines, verapamil and lidocaine. There is less information about other tissues, e.g. muscle, than about plasma protein binding because solid tissue samples require invasive biopsy. Extensive binding to tissues delays elimination from the body and accounts for the long $t_{1/2}$ of chloroquine and amiodarone.

METABOLISM

The body treats most drugs as foreign substances (xenobiotics) and subjects them to various mechanisms for eliminating chemical intruders.

Metabolism is a general term for chemical transformations that occur within the body and its processes change drugs in two major ways by reducing lipid solubility and altering biological activity.

Reducing lipid solubility

Metabolic reactions tend to make a drug molecule progressively more water soluble and so favour its elimination in the urine.

Drug-metabolising enzymes developed during evolution to enable the body to dispose of lipid-soluble substances such as hydrocarbons, steroids and alkaloids that are ingested with food. Some environmental chemicals may persist indefinitely in our fat deposits, e.g. dicophane (DDT), with consequences that are currently unknown.

Altering biological activity

The end-result of metabolism usually is the abolition of biological activity, but various steps in between may have the following consequences:

1. Conversion of a pharmacologically *active* to an *inactive* substance – this applies to most drugs.
2. Conversion of one pharmacologically *active* to another *active* substance – this has the effect of prolonging drug action, as shown below.

Active drug	Active metabolite
amitriptyline	nortriptyline
codeine	morphine
chloroquine	hydroxychloroquine
diazepam	oxazepam
spironolactone	canrenone

3. Conversion of a pharmacologically *inactive* to an *active* substance (then called a prodrug). The process then follows 1 or 2, above.

Inactive substance	Active metabolite(s)	Comment
aciclovir	aciclovir tri-phosphate	
colecalciferol	calcitriol and alfacalcidol	highly active metabolites of vitamin D_3
cyclophos-phamide	phos-phoramide mustard	another metabolite, acrolein, causes the bladder toxicity
perindopril	perindoprilat	less risk of first dose hypotension (applies to all ACE inhibitors except captopril)
levodopa	dopamine	levodopa, but not dopamine, can cross the blood–brain barrier
sulindac	sulindac sul-phide	possibly reduced gastric toxicity
sulfasalazine	5-aminosali-cylic acid	
zidovudine	zidovudine triphosphate	

The metabolic processes

The liver is by far the most important drug-metabolising organ, although a number of tissues, including the kidney, gut mucosa, lung and skin, also contribute. It is useful to think of drug metabolism in two broad phases.

Phase I metabolism brings about a change in the drug molecule by oxidation, reduction or hydrolysis and usually introduces or exposes a chemically active site on it. The new metabolite often has reduced biological activity and different pharmacokinetic properties, e.g. a shorter $t_{1/2}$.

The principal group of reactions is the *oxidations*, in particular those undertaken by the (microsomal) *mixed-function oxidases* which, as the name indicates, are capable of metabolising a wide variety of compounds. The most important of these is a large 'superfamily' of haem proteins, the *cytochrome P450 enzymes*, which metabolise chemicals from the environment, the diet and drugs. By a complex process, the drug molecule incorporates one atom of molecular oxygen (O_2) to form a (chemically active) hydroxyl group and the other oxygen atom converts to water.

The many cytochrome P450 isoenzymes are indicated by the letters CYP (from cytochrome P450) followed by a number denoting a family group, then a subfamily letter, and then a number for the individual enzyme within the family: for example, CYP2E1 is an isoenzyme that catalyses a reaction involved in the metabolism of alcohol, paracetamol, estradiol and ethinylestradiol.

The enzymes of families CYP1, 2 and 3 metabolise 70%–80% of clinically used drugs as well as many other foreign chemicals and, within these, CYP3A, CYP2D and CYP2C are the most important. The very size and variety of the P450 superfamily ensures that we do not need new enzymes for every existing or yet-to-be synthesised drug. Induction and inhibition of P450 enzymes is a fruitful source of drug–drug interactions.

Each P450 enzyme protein is encoded by a separate gene (57 have been identified in humans), and variation in genes leads to differences between individuals, and sometimes between ethnic groups, in the ability to metabolise drugs. Persons who exhibit *polymorphisms* inherit diminished or increased ability to metabolise substrate drugs, predisposing to toxicity or lack of efficacy.

Phase I oxidation of some drugs results in the

formation of *epoxides*, which are short-lived and highly reactive metabolites that bind irreversibly through covalent bonds to cell constituents and are toxic to body tissues. Glutathione is a tripeptide that combines with epoxides, rendering them inactive, and its presence in the liver is part of an important defence mechanism against hepatic damage by halothane and paracetamol.

Note that some drug oxidation reactions do not involve the P450 system: several biologically active amines are inactivated by monoamine oxidase and methylxanthines; mercaptopurine by xanthine oxidase; ethanol by alcohol dehydrogenase.

Hydrolysis (Phase I) reactions create active sites for subsequent conjugation of, e.g., aspirin, lidocaine, but this does not occur with all drugs.

Phase II metabolism involves combination of the drug with one of several polar (water-soluble) endogenous molecules (products of intermediary metabolism), often at the active site (hydroxyl, amino, thiol) created by Phase I metabolism. The kidney readily eliminates the resulting water-soluble conjugate, or the bile if the molecular weight exceeds 300. Morphine, paracetamol and salicylates form conjugates with glucuronic acid (derived from glucose); oral contraceptive steroids form sulphates; isoniazid, phenelzine and dapsone are acetylated. Conjugation with a more polar molecule is also an elimination mechanism for natural substances, e.g. bilirubin as glucuronide, oestrogens as sulphates.

Phase II metabolism almost invariably terminates biological activity.

Transporters. It is convenient here to introduce the subject of *carrier-mediated transporter processes* whose physiological functions include the passage of amino acids, lipids, sugars, hormones and bile acids across cell membranes, and the protection of cells against environmental toxins.

There is an emerging understanding that membrane transporters have a key role in the overall disposition of drugs to their targeted organs. There are broadly two types: *uptake transporters*, which facilitate, for example, the passage of organic anions and cations into cells, and *efflux transporters*, which transport substances out of cells, often against high concentration gradients. Some transporters possess both influx and efflux properties.

Most efflux transporters are members of the ATP-binding cassette (ABC) superfamily that utilises energy derived from the hydrolysis of ATP; they include the P-glycoprotein family that expresses multidrug resistance protein 1 (MDR1).

Their varied locations illustrate the potential for transporters widely to affect the distribution of drugs, namely in:

- Enterocytes of the small intestine, controlling absorption and thus bioavailability, e.g. of ciclosporin, digoxin.
- Liver cells, controlling uptake from the blood and excretion into the bile, e.g. of pravastatin.
- Renal tubular cells, controlling uptake from the blood, secretion into tubular fluid (and thus excretion) of organic anions, e.g. β-lactam antibiotics, diuretics, non-steroidal anti-inflammatory drugs.
- Brain capillary endothelial cells, controlling passage across the blood–brain barrier, e.g. of levodopa (but not dopamine) for benefit in Parkinson's disease.

In time, it is likely that drug occupancy of transporter processes will provide explanations for some drug-induced toxicities and for a number of drug–drug interactions.

Enzyme induction

The mechanisms that the body evolved over millions of years to metabolise foreign substances now enable it to meet the modern environmental challenges of tobacco smoke, hydrocarbon pollutants, insecticides and drugs. At times of high exposure, our enzyme systems respond by increasing in amount and so in activity, i.e. they become *induced*; when exposure falls off, enzyme production gradually lessens.

A first alcoholic drink taken after a period of abstinence from alcohol may have a noticeable effect on behaviour, but the same drink taken at the end of 2 weeks of regular drinking may pass almost unnoticed because the individual's liver enzyme activity is increased (induced), and alcohol is metabolised more rapidly, having less effect, i.e. tolerance is acquired. There is, nevertheless, a ceiling above which alcohol metabolising enzymes are not further induced.

Inducing substances in general share some important properties: they tend to be lipid soluble, are substrates, though sometimes only minor ones, e.g. DDT, for the enzymes they induce, and generally have a long $t_{1/2}$. The time for onset and offset of induction depends on the rate of enzyme turnover, but significant induction generally occurs within a few days and it passes off over 2–3 weeks following withdrawal of the inducer. Thus, certain drugs can alter the capacity of the body to metabolise other substances including drugs, especially in long-term use; this phenomenon has implications for drug therapy. More than 200 substances induce enzymes in animals but the list of proven enzyme inducers in humans is more restricted.

Enzyme inhibition

The consequences of inhibiting drug metabolism can be more profound and more selective than enzyme induction because the outcome is prolongation of action of a drug or metabolite. Consequently, enzyme inhibition offers more scope for therapy. Enzyme inhibition by drugs is also the basis of a number of clinically important drug interactions.

ELIMINATION

The body eliminates drugs following their partial or complete conversion to water-soluble metabolites or, in some cases, without their being metabolised. To avoid repetition the following account refers to the drug whereas the processes deal with both drug and metabolites.

Renal elimination

The following mechanisms are involved.

Glomerular filtration. The rate at which a drug enters the glomerular filtrate depends on the concentration of free drug in plasma water and on its molecular weight. Substances having a molecular weight in excess of 50 000 do not cross into the glomerular filtrate, whereas those of molecular weight less than 10 000 (which includes almost all drugs) pass easily through the pores of the glomerular membrane.

Renal tubular transport. Uptake and efflux transporters in proximal renal tubule cells transfer organic anions and cations between the plasma and the tubular fluid. Renal tubular diffusion. The glomerular filtrate contains drug at the same concentration as it is free in the plasma, but the fluid is concentrated progressively as it flows down the nephron so that a gradient develops, drug in the tubular fluid becoming more concentrated than in the blood perfusing the nephron. As the tubular epithelium has the properties of a lipid membrane, the extent to which a drug diffuses back into the blood will depend on its lipid solubility, i.e. on its pK_a in the case of an electrolyte, and on the pH of tubular fluid. If the fluid becomes more alkaline, an acidic drug ionises, becomes less lipid soluble and its reabsorption diminishes, but a basic drug becomes un-ionised (and therefore more lipid soluble) and its reabsorption increases. Manipulation of urine pH gains useful expression with sodium bicarbonate given to alkalinise the urine for salicylate overdose.

Faecal elimination

When any drug intended for systemic effect is taken by mouth a proportion may remain in the bowel and be excreted in the faeces. Some drugs are intended not be absorbed from the gut, as an objective of therapy, e.g. neomycin. The cells of the intestinal epithelium contain several carrier-mediated transporters that control the absorption of drugs. The efflux transporter MDR1, for example, drives drug from the enterocyte into the gut lumen, limiting its bioavailability. Drug in the blood may also diffuse passively into the gut lumen, depending on its pK_a and the pH difference between blood and gut contents. The effectiveness of activated charcoal by mouth for drug overdose depends partly on its adsorption of such diffused drug, and subsequent elimination in the faeces.

Biliary excretion. Transporters regulate the uptake of organic cations and anions from portal blood to hepatocyte, and thence to the bile. The bile canaliculi tend to reabsorb small molecules and in general, only compounds having a molecular weight greater than 300 pass into bile.

Pulmonary elimination

The lungs are the main route of elimination (and of uptake) of volatile anaesthetics. Apart from this, they play only a trivial role in drug elimination. The route, however, acquires notable medicolegal significance when ethanol concentration is measured in the air expired by vehicle drivers involved in road traffic accidents (via the breathalyser).

Clearance

Elimination of a drug from the plasma is quantified in terms of its clearance. The term has the same meaning as the familiar renal creatinine clearance, which is a measure of removal of endogenous creatinine from the plasma. Clearance values can provide useful information about the biological fate of a drug. There are pharmacokinetic methods for calculating *total body* and *renal* clearance, and the difference between these represents *hepatic* clearance. The renal clearance of a drug eliminated only by filtration by the kidney obviously cannot exceed the glomerular filtration rate (adult male 124 mL/min, female 109 mL/min). If a drug has a renal clearance in excess of this, then the kidney tubules must actively secrete it, e.g. benzylpenicillin (renal clearance 480 mL/min).

Breast milk

Most drugs that are present in a mother's plasma appear to some extent in her milk, although the amounts are so small that loss of drug in milk is of no significance as a mechanism of elimination. Even small amounts, however, may sometimes be of significance for the suckling child, whose drug metabolic and eliminating mechanisms are immature.

While most drugs taken by the mother pose no hazard to the child, exceptions to this observation occur because some drugs are inherently toxic, or transfer to milk in significant amounts, or there are known adverse effects, as below.

Part 4. Drug dosage

Drug dosage can be of five main kinds.

Fixed dose. The effect that is desired can be obtained at well below the toxic dose (many mydriatics, analgesics, oral contraceptives, antimicrobials) and enough drug can be given to render individual variation clinically insignificant.

Variable dose – with crude adjustments. Here fine adjustments make comparatively insignificant differences and the therapeutic endpoint may be hard to measure (depression, anxiety), may change only slowly (thyrotoxicosis), or may vary because of pathophysiological factors (analgesics, adrenal corticosteroids for suppressing disease).

Variable dose – with fine adjustments. Here a vital function (blood pressure, blood sugar level), which often changes rapidly in response to dose changes and can easily be measured repeatedly, provides the endpoint. Adjustment of dose must be accurate. Adrenocortical *replacement* therapy falls into this group, whereas adrenocortical *pharmacotherapy* falls into the group above.

Maximum tolerated dose is used when the ideal therapeutic effect cannot be achieved because of the occurrence of unwanted effects (anticancer drugs; some antimicrobials). The usual way of finding this is to increase the dose until unwanted effects begin to appear and then to reduce it slightly, or to monitor the plasma concentration.

Minimum tolerated dose. This concept is less common than the one above, but it applies to long-term adrenocortical steroid therapy against inflammatory or immunological conditions, e.g. in asthma and some cases of rheumatoid arthritis, when the dose that provides symptomatic relief may be so high that serious adverse effects are inevitable if it is continued indefinitely. The compromise is incomplete relief on the grounds of safety. This can be difficult to achieve.

DOSING SCHEDULES

Dosing schedules are simply schemes aimed at achieving a desired effect while avoiding toxicity. The following discussion assumes that drug effect relates closely to plasma concentration, which in turn relates closely to the amount of drug in the body. The objectives of a dosing regimen where continuing effect is required are:

To specify an initial dose that attains the desired effect rapidly without causing toxicity. Often the dose that is capable of initiating drug effect is the same as that which maintains it. On repeated dosing, however, it takes $5 \times t_{1/2}$ periods to reach steady-state concentration in the plasma and this lapse of time may be undesirable. The effect may be achieved earlier by giving an initial dose that is larger than the maintenance dose; the initial dose is then called the *priming* or *loading* dose, i.e. the dose that will achieve a therapeutic effect in an individual whose body does not already contain the drug.

To specify a maintenance dose: amount and frequency. Intuitively the maintenance dose might be half of the initial/priming dose at intervals equal to its plasma $t_{1/2}$, for this is the time by which the plasma concentration that achieves the desired effect, declines by half. Whether or not this approach is satisfactory or practicable, however, depends very much on the $t_{1/2}$ itself.

Dose calculation by body-weight and surface area

A uniform, fixed drug dose is likely to be ineffective or toxic in several circumstances, e.g. cytotoxic chemotherapy, aminoglycoside antibiotics. It is usual then to calculate the dose according to body-weight. Adjustment according to body surface area is also used and may be more appropriate, for this correlates better with many physiological phenomena, e.g. metabolic rate.

The relationship between body surface area and weight is curvilinear, but a reasonable approximation is that a 70-kg human has a body surface area of 1.8 m^2. A combination of body-weight and height gives a more precise value for surface area (obtained from standard nomograms) and other more sophisticated methods.

The issue takes on special significance for children, if the only dose known is that for the adult; adjustment is then commonly made by body-weight, or body surface area, among other factors.

Prolongation of drug action

Giving a larger dose is the most obvious way to prolong a drug action but this is not always feasible, and other mechanisms are used:

- *Vasoconstriction* will reduce local blood flow so that distribution of drug away from an injection site is retarded, e.g. combination with adrenaline/epinephrine prolongs local anaesthetic action.
- *Slowing of metabolism* may usefully extend drug action, as when a dopa decarboxylase inhibitor, e.g. carbidopa, is combined with levodopa (as co-careldopa) for parkinsonism.
- *Delayed excretion* is seldom practicable, the only important example being the use of probenecid to block renal tubular excretion of penicillin for single-dose treatment of gonorrhoea.
- *Altered molecular structure* can prolong effect, e.g. the various benzodiazepines.
- *Pharmaceutical formulation*. Manipulating the form in which a drug is presented by modified-release systems can achieve the objective of an even as well as a prolonged effect.

Sustained-release (oral) preparations can reduce the frequency of medication to once a day, and compliance becomes easier for the patient. The elderly can now receive most long-term medication as a single morning dose. In addition, sustained-release preparations may avoid bowel toxicity due to high local concentrations, e.g. ulceration of the small intestine with potassium chloride tablets; they may also avoid the toxic peak plasma concentrations that can occur when dissolution of the formulation, and so absorption of the drug, is rapid. Some sustained-release formulations also contain an immediate-release component to provide rapid, as well as sustained, effect.

Depot (injectable) preparations are more reliable

because the environment in which they are deposited is more constant than can ever be the case in the alimentary tract, and medication can be given at longer intervals, even weeks. In general, such preparations are pharmaceutical variants, e.g. micro-crystals, or the original drug in oil, wax, gelatin or synthetic media. They include phenothiazine neuroleptics, the various insulins and penicillins, preparations of vasopressin, and medroxyprogesterone (intramuscular, subcutaneous). Tablets of hormones can be implanted subcutaneously. The advantages of infrequent administration and better patient adherence in a variety of situations are obvious.

Reduction of absorption time

A soluble salt of the drug may be effective by being rapidly absorbed from the site of administration. In the case of subcutaneous or intramuscular injections, the same objective may be obtained with hyaluronidase, an enzyme that depolymerises hyaluronic acid, a constituent of connective tissue that prevents the spread of foreign substances, e.g. bacteria, drugs. Hyaluronidase combined with an intramuscular injection, e.g. a local anaesthetic, or a subcutaneous infusion leads to increased permeation with more rapid absorption. Hyaluronidase also promotes resorption of tissue accumulation of blood and fluid.

Fixed-dose drug combinations

This refers to combinations of drugs in a single pharmaceutical formulation. It does not mean concomitant drug therapy, e.g. in infections, hypertension and in cancer, when several drugs are given separately. Therapeutic aims should be clear. Combinations are logical if there is good reason to consider that the patient needs all the drugs in the formulation and that the doses are appropriate and will not need adjustment separately.

Part 5. Chronic pharmacology

The pharmacodynamics and pharmacokinetics of many drugs differ according to whether their use is in a single dose, or over a brief period (acute pharmacology), or long term (chronic pharmacology). An increasing proportion of the population take drugs continuously for large portions of their lives, as tolerable suppressive and prophylactic remedies for chronic or recurrent conditions are developed; e.g. for arterial hypertension, diabetes mellitus, mental diseases, epilepsies. In general, the dangers of a drug therapy are not markedly greater if therapy lasts for years rather than months, but long-term treatment can introduce significant hazard into patients' lives unless management is skilful.

INTERFERENCE WITH SELFREGU-LATING SYSTEMS

When self-regulating physiological systems (generally controlled by negative feedback systems, e.g. endocrine, cardiovascular) are subject to interference, their control mechanisms respond to minimise the effects of the interference and to restore the previous steady state or rhythm; this is *homeostasis*. The previous state may be a normal function, e.g. ovulation (a rare example of a positive feedback mechanism), or an abnormal function, e.g. high blood pressure. If the body successfully restores the previous steady state or rhythm then the subject has become tolerant to the drug, i.e. needs a higher dose to produce the desired previous effect.

In the case of arterial hypertension, tolerance to a single drug commonly occurs, e.g. reduction of peripheral resistance by a vasodilator is compensated by an increase in blood volume that restores the blood pressure; this is why a diuretic is commonly used together with a vasodilator in therapy.

Feedback systems. The endocrine system serves fluctuating body needs. Glands are therefore capable either of increasing or decreasing their output by means of negative (usually) feedback systems. An administered hormone or hormone analogue activates the receptors of the feedback system so that high doses cause suppression of natural production of the hormone. On withdrawal of the administered hormone, restoration of the normal control mechanism takes time, e.g. the hypothalamic–pituitary–

adrenal cortex system can take months to recover full sensitivity, and sudden withdrawal of administered corticosteroid can result in an acute deficiency state that may be life endangering.

Regulation of receptors. The number (density) of receptors on cells (for hormones, autacoids or local hormones, and drugs), the number occupied (receptor occupancy) and the capacity of the receptor to respond (affinity, efficacy) can change in response to the concentration of the specific binding molecule or ligand, whether this be agonist or antagonist (blocker). The effects always tend to restore cell function to its normal or usual state. Prolonged high concentrations of agonist (whether administered as a drug or over-produced in the body by a tumour) cause a reduction in the number of receptors available for activation (*down-regulation*); changes in receptor occupancy and affinity and the prolonged occupation of receptors antagonists lead to an increase in the number of receptors (*up-regulation*). At least some of this may be achieved by receptors moving inside the cell and out again (internalisation and externalisation).

Down-regulation, and the accompanying receptor changes, may explain the 'on–off' phenomenon in Parkinson's disease. and the action of luteinising hormone releasing hormone (LHRH) super-agonists in reducing follicle stimulating hormone (FSH) concentrations for treating endocrine-sensitive prostate cancer.

Up-regulation. The occasional exacerbation of ischaemic cardiac disease on sudden withdrawal of a β-adrenoceptor blocker may be explained by up-regulation during its administration, so that, on withdrawal, an above-normal number of receptors suddenly become accessible to the normal transmitter, i.e. noradrenaline/norepinephrine.

Up-regulation with rebound sympathomimetic effects may be innocuous to a moderately healthy cardiovascular system, but the increased oxygen demand of these effects can have serious consequences where ischaemic disease is present and increased oxygen need cannot be met (angina pectoris, arrhythmia, myocardial infarction). Unmasking of a disease process that has worsened during prolonged suppressive use of the drug, i.e. resurgence, may also contribute to such exacerbations.

The rebound phenomenon is plainly a potential hazard and the use of a β-adrenoceptor blocker in the presence of ischaemic heart disease would be safer if rebound is eliminated. β-Adrenoceptor blockers that are not pure antagonists but have some agonist (sympathomimetic ischaemic) activity, i.e. partial agonists, may prevent the generation of additional adrenoceptors (up-regulation). Indeed, there is evidence that rebound is less or is absent with pindolol, a partial agonist β-adrenoceptor blocker.

Sometimes a distinction is made between *rebound* (recurrence at intensified degree of the symptoms for which the drug was given) and *withdrawal syndrome* (appearance of new additional symptoms). The distinction is quantitative and does not imply different mechanisms.

Rebound and withdrawal phenomena occur erratically. In general, they are more likely with drugs having a short $t_{1/2}$ (abrupt drop in plasma concentration) and pure agonist or antagonist action. They are less likely to occur with drugs having a long $t_{1/2}$ and (probably) with those having a mixed agonist–antagonist (partial agonist) action on receptors.

Abrupt withdrawal

Clinically important consequences occur, and might occur for a variety of reasons, e.g. a patient interrupting drug therapy to undergo surgery.

Resurgence of chronic disease, which has progressed in severity although its consequences have been wholly or partly suppressed, i.e. a catching-up phenomenon, is a possible outcome of discontinuing effective therapy, e.g. levodopa in Parkinson's disease. Corticosteroid withdrawal in autoimmune disease may cause both resurgence and rebound. The exact mechanisms may remain obscure but clinicians have no reason to be surprised when they occur, and in the case of rebound they may wish to use gradual withdrawal wherever drugs are used to modify complex self-adjusting systems, and to suppress (without cure) chronic diseases.

Conclusions

> Drugs not only induce their known listed primary actions, but may:
>
> - evoke compensatory responses in the complex interrelated physiological systems they affect, and these systems need time to recover on withdrawal of the drug (gradual withdrawal is sometimes mandatory and never harmful)
> - induce metabolic changes that may be trivial in the short term, but serious if they persist for a long time
> - produce localised effects in specially susceptible tissues and induce serious cell damage or malfunction
> - increase susceptibility to intercurrent illness and to interaction with other drugs that may be taken for new indications

That such consequences occur with prolonged drug use need evoke no surprise. But a knowledge of physiology, pathology and pharmacology, combined with awareness that the unexpected can occur, will allow patients who require long-term therapy to be managed safely, or at least with minimum risk of harm.

Part 6. Individual or biological variation

PRESCRIBING FOR SPECIAL RISK GROUPS

That individuals respond differently to drugs, both from time to time and from other individuals, is a matter of everyday experience. Doctors need to accommodate for individual variation, as it may explain both adverse response to a drug and failure of therapy. Sometimes there are obvious physical characteristics such as age, ethnicity (genetics) or disease that warn the prescriber to adjust drug dose, but there are no external features that signify, e.g. pseudocholinesterase deficiency, which causes prolonged paralysis after suxamethonium. An understanding of the reasons for individual variation in response to drugs is relevant to all who prescribe. Both pharmacodynamic and pharmacokinetic effects are involved, and the issues fall in two general categories: inherited influences and environmental and host influences.

Part 7. Pharmacogenomics

Introduction

The response to drugs varies widely among patients – for example, it has been estimated that only about 30% of patients respond to antidepressants. Adverse drug reactions are also common, accounting for 6.5% of admissions to hospital. Part of this variability is due to patient-related factors (non-compliance, smoking, alcohol, co-morbidities) and poor prescribing. However, a significant proportion of the variability, which varies from drug to drug, is due to genetic factors. This area of study is termed *pharmacogenomics*.

> Pharmacogenomics can be defined as the study of the genomic basis of why individuals vary in their response (efficacy and/or toxicity) to drugs. This term is used interchangeably with pharmacogenetics. The first example can be traced back to the time of Pythagoras who described the phenomenon ascribed to red cell haemolysis in some Mediterranean populations eating fava beans (favism), which we now know to be due to glucose-6-phosphate dehydrogenase deficiency, the most common enzyme deficiency in man.

Sources of variability

In general, variability in drug response can be due to pharmacokinetic and/or pharmacodynamic factors (Fig. 5.4). Variability in the expression of the cytochrome P450 enzymes, which are responsible for Phase I drug metabolism, has been the focus of most of the work in pharmacokinetics. Cytochrome P450 2D6 (CYP2D6), for example, is one of the most variable P450 enzymes in man, is absent in 8% of the UK population, and is responsible for the metabolism of 25% of drugs, including CNS (antidepressants and antipsychotics) and cardiovascular (β-blockers and anti-arrhythmics) drugs. Much less work has been done on pharmacodynamic factors causing variation in drug response, but as drugs can affect almost any protein in the body, almost every gene may have an effect on how individual drugs vary in their response. It is important to note, however, that for most drugs variability in response is due to a combination of both pharmacokinetic and pharmacodynamic factors, both of which can be affected by environmental or genetic factors. Specific examples are provided below.

Identifying genetic variation. Much of the work in pharmacogenomics has been based on a study of candidate genes, i.e. a study of genes known to be involved in the pharmacokinetics of the drug and its mechanism of action. Specifically the focus has been on single nucleotide polymorphisms (SNPs), which are base substitutions occurring with a frequency of at least 1% in the human population. With the advances in technologies, more recent work has focused on genome-wide association stud-

ies (GWAS), i.e. a study of all genes in the human genome without any prior knowledge of the pharmacokinetic and pharmacodynamic parameters of the drug. GWAS is also likely to be surpassed by next generation sequencing technologies in the near future, which will provide an evaluation of common and rare variants in the human genome.

EXAMPLES OF PHARMACOGENOMIC VARIATION

Drug efficacy

Cancer therapy. Cancer is essentially a genetic disease with approximately 30–80 mutations per cancer. These mutations within the cancer genome (the somatic genome) also change the responsiveness of the cancer to therapy. The best example is that of trastuzumab (Herceptin) in breast cancer; this drug improves disease-free and overall survival in patients with HER2 gene amplification or over-expression of the protein on breast cancer cells. This adverse prognostic factor occurs in 20% of newly diagnosed breast cancers. In patients with colon cancer, the proto-oncogene KRAS acts as a downstream signal transducer of epidermal growth factor receptor (EGFR), but can undergo activation independently of EGFR in the presence of mutations. Inhibition of EGFR, for example using inhibitory monoclonal antibodies such as panitumumab and cetuximab, is better in patients with the wild-type KRAS gene than in those with mutations.

Warfarin. Warfarin is a narrow therapeutic index drug where individual daily dose requirements vary by at least 40-fold. Inability to maintain an INR between 2 and 3 can predispose to either thrombosis (INR<2) or haemorrhage (INR>3). Warfarin is metabolised by various P450 enzymes, the most important being CYP2C9. Two variants in the CYP2C9 gene (termed CYP2C9*2 and CYP2C9*3) reduce the activity of the enzyme and overall rate of the metabolic turnover of warfarin. The mode of action of warfarin is through interruption of the vitamin K cycle specifically by inhibiting the enzyme vitamin K epoxide reductase

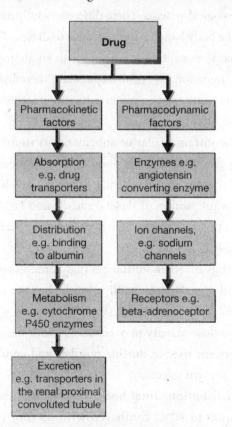

Fig. 5.4 Variation in drug response can be due to genetically determined factors in pharmacokinetic and pharmacodynamic processes in the body. Some examples are given in each box.

complex 1 (VKORC1) – variation in this gene can affect the daily requirements for warfarin. In most global populations, it has now been shown that age and body mass index, together with genetic variation in CYP2C9 and VKORC1, can account for at least 50% of the variation in daily dose requirements for warfarin. This has resulted in the development of dosing algorithms in an attempt to improve the accuracy and prediction of individual dose requirements for warfarin.

Immune-mediated adverse drug reactions. Many type B or idiosyncratic adverse drug reactions are immunologically mediated. Immune response to antigens, including those derived from drugs, is partly under the control of the HLA genes on chromosome 6, which is the polymorphic region of the human genome. Not surprisingly, HLA genes are now being found to be important determinants of susceptibility to these immune-mediated adverse reactions. The best example of this is with abacavir, a drug used to treat HIV, which causes hypersensitivity (skin rash, fever, gastrointestinal and respiratory manifestations) in 5% of patients. A strong association of abacavir hypersensitivity with the HLA allele, HLA-B*5701, has now been shown in several populations. In Europe, it is now mandatory to undertake HLA-B*5701 testing before the prescription of abacavir. Very strong genetic associations between the HLA genes and different forms of hypersensitivity, including those affecting the skin and liver, occur with a number of drugs.

Statin myopathy. Statins are among the most widely used drugs in the world, with marked benefits in terms of reduction of cardiovascular morbidity and mortality. Although generally well tolerated, statins can occasionally cause muscle damage, which can range from muscle pains to rhabdomyolysis (associated with renal failure which can be fatal). A genome-wide approach in patients on simvastatin showed that a variant in an influx drug transporter called SLCO1B1 (also known as OATP1B1) increased the risk of statin-related myopathy. This transporter is highly expressed in the liver and is responsible for the transport of some statins from the blood into the hepatocyte. In patients expressing this variant, the activity of the transporter is reduced which leads to a decrease in hepatocyte uptake and an increase in plasma concentrations of the statin. However, the mechanism by which the statin leads to muscle damage is unknown.

ENVIRONMENTAL AND HOST INFLUENCES

A multitude of factors related to both individuals and their environment contribute to differences in drug response. Some of the more relevant influences are the following:

Age

The neonate, infant and child

Young human beings differ greatly from adults, not merely in size but also in the proportions and constituents of their bodies and the functioning of their physiological systems. These differences influence the way the body handles and responds to drugs:

- Rectal absorption is efficient with an appropriate formulation, e.g. of diazepam and theophyllines; this route may be preferred with an uncooperative infant.

- The intramuscular or subcutaneous routes tend to give unpredictable plasma concentrations, e.g. of digoxin or gentamicin, because of the relatively low proportion of skeletal muscle and fat. Intravenous administration is preferred in the seriously ill newborn.

- Drugs or other substances that come in contact with the skin are readily absorbed as the skin is well hydrated and the stratum corneum is thin; overdose toxicity may result, e.g. with hexachlorophene used in dusting powders and emulsions to prevent infection.

Distribution. Total body water in the neonate amounts to 80%, compared with 65% of bodyweight in older children. Consequently:

- Weight-related loading doses of aminoglycosides, aminophylline, digoxin and furosemide need to be larger for neonates than for older children.

- Less extensive binding of drugs to plasma proteins is generally without clinical importance but there is a risk of kernicterus in the jaundiced neonate following displacement of bilirubin from protein-binding sites by vitamin K, X-ray contrast media or indometacin.

Metabolism. Drug-inactivating enzyme systems are present at birth but are functionally immature (particularly in the preterm baby), especially for oxidation and for conjugation with glucuronic acid. Inadequate conjugation and thus inactivation of chloramphenicol by neonates causes the fatal 'grey' syndrome, but this is not a widely used antibiotic. After the initial weeks of life, because their drug metabolic capacity increases rapidly, young children may require a higher weight-related dose than adults.

Elimination. Glomerular filtration, tubular secretion and reabsorption are low in the neonate (even lower in preterm babies), reaching adult values in relation to body surface area only at 2–5 months. Drugs that the kidney excretes, e.g. aminoglycosides, penicillins, diuretics, require reduced dose; after about 6 months, body-weight- or surface area-related daily doses are the same for all ages.

Pharmacodynamic responses. There is scant information about developmental effects of interaction between drugs and receptors. Other sources suggest possible effects: e.g. thalidomide causes phocomelia only in the forming limb; tetracyclines stain only developing enamel; young children are particularly sensitive to liver toxicity from valproate.

Dosage in the young. No single rule or formula is suitable for all cases. Computation by body-weight may overdose an obese child, for whom calculation of ideal weight from age and height is preferred. Doses based on body surface area are generally more accurate, and preferably should take into account both body-weight and height. The fact that the surface area of a 70kg adult human is 1.8 m^2 then allows adjustment, as follows:

$$\text{Approximate dose} = \text{Surface area of child (m}^2)/ \\ 1.8 \times \text{adult dose}$$

General guidance is available from formularies, e.g.

the *British National Formulary*, and specialist publications.

The elderly

The incidence of adverse drug reactions rises with age in the adult, especially after 65 years, because of the increasing number of drugs that the elderly need because they tend to have multiple diseases, poor compliance with dosing regimens and bodily changes of ageing that require modified dosage regimens.

Absorption of drugs administered orally may be slightly slower because of reduced gastrointestinal blood flow and motility but the effect is rarely important.

Distribution reflects the following changes:

- Lean body mass is less and standard adult doses provide a greater amount of drug per kilogram.
- Body fat increases and may act as a reservoir for lipid-soluble drugs.
- Total body water is less and, in general, water-soluble drugs have a lower distribution volume. Standard doses of drugs, especially the loading doses of those that are water soluble, may thus exceed the requirement.
- Plasma albumin concentration is well maintained in the healthy elderly but may fall with chronic disease, giving scope for a greater proportion of unbound (free) drug, which may be important when priming doses are given.

Metabolism reduces as liver mass and liver blood flow decline. Consequently:

- Metabolic inactivation of drugs is slower, mostly for Phase I (oxidation) reactions; the capacity for Phase II (conjugation) is better preserved.
- Drugs normally extensively eliminated in first pass through the liver appear in higher concentration in the systemic circulation and persist in it for longer. There is, therefore, particular need initially to use lower doses of most neuroleptics, tricyclic antidepressants and cardiac anti-arrhythmic agents.
- Capacity for hepatic enzyme induction appears less.

Elimination. Renal blood flow, glomerular filtration and tubular secretion decrease with age above

55 years, a decline that raised serum creatinine concentration does not signal because production of this metabolite is diminished by the age-associated diminution of muscle mass. Indeed, in the elderly, serum creatinine may be within the concentration range for normal young adults even when the creatinine clearance is 50 mL/min (compared with 127 mL/min in adult males). Particular risk of adverse effects arises with drugs that are eliminated mainly by the kidney and that have a small therapeutic ratio, e.g. aminoglycosides, digoxin, lithium.

Phmacodynamic response may alter with age, to produce either a greater or a lesser effect than is anticipated in younger adults, for example:

- Drugs that act on the CNS appear to produce an exaggerated response in relation to that expected from the plasma concentration, and sedatives and hypnotics may have a pronounced hangover effect. These drugs are also more likely to depress respiration because of reduced vital capacity and maximum breathing capacity in the elderly.
- Response to β-adrenoceptor agonists and antagonists may diminish in old age, possibly through reduced affinity for adrenoceptors, or smaller number of receptors.
- Baroreceptor sensitivity reduces, leading to greater potential for orthostatic hypotension with drugs that reduce blood pressure.

The old (80 + years) are particularly intolerant of neuroleptics (given for confusion) and of diuretics (given for ankle swelling that is postural and not due to heart failure), which cause adverse electrolyte changes. Both classes of drug may result in admission to hospital of semi-comatose 'senior citizens' who deserve better treatment from their juniors.

Pregnancy

As pregnancy evolves, profound changes occur in physiology, including fluid and tissue composition.

Absorption. Despite reduced gastrointestinal motility, there appears to be no major defect in drug absorption except that slow gastric emptying delays the appearance in the plasma of orally administered drugs, especially during labour. Absorption from an intramuscular site is likely to be efficient because vasodilatation increases tissue perfusion.

Distribution. Total body water increases by up to 8 L, creating a larger space within which water-soluble drugs may distribute. Plasma albumin (normal 33–55 g/L) declines by some 10 g/L from haemodilution. While this gives scope for increased free concentration of drugs that normally bind to albumin, unbound drug is also available to distribute, be metabolised and excreted. With phenytoin, for example, the free (and pharmacologically active) concentration does not alter, despite the dilutional fall in the total plasma concentration.

Hepatic metabolism increases, although not blood flow to the liver. There is increased clearance of drugs such as phenytoin and theophylline, whose elimination depends on liver enzyme activity. Drugs that are so rapidly metabolised that elimination depends on delivery to the liver, i.e. on hepatic blood flow, have unaltered clearance, e.g. pethidine.

Elimination. Renal plasma flow almost doubles and there is more rapid loss of renally excreted drugs, e.g. amoxicillin, the dose of which should be doubled for systemic infections (but not for urinary tract infections as penicillins are highly concentrated in the urine).

Placenta. See *Part 2. Pharmacokinetics*

Disease

Pharmacokinetic changes

Absorption. Resection and reconstruction of the gut may lead to malabsorption, e.g. of iron, folic acid and fat-soluble vitamins after partial gastrectomy, and of vitamin B_{12} after ileal resection. Delayed gastric emptying and intestinal stasis during an attack of migraine interfere with drug absorption. Severe low-output cardiac failure or shock (with peripheral vasoconstriction) delays absorption from subcutaneous or intramuscular sites; reduced hepatic blood flow prolongs the presence in the plasma of drugs that are so rapidly extracted by the liver that removal depends on their rate of presentation to it, e.g. lidocaine.

Distribution. Hypoalbuminaemia from any cause, e.g. burns, malnutrition, sepsis, allows a higher proportion of free (unbound) drug in plasma. Although free drug is available for metabolism and excretion, there remains a risk of enhanced or adverse responses especially with initial doses of those that are highly protein bound, e.g. phenytoin.

Metabolism. Acute inflammatory disease of the liver (viral, alcoholic) and cirrhosis affect both the functioning of the hepatocytes and blood flow through the liver. Reduced extraction from the plasma of drugs that are normally highly cleared in first pass through the liver results in increased systemic availability of drugs such as metoprolol, labetalol and clomethiazole. Many other drugs exhibit prolonged $t_½$ and reduced clearance in patients with chronic liver disease, e.g. diazepam, tolbutamide, rifampicin. Thyroid disease has the expected effects, i.e. drug metabolism accelerates in hyperthyroidism and decelerates in hypothyroidism.

Elimination. Renal disease has profound effects on the elimination and hence duration of action of drugs eliminated by the kidney.

Food

- The presence of food in the stomach, especially if it is fatty, delays gastric emptying and the absorption of certain drugs, e.g. ampicillin and rifampicin. More specifically, calcium, for instance in milk, interferes with absorption of tetracyclines and iron (by chelation).

- Substituting protein for fat or carbohydrate in the diet is associated with an increase in drug oxidation rates. Some specific dietary factors induce drug metabolising enzymes, e.g. alcohol, charcoal grilled (broiled) beef, cabbage and Brussels sprouts.

Protein malnutrition causes changes that are likely to influence pharmacokinetics, e.g. loss of body-weight, reduced hepatic metabolising capacity, hypoproteinaemia.

Citrus flavinoids in grapefruit (but not orange) juice decrease hepatic metabolism and may lead to toxicity from amiodarone, terfenadine (cardiac arrhythmia), benzodiazepines (increased sedation), ciclosporin, felodipine (reduced blood pressure).

DRUG INTERACTIONS

When a drug is administered, a response occurs; if a second drug is given and the response to the first drug is altered, a drug–drug interaction is said to have occurred.

Dramatic *unintended* interactions excite most notice but they should not distract attention from the many *intended* interactions that are the basis of rational polypharmacy, e.g. multi-drug treatment of tuberculosis, naloxone for morphine overdose.

For completeness, alterations in drug action caused by diet (above) are termed *drug–food* interactions, and those by herbs *drug–herb* interactions.

Clinical importance of drug interactions

The quantity of drugs listed in any national formulary provides ample scope for possible alteration in the disposition or effect of one drug by another drug. But, in practice, *clinically important adverse drug–drug interactions* become likely with:

- Drugs that have a steep dose–response curve and a small therapeutic index because small quantitative changes at the target site, e.g. receptor or enzyme, lead to substantial changes in effect, e.g. digoxin or lithium.

- Drugs that are known enzyme inducers or inhibitors.

- Drugs that exhibit saturable metabolism (zero-order kinetics), when small interference with kinetics may lead to large alteration of plasma concentration, e.g. phenytoin, theophylline.

- Drugs that are used long term, where precise plasma concentrations are required, e.g. oral contraceptives, antiepilepsy drugs, cardiac antiarrhythmia drugs, lithium.

- Severely ill patients, for they may be receiving several drugs; signs of iatrogenic disease may be difficult to distinguish from those of existing disease and the patient's condition may be such that they cannot tolerate further adversity.

- Patients who have significantly impaired liver or kidney function, for these are the principal organs that terminate drug action.
- The elderly, for they tend to have multiple pathology, and may receive several drugs concurrently.

Pharmacological basis of drug interactions

Listings of recognised or possible adverse drug–drug interactions are now readily available in national formularies, on compact disk or as part of standard prescribing software. We provide here an overview of the pharmacological basis for wanted and unwanted, expected and unexpected effects when drug combinations are used.

Drug interactions are of two principal kinds:

- *Pharmacodynamic interaction*: both drugs act on the target site of clinical effect, exerting synergism (below) or antagonism. The drugs may act on the same or different receptors or processes, mediating similar biological consequences. Examples include: alcohol + benzodiazepine (to produce enhanced sedation), atropine + β-adrenoceptor blocker (to indirectly reverse β-adrenoceptor blocker overdose).
- *Pharmacokinetic interaction*: the drugs interact remotely from the target site to alter plasma (and other tissue) concentrations so that the amount of the drug at the target site of clinical effect is altered, e.g. enzyme induction by rifampicin reduces the plasma concentration of warfarin; enzyme inhibition by ciprofloxacin increases the concentration of theophylline.

SUMMARY

How drugs act and interact, how they enter the body, what happens to them inside the body, how they are eliminated from it; the effects of genetics, age, and disease on drug action – these topics are important even if they are not prominent in the mind of the prescriber, since an understanding of them will enhance rational decision taking.

Knowledge of the requirements for success and the explanations for failure and for adverse events will enable the doctor to maximise the benefits and minimise the risks of drug therapy.

Pharmacodynamics

- Qualitative aspects: receptors, enzymes, selectivity.
- Quantitative aspects: dose response, potency, therapeutic efficacy, tolerance.

Pharmacokinetics

- Time course of drug concentration: drug passage across cell membranes; order of reaction; plasma half-life and steady-state concentration; therapeutic drug monitoring.
- Individual processes: absorption, distribution, metabolism, elimination.
- Drug dosage: dosing schedules.
- Chronic pharmacology: the consequences of prolonged drug administration and drug discontinuation syndromes.

Individual or biological variation

- Pharmacogenomics: variability due to inherited influences.
- Variability due to environmental and host influences.
- Drug interactions: outside the body, at site of absorption, during distribution, directly on receptors, during metabolism, during excretion.

In a word, pharmacodynamics is what drugs do to the body while pharmacokinetics is what the body does to drugs. The practice of drug therapy entails more than remembering an apparently arbitrary list of actions or indications. Scientific incompetence in the modern doctor is inexcusable and, contrary to some assertions, scientific competence is wholly compatible with a humane approach.

IMPORTANT TERMINOLOGY

pharmacodynamics　药效学
pharmacokinetics　药动学
absorption　吸收
distribution　分布
metablism　代谢
elimaniation　消除

receptor　受体
enzyme　酶
tolerance　耐受性
passive diffusion　被动扩散
pharmacogenomics　药物基因组学

CHALLENGE YOURSELVES

1. Could you please tell us what factors can affect absorption of drugs?
2. Could you please give some examples of pharmacogenomics of drug in clinics?
3. How to give individuals adjustment of dug dose? What should you think about in the adjustment?

Hengjie Yuan

Chapter | 6 |

The principle of drug therapy

Drug therapy involves considerations beyond the strictly scientific pharmacological aspects of medicines. These include numerous issues relating to prescribers and to patients: practical prescribing, the therapeutic situation, treating patients with drugs, iatrogenic disease, benefits and risks, public view of drugs and prescribers, criticisms of modern drugs, drug-induced injury, complementary and alternative medicine, placebo medicines, guidelines, 'essential' drugs and prescribing, compliance – patient and doctor, pharmacoeconomics.

PRACTICAL PRESCRIBING

The prescription

The prescription is the means by which patients receive medicines that are considered unsafe for sale directly to the public. Its format is officially regulated to ensure precision in the interests of safety and efficacy, and to prevent fraudulent misuse; full details appear in national formularies, and prescribers have a responsibility to comply with these.

The elementary requirements of a prescription [now usually viewed on screen by a computer programme] are that it should state what is to be given to whom and by whom prescribed, dispensing pharmacist and checking pharmacist, and give instructions on how much should be taken, how often, by what route and for how long, or the total quantity to be supplied.

Prescribing

Prescribing is a task carried out many times each day and can seem mundane – a technical process that is far less stimulating and interesting than reaching a diagnosis. However, there is no such thing as a safe drug and prescribing has the potential to cause harm or death as well as good. This section includes some practical advice aimed at identifying common pitfalls and reducing risk.

Good prescribing means: ① Making a diagnosis – or at least having a range of possibilities. Know what it is you are wishing to achieve and the evidence for the likely efficacy of the drug treatment you wish to give. ②Knowing your patient's kidney and liver function – most drugs are eliminated by these organs; and some drugs can damage them. ③ Getting the dose right. For many drugs you will not know the dose, so do not pretend you do. Never, ever guess. Never be afraid to ask. Never be too busy to look up a dose – better to check now than make a trip to the Coroner's Court later. ④ Explaining to your patient why you think this treatment will work, the likelihood of it working, the more common side-effects and what your plans are if it does not work. ⑤Being alert to the development of adverse drug reactions. If a patient develops new symptoms after starting a drug, it is probably because of the drug. If the adverse effect is in a fairly new drug – or is not already well known – you should report the event to the national body responsible for monitoring and recording adverse drug reactions. ⑥ Being very clear about what it is you are prescribing. ⑦If using a hand-written prescription, write clearly.⑧ If working in a different hospital, remember that the prescription chart may not be the same as where you have just been. ⑨ If using electronic prescribing, beware drop-down menus and drugs with similar looking names, e.g. carbimazole and carbamazepine.

Good prescribing starts with taking a good history: ① Does your patient have other medical conditions – some may be worsened by treatment you would normally give for their presenting complaint. ②What drugs is your patient taking now? What are they for? Are they all still needed? Could they be causing the symptoms or signs that have brought the patient to you? Could they interact with whatever you might think of prescribing? ③What drugs has your patient taken in the past? Why were they stopped? Did they cause side-effects? ④Is the patient allergic to any drugs? ⑤ Are they taking any non-prescription (over-the-counter) drugs? If so, could they interact with whatever you might prescribe (for example, St John's wort is an enzyme inducer)?

Examples of when things went wrong

Focusing on the presenting complaint and forgetting other medical conditions

A 79-year-old man was admitted to a surgical ward. He told the admitting doctor that he had long-standing arthritis which had got worse since his doctor stopped diclofenac and he asked for it to be re-started. The doctor did so, but did not notice the patient's significant renal impairment. The patient went into renal failure and died. A drug which helps one condition may worsen another.

Forgetting that women get pregnant

A 40-year-old woman is found to be hypertensive. She has three children, the youngest being 15. Her GP commences ramipril. Neither the patient nor the doctor suspected that she was, in fact, in the second trimester of pregnancy. The baby died at birth from major renal and other abnormalities. Subsequent liti-gation was settled out of court in the patient's favour. Remember that pregnancy is always a possibility in women of child-bearing age

Not knowing what you are prescribing

A 29-year-old woman came to the hospital with a urinary tract infection. The consultant told a young doctor looking after her to prescribe Penbritin. She did so and the patient died from penicillin anaphylaxis despite having a bracelet warning of the allergy. Neither the young doctor nor the nurse who administered the drug had bothered to find out what they were giving, namely ampicillin. Know what you are prescribing.

Forgetting that a newly prescribed drug can interact with long-term drug treatment

A 64-year-old man had been taking warfarin for many years. He developed a chest infection and an out of hours doctor prescribed amoxicillin. Later that week he was admitted with a large, painful right knee haemarthrosis and an INR >10. New drugs may interact with those the patient has been taking for a long time!

DRUG THERAPY

Drug therapy involves a great deal more than matching the name of the drug to the name of a disease; it requires knowledge, judgement, skill and wisdom, but above all a sense of responsibility.

Uses of drugs/medicines

Drugs are used in three principal ways: To cure disease: primary and auxiliary, to suppress disease and to prevent disease (prophylaxis) including primary and secondary one.

Cure implies primary therapy, as in bacterial and parasitic infections, that eliminates the disease and the drug is withdrawn; or auxiliary therapy, as with an anesthetics and with ergometrine and oxytocin in obstetrics.

Suppression of diseases or symptoms is used continuously or intermittently to avoid the effects of disease without attaining cure (as in hypertension, diabetes mellitus, epilepsy, asthma), or to control symptoms (such as pain and cough) while awaiting recovery from the causative disease.

Prevention (prophylaxis). In primary prevention, the person does not have the condition and avoids getting it. For malaria, vaccinations and contraception, the decision to treat healthy people is generally easy. In secondary prevention, the patient has the disease and the objective is to reduce risk factors, so as to retard progression or avoid repetition of an event, e.g. aspirin and lipid lowering drugs in atherosclerosis and after myocardial infarction, antihypertensives to prevent recurrence of stroke. Taking account of the above, a doctor might ask the following questions before treating a patient with drugs: ① Should I interfere with the patient at all? ② If so, what alteration in the patient's condition do I hope to achieve? ③ Which drug is most likely to bring this about? ④ How can I administer the drug to attain the right concentration in the right place at the right time and for the right duration? ⑤ How will I know when I have achieved the objective? ⑥ What other effects might the drug produce, and are these harmful? ⑦ How will I decide to stop the drug? ⑧ Does the likelihood of benefit, and its importance, outweigh the likelihood of damage, and its importance, i.e. the benefit versus risk, or efficacy against safety?

Drugs can do good

Medically, this good may sometimes seem trivial, as in the avoidance of a sleepless night in a noisy hotel or of social embarrassment from a profusely running nose due to seasonal pollen allergy (hay fever). Such benefits are not necessarily trivial to recipients, concerned to be at their best in important matters, whether of business, pleasure or passion, i.e. with quality of life. Or the good may be literally life-saving, as in serious acute infections (pneumonia, septicaemia) or in the prevention of life-devastating disability from severe asthma, from epilepsy or from blindness due to glaucoma.

Drugs can do harm

This harm may be relatively trivial, as in hangover from a hypnotic or transient headache from glyceryl trinitrate used for angina. The harm may be life-destroying, as in the rare sudden death following an injection of penicillin, rightly regarded as one of the safest of antibiotics, or the destruction of the quality of life that occasionally attends the use of drugs that are effective in rheumatoid arthritis (adrenocortical steroids, penicillamine) and Parkinson's disease (levodopa). There are risks in taking medicines, just as there are risks in food and transport. There are also risks in declining to take medicines when they are needed, just as there are risks in refusing food or transport when they are needed. Efficacy and safety do not lie solely in the molecular structure of the drug. Doctors must choose which drugs to use and must apply them correctly in relation not only to their properties, but also to those of the patients and their disease. Then patients must use the prescribed medicine correctly.

PHYSICIAN-INDUCED (IATROGENIC) DISEASE

Among inpatients in the USA and Australia, about half of the injuries caused by medical mismanagement result from surgery, but therapeutic mishaps and diagnostic errors are the next most common. In one survey of adverse drug events, 1% were fatal, 12% life-threatening, 30% serious and 57% significant. About half of the life-threatening and serious events were preventable. Errors of prescribing account for one-half and those of administering drugs for one-quarter of these. Inevitably, a proportion of lapses result in litigation, and in the UK 20%–25% of complaints received by the medical defence organisations about general practitioners follow medication errors. The most shameful act in therapeutics, apart from actually killing a patient, is to injure a patient who is but little disabled or who is suffering from a self-limiting disorder. Such iatrogenic disease, induced by misguided treatment, is far from rare.

BENEFITS AND RISKS OF MEDICINES

Whenever a drug is taken a risk is taken

The risk comprises the properties of the drug, the prescriber, the patient and the environment; it is often so small that second thoughts are hardly necessary, but sometimes it is substantial. The doctor must weigh the likelihood of gain for the patient against the likelihood of loss. There are often insufficient data for a rational decision to be reached, but a decision must yet be made, and this is one of the greatest difficulties of clinical practice. Its effect on the attitudes of doctors is often not appreciated by those who have never been in this situation. The patient's protection lies in the doctor's knowledge of the drug and of the disease, and experience of both, together with knowledge of the patient. We continue to use drugs that are capable of killing or disabling patients at doses within the therapeutic range where the judgement of overall balance of benefit and risk is favourable. This can be very difficult for the patient who has suffered a rare severe adverse reaction to understand and to accept. In some chronic diseases that ultimately necessitate suppressive drugs, the patient may not experience benefit in the early stages. Patients with early Parkinson's disease may experience little inconvenience or hazard from the condition, and premature exposure to drugs can exact such a price in unwanted effects that they prefer the untreated state. What patients will tolerate depends on their personality, their attitude to disease, their occupation, mode of life and relationship with their doctor.

Three major grades of risk

These are: unacceptable, acceptable and negligible. Where disease is life-threatening and there is reliable information on both the disease and the drug, then decisions, though they may be painful, present relatively obvious problems. But where the disease risk is remote, e.g. mild hypertension, or where drugs are to be used to increase comfort or to suppress symptoms that are, in fact, bearable, or for convenience rather than for need, then the issues of risk acceptance are less obvious. Risks should not be weighed without reference to benefits any more than benefits should be weighed without reference to risks. Risks are among the facts of life. In whatever we do and in whatever we refrain from doing, we are accepting risk. Some risks are obvious, some are unsuspected and some we conceal from ourselves. But risks are universally accepted, whether willingly or unwillingly, whether consciously or not.

Unavoidable risks

The features that a completely risk-free drug would exhibit: ① the physician would know exactly what action is required and use the drug correctly; ② the drug would deliver its desired action and nothing else, either by true biological selectivity or by selective targeted delivery; ③ the drug would achieve exactly the right amount of action – neither too little, nor too much.

Some reasons why drugs fail to meet the criteria of being risk-free include the following:

Drugs may be insufficiently selective. As the concentration rises, a drug that acts at only one site at low concentrations begins to affect other target sites (receptors, enzymes) and recruit new (unwanted) actions; or a disease process (cancer) is so close to normal cellular mechanisms that perfectly selective cell kill is impossible.

Drugs may be highly selective for one pathway but the mechanism affected has widespread functions and interference with it cannot be limited to one site only, e.g. atenolol on the β-adrenoceptor, aspirin on cyclo-oxygenase.

Prolonged modification of cellular mechanisms can lead to permanent change in structure and function, e.g. carcinogenicity.

Insufficient knowledge of disease processes (some cardiac arrhythmias) and of drug action can lead to interventions that, although undertaken with the best intentions, are harmful.

Patients are genetically heterogeneous to a high degree and may have unpredicted responses to drugs.

Dosage adjustment according to need is often unavoidably imprecise, e.g. in depression.

Prescribing without due care and attention.

Reduction of risk

Strategies that can limit risk include those directed at achieving: ① Better knowledge of disease (research)– as much as 40% of useful medical advances derive from basic research that was not funded towards a specific practical outcome; ② Site-specific effect – by molecular manipulation; ③ Site-specific delivery – drug targeting: by topical (local) application and by target-selective carriers; ④ Informed, careful and responsible prescribing.

PUBLIC VIEW OF DRUG AND PRE-SCRIBERS

The public wants benefits without risks and without having to alter its unhealthy ways of living; a deeply irrational position, but then humans are not perfectly rational. It is easy to understand that a person who has taken into his body a chemical with intent to relieve suffering, whether or not it is self-induced, can feel profound anger when harm ensues.

There are obvious areas where some remedial action is possible: ① improvement of prescribing by doctors, including better communication with patients, i.e. doctors must learn to feel that introduction of foreign chemicals into their patients' bodies is a serious matter, which many or most do not seem to feel at present; ② introduction of no-fault compensation schemes for serious drug injury (some countries already have these); ③ informed public discussion of the issues between the medical profession, industrial drug developers, politicians and other 'opinion-formers' in society, and patients (the public); ④restraint in promotion by the pharmaceutical industry including self-control by both industry and doctors in their necessarily close relationship, which the public is inclined to regard as a conspiracy, especially when the gifts and payments made to doctors get into the news.

CRITICISMS OF MODERN DRUGS

Extremist critics have attracted public attention for their view that modern drug therapy, indeed modern medicine in general, does more harm than good; others, while admitting some benefits from drugs, insist that this is medically marginal. These opinions rest on the undisputed fact that favourable trends in many diseases preceded the introduction of modern drugs and were due to economic and environmental changes, sanitation, nutrition and housing. They also rest on the claim that drugs have not changed expectation of life or mortality (as measured by national mortality statistics), or at least it is very difficult to show that they have, and that drugs indisputably can cause illness (adverse reactions). And this is often due to the irrelevant measure of the effects of drugs. Following are two examples of inappropriate measurements: ① In the case of many infections it is not disputed that environmental changes have had a greater beneficial effect on health than the subsequently introduced antimicrobials. But this does not mean that environmental improvements alone are sufficient in the fight against infections. Environmental changes achieved their results when mortality from infections was high and antimicrobials were not available; antimicrobials were introduced later against a background of low mortality as well as of environmental change; decades separate the two parts of the comparison, and observers, diagnostic criteria and data recording changed during this long period. It is evident that determining the value of antimicrobials is not simply a matter of looking at mortality rates. ② About 1% of the UK population has diabetes mellitus, a figure which is increasing rapidly, and about 1% of death certificates mention diabetes. This is no surprise because all must die and insulin is no cure for this lifelong disease. A standard medical textbook of 1907 stated that juvenile-onset 'diabetes is in all cases a grave disease, and the subjects are regarded by all assurance companies as uninsurable lives: life seems to hang by a thread, a thread often cut by a very trifling accident'. Most, if not all, life insurance companies now accept young people with diabetes with no or only modest financial penalty, the premium of a person 5–10 years older. Before insulin replacement therapy was available few survived beyond 3 years after diagnosis; they died for lack of insulin. It is unjustified to assert that a treatment is worthless just because its mention on death certificates (whether as a prime or as a contributory cause) has not declined. The relevant criteria for juvenile-onset diabetes are change in the age at which the subjects die and the quality of life between diagnosis and death, and both of these have changed enormously.

DRUG-INDUCED INJURY

Responsibility for drug-induced injury raises important issues affecting medical practice and development of needed new drugs, as well as of law and of social justice.

Negligence and strict and no-fault liability

All civilised legal systems provide for compensation to be paid to a person injured as a result of using a product of any kind that is defective due to negligence (fault: failure to exercise reasonable care). But there is a growing opinion that special compensation for serious personal injury, beyond the modest sums that general social security systems provide, should be automatic and not dependent on fault and proof of fault of the producer, i.e. there should be 'liability irrespective of fault', 'no-fault liability' or 'strict liability'.

Many countries are now revising their laws on liability for personal injury due to manufactured products and are legislating Consumer Protection Acts (Statutes) which include medicines, for 'drugs represent the class of product in respect of which there has been the greatest pressure for surer compensation in cases of injury'.

Issues that are central to the debate include: ① Capacity to cause harm is inherent in drugs in a way that sets them apart from other manufactured products; and harm often occurs in the absence of fault. ②Safety, i.e. the degree of safety that a person is entitled to expect, and adverse effects that should be accepted without complaint, must often be a matter of opinion and will vary with the disease being treated, e.g. cancer or insomnia. ③ Causation, i.e. proof that the drug in fact caused the injury, is often impossible, particularly where it increases the incidence of a disease that occurs naturally. ④ Contributory negligence. Should compensation be reduced in smokers and drinkers where there is evidence that these pleasure drugs increase liability to adverse reactions to therapeutic drugs? ⑤ The concept of defect, i.e. whether the drug or the prescriber or indeed the patient can be said to be 'defective' so as to attract liability, is a highly complex matter and indeed is a curious concept as applied to medicine.

Nowhere has a scheme that meets all the major difficulties yet been implemented. This is not because there has been too little thought, it is because the subject is so difficult. The following principles might form the basis of a workable compensation scheme for injury due to drugs: ① New unlicensed drugs undergoing clinical trial in small numbers of subjects (healthy or patient volunteers): the developer should be strictly liable for all adverse effects. ② New unlicensed drugs undergoing extensive trials in patients who may reasonably expect benefit: the producer should be strictly liable for any serious effect. ③ New drugs after licensing by an official body: the manufacturer and the community should share liability for serious injury, as new drugs provide general benefit. An option might be to institute a defined period of formal prospective drug surveillance monitoring, in which both doctors and patients agree to participate. ④ Standard drugs in day-to-day therapeutics: there should be a no-fault scheme, operated by or with the assent of government that has authority, through tribunals, to decide cases quickly and to make awards. This body would have authority to reimburse itself from others – manufacturer, supplier, prescriber – wherever that was appropriate. An award must not have to wait on the outcome of prolonged, vexatious, adversarial, expensive court proceedings. Patients would be compensated where: ① causation was proven on 'balance of probability'; ② the injury was serious; ③ the event was rare and remote and not reasonably taken into account in making the decision to treat.

COMPLEMENTARY, ALTERNATIVE AND TRADITIONAL MEDICINE

The term 'complementary and alternative medicine (CAM)' covers a broad range of heterogeneous systems of therapy (from acupuncture to herbalism to yoga), and diagnosis (from bioresonance to pulse and tongue diagnosis). This comprises a mass of practices varying from the worthless to highly effective remedies, such as digitalis (England), quinine (South America), reserpine (India), atropine (various countries). There is no doubt that the domain of CAM has grown in popularity in recent years; a survey estimated that about 20% of the UK population had consulted a CAM practitioner in the previous year. In Germany, the figure exceeds 60%, with $2.06 billion in over-the-counter sales in 2003. Usage rises sharply among those with chronic, relapsing conditions such as cancer, multiple sclerosis, human immunodeficiency virus (HIV) infection, psoriasis and rheumatological diseases. It is difficult to resist the conclusion that when scientific medicine neither guarantees happiness nor wholly eliminates the disabilities of degenerative diseases in long-lived populations, and when drugs used in modern medicine cause serious harm, public disappointment naturally leads to a revival of interest in alternatives that alluringly promise efficacy with complete safety. These range from a revival of traditional medicine to adoption of the more modern cults.

Some common false beliefs of CAM practitioners are that synthetic modern drugs are toxic, but products obtained in nature are not. Scientific medicine is held to accept evidence that remedies are effective only where the mechanism is understood, that it depends on adherence to rigid and unalterable dogmas, and recognises no form of evaluation other than the strict randomised controlled trial. Traditional (prescientific) medicine is deemed to have special virtue, and the collection and formal analysis of data on therapeutic outcomes, failures as well as successes, is deemed inessential. There is also a tenet that if the patient gets better when treated in accordance with certain beliefs, this provides evidence for the truth of these beliefs. Exponents of CAM often state that comparative controlled trials of their medicines against conventional medicines are impracticable because the classic double-blind randomised controlled designs are inappropriate and in particular do not allow for the individual approach characteristic of complementary medicine. But modern therapeutic trial designs can cope with this. There remain extremists who contend that they understand scientific method, and reject it as invalid for what they do and believe, i.e. their beliefs are not, in principle, refutable. This is the position taken up by magic and religion where subordination of reason to faith is a virtue.

CAM particularly charges that conventional medicine seriously neglects patients as whole integrated human beings (body, mind, spirit) and treats them too much as machines. Conventional practitioners may well feel uneasily that there has been and still is truth in this, that with the development of specialisation some doctors have been seduced by the enormous successes of medical science and technology and have become liable to look too narrowly at their patients where a much broader (holistic) approach is required. It is evident that such an approach is likely to give particular satisfaction in psychological and psychosomatic conditions for which conventional doctors in a hurry have been all too ready to think that a prescription meets all the patients' needs.

CAM does not compete with the successful mainstream of scientific medicine. Users of CAM commonly have chronic conditions and have tried conventional medicine but found that it has not offered a satisfactory solution, or has caused adverse effects. The problems, when they occur, are often at the interface between CAM and mainstream medicine. A doctor prescribing a conventional medicine may be unaware that a patient is taking herbal medicine, and there is ample scope for unwanted herb– drug interaction by a variety of mechanisms. These include the following: CYP450 enzyme induction, CYP450 enzyme inhibition and additive action. More troubling is the issue of conflicting advice between CAM and mainstream drugs, as witnessed by the advice to travelers from some homoeopathic pharmacies to use their products for malaria prophylaxis in place of conventional drugs (an action that drew criticism from the Society of Homoeopaths).

The following will suffice to give the flavour of homoeopathy, the principal complementary medicine system involving medicines, and the kind of criticism with which it has to contend.

Conclusion

There is a single fundamental issue between conventional scientific medicine and traditional, complementary and alternative medicine (although it is often obscured by detailed debates on individual practices); the issue is: what constitutes acceptable evidence, i.e. what is the nature, quality and interpretation of evidence that can justify general adoption of modes of treatment and acceptance of hypotheses? When there is agreement that a CAM treatment works, it becomes conventional and, in respect of that treatment, there is no difference between CAM and orthodox scientific medicine.

PLACEBO MEDICINES

A placebo is any component of therapy that is without specific biological activity for the condition being treated. Placebo medicines are used for two purposes: ① As a control in scientific evaluation of drug; ② To benefit or please a patient, not by any pharmacological actions, but for psychological reasons.

A placebo medicine is a vehicle for 'cure' by suggestion, and is surprisingly often successful, if only temporarily. The deliberate use of drugs as placebos is a confession of therapeutic failure by the doctor. Failures, however, are sometimes inevitable and an absolute condemnation of the use of placebos on all occasions would be unrealistic.

A placebo-reactor is an individual who reports changes of physical or mental state after taking a pharmacologically inert substance. Placebo reaction is an inconstant attribute: a person may respond at one time in one situation and not at another time under different conditions. In one study on medical students, psychological tests revealed that those who reacted to a placebo tended to be extroverted, sociable, less dominant, less self-confident, more appreciative of their teaching, more aware of their autonomic functions and more neurotic than their colleagues who did not react to a placebo under the particular conditions of the experiment. Placebo-reactors are suggestible people who are likely to respond favourably to any treatment. They have misled doctors into making false therapeutic claims. Negative reactors, who develop adverse effects when given a placebo, exist but, fortunately, are fewer.

Modern brain-scanning techniques provide evidence that the placebo effect has a physiological basis. Positron emission tomography showed that both opioid and placebo analgesia were associated with increased activity in the same cortical area of the brain, the greatest responses occurring in high placebo responders. Functional magnetic resonance imaging demonstrated that strong cortical activation correlated with greater placebo-induced pain relief. It is important that all who administer drugs should be aware that their attitudes to the treatment may greatly influence the outcome. Undue scepticism may prevent a drug from achieving its effect, and enthusiasm or confidence may potentiate the actions of drugs. Some 30%–80% of patients with chronic stable angina pectoris and 30%–50% with depression respond to placebos.

GUIDELINES, 'ESSENTIAL' DRUGS AND PRESCRIBING

Doctors recognise that they need guidance through the bountiful menu (thousands of medicines) so seductively served to them by the pharmaceutical industry. Principal sources of guidance are the pharmaceutical industry ('prescribe my drug') and governments ('spend less'), and also the developing (profit-making) managed care/ insurance bodies ('spend less') and the proliferating drug bulletins offering independent, and supposedly unbiased advice ('prescribe appropriately').

It may be restricted to what a third-party payer will reimburse, or to the range of formulations stocked in a hospital (and chosen by a local drugs and therapeutics committee, which all hospitals or groups of hospitals should have), or the range agreed by a partnership of general practitioners or primary care health centre. All restricted formularies are heavily motivated to keep costs down without impairing appropriate prescribing. They should make provision for prescribing outside their range in cases of special need with an 'escape clause'. Thus, restricted formularies are in effect guidelines for prescribing. There is a profusion of these from national sources, hospitals, group practices and specialty organisations (epilepsy, diabetes mellitus).

'Essential' drugs

Economically disadvantaged countries may seek help to construct formularies from the World Health Organization (WHO) with its 'Model List of Essential Medicines', i.e. drugs (representatives of classes of drugs) 'that satisfy the health care needs of the majority of the population; they should therefore be available at all times in adequate amounts and in the appropriate dosage forms'. Countries seeking such advice can use the list as a basis for their own choices (the WHO also publishes model prescribing information). The list, updated regularly, contains about 300 items.

Cost-containment

Cost-containment in prescription drug therapy attracts increasing attention. It may involve two particularly contentious activities: **Generic substitution**, where a generic formulation is substituted (by a pharmacist) for the proprietary formulation prescribed by the doctor. **Therapeutic substitution**, where a drug of different chemical structure is substituted for the drug prescribed by the doctor.

The substitute is of the same chemical class and is deemed to have similar pharmacological properties and to give similar therapeutic benefit. Therapeutic substitution is a particularly controversial matter where it is done without consulting the prescriber, and legal issues may be raised in the event of adverse therapeutic outcome.

The following facts and opinions are worth some thought: ① UK National Health Service (NHS) spending on drugs has been 9%–11% per year (of the total cost) for nearly 50 years; ② general practitioners (i.e. primary care) spend some 80% of the total cost of drugs; ③ in the past 25 years, the number of NHS prescriptions has risen from 5.5 to over 13 per person; ④ the average cost per head of medicines supplied to people aged over 75 years is nearly five times that of medicines supplied to those below pensionable age (in the UK: women 62 years, men 65 years, but under revision); ⑤ under-prescribing can be just as harmful to the health of patients as over-prescribing.

It is crucially important that incentives and sanctions address quality of prescribing as well as quantity: 'it would be wrong if too great a preoccupation with the cost issue in isolation were to encourage under-prescribing or have an adverse effect on patient care'.

Reasons for under-prescribing include: lack of information or lack of the will to use available information (in economically privileged countries there is, if anything, a surplus of information); fear of being blamed for adverse reactions (affecting doctors who lack the confidence that a knowledge of pharmacological principles confers); fear of sanctions against over-costly prescribing. Prescription frequency and cost per prescription are lower for older than for younger doctors. There is no evidence that the patients of older doctors are worse off as a result.

Taking a drug history

The reasons for taking a drug history from patients are: ① Drugs are a cause of disease. Withdrawal of drugs, if abrupt, can also cause disease, e.g. benzodiazepines, antiepilepsy drugs. ② Drugs can conceal disease, e.g. adrenal steroid. ③ Drugs can interact, producing a positive adverse effect or a negative adverse effect, i.e. therapeutic failure. This is an increasing problem with polypharmacy, especially in the elderly. ④ Drugs can give diagnostic clues, e.g. ampicillin and amoxicillin causing rash in infectious mononucleosis – a diagnostic adverse effect, not a diagnostic test. ⑤ Drugs can cause false results in clinical chemistry tests, e.g. plasma cortisol, urinary catecholamine, urinary glucose, serum renin and aldosterone. ⑥ Drug history can assist choice of drugs in the future. ⑦ Drugs can leave residual effects after administration has ceased, e.g. chloroquine, amiodarone. ⑧ Drugs available for independent patient self-medication are increasing in range and importance.

Appropriate prescribing is that which bases the choice of a drug on its effectiveness, safety and convenience relative to other drugs or treatments (e.g. surgery or psychotherapy), and considers cost only when those criteria for choice have been satisfied. In some circumstances appropriateness will require the use of more costly drugs.

Prescribing that is inappropriate is the result of several factors: ① Giving in to patient pressure to write unnecessary prescriptions. ② Continuing patients, especially the elderly, on courses of medicinal treatment over many months without proper review of their medication. ③ Doctors may 'prescribe brand-name drugs rather than cheaper generic equivalents, even where there is no conceivable therapeutic advantage in so doing. ④ 'Insufficient training in clinical pharmacology. Many of the drugs on the market may not have been available when a general practitioner was at medical school. The sheer quantity of new products may lead to a practitioner becoming over-reliant on drugs companies' promotional material, or sticking to "tried and tested" products out of caution based on ignorance'. ⑤ Failure of doctors to keep up to date. Computerising prescribing addresses some of these issues, for example by prompting regular review of a patient's medication, by instantly providing generic names from brand names, by giving ready access to formularies and prescribing guidelines.

Repeat prescriptions

About two-thirds of general (family) practice prescriptions are for repeat medication. Some 95% of patients' requests are acceded to without further discussion; 25% of patients who receive repeat prescriptions have had 40 or more repeats; and 55% of patients aged over 75 years are on repeat medication. Many patients taking the same drug for years are doing so for the best reason, i.e. firm diagnosis for which effective therapy is available, such as epilepsy, diabetes, hypertension, but some are not.

Warnings and consent

Doctors have a professional duty to inform and to warn, so that patients, who are increasingly informed and educated, may make meaningful personal choices. Patients now have access to a potentially confusing quantity of detail about the unwanted effects of drugs (information sheet, the internet, the media) but without the balancing influence of data on their frequency of occurrence. It would be prudent for doctors to draw attention at least to adverse effects that are common, serious (even if uncommon), or avoidable or mitigated if recognised.

Warnings to patients are of two kinds: ① warnings that will affect the patient's choice to accept or reject the treatment; ② warnings that will affect the safety of the treatment once it has begun, e.g. risk of stopping treatment, occurrence of drug toxicity.

If drugs are not safe then plainly patients are entitled to be warned of their hazards, which should be explained to them, as to probability, nature and severity. If there is a 'real' (say 1%–2%) risk inherent in a procedure of some misfortune occurring, then doctors should warn patients of the possibility that the injury may occur, however well the treatment is performed. Doctors should take into account the personality of the patient, the likelihood of any misfortune arising and what warning was necessary for each particular patient's welfare.

Legal hazards for prescribers

The provision of information to patients is treated

by (English) law as but one part of the way a doctor discharges the obligation he owes to a patient to take reasonable care in all aspects of his treatment of that patient. The provision of information is a corollary of the patient's right to self-determination which is a right recognised by law. Failure to provide appropriate information will usually be a breach of duty and if that breach leads to the patient suffering injury then the basis for a claim for compensation exists. The keeping of appropriate medical records, written at the time of consultation (and which is so frequently neglected), is not only good medical practice, it is the best way of ensuring that there is an answer to unjustified allegations, made later, when memory has faded. At the very least, these should include records of warning about treatments that are potentially hazardous.

COMPLIANCE

Successful therapy involves patient and doctor compliance. The latter is liable to be overlooked (by doctors), for doctors prefer to dwell on the deficiencies of their patients rather than of themselves.

Patient compliance

Patient compliance is the extent to which the actual behavior of the patient coincides with medical advice and instructions; it may be complete, partial, erratic, nil, or there may be over-compliance. To make a diagnosis and to prescribe evidence-based effective treatment is a satisfying experience for doctors, but too many assume that patients will gratefully or accurately do what they are told, i.e. obtain the medicine and consume it as instructed. This assumption is wrong. The rate of non-presentation (redemption) of prescriptions in the UK is around 5%, but is up to 20% or even more in the elderly (who pay no prescription charge). Where lack of money to pay for the medicine is not the cause, this is due to lack of motivation or apprehension about drugs. Having obtained the medicine, some 25%–50% (sometimes even more) of patients either fail to follow the instruction to a significant extent (taking

50%–90% of the prescribed dose), or they do not take it at all.

Patient non-compliance or non-adherence is identified as a major factor in therapeutic failure in both routine practice and in scientific therapeutic trials; but, sad to say, doctors are too often non-compliant about remedying this. All patients are potential non-compliers; clinical criteria cannot reliably predict good compliance, but non-compliance often can be predicted. In addition to therapeutic failure, undetected noncompliance may lead to rejection of the best drug when it is effective, leading to substitution by second-rank medicines.

Non-compliance may occur because: ① the patient has not understood the instructions, so can not comply; ② the patient understands the instructions, but fails to carry them out.

Prime factors for poor patient compliance are: ① Frequency and complexity of the drug regimen. Many studies attest to polypharmacy as an inhibitor of compliance, i.e. more than three drugs taken concurrently or more than three drug-taking occasions in the day (the ideal of one occasion only is often unattainable). ② Unintentional non-compliance, or forgetfulness, may be addressed by associating drug-taking with cues in daily life (breakfast, bedtime), by special packaging (e.g. calendar packs) and by enlisting the aid of others (e.g. carers, teachers). ③ 'Intelligent' or wilful non-compliance. Patients decide they do not need the drug (asymptomatic disease) or they do not like the drug (unwanted effects), or take 2–3-day 'drug holidays'. ④ Illness. This includes cognitive impairment and psychological problems, with depression being a particular problem. ⑤ Lack of information. Oral instructions alone are not enough; one-third of patients are unable to recount instructions immediately on leaving the consulting room. Lucid and legible labelling of containers is essential, as well as patient-friendly information leaflets, which are increasingly available via doctors and pharmacists, and as package inserts. ⑥ Poor patient–doctor relationship and lack of motivation to take medicines as instructed offer a major challenge to the prescriber whose diagnosis and prescription maybe perfect, yet loses efficacy by patient non-compliance. The best way to achieve compliance is to cultivate the patient–doctor relationship. Doctors cannot be expected actually to like all their patients, but it is a great help (where liking does not come naturally) if they make a positive effort to understand how individual patients must feel about their illnesses and their treatments, i.e. to empathise with their patients. This is not always easy, but its achievement is the action of the true professional, and indeed is part of their professional duty of care.

Suggestions for doctors to enhance patient compliance/adherence

①Form a non-judgemental alliance or partnership with the patient, giving the patient an opportunity to ask questions. ② Plan a regimen with the minimum number of drugs and drug-taking occasions, adjusted to fit the patient's lifestyle. Use fixed-dose combinations, sustained release (or injectable depot) formulations, or long $t_{1/2}$ drugs as appropriate; arrange direct observation of each dose in exceptional cases. ③ Provide clear oral and written information adapted to the patient's understanding and medical and cultural needs. ④ Use patient-friendly packaging, e.g. calendar packs, where appropriate; or monitored-dose systems, e.g. boxes compartmented and labelled (Dosette boxes). ⑤ See the patient regularly and not so infrequently that the patient feels the doctor has lost interest. ⑥ Enlist the help of family members, carers, friends. ⑦ Use computer-generated reminders for repeat prescriptions.

Factors that are insignificant for compliance are: age (except at extremes), sex, intelligence (except at extreme deficiency) and educational level (probably).

Directly observed therapy (DOT) (where a reliable person supervises each dose). In addition to the areas where supervision is obviously in the interest of patients, e.g. a child, DOT is employed (even imposed) among free-living uncooperative patients who may be a menace to the community, such as those with multiple drug-resistant tuberculosis.

What every patient needs to know
① An account of the disease and the reason for prescribing. ② The name of the medicine. ③ The objective: to treat the disease and/or to relieve symptoms, i.e. how important the medicine is, whether the patient can judge its efficacy and when benefit can be expected to occur. ④ How and when to take the medicine. ⑤ Whether it matters if a dose is missed and what, if anything, to do about it. ⑥ For how long the medicine is likely to be needed. ⑦ How to recognise adverse effects and any action that should be taken, including effects on car driving. ⑧ Any interaction with alcohol or other medicines.

Over-compliance. Patients (up to 20%) may take more drug than is prescribed, even increasing the dose by 50%. In diseases where precise compliance with frequent or complex regimens is important, for example in glaucoma where sight is at risk, there have been instances of obsessional patients responding to their doctors' overemphatic instructions by clock-watching in a state of anxiety to avoid the slightest deviance from timed administration of the correct dose, to the extent that their daily (and nightly) life becomes dominated by this single purpose.

Evaluation of patient compliance. Merely asking patients whether they have taken the drug as directed is not likely to provide reliable evidence. It is safest to assume that any event that can impair compliance will sometimes happen.

Estimations of compliance come from a variety of measures. DOT (above) is the most accurate, and identification of the drug or metabolites in plasma (or an artificial biological marker in the case of a clinical trial) is persuasive at least of recent compliance.

Some pharmacodynamic effects, such as heart rate with a b-adrenoceptor blocker, provide a physiological marker as an indicator of the presence of drug in the body. Monitoring plasma drug concentrations is possible but to do so without informing the patient raises ethical issues.

Doctor compliance

Doctor compliance is the extent to which the behaviour of doctors fulfils their professional duty: ① not to be ignorant; ② to adopt new advances when they are sufficiently proved (which doctors are often slow to do); ③ to prescribe accurately; ④ to tell patients what they need to know; ⑤ to warn, i.e. to recognise the importance of the act of prescribing.

Underdosing

Use of suboptimal doses of drugs in serious disease occurs, sacrificing therapeutic efficacy to avoid serious adverse effects. Instances are commonest with drugs of low therapeutic index, i.e. where the effective and toxic dose ranges are close, or even overlap, e.g. heparin, anticancer drugs, aminoglycoside antimicrobials. In these cases dose adjustment to obtain maximum benefit with minimum risk requires both knowledge and attentiveness.

The clinical importance of missed dose(s)

Even the most conscientious of patients will miss a dose or doses occasionally. Patients should therefore be told whether this matters and what they should do about it, if anything. Missed dose(s) may lead to: ① Loss of therapeutic efficacy (acute disease); ② Resurgence (chronic disease); ③ Rebound or withdrawal syndrome.

Loss of therapeutic efficacy involves the pharmacokinetic properties of drugs. With some drugs of short $t_{1/2}$, the issue is simply a transient drop in plasma concentration below a defined therapeutic concentration. The issues are more complex where therapeutic effect may not decline in parallel with plasma concentration, as with recovery of negative feedback homoeostatic mechanisms (adrenocortical steroids).

A single missed dose may be important with some drugs, e.g. oral contraceptives, but with others (long $t_{1/2}$), omission of several doses is tolerated without any serious decline in efficacy, e.g. levothyroxine.

These pharmacokinetic considerations are complex and important, and are, or should be, taken into account by drug manufacturers in devising dosage schedules and informative data sheets. Manufac-turers should aim at one or two doses per day (not more), and this is generally best achieved with drugs with relatively long biological effect $t_{1/2}$ or, where the biological effect $t_{1/2}$ is short, by using sustained-release formulations. Discontinuation syndrome (recurrence of disease, rebound, or withdrawal syndrome) may occur due to a variety of mechanisms.

PHARMACOECONOMICS

Even the richest societies cannot satisfy the appetite of their citizens for health care based on their real needs, on their wants and on their (often unrealistic) expectations.

Health-care resources are rationed in one way or another, whether according to national social policies or to individual wealth. The debate on supply is not about whether there should be rationing, but about what form rationing should take; whether it should be explicit or concealed (from the public).

Economics is the science of the distribution of wealth and resources. Prescribing doctors, who have a duty to the community as well as to individual patients, cannot escape involvement with economics.

The economists' objective

The objective is to define needs, thereby enabling the deployment of resources according to priorities set by society, which has an interest in fairness between its members.

Economists are often portrayed as people who want to focus on cost, whereas in reality they see everything in terms of a balance between costs and benefits.

Four economic concepts have particular importance to the thinking of every doctor who makes a decision to prescribe:

- **Opportunity cost** means that which has to be sacrificed in order to carry out a certain course of action, i.e. costs are benefits foregone elsewhere. Money spent on prescribing is not available for another purpose; wasteful prescribing is as an affront to those who are in serious need, e.g. institutionalised mentally handicapped citizens who everywhere would benefit from increased resources, or patients requiring hip replacement.

- **Cost–effectiveness analysis** is concerned with how to attain a given objective at minimal financial cost, e.g. prevention of post-surgical venous thromboembolism by heparins, warfarin, aspirin, external pneumatic compression. Analysis includes the cost of materials, adverse effects, any tests, nursing and doctor time, duration of stay in hospital (which may greatly exceed the cost of the drug).

- **Cost–benefit analysis** is concerned with issues of whether (and to what extent) to pursue objectives and policies; it is thus a broader activity than cost–effectiveness analysis and puts monetary values on the quality as well as on the quantity (duration) of life.

- **Cost–utility analysis** is concerned with comparisons between programmes, such as an antenatal drug treatment which saves a young life, or a hip replacement operation which improves mobility in a man of 60 years. Such differing issues are also the basis for comparison by computing quality-adjusted life years.

An allied measure is the cost–minimisation analysis, which finds the least costly programme among those shown or assumed to be of equal benefit. Economic analysis requires that both quantity and quality of life be measured. The former is easy, the latter is hard to determine.

Quality of life

Life may be extended and yet have a low quality, even to the point that it is not worth having at all. It is therefore useful to have a unit of health measurement that combines the quantity of life with its quality, to place individual and social decision-making on a sounder basis than mere intuition. Economists met this need by developing the quality-adjusted life year (QALY) whereby estimations of years of life expectancy are modified according to estimations of quality of life. Quality of life has four principal dimensions: ① physical mobility; ② freedom from pain and distress; ③ capacity for self-care; ④ ability to engage in normal work and social interactions. The assessments are refined to provide improved assessment of the benefits and risks of medicines to the individual and to society.

SUMMARY

Prescribing is a task carried out many times each day and has the potential to cause harm or death as well as good. Drug therapy requires knowledge, judgement, skill and wisdom, but above all a sense of responsibility. Drugs are used in three principal ways: to cure disease, to suppress disease and to prevent disease (prophylaxis). There is general agreement that drugs prescribed for disease are themselves the cause of a significant amount of disease (adverse reactions), of death, of permanent disability of recoverable illness and of minor inconvenience.

Whenever a drug is taken a risk is taken. Three major grades of risk of drugs are unacceptable, acceptable and negligible. Responsibility for drug-induced injury raises important issues affecting medical practice and development of needed new drugs, as well as of law and of social justice. Practitioners of complementary and alternative medicine (CAM) are severely critical of modern drugs. Users of CAM commonly have chronic conditions and have tried conventional medicine but found that it has not offered a satisfactory solution, or has caused adverse effects. When there is agreement that a CAM treatment works, it becomes conventional and, in respect of that treatment, there is no difference between CAM and orthodox scientific medicine.

A placebo is any component of therapy that is without specific biological activity for the condition being treated. Placebo medicines are used for two purposes: ① as a control in scientific evaluation of drugs; ② to benefit or please a patient, not by any pharmacological actions, but for psychological reasons.

Appropriate prescribing is that which bases the choice of a drug on its effectiveness, safety and convenience relative to other drugs or treatments (e.g. surgery or psychotherapy), and considers cost only when those criteria for choice have been satisfied. In some circumstances appropriateness will require the use of more costly drugs. Successful therapy involves patient and doctor compliance. The latter is liable to be overlooked (by doctors), for doctors prefer to dwell on the deficiencies of their patients rather than of themselves.

IMPORTANT TERMINOLOGY

prescription 处方
prescribing 开处方
complaint 主诉
prophylaxis 预防
iatrogenic 医源性
complementary 互补的
alternative 替代的

placebo 安慰剂
compliance 依从性
pharmacoeconomics 药物经济学
cost–effectiveness analysis 成本 - 效果分析
cost–benefit analysis 成本 - 效益分析
cost–utility analysis 成本 - 效用分析

CHALLENGE YOURSELF

1. What is prescription?
2. In which ways drugs are used?
3. Please describe the reasons why drugs fail to meet the criteria of being risk-free.
4. What are the prime factors for poor patient compliance?

Huijun Sun

Adverse drug reactions and pharmacovigilance

BACKGROUND

"Cured yesterday of my disease, I died last night of my physician."

Nature is neutral, *i.e.* it has no "intentions" towards humans, though it is often unfavorable to them. It is humans, in their desire to avoid suffering and death, who decide that some of the biological effects of drugs are desirable (therapeutic) and others undesirable (adverse). In addition to this arbitrary division, which has no fundamental biological basis, numerous non-drug factors promote or even cause unwanted effects. Because of the variety of these factors, attempts to make a simple account of the unwanted effects of drugs must be imperfect.

There is general agreement that drugs prescribed for disease are themselves the cause of a serious amount of disease (adverse reactions), ranging from mere inconvenience to permanent disability and death.

It is not enough to measure the incidence of adverse reactions to drugs, their nature and their severity, although accurate data are obviously useful. It is necessary to take, or to try to take, into account which effects are avoidable (by skilled choice and use) and which unavoidable (inherent in drug or patient).

As there can be no hope of eliminating all adverse effects of drugs, it is necessary to evaluate patterns of adverse reaction against one another. One drug may frequently cause minor ill-effects but pose no threat to life, though patients do not like it and may take it irregularly, to their own long-term harm. Another drug may be pleasant to take, so that patients take it consistently, with benefit, but on rare occasions it may kill someone. It is not obvious which drug is to be preferred.

Some patients, *e.g.* those with a history of allergy or previous reactions to drugs, are up to four times more likely to have another adverse reaction, so that the incidence does not fall evenly. It is also useful to discover the causes of adverse reactions (*e.g.* individuals who lack certain enzymes), for use of such knowledge can render avoidable what are at present unavoidable reactions.

More skilful prescribing will reduce avoidable adverse effects and this means that doctors, among all the other claims on their time, must find time better to understand drugs, as well as understanding patients and their diseases.

DEFINITIONS

Many unwanted effects of drugs are medically trivial and, in order to avoid inflating the figures of drug-induced disease, it is convenient to retain the widely-used term side-effects for minor reactions that occur at normal therapeutic doses, and that are predictable and usually dose related.

The term adverse drug reaction (ADR) should be confined to harmful or seriously unpleasant effects occurring at doses intended for therapeutic (including prophylactic or diagnostic) effect and which call for reduction of dose or withdrawal of the drug and/or forecast hazard from future administration; it is effects of this order that are of importance in evaluating drug-induced disease in the community.

The term adverse "reaction" is almost synonymous with adverse "effect", except that an "effect" relates to the drug and a "reaction" to the patient. Both terms should be distinguished from an adverse "event", which is an adverse happening that occurs during exposure to a drug without any assumption being made about its cause.

CLASSIFICATIONS

Toxicity implies a direct action of the drug, often at high dose, damaging cells, *e.g.* liver damage from paracetamol overdose, eighth cranial nerve damage from gentamicin. All drugs, for practical purposes, are toxic in overdose and overdose can be absolute or relative; in the latter case an ordinary dose may be administered but may be toxic due to an underlying abnormality in the patient, *e.g.* disease of the kidney. Mutagenicity, carcinogenicity and teratogenicity are special cases of toxicity.

The above principle of drug dose appreciated by Paracelsus 500 years ago, who stated that "All things are poisons and there is nothing that is harmless; the dose alone decides that something is no poison". The physician, alchemist and philosopher are regarded as the founders of chemical therapeutics; they were the first to use carefully measured doses of mercury to treat syphilis.

Secondary effects are the indirect consequences of a primary drug action. Examples are: vitamin deficiency or opportunistic infection in patients whose normal bowel flora has been altered by antimicrobials; diuretic-induced hypokalaemia causing digoxin toxicity.

Intolerance means a low threshold to the normal pharmacodynamic action of a drug. Individuals vary greatly in their susceptibility to drugs, those at one extreme of the normal distribution curve being intolerant of the drugs, those at the other, tolerant.

Idiosyncrasy implies an inherent qualitative abnormal reaction to a drug, usually due to genetic abnormality, *e.g.* porphyria.

ATTRIBUTION AND DEGREES OF CERTAINTY

When an unexpected event, for which there is no obvious cause, occurs in a patient already taking a drug, the possibility that it is drug attributable must always be considered. Distinguishing between natural progression of a disease and drug-induced deterioration is particularly challenging, *e.g.* sodium in antacid formulations may aggravate cardiac failure, tricyclic antidepressants may provoke epileptic seizures, and aspirin may cause bronchospasm in some asthmatics.

The following elements are useful in attributing the cause of an adverse event to a drug:

1. The time sequence in relation to taking the drug. The majority of reactions develop soon after exposure. Anaphylactic reactions (within minutes or hours) and hypersensitivity reactions (within weeks) may readily suggest an association, but delayed effects such as carcinogenesis or tardive dyskinesia (after years or even decades) present more difficulty.

2. The effects of withdrawing or reintroducing the drug. Most reactions subside when the drug is discontinued, unless an autoimmune reaction is established, when effects persist. Planned re-exposing a patient to a drug is rarely indicated unless treatment with it is essential and there is no reliable alternative.

3. The relationship to what is already known about the drug. This of course invites questions about consistency with the established pharmacology and toxicology of the drug or related substances.

Degrees of conviction for attributing adverse reactions to drugs may be ascribed as:

• *Definite:* time sequence from taking the drug is reasonable; event corresponds to what is known of the drug and is not explicable by concurrent disease or drugs; event ceases on stopping the drug; event returns on restarting the drug (rarely advisable).

- *Probable:* time sequence is reasonable; event corresponds to what is known of the drug; event ceases on stopping the drug; event not reasonably explained by patient's disease or other drugs.
- *Possible:* time sequence is reasonable; event corresponds to what is known of the drug; uncertain relationship to effect of stopping the drug; event could readily have been result of the patient's disease or other therapy.
- *Conditional:* time sequence is reasonable; event does not correspond to what is known of the drug; event could not reasonably be explained by the patient's disease or other drugs.
- *Doubtful:* event not meeting the above criteria.

Caution. About 80% of well people not taking any drugs admit on questioning to symptoms (often several) such as are commonly experienced as lesser adverse reactions to drugs. Administration of a placebo intensifies (or diminishes) these symptoms. Thus, many (minor) symptoms may be wrongly attributed to drugs. Similarly, minor and possibly transient abnormalities in laboratory results, *e.g.* liver function tests, occur in apparently healthy people.

SOURCES OF ADVERSE DRUG REACTIONS

The reasons why patients experience ADRs are varied and numerous, but reflection on the following may help a prescriber to anticipate and avoid unwelcome events:

- **The patient may be predisposed to an ADR** by age, sex, genetic constitution, known tendency to allergy, disease of drug eliminating organs, or social habits, *e.g.* use of tobacco, alcohol, other recreational drugs.
- **The known nature of the drug may forewarn.** Some drugs, *e.g.* digoxin, have steep dose-response curves and small increments of dose are more likely to induce adverse or toxic reactions. The capacity of the body to eliminate certain drugs, *e.g.* phenytoin, may saturate within the

therapeutic dose range so that standard increases cause a disproportionate rise in plasma concentration, risking toxic effects. Some drugs, *e.g.* antimicrobials and particularly penicillins, have a tendency to cause allergy. Anticancer agents warrant special care as they are by their nature cytotoxic. Use of these and other drugs may raise longer-term issues of mutagenicity, carcinogenicity and teratogenicity. Ingredients of a formulation, rather than the active drug, may also cause adverse reactions. Examples include the high sodium content of some antacids, and coloring and flavoring agents.

- **The prescriber** needs to be aware that adverse reactions may occur after a drug has been used for a long time, at a critical phase in pregnancy, is abruptly discontinued or given with other drugs.

Aspects of the above appear throughout the book as is indicated. Selected topics are:

Age

The very old and the very young are liable to be intolerant of many drugs, largely because the mechanisms for disposing of them in the body are less efficient. The young are not simply "small adults" and "respect for their pharmacokinetic variability should be added to the list of our senior citizens' rights". Multiple drug therapy is commonly found in the old, which further predisposes to adverse effects.

Sex

Females are more likely to experience adverse reactions to certain drugs, *e.g.* mefloquine (neuropsychiatric effects).

Genetic constitution

Inherited factors that influence response to drugs appear in general under Pharmacogenomics. For convenience, we describe here the porphyrias, a specific group of disorders for which careful prescribing in a subgroup, the acute porphyrias, is vital.

Healthy people need to produce haem, *e.g.* for erythrocytes and haem-dependent enzymes. Haem is synthesized by a sequence of enzymes and in non-erythroid cells (including the liver) the rate of the synthetic process is controlled by the first of these, D-aminolaevulinic acid (D-ALA) synthase, on which haem provides a negative feedback.

The porphyrias comprise a number of rare, genetically determined, single-enzyme defects in haem biosynthesis and give rise to two main clinical manifestations: acute neurovisceral attacks and/or skin lesions. Non-acute porphyrias (porphyria cutanea tarda, erythropoietic protoporphyria and congenital erythropoietic porphyria) present with cutaneous photosensitivity that result from the overproduction of porphyrins, which are photosensitizing. In porphyria cutanea tarda, a mainly acquired disorder of hepatic enzyme function, one of the main provoking agents is alcohol (and prescribed oestrogens in women).

The acute hepatic porphyrias (acute intermittent porphyria, variegate porphyria and hereditary coproporphyria) are characterized by severe attacks of neurovisceral dysfunction precipitated principally by a wide variety of drugs (also by alcohol, fasting and infection). Clinical effects arise from the accumulation of the precursors of haem synthesis, D-ALA, porphobilinogen.

Induction of the haem-containing hepatic oxidising enzymes of the cytochrome P450 group causes an increased demand for haem. Therefore drugs that induce these enzymes would be expected to precipitate acute attacks of porphyria, and they do so: tobacco smoking and alcohol excess may also act *via* this mechanism. Apparently unexplained attacks of porphyria should be an indication for close enquiry into all possible chemical intakes, including recreational substances such as marijuana, cocaine, amfetamines and ecstasy. Patients must be educated to understand their condition, to possess a list of safe and unsafe drugs, and to protect themselves from themselves and from others, including, especially, prescribing doctors.

Great care in prescribing for these patients is required if serious illness is to be avoided and it is therefore essential that patients and their clinicians have access to information concerning the safe use of prescription medication. If no recognized safe option is available, the clinician should assess the severity of the condition and the activity of the porphyria and make a risk versus benefit assessment. In these circumstances the clinician recommends that the patient be monitored as follows:

1. Measure porphyrin and porphobilinogen before starting treatment.
2. Repeat the measurement at regular intervals or if the patient has symptoms in keeping with an acute attack. If there is an increase in the precursor levels, stop the treatment and consider giving haem arginate for acute attack.

In treatment of the acute attack the rationale is to use means of reducing d-ALA synthase activity. Haem arginate (human haematin) infusion, by replenishing haem and so removing the stimulus to D-ALA synthase, is effective if given early, and may prevent chronic neuropathy.

The environment and social habits

Drug metabolism may be increased by hepatic enzyme induction from insecticide accumulation, *e.g.* dicophane (DDT), and from alcohol use and the tobacco habit, *e.g.* smokers require a higher dose of theophylline. Antimicrobials used in feeds of animals for human consumption have given rise to concern in relation to the spread of resistant bacteria that may affect man. Penicillin in the air of hospitals or in milk may cause allergy.

PHARMACOVIGILANCE AND PHARMACOEPIDEMIOLOGY

The principal methods of collecting data on ADRs (pharmacovigilance) are:

Experimental studies, *i.e.* formal therapeutic trials of Phases 1–3. These provide reliable data on only the commoner events as they involve relatively small numbers of patients (hundreds); they detect an incidence of up to about 1 in 200.

Observational studies, where the drug is observed epidemiologically under conditions of normal use in the community, *i.e.* pharmacoepidemiology and pharmacovigilance. Techniques used for postmarketing (Phase 4) studies include the observational cohort study and the case-control study.

Drug-induced illness

The discovery of drug-induced illness can be analysed as follows:

A drug commonly induces an otherwise rare illness: this effect is likely to be discovered by clinical observation in the licensing (pre-marketing) formal therapeutic trials and the drug will almost always be abandoned; but some patients are normally excluded from such trials, *e.g.* pregnant women, and detection will then occur later.

A drug rarely or uncommonly induces an otherwise common illness: this effect is likely to remain undiscovered. Cardiovascular risk from coxibs (e.g. rofecoxib, Vioxx) approximates as an example, but the degree of increased risk did become apparent after meta-analysis of several clinical trials and observational studies.

A drug rarely induces an otherwise rare illness: this effect is likely to remain undiscovered before the drug is released for general prescribing. The effect could be detected by informal clinical observation or during any special post-registration surveillance and confirmed by a case-control study; aplastic anaemia with chloramphenicol and the oculomucocutaneous syndrome with practolol were uncovered in this way.

A drug commonly induces an otherwise common illness: this effect will not be discovered by informal clinical observation. If very common, it may be discovered in formal therapeutic trials and in case-control studies, but if only moderately common it may require observational cohort studies, *e.g.* proarrhythmic effects of anti-arrhythmic drugs.

Drug adverse effects and illness incidence in an intermediate range: both case-control and cohort studies may be needed.

Some impression of the features of drug-induced illness can be gained from the following statistics:

1. In a large UK study, the prevalence of ADRs as a cause of admission to hospital was 6.5%, with a median bed stay of 8 days (4% of hospital bed capacity); most reactions were definitely or possibly avoidable; the commonest drugs were: low-dose aspirin, diuretics, warfarin, non-steroidal anti-inflammatory drugs (other than aspirin); the commonest adverse reaction was gastrointestinal bleeding.

2. Overall incidence in hospital inpatients is 10%–20%, with possible prolongation of hospital stay in 2%–10% of patients in acute medical wards.

3. ADRs cause 2%–3% of consultations in general practice.

4. A study of 661 ambulatory patients found that 25% experienced adverse events, of which 13% were serious and 11% were preventable.

5. Predisposing factors for ADRs are: age over 60 years or under 1 month, female sex, previous history of adverse reaction, hepatic or renal disease, number of medications taken.

It is important to avoid alarmist or defeatist reactions. Many treatments are dangerous, *e.g.* surgery, electroshock, drugs, and it is irrational to accept the risks of surgery for biliary stones or hernia and to refuse to accept any risk at all from drugs for conditions of comparable severity.

Many patients, whose death is deemed to be partly or wholly caused by drugs, are dangerously ill already; justifiable risks may be taken in the hope of helping them; ill-informed criticism in such cases can act against the interest of the sick. On the other hand, there is no doubt that some of these accidents are avoidable. This is often more obvious when reviewing the conduct of treatment after the event, *i.e.* with the benefit of hindsight.

Sir Anthony Carlisle, in the first half of the 19th century, said that "medicine is an art founded on conjecture and improved by murder". Although medicine has advanced rapidly, there is still a ring of truth in that statement, as witness anyone who follows the introduction of new drugs and observes how, after the early enthusiasm, there follow reports of serious toxic effects, and withdrawal of the drug may then follow. The challenge is to find and avoid these, and, indeed, the present systems for detecting adverse reactions came into being largely in the wake of the thalidomide, practolol and benoxaprofen disasters; they are now an increasingly sophisticated and effective part of medicines development.

Drugs and skilled tasks

Many medicines affect performance, and it is relevant to review here some examples with their mechanisms of action. As might be expected, centrally acting and psychotropic drugs are prominent, *e.g.* the sedative antidepressants, benzodiazepines, non-benzodiazepine and other hypnotics, and antipsychotics (the "classical" type more so than the "atypical"). Many drugs possess anticholinergic activity either directly (atropine, oxybutynin) or indirectly (tricyclic antidepressants, antipsychotics), the central effects of which cause confusion and impaired ability to process information. The first-generation H_1-receptor antihistamines (chlorphenamine, diphenhydramine) are notably sedating and impair alertness and concentration, which features the recipient may not recognise. Drugs may also affect performance through cerebral depression (antiepileptics, opioids), hypoglycaemia (antidiabetics) and hypotension (antihypertensives).

ALLERGY IN RESPONSE TO DRUGS

Allergic reactions to drugs are the result of the interaction of drug or metabolite (or a non-drug element in the formulation) with patient and disease, and subsequent re-exposure.

Lack of previous exposure is not the same as lack of history of previous exposure, and "first dose reactions" are among the most dramatic. Exposure is not necessarily medical, *e.g.* penicillins may occur in dairy products following treatment of mastitis in cows (despite laws to prevent this), and penicillin antibodies are commonly present in those who deny ever having received the drug. Immune responses to drugs may be harmful in varying degrees (allergy) or harmless; the fact that antibodies are produced does not mean a patient will necessarily respond to re-exposure with clinical manifestations; most of the UK population has antibodies to penicillins but, fortunately, comparatively few react clinically to penicillin administration.

While macromolecules (proteins, peptides, dextran polysaccharides) can act as complete antigens, most drugs are simple chemicals (mol. wt. less than 1 000) and act as incomplete antigens or haptens, which become complete antigens in combination with a body protein.

The chief target organs of drug allergy are the skin, respiratory tract, gastrointestinal tract, blood and blood vessels.

Classification of allergic reactions

Allergic reactions in general may be classified according to four types of hypersensitivity, and drugs can elicit reactions of all types.

Type I reactions: immediate or anaphylactic type. The drug causes formation of tissue-sensitising immunoglobulin (Ig) E antibodies that are fixed to mast cells or leucocytes. On subsequent administration the allergen (conjugate of drug or metabolite with tissue protein) reacts with these antibodies, activating but not damaging the cell to which they are fixed and causing release of pharmacologically active substances, *e.g.* histamine, leukotrienes, prostaglandins, *platelet activating factor*, and causing effects such as urticaria, anaphylactic shock and asthma. Allergy develops within minutes and lasts for 1–2h: it may of course be fatal.

Type II reactions: antibody-dependent cytotoxic type. The drug or metabolite combines with a protein in the body so that the body no longer recognises the protein as self, treats it as a foreign protein and forms antibodies (IgG, IgM) that combine with the antigen and activate complement which damages cells, *e.g.* penicillin- or methyl- dopa-induced haemolytic anaemia.

Type III reactions: immune complex-mediated type. Antigen and antibody form large complexes and activate complement. Small blood vessels are damaged or blocked. Leucocytes attracted to the site of reaction engulf the immune complexes and release pharmacologically active substances (including lysosomal enzymes), starting an inflammatory process. These reactions include serum sickness, glomerulonephritis, vasculitis and pulmonary disease.

Type IV reactions: lymphocyte-mediated type. Antigen-specific receptors develop on T lymphocytes. Subsequent administration leads to a local or tissue allergic reaction, *e.g.* contact dermatitis.

Cross-allergy within a group of drugs is usual, *e.g.* the penicillins. (The extent of cross-reaction with cephalosporins is highly controversial). When allergy to a particular drug is established, select a substitute from a chemically different group. Patients with allergic diseases (atopy), *e.g.* eczema, are more likely to develop allergy to drugs.

The distinctive features of allergic reactions are:

- Lack of correlation with known pharmacological properties of the drug.
- Lack of linear relation with drug dose (very small doses may cause very severe effects).
- Rashes, angioedema, serum sickness syndrome, anaphylaxis or asthma; characteristics of classic protein allergy.
- Requirement of an induction period on primary exposure, but not on re-exposure.
- Disappearance on cessation of administration and reappearance on re-exposure to a small dose.
- Occurrence in a minority of patients receiving the drug.
- Possible response to desensitisation.

Principal clinical manifestations and treatment

1. **Urticarial rashes and angioedema (types I, III)** These are probably the commonest type of drug allergy. Reactions may be generalised, but frequently are worst in and around the external area of administration of the drug. The eyelids, lips and face are usually most affected and itching is usual; edema of the larynx is rare but may be fatal. They respond to adrenaline/epinephrine, ephedrine, H_1- receptor antihistamine and adrenal steroid.

2a.**Non-urticarial rashes (types I, II, IV)** These occur in great variety; frequently they are weeping exudative lesions. It is often difficult to be sure when a rash is due to a drug. Apart from stopping

the drug, treatment is non-specific; in severe cases an adrenal steroid should be used. Skin sensitisation to antimicrobials may be very troublesome, especially among those who handle them.

2b.**Diseases of the lymphoid system** Infectious mononucleosis (and lymphoma, leukaemia) is associated with an increased incidence (>40%) of a characteristic maculopapular, sometimes purpuric, rash which is probably allergic, when an aminopenicillin (ampicillin, amoxicillin) is taken; patients may not be allergic to other penicillins. Erythromycin may cause a similar reaction.

3. **Anaphylactic shock (type I)** It occurs with penicillin, anaesthetics (intravenous), iodine-containing radio-contrast media and a huge variety of other drugs. A severe fall in blood pressure occurs, with bronchoconstriction, angioedema (including larynx) and sometimes death due to loss of fluid from the intravascular compartment and respiratory obstruction. Anaphylactic shock usually occurs suddenly, in less than an hour after the drug, but within minutes if it has been given intravenously.

Treatment is urgent. According to the comments on the action of the drugs used, advice on the management of anaphylactic shock is altered.

- In adults, 500 micrograms of adrenaline/epinephrine injection (1mg/mL) should be given intramuscularly to raise the blood pressure and dilate the bronchi (vasoconstriction renders the subcutaneous route less effective). If there is no clinical improvement, further intramuscular injections of adrenaline/epinephrine 500 micrograms should be given at 5-min intervals according to blood pressure, pulse and respiration.
- If shock is profound, cardiopulmonary resuscitation/advanced life support are necessary. Consider also giving adrenaline/epinephrine 1:10 000 by slow intravenous infusion, at a rate of 100 micrograms/min (1 mL/min of 20 micrograms/mL over 5 min), preferably with continuous ECG monitoring, stopping when a response has been obtained. This procedure is hazardous and should be undertaken only by an experienced practitio-

ner who can obtain immediate intravenous access and where other resuscitation facilities are available.

- The adrenaline/epinephrine should be accompanied by an H_1-receptor antihistamine, *e.g.* chlorphenamine 10–20 mg intramuscularly or by slow intravenous injection, and by hydrocortisone 200–500 mg intramuscularly or by slow intravenous injection. The adrenal steroid acts by reducing vascular permeability and by suppressing further response to the antigen-antibody reaction. Benefit from an adrenal steroid is not immediate; it is unlikely to begin for 30 min and takes hours to reach its maximum.

- In severe anaphylaxis, hypotension is due to vasodilatation and loss of circulating volume through leaky capillaries. Thus, when there is no response to drug treatment, 1–2 L of plasma substitute should be infused rapidly. Crystalloid may be safer than colloid, which causes more allergic reactions.

- Where bronchospasm is severe and does not respond rapidly to other treatment, a β_2-adrenoceptor agonist is a useful adjunctive measure.

- Where susceptibility to anaphylaxis is known, *e.g.* in patients with allergy to bee or wasp stings, preventive self-management is feasible. The patient is taught to administer adrenaline/epinephrine intramuscularly from a pre-filled syringe (EpiPen Auto-injector, delivering adrenaline/epinephrine 300 micrograms per dose).

- Half of the above doses of adrenaline/epinephrine may be safer for patients who are receiving amitriptyline or imipramine.

4a. **Pulmonary reactions: asthma (type I)** Aspirin and other non-steroidal anti-inflammatory drugs may cause bronchoconstriction, and not only in asthmatic patients. Abnormal levels of leukotrienes synthesis following blockade of cyclo-oxygenase maybe causal; this is a pseudo-allergic reaction. Another such reaction is the well-known occurrence of cough due to angiotensin-converting enzyme inhibitors: in this case, pro-inflammatory peptides such as bradykinin accumulate and trigger cough.

4b. **Other types of pulmonary reaction (type III)** include syndromes resembling acute and chronic lung infections, pneumonitis, fibrosis and eosinophilia.

5. **The serum sickness syndrome (type III)** This occurs about 1–3 weeks after administration. Treatment is by an adrenal steroid, and as above if there is urticaria.

6. Blood disorders

6a. **Thrombocytopenia (type II, but also pseudo-allergic)** may occur after exposure to any of a large number of drugs, including: gold, quinine, quinidine, rifampicin, heparin, thionamide derivatives, thiazide diuretics, sulphonamides, oestrogens, indometacin. Adrenal steroid may help.

6b. **Granulocytopenia (type II, but also pseudo-allergic)** sometimes leading to agranulocytosis, is a very serious reaction which may occur with many drugs, *e.g.* clozapine, carbamazepine, carbimazole, chloramphenicol, sulphonamides (including diuretic and hypoglycaemic derivatives), colchicine, gold.

The value of precautionary leucocyte counts for drugs having special risk remains uncertain. Weekly counts may detect presymptomatic granulocytopenia from antithyroid drugs, but onset can be sudden and an alternative view is to monitor only with drugs having special risk, *e.g.* clozapine, where it is mandatory. The chief clinical manifestation of agranulocytosis is sore throat or mouth ulcers, and patients should be warned to report such events immediately and to stop taking the drug, but they should not be frightened into non-compliance with essential therapy. Treatment of the agranulocytosis involves both stopping the drug responsible and giving a bactericidal drug, *e.g.* penicillin, to prevent or treat infection.

6c. **Aplastic anaemia (type II, but not always allergic)** Causal agents include chloramphenicol, sulphonamides and derivatives (diuretics, antidiabetics), gold, penicillamine, allopurinol, felbamate, phenothiazines and some insecticides, *e.g.* dicophane (DDT). In the case of chloramphenicol, bone marrow depression is a normal pharmacodynamic effect, although aplastic anaemia may also be due to idiosyncrasy or allergy.

Death occurs in about 50% of cases, and treatment is as for agranulocytosis, with, obviously, blood transfusion.

6d. **Haemolysis of all kinds** is included here for convenience. There are three principal categories:

- Allergy (type II) occurs with penicillins, methyldopa, levodopa, quinine, quinidine, sulfasalazine and organic antimony. In some of these cases a drug-protein-antigen/antibody interaction may involve erythrocytes only casually, *i.e.* a true "innocent bystander" phenomenon.

- Dose-related pharmacodynamic action on normal cells, *e.g.* lead, benzene, phenylhydrazine, chlorates (weed-killer), methyl chloride (refrigerant), some snake venoms.

- Idiosyncrasy. Precipitation of a haemolytic crisis may also occur with the above drugs in the rare genetic haemoglobinopathies. Treatment is to withdraw the drug, and an adrenal steroid is useful in severe cases if the mechanism is immunological. Blood transfusion may be needed.

7. **Fever** is common; a mechanism is the release of interleukin-1 by leucocytes into the circulation; this acts on receptors in the hypothalamic thermoregulatory centre, releasing prostaglandin E_1.

8. **Collagen diseases (type II)** and syndromes resembling them. Systemic lupus erythematosus is sometimes caused by drugs, *e.g.* hydralazine, procainamide, isoniazid, sulphonamides. Adrenal steroid is useful.

9. **Hepatitis and cholestatic jaundice** are sometimes allergic. Adrenal steroid may be useful.

10. **Nephropathy** of various kinds (types II, I) occurs, as does damage to other organs, *e.g.* myocarditis. Adrenal steroid may be useful.

Diagnosis of drug allergy

This still depends largely on clinical criteria, history, type of reaction, response to withdrawal and systemic re-challenge (if thought safe to do so).

Simple patch skin testing is naturally most useful in diagnosing contact dermatitis, but it is unreliable for other allergies. Skin prick tests are helpful in specialist hands for diagnosing IgE-dependent drug reactions, notably due to penicillin, cephalosporins, muscle relaxants, thiopental, streptokinase, cisplatin, insulin and latex. They can cause anaphylactic shock. False-positive results occur.

Development of reliable *in vitro* predictive tests, *e.g.* employing serum or lymphocytes, is a matter of considerable importance, not merely to remove hazard but also to avoid depriving patients of a drug that may be useful. Detection of drug-specific circulating IgE antibodies by the radioallergosorbent test (RAST) is best developed for many drugs and other allergens.

Drug allergy, once it has occurred, is not necessarily permanent, *e.g.* less than 50% of patients giving a history of allergy to penicillin have a reaction if it is given again, but re-challenging is best avoided if possible!

Desensitisation

Once patients become allergic to a drug, it is better that they should never again receive it. Desensitisation may be considered (in hospital) where a patient has suffered an IgE-mediated reaction to penicillin and requires the drug for serious infection, *e.g.* meningitis or endocarditis. Such people can be desensitized by giving very small amounts of allergen, which are then gradually increased (usually every few hours) until a normal dose is tolerated.

The procedure may necessitate cover with a corticosteroid and a β-adrenoceptor agonist (both of which inhibit mediator synthesis and release), and an H_1-receptor antihistamine maybe added if an adverse reaction occurs. A full kit for treating anaphylactic shock should be at hand. Desensitisation may also be carried out for other antimicrobials, *e.g.* antituberculous drugs.

The mechanism underlying desensitisation may involve the production by the patient of blocking antibodies that compete successfully for the allergen but whose combination with it is innocuous; or the threshold of cells to the triggering antibodies may be raised. Sometimes allergy is to an ingredient of the preparation other than the essential drug, and merely changing the preparation is sufficient. Impurities are sometimes responsible, and purified penicillins and insulins reduce the incidence of reactions.

Prevention of allergic reactions

Prevention is important because these reactions are unpleasant and may be fatal; it provides good reason for taking a drug history. Patients should always be told if there is reason to believe they are allergic to a drug.

When looking for an alternative drug to avoid an adverse reaction, it is important not to select one from the same chemical group, as may inadvertently occur because the proprietary name gives no indication of the nature of the drug. This is another good reason for using the non-proprietary (generic) names as a matter of course.

> If a patient claims to be allergic to a drug then that drug should not be given without carefulenquiry that may include testing (above).

Pseudo-allergic reactions

These are effects that mimic allergic reactions but have no immunological basis and are largely genetically determined. They are due to release of endogenous, biologically active substances, *e.g.* histamine and leukotrienes, by the drug. A variety of mechanisms is probably involved, direct and indirect, including complement activation leading to formation of polypeptides that affect mast cells, as in true immunological reactions. Some drugs may produce both allergic and pseudo-allergic reactions.

Pseudo-allergic effects mimicking type I reactions (above) are called anaphylactoid; they occur with aspirin and other non-steroidal anti-inflammatory drugs and with N-acetylcysteine (indirect action as above); corticotropin (direct histamine release); intravenous anaesthetics and a variety of other drugs given intravenously (morphine, tubocurarine, dextran, radiographic contrast media) and inhaled (cromoglicate). Severe cases are treated as for true

allergic anaphylactic shock (above), from which, at the time, they are not distinguishable.

Type II reactions are mimicked by the haemolysis induced by drugs (some antimalarials, sulphonamides and oxidising agents) and food (broad beans) in subjects with inherited abnormalities of erythrocyte enzymes or haemoglobin.

Type III reactions are mimicked by nitrofurantoin (pneumonitis) and penicillamine (nephropathy). Lupus erythematosus due to drugs (procainamide, isoniazid, phenytoin) may be pseudo-allergic.

MISCELLANEOUS ADVERSE REACTIONS

Transient reactions to intravenous injections are fairly common, resulting in hypotension, renal pain, fever or rigors, especially if the injection is very rapid.

EFFECTS OF PROLONGED ADMINISTRATION: CHRONIC ORGAN TOXICITY

Although the majority of adverse events occur within days or weeks after a drug is administered, some reactions develop only after months or years of exposure. In general, pharmacovigilance programmes reveal such effects; once recognised, they demand careful monitoring during chronic drug therapy for their occurrence may carry serious consequences for the patient (and the non-vigilant doctor, medicolegally). Descriptions of such reactions appear with the accounts of relevant drugs; some examples are given.

Eye. Toxic cataract can be due to chloroquine and related drugs, adrenal steroids (topical and systemic), phenothiazines and alkylating agents. Corneal opacities occur with phenothiazines and chloroquine. Retinal injury develops with thioridazine (particularly, of the antipsychotics), chloroquine and indometacin, and visual field defects with vigabatrin.

Nervous system. Tardive dyskinesias occur with neuroleptics; polyneuritis with metronidazole; optic neuritis with ethambutol.

Lung. Amiodarone may cause pulmonary fibrosis. Sulfasalazine is associated with fibrosing alveolitis.

Kidney. Gold salts may cause nephropathy; see also analgesic nephropathy.

Liver. Methotrexate may cause liver damage and hepatic fibrosis; amiodarone may induce steatohepatitis (fatty liver).

Carcinogenesis. Mechanisms of carcinogenesis are complex; prediction from animal tests is uncertain and causal attribution in humans has finally to be based on epidemiological studies. The principal mechanisms are:

- **Alteration of DNA** (genotoxicity, mutagenicity). Many chemicals or their metabolites act by causing mutations, activating oncogenes; those substances that are used as medicines include griseofulvin and alkylating cytotoxics. Leukaemias and lymphomas are the most common malignancies.
- **Immunosuppression.** Malignancies develop in immunosuppressed patients, *e.g.* after organ transplantation and cancer chemotherapy. There is a high incidence of lymphoid neoplasm. Chlorambucil, melphalan and thiotepa present particular high relative risks. The use of immunosuppression in, *e.g.*, rheumatoid arthritis, also increases the incidence of neoplasms.
- **Hormonal.** Long-term use of oestrogen replacement in postmenopausal women induces endometrial cancer. Combined oestrogen/progestogenoral contraceptives may both suppress and enhance cancers. Diethylstilbestrol caused vaginal adenosis and cancer in the offspring of mothers who took it during pregnancy in the hope of preventing miscarriage. It was used for this purpose for decades after its introduction in the 1940s, on purely theoretical grounds. Controlled therapeutic trials were not done and there was no valid evidence of therapeutic efficacy. Male fetuses developed non-malignant genital abnormalities.

Carcinogenesis due to medicines follows prolonged drug exposure, *i.e.* months or years; the cancers develop most commonly over 3–5 years, but sometimes years after treatment has ceased. There is a higher incidence of secondary cancers in patients treated for a primary cancer.

ADVERSE EFFECTS ON REPRODUCTION

Adverse effects on female reproduction

The medical profession has a grave duty to refrain from all unessential prescribing for women of childbearing potential of drugs with, say, less than 10–15 years of widespread use behind them. It is not sufficient safeguard merely to ask a woman if she is, or may be, pregnant, for it is also necessary to consider the possibility that a woman who is not pregnant at the time of prescribing may become so while taking the drug.

Testing of new drugs on animals for reproductive effects has been mandatory since the thalidomide disaster, even though the extrapolation of the findings to humans is uncertain. The placental transfer of drugs from the mother to the fetus is considered and the actions of drugs on embryo and fetus are as follow.

Drugs may act on the embryo and fetus:

- **Directly** (thalidomide, cytotoxic drugs, antithyroid drugs, aromatic retinoids, *e.g.* isotretinoin): any drug affecting cell division, enzymes, protein synthesis or DNA synthesis is a potential teratogen, *e.g.* many antimicrobials.
- **Indirectly:** Drugs act on the uterus (vasoconstrictors reduce blood supply and cause fetal anoxia, misoprostol causes uterine contraction leading to abortion).

Drugs act on the mother's hormone balance.

Early pregnancy. During the first week after fertilisation, exposure to antimetabolites, misoprostol, ergot alkaloids or diethylstilbestrol can cause abortion, which may not be recognized as such. The most vulnerable period for major anatomical abnormality is that of organogenesis which occurs during weeks 2–8 of intrauterine life (4–10 weeks after the first day of the last menstruation). After the organs are formed, abnormalities are less anatomically dramatic. Thus, the activity of a teratogen (teratos, monster) is most devastating soon after implantation, at doses that may not harm the mother and at a time when she may not know she is pregnant.

Drugs known to be teratogenic include cytotoxics, warfarin, alcohol, lithium, methotrexate, phenytoin, sodium valproate, angiotensin-converting enzyme (ACE) inhibitors and isotretinoin. Selective interference can produce characteristic anatomical abnormalities; the phocomelia (flipper-like) limb defect was one factor that caused the effects of thalidomide to be recognized so readily.

Innumerable drugs have come under suspicion. Those subsequently found to be safe include diazepam, oral contraceptives, spermicides and salicylates. Naturally, the subject is a highly emotional one for prospective parents. A definitive list of unsafe drugs is not practicable. Much depends on the dose taken and at what stage of pregnancy.

Late pregnancy. Because the important organs are well formed, drugs will not cause the gross anatomical defects that can occur following exposure in early pregnancy. Administration of hormones, androgens or progestogens can cause fetal masculinisation; iodide and antithyroid drugs in high dose can cause fetal goitre, as can lithium; tetracyclines can interfere with tooth and bone development, ACE inhibitors are associated with renal tubular dysgenesis and a skull ossification defect. Tobacco smoking retards fetal growth; it does not cause anatomical abnormalities in humans as far as is known.

Inhibitors of prostaglandin synthesis (aspirin, indometacin) may delay onset of labour and, in the fetus, cause closure of the ductus arteriosus, patency of which is dependent on prostaglandins.

The suggestion that congenital cataract (due to denaturation of lens protein) might be due to drugs has some support in humans. Chloroquine and chlorpromazine are concentrated in the fetal eye. As both can cause retinopathy, it would seem wise to avoid them in pregnancy if possible.

Drugs given to the mother just prior to labour can cause postnatal effects. CNS depressants may persist in and affect the baby for days after birth; vasoconstrictors can cause fetal distress by reducing uterine blood supply; β-adrenoceptor blockers may impair fetal response to hypoxia; sulphonamides displace bilirubin from plasma protein (risk of kernicterus).

Babies born to mothers dependent on opioids may show a physical withdrawal syndrome.

Drugs given during labour. Any drug that acts to depress respiration in the mother can cause respiratory depression in the newborn; opioid analgesics are notorious in this respect, but there can also be difficulty with any sedatives and general anaesthetics; they may also cause fetal distress by reducing uterine blood flow, and prolong labor by depressing uterine muscle.

Diazepam (and other depressants) in high doses may cause hypotonia in the baby and possibly interfere with suckling. There remains the possibility of later behavioral effects due to impaired development of the central nervous system from psychotropic drugs use during pregnancy; such effects are known in animals.

Detection of teratogens. Anatomical abnormalities are the easiest to detect. Non-anatomical (functional) effects can also occur; they include effects on brain biochemistry that may have late behavioral consequences.

There is a substantial spontaneous background incidence of birth defect in the community (up to 2%), so the detection of a low-grade teratogen that increases the incidence of one of the commoner abnormalities presents an intimidating task. In addition, most teratogenic effects are probably multifactorial. In this emotionally charged area it is indeed hard for the public, and especially for parents of an affected child.

Adverse effects on male reproductive function

Impotence may occur with drugs affecting autonomic sympathetic function, *e.g.* many antihypertensives.

Spermatogenesis is reduced by a number of drugs including sulfasalazine and mesalazine (reversible), cytotoxic anticancer drugs (reversible and irreversible) and nitrofurantoin. There has been a global decline in sperm concentration and an environmental cause, *e.g.* chemicals that possess oestrogenic activity, seems likely.

Causation of birth defects due to abnormal sperm remains uncertain.

SUMMARY

As drugs are intended to relieve suffering, patients find it peculiarly offensive that they can also cause disease (especially if they are not forewarned). Therefore, it is important to know how much disease drugs do cause and why they cause it, so that preventive measures can be taken. This chapter examines the definitions of ADR; Attribution and degrees of certainty; Sources of adverse drug reactions; Pharmacovigilance and pharmacoepidemiology; Allergy in response to drugs; Chronic organ toxicity induced by prolonged administration; Adverse effects on reproduction.

IMPORTANT TERMINOLOGY

adverse drug reaction   药物不良反应
pharmacovigilance   药物警戒
pharmacoepidemiology   药物流行病学
allergy reaction   变态反应
desensitization   脱敏作用
toxicity   毒性
secondary effects   继发性反应

intolerance   不耐受
idiosyncrasy   特异质
mutagenicity   致突变性
carcinogenicity   致癌性
teratogenicity   致畸性
cohort study   队列研究
case-control study   病例对照研究
porphyria   卟啉症
aplastic anemia   再生障碍性贫血
urticaria   荨麻疹
thrombocytopenia   血小板减少症
granulocytopenia   粒细胞减少症
fetal distress   胎儿窘迫

CHALLENGE YOURSELF

1. Definitions: adverse drug reaction (ADR), toxicity, second effects, intolerance, idiosyncrasy, pharmacovigilance, pharmacoepedemiology, ADR surveillance.
2. Reviewing factors related to ADR, including patients, drugs, circumstances, etc.
3. State evaluation criteria of attribution of ADR and purpose of ADR surveillance.
4. Besides allergy inresponse to drugs or adverse effects on reproduction, are there any important drugs-induced diseases? State the inducement, feature and prophylaxis and treatment of these diseases.
5. The similarities and differences between ADR surveillance and pharmacovigilance.

Xiuli Guo

Chapter | 8 |

Drug dependence

INTRODUCTION

The dividing line between legitimate use of drugs for social purposes and their abuse is indistinct, for it is not only a matter of which drug, but of the amount of drug and of whether the effect is antisocial or not. The classification of drugs of abuse continues to be subject to controversy.

'Normal' people seem to be able to use alcohol for their occasional purposes without harm but, given the appropriate personality and/or environmental adversity, many may turn to it for relief and become dependent on it, both psychologically and physically. But drug abuse is not primarily a pharmacological problem; it is a social problem with important pharmacological aspects.

Abuse of drugs to improve performance in sport stems from a distinct and different motivation, namely, the obtaining of advantage in competition, but the practice yet has major implications for the health of the individual and for the participating and spectating sporting community.

DEFINITION

Substance (drug) dependence is defined as: when an individual persists in use of alcohol or other drugs despite problems related to use of the substance, substance dependence may be diagnosed. Compulsive and repetitive use may result in tolerance to the effect of the drug and withdrawal symptoms when use is reduced or stopped.

Substance (drug) abuse is a term that is less clearly defined and becoming less used, in favour of the term substance dependence. Nevertheless, the terms 'addict' or 'addiction' have not been completely abandoned in this book because they remain convenient. The WHO Expert Committee on Addiction Producing Drugs 1957 defined substance abuse in the context of two components:

Substance (drug) addiction is a state of periodic or chronic intoxication produced by the repeated consumption of a drug (natural or synthetic). Its characteristics include: ① an overpowering desire or need (compulsion) to continue taking the drug and to obtain it by any means; ② a tendency to increase the dose; ③ a psychic (psychological) and generally a physical dependence on the effects of the drug; ④ detrimental effects on the individual and on society.

Substance (drug) habituation is a condition resulting from the repeated consumption of a drug. Its characteristics include ① a desire (but not a compulsion) to continue taking the drug for the sense of improved well-being which it engenders; ② little or no tendency to increase the dose; ③ some degree of psychic dependence on the effect of the drug, but absence of physical dependence and hence of an abstinence syndrome (withdrawal);④ detrimental effects, if any, primarily on the individual.

Psychological (psychic) dependence is characterised by emotional distress if the drug of dependence is withdrawn. The subject may develop craving for the drug with anxiety, insomnia and dysphoria. It develops before physical dependence.

Physical (physiological) dependence implies that continued exposure to a drug induces adaptive changes in body tissues so that *tolerance* occurs, and that abrupt withdrawal of the drug leaves these changes unopposed, resulting generally in a *discontinuation (withdrawal) syndrome*, usually of rebound overactivity.

Tolerance follows the operation of homeostatic adaptation, e.g. to continued high occupancy of opioid receptors. Changes of similar type may occur with γ-aminobutyric acid (GABA) transmission, involving benzodiazepines. It also results from metabolic changes (enzyme induction) and physiological or behavioural adaptation to drug effects, e.g. opioids. Physiological adaptation develops to a substantial degree with cerebral depressants, but is minor or absent with excitant drugs. There is commonly cross-tolerance between drugs of similar, and sometimes even of dissimilar, chemical groups, e.g. alcohol and benzodiazepines.

A discontinuation (withdrawal) syndrome occurs, for example, when administration of an opioid is suddenly stopped. Morphine-like substances (endomorphins, dynorphins) act as CNS neurotransmitters, and exogenously administered opioid suppresses their endogenous production by a feedback mechanism. Abrupt discontinuation results in an immediate deficiency of endogenous opioid, which thus causes the withdrawal syndrome.

Drugs of dependence are often divided into two groups, hard and soft. There are again no absolute definitions of these categories.

Hard drugs are those that are liable seriously to disable the individual as a functioning member of society by inducing severe psychological and, in the case of cerebral depressants, physical dependence. The group includes heroin and cocaine.

Soft drugs are less dependence producing. There may be psychological dependence, but there is little or no physical dependence except with heavy doses of depressants (alcohol). The group includes sedatives and tranquillisers, amfetamines, cannabis, hallucinogens, alcohol, tobacco and caffeine.

This classification fails to recognise individual variation in drug use. Alcohol can be used in heavy doses that are gravely disabling and induce severe physical dependence with convulsions on sudden withdrawal; i.e. for the individual the drug is 'hard'. But there are many people mildly psychologically dependent on it who retain their position in the home and society.

Hard use, where the drug is central in the user's life, and soft use, where it is merely incidental, are terms of assistance in making this distinction, i.e. what is classified is not the drug but the effect it has on, or the way it is used by, the individual. The term '*recreational*' is often applied to such use, conferring an apparent sanction that relates more to the latter category.

Dependence/abuse liability of a drug is related to its capacity to produce immediate gratification, which may be a feature of the drug itself (amfetamine and heroin give rapid effect whereas tricyclic antidepressants do not), and its route of administration, in descending order: inhalation/intravenous, intramuscular/subcutaneous. Those drugs with high dependence/abuse liability are subject to regulation and non-medicinal use may be a criminal offence.

Drug abuse use has two principal forms: *continuous use* describes a true dependence, e.g. opioids, alcohol, benzodiazepines; *intermittent or occasional use* describes either a recreational experience, e.g. 'ecstasy' (tenamfetamine), LSD, cocaine, cannabis, solvents, or use to relieve stress, e.g. alcohol. Some drugs, e.g. alcohol, are used in both ways, but others, e.g. ecstasy, LSD, cannabis, are virtually confined to intermittent use.

Drives to drug abuse can be grouped as follows:

1. Relief of anxiety, tension and depression; escape from personal psychological problems; detachment from harsh reality; ease of social intercourse.
2. Rebellion against or despair about orthodox social values and the environment. Fear of missing something, and conformity with own social subgroup (the young, especially).
3. Fun, amusement, recreation, excitement, curiosity (the young, especially).

4. Improvement of performance in competitive sport (a distinct motivation).

SITES AND MECHANISMS OF ACTION

Drugs of abuse are extremely diverse in their chemical structures, mechanisms of action and anatomical and cellular targets. Nevertheless, there is an emerging consensus that addictive drugs possess a parallel ability to modulate the brain reward system that is key to activities that are vital for survival (e.g. eating and sexual behaviour). Of particular relevance is the medial forebrain bundle (MFB) that connects the ventral tegmental area and the nucleus accumbens. Natural and artificial rewards (including drugs of abuse) have been shown to activate the dopaminergic neurones within the MFB. It seems that drugs of abuse can converge on common neural mechanisms in these areas to produce acute reward and chronic alterations in reward systems that lead to addiction. This is summarised in Figure 8.1.

> Increasing evidence suggests that drugs of addiction all act by modulating dopaminergic transmission in the medial forebrain bundle.

ROUTE OF ADMINISTRATION AND EFFECT

With the intravenous route or inhalation, much higher peak plasma concentrations can be reached than with oral administration. This accounts for the 'kick' or 'flash' that abusers report and which many seek, likening it to sexual orgasm or better. As an addict said, 'The ultimate high is death', and it has been reported that, when hearing of someone dying from an overdose, some addicts will seek out the vendor as it is evident he is selling 'really good stuff'.

PRESCRIBING FOR DRUG DEPENDENCE

In the UK, supply of certain drugs for the purpose of sustaining addiction or managing withdrawal is permitted under strict legal limitations, usually by designated doctors. Guidance about the responsibilities and management of addiction is available. By such procedures it is hoped to limit the expansion of the illicit market, and its accompanying crime and dangers to health, e.g. from infected needles and syringes. The object is to sustain young (usually)

Fig. 8.1 Common pathway of drugs of addiction on the dopaminergic neurones.

addicts, who cannot be weaned from drug use, in reasonable health until they relinquish their dependence (often over about 10 years).

When injectable drugs are prescribed there is currently no way of assessing the truth of an addict's statement that he or she needs x mg of heroin (or other drug), and the dose has to be assessed intuitively by the doctor. This has resulted in addicts obtaining more than they need and selling it, sometimes to initiate new users. The use of oral methadone or other opioid for maintenance by prescription is devised to mitigate this problem.

TREATMENT OF DEPENDENCE

The majority are dependent on heroin. These are managed by either abstinence or, more commonly, maintenance on prescribed alternatives such as methadone.

Withdrawal of the drug. While obviously important, this is only a step on what can be a long and often disappointing journey to psychological and social rehabilitation, e.g. in 'therapeutic communities'. A heroin addict may be given methadone as part of a gradual withdrawal programme, for this drug has a long duration of action and blocks access of injected opioid to the opioid receptor so that if, in a moment of weakness, the subject takes heroin, the 'kick' is reduced. More acutely, the physical features associated with discontinuing high alcohol use may be alleviated by chlordiazepoxide given in decreasing doses for 7–14 days. Sympathetic autonomic overactivity can be treated with a β-adrenoceptor blocker.

Maintenance and relapse. Relapsed addicts who live a fairly normal life are sometimes best treated by supplying drugs under supervision. A less harmful drug by a less harmful route may be substituted, e.g. oral methadone for intravenous heroin. Addicts are often particularly reluctant to abandon the intravenous route, which provides the 'immediate high' that they find, or originally found, so desirable.

Severe pain in an opioid addict presents a special problem. High-efficacy opioid may be ineffective (tolerance) or overdose may result; low-efficacy opioids will not only be ineffective but may induce withdrawal symptoms, especially if they have some antagonist effect, e.g. pentazocine. This leaves as drugs of choice non-steroidal anti-inflammatory drugs (NSAIDs), e.g. indometacin, and nefopam (which is neither opioid nor NSAID).

MORTALITY

Young illicit users by intravenous injection (heroin, benzodiazepines, amfetamine) have a high mortality rate. Death follows either overdose or the occurrence of septicaemia, endocarditis, hepatitis, AIDS, gas gangrene, tetanus or pulmonary embolism from the contaminated materials used without aseptic precautions (schemes to provide clean equipment mitigate this). Smugglers of illicit cocaine or heroin sometimes carry the drug in plastic bags concealed by swallowing or in the rectum ('body packing'). Leakage of the packages, not surprisingly, may have a fatal result.

ESCALATION

A variable proportion of subjects who start with cannabis eventually take heroin. This disposition to progress from occasional to frequent soft use of drugs through to hard drug use, when it occurs, is less likely to be due to pharmacological actions than to psychosocial factors, although increased suggestibility induced by cannabis may contribute.

De-escalation also occurs as users become disillusioned with drugs over about 10 years.

'DESIGNER DRUGS'

This unhappily chosen term has been generally taken to refer to molecular modifications produced in secret for profit by skilled and criminally minded chemists to produce drugs which are structurally and pharmacologically very similar to a controlled substance but are not themselves controlled substances. Increasingly the production of such agents is becoming more sophisticated. The World Wide

Web enables customers to order such 'research chemicals' online from large laboratories based in countries where the production of such compounds is not legally restricted. It is then hard to detect such compounds entering the country through the postal system. Popularity trends of such agents develop. As ecstasy use in the UK has fallen, designer drugs of the phenylethylamine class have arrived on the club scene. These drugs are structurally similar to mescaline and MDMA. They have similar effects to ecstasy but in addition, mild LSD-like perceptional distortions.

Part 1. Types Of Drug Dependence

The World Health Organization recommends that drug dependence be specified by type for purposes of detailed discussion. The subject can be treated according to the following principal types:

- opioids (see chapter 23)
- alcohol and other cerebral depressants (benzodiazepines, γ-hydroxybutyrate)
- tobacco
- psychodysleptics (LSD, mescaline, tenamfetamine, phencyclidine, cannabis)
- psychostimulants (cocaine, amfetamines, methylxanthines, khat)
- volatile substances

Part 2. Ethyl Alcohol (Ethanol)

Alcohol is important in medicine chiefly because of the consequences of its misuse/abuse. Alcohol-related mortality has increased steadily since the 1990s, with over 9 000 deaths attributed to alcohol in 2008. Alcohol-related deaths are over twice as common in men as in women.

Pharmacokinetics

Absorption. The gastrointestinal absorption of alcohol taken orally is rapid as it is highly lipid soluble and diffusible. The major site of absorption is the small intestine; solutions above 20% are absorbed more slowly because high concentrations of alcohol

inhibit gastric peristalsis, thus delaying the arrival of the alcohol in the small intestine. Absorption is delayed by food, especially milk, the effect of which is probably due to the fat it contains. Carbohydrate also delays absorption of alcohol.

Distribution. It is distributed rapidly and throughout the body water (dist. vol. 0.7 L/kg men; 0.6 L/kg women) with no selective tissue storage. Maximum blood concentrations after oral alcohol therefore depend on numerous factors including: the total dose; sex; the strength of the solution; the time over which it is taken; the presence or absence of food in the stomach; the time relations of taking food and alcohol, and the kind of food eaten; the speed of metabolism and excretion.

Alcoholic drinks taken on an empty stomach will probably produce maximal blood concentration at 30–90 min and will not all be disposed of for 6–8 h or even more. There are very great individual variations.

Metabolism About 95% of absorbed alcohol is metabolised by the liver, the remainder being excreted in the breath, urine and sweat; convenient methods of estimation of alcohol in all these media are available (Fig. 8.2).

Alcohol metabolism by alcohol dehydrogenase follows first-order kinetics after the smallest doses. Once the blood concentration exceeds about 10 mg/100 mL the enzymatic processes are saturated and elimination rate no longer increases with increasing concentration but becomes steady at 10–15 mL/h in occasional drinkers. Thus alcohol is subject to dose-dependent kinetics, i.e. saturation or zero-order kinetics, with potentially major consequences for the individual.

Induction of hepatic drug-metabolising enzymes occurs with repeated exposure to alcohol. This contributes to tolerance in habitual users, and to toxicity. Increased formation of metabolites causes organ damage in chronic over-consumption (acetaldehyde in the liver and probably fatty ethyl esters in other organs) and increases susceptibility to liver injury when heavy drinkers are exposed to anaesthetics, industrial solvents and drugs. But chronic use of large amounts reduces hepatic metabolic capacity by

Catalase

Ethanol

Cytochrome P450 oxidase system

Alcohol dehydrogenase (90%)

Ethanal (acetaldehyde)

Aldehyde dehydrogenase

Ethanoate (acetate)

AcetylCoA sythetase

Acetyl CoA

Tricarboxylic acid cycle

Protein and fat biosynthesis

Is inducible by ethanol

Fig. 8.2 Metabolism of ethanol by the liver.

causing cellular damage. An acute substantial dose of alcohol (binge drinking) inhibits hepatic drug metabolism.

The blood concentration of alcohol (Fig. 8.3) has great medicolegal importance. Alcohol in alveolar air is in equilibrium with that in pulmonary capillary blood, and reliable, easily handled measurement devices (breathalysers) are used by police at the roadside on both drivers and pedestrians.

Pharmacodynamics

Alcohol exerts on cells in the CNS a generally depressant effect that is probably mediated through particular membrane ion channels and receptors. It seems likely that acetaldehyde acts synergistically with alcohol to determine the range of neurochemical and behavioural effects of alcohol consumption. There is considerable evidence that ethanol affects neurotransmitter release and activity. Alcohol enhances dopamine release, inhibits the reuptake of brain amines and enhances (inhibitory) $GABA_A$-stimulated flux of chloride through receptor-gated membrane ion channels, a receptor subtype effect that may be involved in the motor impairment caused by alcohol. Other possible modes of action include inhibition of the (excitatory) N-methyl-d-aspartate (NMDA) receptor and inhibition of calcium entry via voltage-gated (L type) calcium channels.

Alcohol is not a stimulant; hyperactivity, when it occurs, is due to removal of inhibitory effects. Psychic effects are the most important socially, and it is to obtain these that the drug is habitually used in so many societies, to make social intercourse not merely easy but even pleasant. Environment, personality, mood and dose of alcohol are all relevant to the final effect on the individual.

Alcohol in ordinary doses may act chiefly on the arousal mechanisms of the brainstem reticular formation, inhibiting polysynaptic function and enhancing presynaptic inhibition. Direct cortical

Fig. 8.3 Stimulatory and depressant effects of acute alcohol ingestion.

depression probably occurs only with large amounts. With increasing doses the subject passes through all the stages of general anaesthesia and may die from respiratory depression. Loss of consciousness occurs at blood concentrations around 300mg/100mL, death at about 400mg/100mL. The usual cause of death in acute alcohol poisoning is inhalation of vomit.

Innumerable tests of physical and mental performance have been used to demonstrate the effects of alcohol. Results show that alcohol reduces visual acuity and delays recovery from visual dazzle, impairs taste, smell and hearing, muscular coordination and steadiness, and prolongs reaction time. It also causes nystagmus and vertigo. It commonly increases subjects' confidence in their ability to perform well when tested and tendency to underestimate their errors, even after quite low doses. There is a decline in attentiveness and ability to assimilate, sort and take quick decisions on continuously changing information input; an example is inattentiveness to the periphery of the visual field, which is important in motoring. All of these are clearly highly undesirable effects when a person is in a position where failure to perform well may be dangerous.

Acute alcohol poisoning is characterised by behaviour changes, excitement, mental confusion (including 'blackouts'), incoordination and even coma. Numerous other conditions can mimic this presentation and diagnosis can be difficult if a sick or injured patient happens to have taken alcohol as well. Alcohol can cause severe hypoglycaemia; measurement of blood alcohol may clarify the situation. If sedation is essential, diazepam in low dose is least hazardous. Alcohol dialyses well, but dialysis is used only in extreme cases.

Chronic consumption

Tolerance to alcohol can be acquired and the point has been made that it costs the regular heavy drinker 2.5 times as much to get visibly drunk as it would cost the average abstainer. This is probably due both to enzyme induction and to adaptation of the CNS.

CAR DRIVING AND ALCOHOL

The effects of alcohol and psychotropic drugs on motor car driving have been the subject of well-deserved attention, and many countries have passed laws designed to prevent motor accidents caused by alcohol.

Alcohol is a factor in as many as 50% of motor accidents. For this reason, the compulsory use of a roadside breath test is acknowledged to be in the public interest. In the UK (also in China), having a blood concentration exceeding 80 mg alcohol per 100 mL blood (17.4 mmol/L) while in charge of a car is a statutory offence. At this concentration, the liability to accident is about twice normal. Other countries set lower limits, e.g. Nordic countries, some states of the USA, Australia, Greece.

Where blood or breath analysis is not immediately available after an accident, it may be measured hours later and 'back calculated' to what it would have been at the time of the accident. It is usual to assume that the blood concentration falls at about 15mg/100mL·h. Naturally, the validity of such calculations leads to acrimonious disputes in the courts of law.

ALCOHOL-DEPENDENCE SYNDROME

Alcohol dependence is a complex disorder with environmental, drug-induced and genetic components with multiple genes probably contributing to vulnerability to the condition. The major factors determining physical dependence are dose, frequency of dosing, and duration of abuse. Development involves alterations in CNS neurotransmission:

- *Acute* effect of alcohol appears to be blockade of NMDA receptors for which the normal agonist is glutamate, the main excitatory transmitter in the brain.
- *Chronic* exposure increases the number of (excitatory) NMDA receptors and also 'L type' calcium channels, while the action of the (inhibitory) GABA$_A$ neurotransmitter is reduced.
- *The resulting excitatory effects* may explain the anxiety, insomnia and craving that accompanies

sudden withdrawal of alcohol (and may explain why resumption of drinking brings about relief, perpetuating dependence).

Withdrawal of alcohol

Abrupt withdrawal of alcohol from a person who has developed physical dependence, such as may occur when an ill or injured alcoholic is admitted to hospital, can precipitate withdrawal syndrome (agitation, anxiety and excess sympathetic autonomic activity) in 6–12 h. This may be followed by: alcohol withdrawal seizures (rum fits) in 6–48 h; alcoholic hallucinosis (commonly visual) in 10–72 h; delirium tremens in 3–7 days. Mortality from the last is high.

Generally, withdrawal should be supervised in hospital. Fixed dose regimens have been traditionally used where patients received *chlordiazepoxide* by mouth, 10–50 mg four times daily, gradually reducing over 7–14 days. Due to the risk of over- or under-prescribing, increasingly symptom-triggered prescribing is used to facilitate the inpatient detoxification. Longer exposure to chlordiazepoxide should be avoided as it has the potential to induce dependence. A β-adrenoceptor blocker may be given to attenuate symptoms of sympathetic overactivity. General aspects of care, e.g. attention to fluid and electrolyte balance, are important.

It is usual to administer vitamins, especially thiamine, in which alcoholics are commonly deficient, and intravenous glucose unaccompanied by thiamine may precipitate Wernicke's encephalopathy.

Clomethiazole is an alternative, also for inpatient use, but it carries significant risk of dependence and should not be given if the patient is likely to persist in drinking alcohol. It is now rarely used in the UK. Anticonvulsants, e.g. carbamazepine, topiramate, have also been used to alleviate symptoms of alcohol withdrawal.

> Acute alcohol withdrawal with tremors, sweating and restlessness is common after abstinence in heavy habitual drinkers. Delirium tremens is less common and needs to be recognised early due to very high mortality if not correctly managed.

Treatment of alcohol dependence

Psychosocial support is more important than drugs, which nevertheless may help.

Acamprosate chemically similar to both glutamate and $GABA_A$ appears to reduce the effect of excitatory amino acids such as glutamate, and modifies $GABA_A$ neurotransmission during withdrawal. If taken for 1 year (accompanied by counselling and psychosocial support), acamprosate increases the number of alcohol-free days and also the chance of subsequent complete abstinence. The benefit may last for 1 year after stopping treatment.

Acamprosate may cause diarrhoea, and cutaneous eruptions.

Disulfiram (Antabuse) discourages drinking by inducing immediate unpleasantness. It is an aldehyde dehydrogenase inhibitor, so that acetaldehyde (a toxic metabolite of alcohol) accumulates. It should be administered only under specialist supervision. A typical reaction of medium severity comes on about 5 min after taking alcohol and consists of generalised vasodilatation and fall in blood pressure, sweating, dyspnoea, headache, chest pain, nausea and vomiting. These features may result from even small amounts of alcohol (such as may be present in some oral medicines or mouthwashes).

Severe reactions include convulsions and circulatory collapse, and may last several hours. Some advocate the use of a test dose of alcohol under supervision (after the 5th day of taking), so that patients can be taught what to expect, and also to induce an aversion from alcohol.

There is clinical trial evidence for other drugs to assist with alcohol withdrawal. In particular naltrexone (an opioid antagonist) is registered by the Food and Drug Administration (FDA) in the USA for this indication but not in the UK. This remains an extremely active area of research.

Safe limits for chronic consumption

These cannot be defined accurately. But both patients and non-patients justifiably expect some guidance, and doctors and government departments will wish to be helpful. They may reasonably advise, as a 'safe' or prudent maximum (there being no particular individual contraindication):

For men not more than 21 units per week (and not more than 4 units in any 1 day); *for women* not more than 14 units per week (and not more than 3 units in any 1 day).

Consistent drinking of more than these amounts carries a progressive risk to health. In other societies recommended maxima are higher or lower. Alcoholics with established cirrhosis have usually consumed about 23 units (230 mL; 184 g) daily for 10 years. Heavy drinkers may develop hepatic cirrhosis at a rate of about 2% per annum. The type of drink (beer, wine, spirits) is not particularly relevant to the adverse health consequences; a standard bottle of spirits (750 mL) contains 300 mL (240 g) of alcohol (i.e. 40% by volume). Most people cannot metabolise more than about 170 g/day. On the other hand, regular low alcohol consumption may confer benefit: up to one drink per day appears not to impair cognitive function in women and may actually decrease the risk of cognitive decline, and light-to-moderate alcohol consumption may reduce risk of dementia in people aged 55 years or more.

The curve that relates mortality (vertical axis) to alcoholic drink consumption (horizontal axis) is J-shaped. As consumption rises above zero the all-cause mortality declines, then levels off, and then progressively rises. The benefit is largely a reduction of deaths due to cardiovascular and cerebrovascular disease for regular drinkers of 1–2 units per day for men aged over 40 years and postmenopausal women. Consuming more than 2 units a day does not provide any major additional health benefit. The mechanism may be an improvement in lipoprotein (HDL/LDL) profiles and changes in haemostatic factors. The effect appears to be due mainly to ethanol itself, but non-ethanol ingredients (antioxidants, phenols, flavinoids) may contribute. The rising (adverse) arm of the curve is associated with known harmful effects of alcohol (already described), but also, for example, with pneumonia (which may be secondary to direct alcohol effects, or with the increased smoking of alcohol users).

ALCOHOL IN PREGNANCY AND BREAST FEEDING

There is no level of maternal consumption that can be guaranteed safe for the fetus and fetal injury can occur early in pregnancy (4–10 weeks), often before the pregnancy has been diagnosed (usually 3–8 weeks). The current advice in the UK is therefore that women should abstain from alcohol if they are pregnant or intending to become pregnant. The mechanisms by which alcohol exerts its toxicity on the fetus are complex and involve both ethanol and its metabolite acetaldehyde.

In addition to the fetal alcohol syndrome there is general fetal/embryonic growth retardation (1% for every 10 g alcohol per day) and this is not 'caught up' later.

Fetal alcohol syndrome is a term that covers a spectrum of disorders; it includes the following characteristics: microcephaly, mental retardation, low body-weight, poor coordination, hypotonia, small eyeballs and short palpebral fissures, lack of nasal bridge.

Children of about 10% of alcohol abusers may show the syndrome. In women consuming 12 units of alcohol per day the incidence may be as high as 30%.

Lactation. Even small amounts of alcohol taken by the mother delay motor development in the child; an effect on mental development is uncertain.

Miscellaneous uses of alcohol

- Used as a skin antiseptic, 70% by weight (76% by volume) is most effective. Stronger solutions are less effective.
- Alcohol injections are sometimes used to destroy nervous tissue in cases of intractable pain (trigeminal neuralgia, carcinoma involving nerves).
- As a treatment in ethylene glycol (antifreeze) poisoning.

OTHER CEREBRAL DEPRESSANTS

Alcohol, benzodiazepines, clomethiazole and barbiturates broadly possess the common action of influencing GABA neurotransmission through the GABA$_A$–benzodiazepine receptor complex and all readily induce tolerance and dependence.

γ-Hydroxybutyrate (GHB) is a metabolite of GABA, the major inhibitory transmitter in the CNS. It acts by binding to GABA receptors but additionally affects dopamine, serotonin and endogenous systems. It has euphoric and sedative effects and is popular at dance parties where it has achieved notoriety as a 'date-rape drug'. It is highly addictive and frequent ingestion may induce dependency and a severe withdrawal state.

Clomethiazole and barbiturate are now rarely used, and accordingly opportunity for abuse is limited.

Part 3. Tobacco

In 1492, the explorer Christopher Columbus observed Native Americans using the dried leaves of the tobacco plant (later named *Nicotiana* for pleasure and also to treat ailments.

Following its introduction to Europe in the 16th century, tobacco enjoyed popularity to the extent of being considered a panacea, being called 'holy herb' and 'God's remedy'. Only relatively recently have the harmful effects of tobacco come to light, notably from mortality studies among British doctors. Current estimates hold that there are more than a billion smokers worldwide. In 1990 there were 3 million smoking-related deaths per year, projected to reach 10 million by 2030.

Composition

Tobacco smoke is complex (over 4 000 compounds have been identified) and varies with the type of tobacco and the way it is smoked. The chief pharmacologically active ingredients are nicotine, responsible for acute effects (1–2 mg per cigarette); tars, responsible for chronic effects (10–15 mg per cigarette). Amounts of both can vary greatly (even for the same brand) depending on the country in which cigarettes are sold.

Smoke of cigars and pipes is alkaline (pH 8.5). Nicotine is relatively un-ionised at this pH, and is readily absorbed in the mouth. Cigar and pipe smokers thus obtain nicotine without inhaling, and thus have a lower death rate from lung cancer, which is caused by non-nicotine constituents.

Smoke of cigarettes is acidic (pH 5.3). Nicotine is relatively ionised and insoluble in lipids. Desired amounts are absorbed only if nicotine is taken into the lungs, where the enormous surface area for absorption compensates for the lower lipid solubility. Cigarette smokers therefore inhale (and have a high rate of death from tar-induced lung cancer). The amount of nicotine absorbed from tobacco smoke varies from 90% in those who inhale to 10% in those who do not. Smoke drawn through the tobacco and taken in by the smoker is known as main-stream smoke; smoke that arises from smouldering tobacco and passes directly into the surrounding air is known as side-stream smoke. These differ in composition, partly because of the different temperatures at which they are produced. Side-stream smoke constitutes about 85% of smoke generated in an average room during cigarette smoking.

Environmental tobacco smoke has been classified as a known human carcinogen in the USA since 1992. Although the risks of passive smoking are naturally smaller, the number of people affected is large. One study estimated that breathing other people's smoke increases a person's risk of ischaemic heart disease by a quarter.

TOBACCO DEPENDENCE

The immediate satisfaction of smoking is due to nicotine and also to tars, which provide flavour. Initially the factors are psychosocial; pharmacodynamic effects are unpleasant. But under the psychosocial pressures the subject continues, learns to limit and adjust nicotine intake, so that the pleasant pharmacological effects of nicotine develop and tolerance to the adverse effects occurs. Thus to the psychosocial pressure is now added pharmacological pleasure.

Nicotine possesses all the characteristics of a drug of dependence:

- It modulates dopamine activity in the midbrain,

particularly in the mesolimbic system, which promotes the development and maintenance of reward behaviour.

- Nicotine inhaled in cigarette smoke reaches the brain in 10–19 s.
- Short elimination $t_{1/2}$ requires regular smoking to maintain the effect.
- Inhaling cigarette smoke is thus an ideal drug delivery system to institute behavioural reinforcement and then dependence.

> Nicotine shows all the characteristics of a drug of dependence with both tolerance and some physical dependence.

ACUTE EFFECTS OF SMOKING TOBACCO

- *Increased airways resistance* occurs due to the non-specific effects of submicronic particles, e.g. carbon particles less than 1 micrometre across. The effect is reflex: even inert particles of this size cause bronchial narrowing sufficient to double airways resistance; this is insufficient to cause dyspnoea, though it might affect athletic performance. Pure nicotine inhalations of concentration comparable to that reached in smoking do not increase airways resistance.
- *Ciliary activity*, after transient stimulation, is depressed, and particles are removed from the lungs more slowly.
- *Carbon monoxide absorption* may be clinically important in the presence of coronary heart disease, although it is physiologically insignificant in healthy young adults.

Nicotine pharmacology

Pharmacokinetics

Nicotine is absorbed through mucous membranes in a highly pH-dependent fashion. The $t_{1/2}$ is 2 h. It is metabolised largely by P450 (CYP) 2A6 to inert substances, e.g. cotinine, although some is excreted unchanged in the urine (pH dependent, it is un-ionised at acid pH). Cotinine is used as a marker for nicotine intake in smoking surveys because of its conveniently long $t_{1/2}$ (20 h).

Pharmacodynamics

Large doses. Nicotine is an agonist to receptors at the ends of peripheral cholinergic nerves whose cell bodies lie in the CNS: i.e. it acts at autonomic ganglia and at the voluntary neuromuscular junction. This is what is meant by the term 'nicotine-like' or 'nicotinic' effect. Higher doses paralyse at the same points. The CNS is stimulated, including the vomiting centre, both directly and via chemoreceptors in the carotid body. Tremors and convulsions may occur. As with the peripheral actions, depression follows stimulation.

Doses from/with smoking. Nicotine causes release of CNS catecholamines, serotonin, antidiuretic hormone, corticotropin and growth hormone. The effects of nicotine on viscera are probably largely reflex, from stimulation of sensory receptors (chemoreceptors) in the carotid and aortic bodies, pulmonary circulation and left ventricle. Some of the results are mutually antagonistic.

The following account tells what generally happens after one cigarette, from which about 1 mg of nicotine is absorbed, although much depends on the amount and depth of inhalation and on the duration of end-inspiratory breath-holding.

On the *cardiovascular system* the effects are those of sympathetic autonomic stimulation. There is vasoconstriction in the skin and vasodilatation in the muscles, tachycardia and a rise in blood pressure of about 15 mmHg systolic and 10 mmHg diastolic, and increased plasma noradrenaline/norepinephrine. Ventricular extrasystoles may occur. Cardiac output, work and oxygen consumption rise. Nicotine increases platelet adhesiveness, an effect that may be clinically significant in the development of atheroma and thrombosis.

Metabolic rate. Nicotine increases the metabolic rate only slightly at rest, but approximately doubles it during light exercise (occupational tasks, housework). This may be due to increase in autonomic sympathetic activity. The effect declines over 24 h on stopping smoking and accounts for the characteristic weight gain that is so disliked and which is sometimes given as a reason for continuing or resuming smoking. Smokers weigh 2–4 kg less than non-smokers (not enough to be a health issue).

Tolerance develops to some of the effects of nicotine, taken repeatedly over a few hours; a first experience commonly causes nausea and vomiting, which quickly ceases with repetition of smoking. Tolerance is usually rapidly lost; the first cigarette of the day has a greater effect on the cardiovascular system than do subsequent cigarettes.

Conclusion. The pleasurable effects of smoking are derived from a complex mixture of multiple pharmacological and non-pharmacological factors.

In this account nicotine is represented as being the major (but not the sole) determinant of tobacco dependence after the smoker has adapted to the usual initial unpleasant effects. But there remains some uncertainty as to its role, e.g. intravenous nicotine fails adequately to substitute the effects of smoking. An understanding of the full function of nicotine is important if less harmful alternatives to smoking, such as nicotine chewing gum, are to be exploited.

EFFECTS OF CHRONIC SMOKING

Bronchogenic carcinoma

- The risk of death from lung cancer is related to the number of cigarettes smoked and the age of starting.
- It is similar between smokers of medium (15–21 mg), low (8–14 mg) and very low (<0.5 mg) tar cigarettes.
- Giving up smoking reduces the risk of death progressively from the time of cessation.

Other cancers. The risk of smokers developing cancer of the mouth, throat and oesophagus is 5–10 times greater than that of non-smokers. It is as great for pipe and cigar smokers as it is for cigarette smokers. Cancer of the pancreas, kidney and urinary tract is also commoner in smokers.

Coronary heart disease (CHD). In the UK about 30% of CHD deaths can be attributed to smoking.

Sudden death may be the first manifestation of CHD and, especially in young men, is related to cigarette smoking. Smoking is especially dangerous for people in whom other risk factors (raised blood cholesterol, high blood pressure) are present. Atherosclerotic narrowing of the smallest coronary arteries is enormously increased in heavy and even in moderate smokers; the increased platelet adhesiveness caused by smoking increases the readiness with which thrombi form. Stopping smoking reduces the excess risk of CHD in people under the age of 65 years, and after about 4 years of abstinence the risk approximates to that of non-smokers.

Chronic lung disease. The adverse effects of cigarette smoke on the lungs may be separated into two distinct conditions:

- *Chronic mucus hypersecretion*, which causes persistent cough with sputum and fits with the original definition of simple chronic bronchitis. This condition arises chiefly in the large airways, usually clears up when the subject stops smoking and does not on its own carry any substantial risk of death.
- *Chronic obstructive lung disease*, which causes difficulty in breathing chiefly due to narrowing of the small airways, includes a variable element of destruction of peripheral lung units (emphysema), is progressive and largely irreversible and may ultimately lead to disability and death.

Both conditions can coexist in one person and they predispose to recurrent acute infective illnesses.

Interactions with drug therapy. Induction of hepatic drug metabolising enzymes by non-nicotine constituents of smoke causes increased metabolism of a range of drugs, including oestrogens, theophylline and warfarin.

WOMEN AND SMOKING

Fertility. Women who smoke are more likely to be infertile or take longer to conceive than women who do not smoke:

- Smokers are more liable to have an earlier menopause than are non-smokers.

117

- Increased metabolism of oestrogens may not be the whole explanation.

Complications of pregnancy

- The risks of spontaneous abortion, stillbirth and neonatal death are approximately doubled.
- The placenta is heavier in smoking than non-smoking women and its diameter larger, possibly from adaptations to lack of oxygen due to smoking, secondary to raised concentrations of circulating carboxyhaemoglobin.

The child

- The babies of women who smoke are approximately 200 g lighter than those of women who do not smoke.
- They have an increased risk of death in the perinatal period which is independent of other variables such as social class, level of education, age of mother, race or extent of antenatal care.
- The increased risk rises two-fold or more in heavy smokers and appears to be accounted for entirely by the placental abnormalities and the consequences of low birth-weight.
- Ex-smokers and women who give up smoking in the first 20 weeks of pregnancy have offspring whose birth-weight is similar to that of the children of women who have never smoked.

STARTING AND STOPPING USE

Contrary to popular belief it is not generally difficult to stop, only 14% finding it 'very difficult'. But ex-smoker status is unstable and the long-term success rate of a smoking withdrawal clinic is rarely above 30%. The situation is summed up by the witticism, 'Giving up smoking is easy, I've done it many times'.

Though they are as aware of the risks of smoking as men, women find it harder to stop; they have consistently lower success rates. This trend crosses every age group and occupation. Women particularly dislike the weight gain.

Aids to giving up

For those smoking more than 10 cigarettes per day, nicotine replacement and bupropion can provide effective therapy, particularly if supported by access to a smoking cessation clinic for behavioural support. Ideally, smoking should stop completely before embarking on a cessation regimen.

Nicotine is principally responsible for the addictive effects of tobacco smoking, and is therefore a logical pharmacological aid to quitting. It is available in a number of formulations, including chewing gum, transdermal patch, oral and nasal spray. When used casually without special attention to technique, nicotine formulations have proved no better than other aids but, if used carefully and withdrawn as recommended, the accumulated results are almost two times better than in smokers who try to stop without this assistance.

Restlessness during terminal illness may be due to nicotine withdrawal and go unrecognised; a nicotine patch may benefit a (deprived) heavy smoker. Nicotine transdermal patches may cause nightmares and abnormal dreaming, and skin reactions (rash, pruritus and 'burning' at the application site). Immunotherapy, using a vaccine of antibodies specific for nicotine, holds promises to prevent relapse in abstinent smokers or for adolescents to avoid initiation. **Bupropion** may provide an alternative, or addition, to nicotine. When the drug was being investigated as an antidepressant, researchers noticed that patients gave up smoking, and it was developed as an aid to smoking cessation. Bupropion selectively inhibits neuronal uptake of noradrenaline/norepinephrine and dopamine, and may reduce nicotine craving by an action on the mesolimbic system. Evidence suggests that bupropion may be at least as effective as the nicotine patch, with which it may usefully be combined. It may cause dry mouth and insomnia. It is contraindicated in patients with a history of eating disorder or epilepsy or who are experiencing acute symptoms of alcohol or benzodiazepine withdrawal; where potential for seizure exists, e.g. use of drugs that lower the seizure threshold, this hazard must be weighed against the possible benefits of smoking cessation.

If the patient is heavily tobacco-dependent and severe anxiety, irritability, headache, insomnia and weight gain (about 3 kg) and tension are concomitants of attempts to stop smoking, an anxiolytic sedative (or β-adrenoceptor blocker) may be useful for a short time, but it is important to avoid substituting one drug dependence for another.

Part 4. Psychodysleptics or hallucinogens

These substances produce mental changes that resemble those of some psychotic states in which the subject experiences hallucinations or illusions, i.e. disturbance of perception with the apparent awareness of sights, sounds and smells that are not actually present.

Experiences with these drugs vary greatly with the subject's expectations, existing frame of mind and personality and environment. Subjects can be prepared so that they are more likely to have a good 'trip' than a bad one.

Experiences with psychodysleptics

The following brief account of experiences with LSD (lysergic acid diethylamide, lysergide) in normal subjects will serve as a model. Experiences with mescaline and psilocybin are similar.

Vision may become blurred and there may be hallucinations; these generally do not occur in the blind and are fewer if the subject is blindfolded. Objects appear distorted, and trivial things, e.g. a mark on a wall, may change shape and acquire special significance. Auditory acuity increases, but hallucinations are uncommon. Subjects who do not ordinarily appreciate music may suddenly come to do so. Foods may feel coarse and gritty in the mouth. Limbs may be left in uncomfortable positions. Time may seem to stop or to pass slowly, but usually it gets faster and thousands of years may seem suddenly to go by. The subject may feel relaxed and supremely happy, or may become fearful or depressed. Feelings of depersonalisation and dreamy states occur.

The experience lasts for a few hours, depending on the dose; intervals of normality then occur and become progressively longer.

Somatic symptoms and signs include nausea, dizziness, paraesthesiae, weakness, drowsiness, tremors, dilated pupils, ataxia. Effects on the cardiovascular system and respiration vary and probably reflect fluctuating anxiety.

LYSERGIDE (LSD)

Lysergic acid is a semi-synthetic drug belonging to the ergoline family. An effective oral dose is about 30 micrograms. The $t_{1/2}$ is 3 h. Its mechanisms of action are complex and include agonist effect at pre-synaptic 5-HT receptors in the CNS. Tachyphylaxis (acute tolerance) occurs to LSD. Psychological dependence may occur, but physical dependence does not occur. Serious adverse effects include psychotic reactions (which can be delayed in onset) with suicide.

Mescaline is an alkaloid from the Mexican peyote cactus. It does not induce serious dependence and the drug has little importance except to members of some North and Central American societies and to psychiatrists and biochemists who are interested in the mechanism of induced psychotic states.

Psilocybin is derived from varieties of the fungus *Psilocybe* ('magic mushrooms') that grow in many countries. It is related to LSD.

Tenamfetamine (ecstasy, MDMA: methylenedioxymethamfetamine) is structurally related to both mescaline and amfetamine. It has a $t_{1/2}$ of about 8 h. It is popular as a dance drug at 'rave' parties. An estimated 5% of the American adult population have used tenamfetamine at least once. Popular names reflect the appearance of the tablets and capsules and include White Dove, White Burger, Red and Black, Denis the Menace. Tenamfetamine stimulates central and peripheral α- and β-adrenoceptors; thus the pharmacological effects are compounded by those of physical exertion, dehydration and heat.

In susceptible individuals (poor metabolisers who exhibit the CYP450 2D6 polymorphism) a severe and fatal idiosyncratic reaction may occur with fulminant hyperthermia, convulsions, disseminated intravascular coagulation, rhabdomyolysis, and acute renal and hepatic failure. Treatment includes activated charcoal, diazepam for convulsions, β-blockade (atenolol) for tachycardia, α-blockade (phentolamine) for hypertension, and dantrolene if the rectal temperature exceeds 39°C. In chronic users, positive emission tomographic (PET) brain scans show selective dysfunction of serotonergic neurones, raising concerns that neurodegenerative changes accompany long-term use of MDMA.

Phencyclidine ('angel dust') is structurally related to pethidine. It induces analgesia without unconsciousness, but with amnesia, in humans (dissociative anaesthesia). It acts as an antagonist at NMDA glutamate receptors. It can be insufflated as a dry powder or smoked (cigarettes are dipped in phencyclidine dissolved in an organics solvent). Phencyclidine overdose can cause agitation, abreactions, hallucinations and psychosis, and if severe can result in seizures, coma, hyperthermia, muscular rigidity and rhabdomyolysis.

Ketamine (K, special K) has similar effects to those of phencyclidine. It is used as a short-acting general anaesthetic. It can be injected as liquid or inhaled as powder or swallowed as tablet. It is an NMDA antagonist. It induces perceptual changes and hallucinations similar to LSD, and in addition induces dissociative analgesia, with consequent risk of serious injury. Nausea, vomiting and risk of death can result from inhalation of vomitus. It has been used as a date-rape drug. There is increasing evidence that it can cause serious long-term bladder damage.

METHYLXANTHINES (XANTHINES)

The three xanthines, *caffeine*, *theophylline* and *theobromine*, occur in plants. They are qualitatively similar but differ markedly in potency:
- Tea contains caffeine and theophylline.
- Coffee contains caffeine.
- Cocoa and chocolate contain caffeine and theobromine.
- The cola nut ('cola' drinks) contains caffeine.
- Theobromine is weak and of no clinical importance (although responsible for the toxicity of

chocolate when ingested by dogs).

Pharmacokinetics. Absorption of xanthines after oral or rectal administration varies with the preparation used. It is generally extensive (> 95%). Caffeine metabolism varies much between individuals ($t_{1/2}$ 2–12 h). Xanthines are metabolised (> 90%) by numerous mixed-function oxidase enzymes, and xanthine oxidase.

Pharmacodynamics. Caffeine and theophylline have complex and incompletely elucidated actions, which include inhibition of phosphodiesterase (the enzyme that breaks down cyclic AMP), effects on intracellular calcium distribution, and on noradrenergic function.

Actions on mental performance. Caffeine is more potent than theophylline, but both drugs stimulate mental activity where it is below normal. Thought is more rapid and fatigue is removed or its onset delayed. The effects on mental and physical performance vary according to the mental state and personality of the subject. Reaction time is decreased. Performance that is inferior because of excessive anxiety may become worse. Caffeine can also improve physical performance, both in tasks requiring more physical effort than skill (athletics) and in tasks requiring more skill than physical effort (monitoring instruments and taking corrective action in an aircraft flight simulator). In general, caffeine induces feelings of alertness and well-being, euphoria or exhilaration. Onset of boredom, fatigue, inattentiveness and sleepiness is postponed.

Overdose will certainly reduce performance. Acute overdose, e.g. intravenous aminophylline, can cause convulsions, hypotension, cardiac arrhythmia and sudden death.

OTHER EFFECTS

Respiratory stimulation occurs with substantial doses.

Sleep. Caffeine affects sleep of older people more than it does that of younger people. Onset of sleep (sleep latency) is delayed, bodily movements are increased, total sleep time is reduced and there are increased awakenings. Tolerance to this effect does not occur, as is shown by the provision of decaffeinated coffee.

Skeletal muscle. Metabolism is increased, and this may play a part in the enhanced athletic performance mentioned above. There is significant improvement of diaphragmatic function in chronic obstructive pulmonary disease.

Cardiovascular system. Both caffeine and theophylline directly stimulate the myocardium and cause increased cardiac output, tachycardia, and sometimes ectopic beats and palpitations. This effect occurs almost at once after intravenous injection and lasts for half an hour. Theophylline contributes usefully to the relief of acute left ventricular failure. There is peripheral (but not cerebral) vasodilatation due to a direct action of the drugs on the blood vessels, but stimulation of the vasomotor centre tends to counter this.

Changes in the blood pressure are therefore somewhat unpredictable, but caffeine 250 mg (single dose) usually causes a transient rise of blood pressure of about 14/10 mmHg in occasional coffee drinkers (but has no additional effect in habitual drinkers); this effect can be used advantageously in patients with autonomic nervous system failure who experience postprandial hypotension (two cups of coffee with breakfast may suffice for the day). In occasional coffee drinkers two cups of coffee (about 160 mg caffeine) per day raise blood pressure by 5/4 mmHg. Increased coronary artery blood flow may occur but increased cardiac work counterbalances this in angina pectoris.

When theophylline (aminophylline) is given intravenously, slow injection is essential in order to avoid transient peak concentrations which are equivalent to administering an overdose.

Smooth muscle (other than vascular muscle, which is discussed above) is relaxed. The only important clinical use for this action is in reversible airways obstruction (asthma), when the action of theophylline can be a very valuable addition to therapy.

Kidney. Diuresis occurs in normal people chiefly due to reduced tubular reabsorption of sodium, similar to thiazide action, but weaker.

Preparations and uses of caffeine and theophylline

Aminophylline. The most generally useful preparation is aminophylline, which is a soluble, irritant salt of theophylline with ethylenediamine.

Attempts to make non-irritant, orally reliable preparations of theophylline have resulted in choline theophyllinate and numerous variants. Sustained-release formulations are convenient for asthmatics, but they cannot be assumed to be bio-equivalent and repeat prescriptions should adhere to the formulation of a particular manufacturer. Suppositories are available. Aminophylline is used in the following conditions:

- Asthma. In severe asthma (given intravenously) when β-adrenoceptor agonists fail to give adequate response; and for chronic asthma (orally) to provide a background bronchodilator effect.
- Neonatal apnoea; caffeine is also effective.

Caffeine is used as an additional ingredient in analgesic tablets; about 60 mg potentiates the effects of NSAIDs; also as an aid in hypotension of autonomic failure (above) and to enhance oral ergotamine absorption in migraine.

Xanthine-containing drinks

Coffee, tea and cola drinks in excess can make people tense and anxious. Epidemiological studies indicate either no, or only slight, increased risk (two- to three-fold) of coronary heart disease in heavy (including decaffeinated) coffee consumers (more than four cups daily). Slight tolerance to the effects of caffeine (on all systems) occurs. Withdrawal symptoms, attributable to psychological and perhaps mild physical dependence, occur in habitual coffee drinkers (five or more cups/day) 12–16 h after the last cup; they include headache (lasting up to 6 days), irritability and jitteriness; they may occur with transient changes in intake, e.g. high at work, lower at the weekend.

Chronic overdose. Excessive prolonged consumption of caffeine causes anxiety, restlessness, tremors, insomnia, headache, cardiac extrasystoles and confusion. The cause can easily be overlooked if specific enquiry into habits is not made, including children regarding cola drinks. Of coffee drinkers, up to 25% who complain of anxiety may benefit from reduction of caffeine intake. An adult heavy user may be defined as one who takes more than 300 mg caffeine per day, i.e. four cups of 150 mL of brewed coffee, each containing 80 mg ± 20 mg caffeine per cup or five cups (60 mg ± 20 mg) of instant coffee. The equivalent for tea would be 10 cups at approximately 30 mg caffeine per cup; and of cola drinks about 2 L. Plainly, caffeine drinks brewed to personal taste of consumer or vendor must have an extremely variable concentration according to source of coffee or tea, amount used, method and duration of brewing. There is also great individual variation in the effect of coffee both between individuals and sometimes in the same individual at different times of life.

Decaffeinated coffee contains about 3 mg per cup; cola drinks contain 8–13 mg caffeine per 100 mL; cocoa as a drink, 4 mg per cup; chocolate (solid) 6–20 mg/ 30 g.

In *young people* high caffeine intake has been linked to behaviour disorders and a limit of 125 mg/L has been proposed for cola drinks.

Blood lipids. Drinking five cups of boiled coffee per day increases plasma total cholesterol by up to 10%; this does not occur with coffee made by simple filtration. Cessation of coffee drinking can reduce plasma cholesterol concentration in hypercholesterolaemic men.

Breast-fed infants may become sleepless and irritable if there is high maternal intake. Fetal cardiac arrhythmias have been reported with exceptionally high maternal caffeine intake, e.g. 1.5 L cola drinks per day.

CANNABIS

Cannabis is obtained from the annual plant *Cannabis sativa* (hemp) and its varieties *Cannabis indica* and *Cannabis americana*. The preparations that are smoked are called marijuana (also grass, pot, weed) and consist of crushed leaves and flowers. The resin scraped off the plant is known as hashish (hash). The term cannabis is used to include all the above preparations. As most preparations are illegally prepared it is not surprising that they are impure and of variable potency. The plant grows wild in the Americas, Africa and Asia. It can also be grown successfully in the open in the warmer southern areas of Britain. Some 27% of the adult UK population report having used cannabis in their lifetime.

Pharmacokinetics

Of the scores of chemical compounds that the resin contains, the most important are the oily cannabinoids, including tetrahydrocannabinol (THC), which is the main psychoactive ingredient. Samples of resin vary greatly in the amounts and proportions of these cannabinoids according to their country of origin. As the sample ages, its THC content declines. THC content of samples can vary from 8% to almost zero. Smoke from a cannabis cigarette (the usual mode of use is to inhale and hold the breath to allow maximum absorption) delivers 25%–50% of the THC content to the respiratory tract. THC ($t_{1/2}$ 4 days) and other cannabinoids undergo extensive biotransformation in the body, yielding scores of metabolites, several of which are themselves psychoactive. They are extremely lipid-soluble and are stored in body fat from which they are slowly released. Hepatic drug-metabolising enzymes are inhibited acutely but may also be induced by chronic use of crude preparations.

Pharmacodynamics

Cannabinoid CB_1-receptors (expressed by hypothalamic and peripheral neurones, e.g. sensory terminals in the gastrointestinal tract, and by adipocytes) and CB_2-receptors (expressed only in the periphery by immune cells) together with their endogenous ligands (called endocannabinoids) are components of the *endocannabinoid neuromodulatory system*, which has a role in many physiological processes including food intake and energy homeostasis. Cannabinoids act as agonists at CB_1-receptors (mediating addictive effects) and CB_2-receptors. Understanding this system offers scope for developing novel drug therapies.

Psychological reactions are very varied, being much influenced by the behaviour of the group. They commence within minutes of starting to smoke and last for 2–3 h. Euphoria is common and is believed to follow stimulation of the limbic system reward pathways causing release of dopamine from the nucleus accumbens. There may be giggling or laughter which can seem pointless to an observer. Sensations become more vivid, especially visual, and contrast and intensity of colour can increase, although no change in acuity occurs. Size of objects and distance are distorted. Sense of time can disappear altogether, leaving a sometimes distressing sense of timelessness. Recent memory and selective attention are impaired; the beginning of a sentence may be forgotten before it is finished. The subject is very suggestible and easily distracted. Psychological tests such as mental arithmetic, digit-symbol substitution and pursuit meter tests show impairment. These effects may be accompanied by feelings of deep insight and truth. Memory defect may persist for weeks after abstinence. Once memory is impaired, concentration becomes less effective, because the object of attention is less well remembered. With this may go an insensitivity to danger or the consequences of actions. A striking phenomenon is the intermittent wavelike nature of these effects which affects mood, visual impressions, time sense, spatial sense and other functions.

The desired effects of cannabinoids, as of other psychodysleptics, depend not only on the expectation of the user and the dose, but also on the environmental situation and personality. Genial or revelatory experiences may indeed occur.

Cannabinoids and skilled tasks e.g. car driving. General performance in both motor and psychological tests deteriorates, more in naive than in experienced subjects. Effects may be similar to alcohol, but experiments in which the subjects are unaware that they are being tested (and so do not compensate voluntarily) are difficult to do, as with alcohol. In a placebo-controlled trial of airline pilots in a flight simulator, performance was impaired for up to 50 h after the pilots smoked a joint containing THC 20 mg (a relatively low dose by current standards).

USES

A therapeutic role has been suggested for cannabinoids in a variety of conditions including chronic pain, migraine headaches, muscle spasticity in multiple sclerosis or spinal cord injury, movement disorders, appetite stimulation in patients with AIDS, nausea and vomiting.

THC is currently available as *dronabinol*, a synthetic form and as *nabilone*, a synthetic analogue, and both are approved to alleviate chemotherapy-induced vomiting in patients who have shown inadequate response to conventional antiemetics, and AIDS-related wasting syndrome.

Issues of cannabis and cannabis-based medicines were the subject of a working party report whose main conclusions were:

- Inhibition of cannabinoid action can be used to help obese patients to *lose weight*. The first of a new class of CB_1-receptor antagonists, rimonabant, reduced body-weight and improved cardiovascular risk factors (HDL-cholesterol, triglycerides, insulin resistance) in obese patients over 1 year. It may cause nausea and depression and is contraindicated in pregnancy.
- In *neuropathic pain*, i.e. due to damaged neural tissue, data from well-controlled but limited duration trials suggest that THC is similar to codeine in potency, is safe and is not associated with tolerance or dependence.
- Cannabinoids regulate bone mass, and cannabinoid receptor antagonists may have a role in the treatment of osteoporosis.
- Data on the value of cannabis preparations for multiple sclerosis are not conclusive, although there is some support for a therapeutic effect.

Adverse effects

Acute

The *psychological* effects can be unpleasant, especially in inexperienced subjects. These are: timelessness and the feeling of loss of control of mental processes; feelings of unease, sometimes amounting to anguish and acute panic; 'flashbacks' of previously experienced hallucinations, e.g. on LSD. The effect of an acute dose usually ends in drowsiness and sleep. Increase in appetite is commonly experienced. It has been suggested that acute cannabis use might be associated with acute cardiovascular fatality, but this remains unproven.

Chronic

There is tendency to paranoid thinking. Cognitive defect occurs and persists in relation to the duration of cannabis use. High or habitual use can be followed by a psychotic state; this is usually reversible, quickly with brief periods of cannabis use, but more slowly after sustained exposures. Evidence indicates that chronic use may precipitate psychosis in vulnerable individuals. Continued heavy use can lead to *tolerance*, and a *withdrawal* syndrome (depression, anxiety, sleep disturbance, tremor and other symptoms). Abandoning cannabis is difficult for many users.

In studies of self-administration by monkeys, spontaneous use did not occur but, once use was initiated, drug-seeking behaviour developed. Subjects who have become tolerant to LSD or opioids as a result of repeated dosage respond normally to cannabis but there appears to be cross-tolerance between cannabinoids and alcohol. The term '*amotivational syndrome*' dignifies an imprecisely characterised state, with features ranging from a feeling of unease and sense of not being fully effective, up to a gross lethargy, with social passivity and deterioration. Yet the reversibility of the state, its association with cannabinoid use, and its recognition by cannabis users make it impossible to ignore.

The smoke produces the usual smoker's cough and delivers much more tar than tobacco cigarettes. In terms of damage to the bronchial epithelium, e.g. squamous metaplasia (a pre-cancerous change), three or four cannabis cigarettes are the equivalent of 20 tobacco cigarettes. Cannabinoids are teratogenic in animals, but effect in humans is unproved, although there is impaired fetal growth with repeated use.

MANAGEMENT OF ADVERSE REACTIONS TO PSYCHODYSLEPTICS

Mild and sometimes even severe episodes ('bad trips') can be managed by reassurance including talk, 'talking the patient down' and physical contact, e.g. hand-holding (LSD and mescaline). Sedation of anxious or excited subjects can be effected with diazepam (or haloperidol).

Part 5. Psychostimulants

COCAINE

Cocaine is found in the leaves of the coca plant (*Erythroxylum coca*), a bush commonly found growing wild in Peru, Ecuador and Bolivia, and cultivated in many other countries. A widespread and ancient practice among South American peasants is to chew coca leaves with lime to release the alkaloid which gives relief from fatigue and hunger, and from altitude sickness in the Andes, experienced even by natives of the area when journeying; it also induces a pleasant introverted mental state. What may have been (or even still may be) an acceptable feature of these ancient stable societies has now developed into a massive criminal business for the manufacture and export of purified cocaine to developed societies, where its use constitutes an intractable social problem. An estimated 1 million people abused cocaine in the UK in 2009. This increase in use has been fuelled by falling street prices.

Pharmacokinetics. Cocaine hydrochloride, extracted from the coca leaves, is a fine white powder. It is metabolised by plasma esterases; the $t_{1/2}$ is 50 min. It is taken to obtain the immediate characteristic intense euphoria which is often followed in a few minutes by dysphoria. This leads to repeated use (10–45 min) during 'runs' of usually about 12 h. After the 'run' there follows the 'crash' (dysphoria, irritability, hypersomnia), lasting for hours to days. After the 'crash' there may be depression ('cocaine blues') and decreased capacity to experience pleasure (anhedonia) for days to weeks.

Route of administration. Cocaine can be snorted, swallowed, smoked (below) or injected. Intranasal use causes mucosal vasoconstriction, anosmia and eventually necrosis and perforation of the nasal septum. Smoking involves converting the non-volatile cocaine HCl into the volatile 'free base' or 'crack' (by extracting the HCl with alkali).

For use it is vaporised by heat (it pops or cracks) in a special glass 'pipe'; or mixed with tobacco in a cigarette. Inhalation with breath-holding allows pulmonary absorption that is about as rapid as an intravenous injection. It induces an intense euphoric state. The mouth and pharynx become anaesthetised. Intravenous use gives the expected rapid effect (kick, flash, rush). Cocaine may be mixed with heroin (as 'speedball').

Mode of action. Cocaine binds to and blocks the dopamine reuptake transporter which plays a key role in controlling entry of dopamine into central nerve terminals after release. Dopamine then accumulates in the synapse and acts on adjacent neurones to produce the characteristic 'high'. The psychotropic effects of cocaine are similar to those of amfetamine (euphoria and excitement) but briefer. Psychological dependence with intense compulsive drug-seeking behaviour is characteristic of even short-term use. Physical dependence is arguably slight or absent. Tachyphylaxis, acute tolerance, occurs.

Overdose is common among users. Up to 22% of heavy users report losing consciousness. The desired euphoria and excitement turn to acute fear, with psychotic symptoms, convulsions, hypertension, haemorrhagic stroke, tachycardia, arrhythmias, hyperthermia. Coronary artery vasospasm (sufficient to present as the acute coronary syndrome with chest pain and myocardial infarction) may occur, and acute left ventricular dysfunction.

Treatment is chosen according to the clinical picture (and the known mode of action), from haloperidol (rather than chlorpromazine) for mental disturbance; diazepam for convulsions; a vasodilator, e.g. a calcium channel blocker, for hypertension; glyceryl trinitrate for myocardial ischaemia (but not a β-blocker which aggravates cocaine-induced coronary vasospasm). Fetal growth is retarded by maternal use, but teratogenicity is uncertain.

> Cocaine induced coronary artery spasm and myocardial infarction is an increasingly recognised problem and should be suspected in a young person presenting with cardiac chest pain.

AMFETAMINES

An easily prepared crystalline form of methylamfetamine (known as 'crystal meth' or 'ice') is in widespread illicit use as a psychostimulant. Amfetamine is a racemic compound: the *laevo* form is relatively inactive but dexamfetamine (the *dextro* isomer) finds use in medicine. Amfetamine will be described, and structurally related drugs only in the ways in which they differ.

Pharmacokinetics. Amfetamine ($t_{1/2}$ 12 h) is readily absorbed by any usual route and is largely eliminated unchanged in the urine. Urinary excretion is pH dependent; being a basic substance, elimination will be greater in an acid urine. As well as oral use, intravenous administration (with the pleasurable 'flash' as with opioids) is employed. *Interactions* are as expected from mode of action, e.g. antagonism of antihypertensives; severe hypertension with MAOIs and β-adrenoceptor blocking drugs.

Mode of action. Amfetamine acts centrally by releasing dopamine stored in nerve endings and peripherally by α-and β-adrenoceptor actions common to indirectly acting sympathomimetics. As with all drugs acting on the CNS, the psychological effects vary with mood, personality and environment, as well as with dose. Subjects become euphoric and fatigue is postponed. Although physical and mental performance may improve, this cannot be relied on. Subjects may be more confident and show more initiative, and be better satisfied with a more speedy performance that has deteriorated in accuracy. There may be anxiety and a feeling of nervous and physical tension, especially with large doses, and subjects develop tremors and confusion, and feel dizzy. Time seems to pass with greater rapidity. The sympathomimetic effect on the heart, causing palpitations, may intensify discomfort or alarm. Amfetamine increases the peripheral oxygen consumption and this, together with vasoconstriction and restlessness, leads to hyperthermia in overdose, especially if the subject exercises.

Dependence on amfetamine and similar sympathomimetics is chiefly psychological. There is a withdrawal syndrome, suggesting physical dependence. Tolerance occurs. Severe dependence induces behaviour disorders, hallucinations, even florid psychosis, which can be controlled by haloperidol. Withdrawal is accompanied by lethargy and sleep, desire for food, and sometimes severe depression, which leads to an urge to resume the drug.

Acute poisoning is manifested by excitement and peripheral sympathomimetic effects. Convulsions may occur in acute or chronic overuse; a state resembling hyperactive paranoid schizophrenia with hallucinations develops. Hyperthermia occurs with cardiac arrhythmias, vascular collapse, intracranial haemorrhage and death. Treatment is chlorpromazine with added antihypertensive, e.g. labetalol, if necessary; these provide sedation and β-adrenoceptor blockade (but not a β-blocker alone), rendering unnecessary the optional enhancement of elimination by urinary acidification.

Chronic overdose can cause a psychotic state mimicking schizophrenia. A vasculitis of the cerebral and/or renal vessels can occur, possibly due to release of vasoconstrictor amines from both platelets and nerve endings. Severe hypertension can result from the renal vasculitis.

Structurally related drugs include dexamfetamine, used for narcolepsy and in attention-deficit hyperactivity disorder (ADHD), methylphenidate (used for ADHD), tenamfetamine, phentermine, diethylpropion and pemoline.

KHAT

The leaves of the khat shrub (*Catha edulis*) contain alkaloids (cathinine, cathine, cathidine) that are structurally like amfetamine and produce similar effects. They are chewed fresh (for maximal alkaloid content). The habit was confined to geographical areas favourable to the shrub (Arabia, East Africa) until modern transportation allowed wider distribution. Use in the UK has been increasingly reported. It has been banned in the USA and Canada. Khat chewers (mostly male) became euphoric, loquacious, excited, hyperactive and even manic. As with some other drug dependencies, subjects may give priority to their drug needs above personal, family, and other social and economic responsibilities. Cultivation takes up serious amounts of scarce arable land and irrigation water.

Part 6. Volatile substance abuse

Seekers of the 'self-gratifying high' also inhale any volatile substance that may affect the CNS. These include adhesives ('glue sniffing'), lacquer-paint solvents, petrol, nail varnish, any pressurised aerosol, butane liquid gas (which latter especially may 'freeze' the larynx, allowing fatal inhalation of food, drink, gastric contents, or even the liquid itself to flood the lungs). Even solids, e.g. paint scrapings, solid shoe polish, may be volatilised over a fire.

These substances are particularly abused by the young (13–15 years), no doubt largely because they are accessible at home and in ordinary shops, and these children cannot easily buy alcohol or 'street' drugs (although this may be changing as dealers target the youngest).

CNS effects include confusion and hallucinations, ataxia, dysarthria, coma, convulsions, respiratory failure. Liver, kidney, lung and heart damage occur. Sudden cardiac death may be due to sensitisation of the heart to endogenous catecholamines. If the substance is put in a plastic bag from which the user takes deep inhalations, or is sprayed in a confined space, e.g. cupboard, there is particularly high risk.

Signs of frequent volatile substance abuse include perioral eczema and inflammation of the upper respiratory tract.

SUMMARY

Substance (drug) dependence is defined as *when an individual persists in use of alcohol or other drugs, which* include opioids; cerebral depressants (benzodiazepines, γ-hydroxybutyrate); tobacco; psychodysleptics (LSD, mescaline, tenamfetamine, phencyclidine, cannabis); psychostimulants (cocaine, amfetamines, methylxanthines, khat); volatile substances, *despite problems related to use of the substance, substance dependence may be diagnosed. Compulsive and repetitive use may result in tolerance to the effect of the drug and withdrawal symptoms when use is reduced or stopped.* The WHO Expert Committee on Addiction Producing Drugs 1957 defined **substance (drug) abuse** in the context of two components: **Substance (drug) addiction** *is a state of periodic or chronic intoxication produced by the repeated consumption of a drug (natural or synthetic). Its characteristics include*: ① *an overpowering desire or need (compulsion) to continue taking the drug and to obtain it by any means*; ② *a tendency to increase the dose*; ③ *a psychic (psychological) and generally a physical dependence on the effects of the drug; and* ④ *detrimental effects on the individual and on society.* **Substance (drug) habituation** is a condition resulting from the repeated consumption of a drug. Its characteristics include ① a desire (but not a compulsion) to continue taking the drug for the sense of improved well-being which it engenders; ② little or no tendency to increase the dose; ③ some degree of psychic dependence on the effect of the drug, but absence of physical dependence and hence of an abstinence syndrome (withdrawal), and ④ detrimental effects, if any, primarily on the individual. **Psychological (*psychic*) dependence** is characterised by emotional distress if the drug of dependence is withdrawn. The subject may develop craving for the drug with anxiety, insomnia and dysphoria. It develops before physical dependence. **Physical (physiological) dependence** implies that continued exposure to a drug induces adaptive changes in body tissues so that *tolerance* occurs, and that abrupt withdrawal of the drug leaves these changes unopposed, resulting generally in a *discontinuation (withdrawal) syndrome*, usually of rebound overactivity. **Tolerance** follows the operation of homeostatic adaptation. **A discontinuation (withdrawal) syndrome** occurs when administration of an opioid is suddenly stopped. Because exogenously administered opioid suppresses their endogenous production by a feedback mechanism. Abrupt discontinuation results in an immediate deficiency of endogenous opioid, which thus causes the withdrawal syndrome. **Drugs of dependence** are often divided into two groups, hard and soft. **Hard drugs** are those that are liable seriously to disable the individual as a functioning member of society by inducing severe psychological and, in the case of cerebral depressants, physical dependence. The group includes heroin and cocaine. **Soft drugs** are less dependence producing. There may be psychological dependence, but there is little or no physical dependence except with heavy doses of depressants (alcohol). The group includes sedatives and tranquillisers, amfetamines, cannabis, hallucinogens, alcohol, tobacco and caffeine.

IMPORTANT TERMINOLOGY

substance (drug) dependence　物质(药物)依赖性

substance (drug) abuse　物质(药物)滥用

substance (drug) addiction　物质(药物)成瘾性

substance (drug) habituation　物质(药物)习惯性

psychological (psychic) dependence　心理(精神)
依赖性

physical (physiological) dependence　身体(生理)
依赖性

tolerance　耐受性

a discontinuation (withdrawal) syndrome　停药
(戒断)综合征

hard drugs　硬毒品

soft drugs　软毒品

dependence/abuse liability　依赖 /滥用倾向

cerebral depressants　中枢抑制药

psychodysleptics　精神致幻药

psychostimulants　精神兴奋药 /精神振奋药 /中枢
兴奋剂

opioids　阿片样物质

pentazocine　喷他佐辛

indometacin　吲哚美辛

nefopam　奈福泮

heroin　海洛因

phenylethylamine　苯乙胺

alcohol　醇

benzodiazepines　苯二氮杂䓬类

γ-hydroxybutyrate　γ-羟基丁酸

acamprosate　阿坎酸

disulfiram　戒酒硫（用以治疗慢性酒精中毒）

tobacco　烟草

nicotine　尼古丁

bupropion　安非他酮

lysergic acid diethylamide (lysergide)　酒石酸麦角酰二乙胺（麦角胺）

mescaline　麦斯卡林（一种致幻剂）

psilocybin　裸头草碱（采自墨西哥蘑菇的一种迷幻药）

tenamfetamine　替苯丙胺（中枢兴奋药）

phencyclidine　苯环己哌啶（即"天使粉"，一种麻醉药和致幻剂）

ketamine　氯胺酮

methylxanthines　甲基黄嘌呤类

caffeine　咖啡因

theophylline　茶碱

theobromine　可可碱

aminophylline　氨茶碱

ethylenediamine　乙（撑）二胺

cannabis　大麻

cannabinoids　大麻素类

tetrahydrocannabinol (THC)　四氢大麻醇，四氢大麻酚（大麻树脂的主要成分，麻醉用）

cocaine　可卡因

amfetamine　苯丙胺，安非他明

methylamfetamine　甲基苯丙胺

dexamfetamine　右旋苯丙胺（拟交感神经兴奋药、食欲抑制药）

methylphenidate　利他灵（一种中枢兴奋药）

phentermine　芬特明（苯丁胺）

diethylpropion　安非拉酮（二乙胺苯丙酮）

pemoline　帕吗啉，苯异妥英

khat　阿拉伯茶（产于非洲和阿拉伯）

cathinine (cathine, cathidine)　阿茶碱，阿拉伯茶碱

volatile substances　挥发性物质

CHALLENGE YOURSELF

1. Please explain the term "substance (drug) dependence".
2. Discuss the harms of substance (drug) dependence to individuals and society.
3. Please descript the classification of the substances (drugs) which result in drug dependence.
4. Please detail the mechanisms of drug dependence.
5. Please detail the treatment of drug dependence.

Jian Yang

Chapter | 9 |

Poisoning, overdose, antidotes

INTRODUCTION

The UK has one of the highest rates of deliberate self-harm in Europe. Deliberate self-harm involves intentional self-poisoning or self-injury irrespective of the intended purpose of that act. Self-poisoning is the commonest form of deliberate self-harm after self-mutilation. Poisoning, usually by medicines taken in overdose, is currently responsible for over 150 000 hospital attendances per annum in England and Wales (population 54 million). Prescribed drugs are involved in more than 75% of episodes, but teenagers tend to favour non-prescribed analgesics available by direct sale. In particular, over half of these involve ingestion of paracetamol, with the associated risk of serious toxicity. In order to address this problem the pack size of paracetamol was reduced to 8 g for non-prescription purchase and 16 g for prescription in the UK in 1998. Evidence suggests that this has not so far been effective in reducing paracetamol-related deaths but the mortality rate of self-poisoning overall is very low (less than 1% of acute hospital admissions with poisoning). The total number of deaths related to drug poisoning in England and Wales increased each year from 1993 to a peak in 1999, and then began to decline.

Most patients who die from deliberate ingestion of drugs do so before reaching medical assistance; overall only 11%–28% of those who die following the deliberate ingestion of drugs reach hospital alive. The drugs most frequently implicated in hospital deaths of such individuals in the UK are paracetamol, tricyclic antidepressants and benzodiazepines. In India, deliberate self harm is seen with similar prescribed agents, together with frequent deliberate self-harm with the antimalarial chloroquine and accidental or deliberate injury from pesticides such as the organophosphates or aluminium phosphide. In Sri Lanka deliberate pesticide ingestion is also a serious public health issue.

Accidental self-poisoning, causing admission to hospital, occurs predominantly among children under 5 years old, usually from medicines left within their reach or with commonly available domestic chemicals, e.g. bleach, detergents etc.

> Most patients who die from deliberate ingestion of drugs do so before reaching medical assistance. For those reaching hospital, the overall mortality is very low.

INITIAL ASSESSMENT

It is important to obtain information on the poison that has been taken. The key pieces of information are:

- The identity of the substance(s) taken.
- The dose(s).
- The time that has elapsed since ingestion.
- Whether alcohol was also taken.
- Whether the subject has vomited since ingestion.
  Adults may be sufficiently conscious to give some

indication of the poison or may have referred to it in a suicide note, or there may be other circumstantial evidence e.g. knowledge of the prescribed drugs that the patient had access to, empty drug containers in pocket or at the scene. The ambulance crew attending to the patient at home may have very valuable information and should be questioned for any clues to the ingested drug. Any family or friends attending with the patient should be similarly questioned.

The response to a specific antidote may provide a diagnosis, e.g. dilatation of constricted pupils and increased respiratory rate after intravenous naloxone (opioid poisoning) or arousal from unconsciousness in response to intravenous flumazenil (benzodiazepine poisoning).

Many substances used in accidental or self-poisoning produce recognisable symptoms and signs. Some arise from dysfunction of the central or autonomic nervous systems; other agents produce individual effects. They can be useful diagnostically and provide characteristic toxic syndromes or 'toxidromes'.

In addition, sedatives, opioids and ethanol cause signs that may include respiratory depression, miosis, hyporeflexia, coma, hypotension and hypothermia. Other drugs and non-drug chemicals that produce characteristic effects include: salicylates, methanol and ethylene glycol, iron, selective serotonin reuptake inhibitors. Effects of overdose (and treatment) with other individual drugs or drug groups appear in the relevant accounts throughout the book.

RESUSCITATION

In concert with attempts to define the nature of the overdose, it is essential to carry out standard resuscitation methods. Maintenance of an adequate oxygen supply is the first priority and the airway must be sucked clear of oropharyngeal secretions or regurgitated matter. Shock in acute poisoning is usually due to expansion of the venous capacitance bed and placing the patient in the head-down position to encourage venous return to the heart, or a colloid plasma expander administered intravenously restores blood pressure. External cardiac compression may be

necessary and should be continued until the cardiac output is self-sustaining, which may be a long time when the patient is hypothermic or poisoned with a cardiodepressant drug, e.g. tricyclic antidepressant, β-adrenoceptor blocker.

> External cardiac compression may be required for prolonged periods of cardiac arrest, up to several hours. In young patients the heart is anatomically and physiologically normal and will recover when the poison has been eliminated from the body.

Investigations may include arterial blood gas analysis and examination of plasma for specific substances that would require treatment with an antidote, e.g. with paracetamol, iron and digoxin.

Plasma concentration measurement is also used to quantify the risk. Particular treatments such as haemodialysis or urine alkalinisation may be indicated for overdose with salicylate, lithium and some sedative drugs, e.g. trichloroethanol derivatives, phenobarbital.

Rapid biochemical 'screens' of urine are widely available in hospital emergency departments and will detect a range of drugs.

SUPPORTIVE TREATMENT

The majority of patients admitted to hospital will require only observation combined with medical and nursing supportive measures while they metabolise and eliminate the poison. Some will require specific measures to reduce absorption or to increase elimination. A few will require administration of a specific antidote. A very few will need intensive care facilities. In the event of serious overdose, always obtain the latest advice on management.

In the UK, regional medicines information centres provide specialist advice and information over the telephone throughout the day and night.

> The most efficient eliminating mechanisms are the patient's own physiological processes, which, given time, will inactivate and eliminate all the

poison. Most patients recover from acute poisonings provided they are adequately oxygenated, hydrated and perfused.

Special problems introduced by poisoning are as follows:

- *Airway* maintenance is essential; some patients require a cuffed endotracheal tube but seldom for more than 24 h.
- *Ventilation*: a mixed respiratory and metabolic acidosis is common; the inspired air is supplemented with oxygen to correct the hypoxia. Mechanical ventilation is necessary if adequate oxygenation cannot be obtained or hypercapnia ensues.
- *Hypotension*: this is common in poisoning and, in addition to the resuscitative measures indicated above, conventional inotropic support may be required.
- *In addition*: there is recent interest in the use of high dose insulin infusions with euglycaemic clamping as a positive inotrope in the context of overdose with myocardial depressant agents. The very high insulin doses given (0.5–2 units/kg·h) have so far deterred physicians from the routine use of such therapy. There are, however, a number of case reports that support such an approach. Many of these are in the context of overdosage with non-dihydropyridine calcium channel blockers that are often resistant to conventional inotropic agents.
- *Convulsions* should be treated if they are persistent or protracted. Intravenous benzodiazepine (diazepam or lorazepam) is the first choice.
- *Cardiac arrhythmia* frequently accompanies poisoning, e.g. with tricyclic antidepressants, theophylline, β-adrenoceptor blockers.
- *Acidosis, hypoxia and electrolyte disturbance* are often important contributory factors and it is preferable to observe the effect of correcting these before considering resort to an antiarrhythmic drug. If arrhythmia does lead to persistent peripheral circulatory failure, an appropriate drug may be cautiously justified, e.g. a β-adrenoceptor blocker for poisoning with a sympathomimetic drug.

- *Hypothermia* may occur if CNS depression impairs temperature regulation. A low-reading rectal thermometer is used to monitor core temperature and the patient is nursed in a heat-retaining 'space blanket'.
- *Immobility* may lead to pressure lesions of peripheral nerves, cutaneous blisters, necrosis over bony prominences, and increased risk of thromboembolism warrants prophylaxis.
- *Rhabdomyolysis* may result from prolonged pressure on muscles from agents that cause muscle spasm or convulsions (phencyclidine, theophylline); may be aggravated by hyperthermia due to muscle contraction, e.g. with MDMA ('ecstasy'). Aggressive volume repletion and correction of acid–base abnormality are needed; urine alkalinisation and/or diuretic therapy may be helpful in preventing acute tubular necrosis but evidence is not conclusive.

Patients die from overdose
- *Early*– from direct respiratory depression, fatal cardiac arrhythmias, fatal convulsions.
- *Delayed*– from organ damage consequent upon poorly managed cardiorespiratory support.
- *Late*– from delayed toxicity of the drug causing severe direct end organ damage, e.g. liver failure.

PREVENTING FURTHER ABSORPTION OF THE POISON

From the environment

When a poison has been inhaled or absorbed through the skin, the patient should be taken from the toxic environment, the contaminated clothing should be removed and the skin should be cleansed.

From the alimentary tract ('gut decontamination')

In the United States and European countries, gastric lavage should not be employed routinely, if ever, in the management of poisoned patients. Serious risks of the procedure include hypoxia, cardiac arrhythmias, laryngospasm, perforation of the GI tract or pharynx, fluid and electrolyte abnormalities and aspiration pneumonitis. Clinical studies show no beneficial effect. The procedure may be considered in very extraordinary circumstances for the hospitalised adult who is believed to have ingested a potentially life-threatening amount of a poison within the previous hour, and provided the airways are protected by a cuffed endotracheal tube. It is *contraindicated* for corrosive substances, hydrocarbons with high aspiration potential and where there is risk of haemorrhage from an underlying gastrointestinal condition.

Emesis using syrup of ipecacuanha is no longer practised in hospital, as there is no clinical trial evidence that the procedure improves outcome.

Oral adsorbents. Activated charcoal (Carbomix) consists of a very fine black powder prepared from vegetable matter, e.g. wood pulp, coconut shell, which is 'activated' by an oxidising gas flow at high temperature to create a network of small (10–20 nm) pores with an enormous surface area in relation to weight (1 000 m^2/g). This binds to, and thus inactivates, a wide variety of compounds in the gut. Indeed, activated charcoal comes nearest to fulfilling the long-sought notion of a 'universal antidote'. Thus it is simpler to list the exceptions, i.e. substances that are poorly adsorbed by charcoal:

- Metal salts (iron, lithium).
- Cyanide.
- Alcohols (ethanol, methanol, ethylene glycol).
- Petroleum distillates.
- Clofenotane (dicophane, DDT).
- Malathion.
- Strong acids and alkalis.
- Corrosive agents.

To be most effective, five to ten times as much charcoal as poison, weight for weight, is needed. In the adult an initial dose of 50 g is usual, repeated if necessary. If the patient is vomiting, give the charcoal through a nasogastric tube. Unless a patient has an intact or protected airway, its administration is contraindicated.

Activated charcoal is most effective when given soon after ingestion of a potentially toxic amount of a poison and while a significant amount remains yet unabsorbed. Volunteer studies suggest that administration within 1 h can be expected to prevent up to 40%–50% of absorption. There are no satisfactorily designed clinical trials in patients to assess the benefit of single dose activated charcoal. Benefit after 1 h cannot be excluded and may be sometimes be indicated. Charcoal in repeated doses accelerates the elimination of poison that has been absorbed. Activated charcoal, although unpalatable, appears to be relatively safe but constipation or mechanical bowel obstruction may follow repeated use. In the drowsy or comatose patient there is particular risk of aspiration into the lungs causing hypoxia through obstruction and arteriovenous shunting. Methionine, used orally for paracetamol poisoning, is adsorbed by the charcoal.

Other oral adsorbents have specific uses. Fuller's earth (a natural form of aluminium silicate) binds and inactivates the herbicides paraquat (activated charcoal is superior) and diquat; colestyramine and colestipol will adsorb warfarin.

Whole-bowel irrigation should not be used routinely in the management of the poisoned patient. While volunteer studies have shown marked reductions in the bioavailability of ingested drugs, there is no evidence from controlled clinical trials in patients. It should be used for the removal of sustained-release or enteric-coated formulations from patients who present more than 2 h after ingestion, e.g. iron, theophylline, aspirin. Evidence of benefit is conflicting. Activated charcoal in frequent (50 g) doses is generally preferred. Sustained-release formulations are common, and patients have died from failure to recognise the danger of continued release of drug from such products. Whole-bowel irrigation is also an option for the removal of ingested packets of illicit drugs. It is contraindicated in patients with bowel obstruction, perforation or ileus, with haemodynamic instability and with compromised unprotected airways.

Whole bowel irrigation should be used with

special care in patients who are debilitated or who have significant concurrent medical conditions. The effectiveness of activated charcoal may be reduced by co-administration with whole bowel irrigation.

Cathartics have no routine role in gut decontamination, but a single dose of an osmotic agent (sorbitol, magnesium sulphate) may be justified on occasion.

ACCELERATING ELIMINATION OF THE POISON

Techniques for eliminating absorbed poisons have a role that is limited, but important when applicable. Each method depends, directly or indirectly, on removing drug from the circulation and successful use requires that:

- The poison should be present in high concentration in the plasma relative to that in the rest of the body, i.e. it should have a small volume of distribution.
- The poison should dissociate readily from any plasma protein binding sites.
- The effects of the poison should relate to its plasma concentration.

Methods used are:

Repeated doses of activated charcoal

Activated charcoal by mouth not only adsorbs ingested drug in the gut, preventing absorption into the body, it also adsorbs drug that diffuses from the blood into the gut lumen when the concentration there is lower. As binding is irreversible, the concentration gradient is maintained and drug is continuously removed; this has been called 'intestinal dialysis'. Charcoal may also adsorb drugs that secrete into the bile, i.e. by interrupting an enterohepatic cycle. The procedure is effective for overdose of carbamazepine, dapsone, phenobarbital, quinine, salicylate and theophylline.

Repeated-dose activated charcoal is increasingly preferred to alkalinisation of urine (below) for phenobarbital and salicylate poisoning. In adults, activated charcoal 50 g is given initially, then 50 g every

4 h. Vomiting should be treated with an antiemetic drug because it reduces the efficacy of charcoal treatment. Where there is intolerance, the dose may be reduced and the frequency increased, e.g. 25 g every 2 h or 12.5 g every hour, but efficacy may be compromised.

Alteration of urine pH and diuresis

It is useful to alter the pH of the glomerular filtrate such that a drug that is a weak electrolyte will ionise, become less lipid soluble, remain in the renal tubular fluid, and leave the body in the urine.

Maintenance of a good urine flow (e.g. 100 mL/h) helps this process, but the alteration of tubular fluid pH is the important determinant. The practice of forcing diuresis with furosemide and large volumes of intravenous fluid does not add significantly to drug clearance but may cause fluid overload; it is obsolete.

The objective is to maintain a urine pH of 7.5–8.5 by an intravenous infusion of sodium bicarbonate. Available preparations of sodium bicarbonate vary between 1.2% and 8.4% (1 mL of the 8.4% preparation contains 1 mmol sodium bicarbonate) and the concentration given will depend on the patient's fluid needs.

Alkalinisation may be used for: salicylate (> 500 mg/L + metabolic acidosis, or in any case > 750 mg/L) phenobarbital (75–150 mg/L); phenoxy herbicides, e.g. 2,4-D, mecoprop, dichlorprop; moderately severe salicylate poisoning that does not meet the criteria for haemodialysis.

Acidification may be used for severe, acute poisoning with: amfetamine; dexfenfluramine; phencyclidine. The objective is to maintain a urine pH of 5.5–6.5 by giving an intravenous infusion of arginine hydrochloride (10 g) over 30 min, followed by ammonium chloride (4 g) every 2 h by mouth. It is very rarely indicated. Hypertension due to amfetamine-like drugs, for example, will respond to phenoxybenzamine (by α-adrenoceptor block).

Haemodialysis

The system requires a temporary extracorporeal circulation, e.g. from an artery to a vein in the arm. A semipermeable membrane separates blood from dialysis fluid; the poison passes passively from the blood, where it is present in high concentration, to enter the dialysis fluid, which is flowing and thus constantly replaced.

Haemodialysis significantly increases the elimination of: salicylate (> 750 mg/L + renal failure, or in any case > 900 mg/L); isopropanol (present in aftershave lotions and window-cleaning solutions); lithium; methanol; ethylene glycol; ethanol.

Haemofiltration

An extracorporeal circulation brings blood into contact with a highly permeable membrane. Water is lost by ultrafiltration (the rate being dependent on the hydrostatic pressure gradient across membrane) and solutes by convection; the main change in plasma concentrations results from replacement of ultrafiltrate with an appropriate solution.

Haemofiltration is effective for: phenobarbital (> 100–150 mg/L, but repeat-dose activated charcoal by mouth appears to be as effective) and other barbiturates; ethchlorvynol; glutethimide; meprobamate; methaqualone; theophylline; trichloroethanol derivatives.

Peritoneal dialysis

This involves instilling appropriate fluid into the peritoneal cavity. Poison in the blood diffuses down the concentration gradient into the dialysis fluid, which undergoes repeated drainage and replacement. The technique requires little equipment; it may be worth using for lithium and methanol poisoning.

Haemofiltration and peritoneal dialysis are more readily available but are less efficient (one-half to one-third) than haemodialysis.

> Haemodialysis is invasive, demands skill and experience on the part of the operator, and is costly in terms of staffing. Its use should be confined to cases of severe, prolonged or progressive clinical intoxication, when high plasma concentration indicates a dangerous degree of poisoning, and its effect constitutes a significant addition to natural methods of elimination.

SPECIFIC ANTIDOTES

Specific antidotes reduce or abolish the effects of poisons through a variety of general mechanisms.

PSYCHIATRIC AND SOCIAL ASSESSMENT

Patients require a psychosocial assessment when they have recovered from the medical aspects of the overdose. The immediate risk and subsequent risk of suicide should be assessed. Even 'minor' cases of deliberate self-harm should not be dismissed, as 20%–25% of patients who die from deliberate self-harm will have presented to hospital with an episode of self-harm in the previous year. Interpersonal or social problems precipitate most cases of self-poisoning and require attention. Identify and treat any significant psychiatric illness. Consider the impact of any associated medical problems and their symptom control. Obtain information on associated alcohol and substance abuse. In UK hospitals such assessments are usually performed by the hospital psychiatric liaison service prior to discharge of the patient from the hospital. Most patients can be discharged without psychiatric follow-up. Rarely, patients with a high suicide risk and/or an underlying severe psychiatric illness may require transfer to an inpatient psychiatric facility, either voluntarily or under the appropriate section of the 1983 Mental Health Act. More commonly, patients may benefit from community psychiatric support as outpatients.

POISONING BY (NON-DRUG) CHEMICALS

Heavy metal poisoning and use of chelating agents

Acute or chronic exposure to heavy metals can harm the body. Treatment is with chelating agents which incorporate the metal ions into an inner ring structure in the molecule (Greek: *chele*, claw) by means of structural groups called ligands (Latin: *ligare*, to bind). Effective agents form stable, biologically inert complexes that pass into the urine.

Dimercaprol (British Anti-Lewisite, BAL). Arsenic and other metal ions are toxic in low concentration because they combine with the SH-groups of essential enzymes, thus inactivating them. Dimercaprol provides SH-groups, which combine with the metal ions to form relatively harmless ring compounds that pass from the body, mainly in the urine. As dimercaprol itself is oxidised in the body and excreted renally, repeated administration is necessary to ensure that an excess is available to eliminate all of the metal.

Dimercaprol may be used in cases of poisoning by antimony, arsenic, bismuth, gold and mercury (inorganic, e.g. $HgCl_2$).

Adverse effects are common, particularly with larger doses, and include nausea, vomiting, lachrymation, salivation, paraesthesiae, muscular aches and pains, urticarial rashes, tachycardia and raised blood pressure. Gross overdosage may cause over-breathing, muscular tremors, convulsions and coma.

Unithiol (dimercaptopropanesulphonate, DMPS) effectively chelates lead and mercury; it is well tolerated.

Sodium calcium edetate is the calcium chelate of the disodium salt of ethylenediaminetetra-acetic acid (calcium EDTA). It is effective in acute lead poisoning because of its capacity to exchange calcium for lead: the kidney excretes the lead chelate, leaving behind a harmless amount of calcium. Dimercaprol may usefully be combined with sodium calcium edetate when lead poisoning is severe, e.g. with encephalopathy.

Adverse effects are fairly common, and include hypotension, lachrymation, nasal stuffiness, sneezing, muscle pains and possible nephrotoxicity.

Dicobalt edetate. Cobalt forms stable, non-toxic complexes with cyanide. It is toxic (especially if the wrong diagnosis is made and no cyanide is present), causing hypertension, tachycardia and chest pain. Cobalt poisoning is treated by giving sodium calciumedetate and intravenous glucose.

Penicillamine (dimethylcysteine) is a metabolite of penicillin that contains SH-groups; it may be used to chelate lead and copper. Its principal use is for rheumatoid arthritis.

Desferrioxamine.

Cyanide poisoning results in tissue anoxia by chelating the ferric part of the intracellular respiratory enzyme, cytochrome oxidase. It thus uncouples mitochondrial oxidative phosphorylation and inhibits cellular respiration in the presence of adequate oxygenation. Poisoning may occur as a result of: self-administration of hydrocyanic (prussic) acid; accidental exposure in industry; inhaling smoke from burning polyurethane foams in furniture; ingesting amygdalin which is present in the kernels of several fruits including apricots, almonds and peaches (constituents of the unlicensed anticancer agent, laetrile); excessive use of sodium nitroprusside for severe hypertension.

The symptoms of acute poisoning are due to tissue anoxia, with dizziness, palpitations, a feeling of chest constriction and anxiety. Characteristically the breath smells of bitter almonds. In more severe cases there is acidosis and coma. Inhaled hydrogen cyanide may lead to death within minutes, but with the ingested salt several hours may elapse before the patient is seriously ill.

> Cyanide toxicity is suggested by a metabolic acidosis, reduced arterial/venous oxygen saturation difference and markedly elevated plasma lactate. The presence of these findings in the context of smoke inhalation should alert the physician to the possibility that cyanide poisoning has occurred and needs urgent treatment.

The principles of specific therapy are as follows:

Hydroxocobalamin (5 g for an adult) combines with cyanide to form cyanocobalamin and is excreted by the kidney. Adverse effects include transient hypertension (may be beneficial) and rare anaphylactic and anaphylactoid reactions. Co-administration with sodium thiosulphate (through a separate intravenous line or sequentially) may have added benefit. The use of hydroxocobalamin has largely superseded that of the alternative, dicobalt edetate.

135

- *Dicobalt edetate*. The dose is 300 mg given intravenously over 1 min (5 min if condition is less serious), followed immediately by a 50 mL intravenous infusion of 50% glucose; a further 300 mg dicobalt edetate should be given if recovery is not evident within 1 min.
- Alternatively, a two-stage procedure may be followed by intravenous administration of: *Sodium nitrite*, which rapidly converts haemoglobin to methaemoglobin, the ferric ion of which takes up cyanide as cyanmethaemoglobin (up to 40% methaemoglobin can be tolerated).
- *Sodium thiosulphate*, which more slowly detoxifies the cyanide by permitting the formation of thiocyanate. When the diagnosis is uncertain, administration of thiosulphate plus oxygen is a safe course.

The increasing use of hydroxocobalamin as a first-line treatment is based upon animal studies that have shown a faster improvement of arterial blood pressure compared to sodium nitrate. No benefit in terms of mortality was seen in these studies.

There is evidence that *oxygen*, especially if at high pressure (hyperbaric), overcomes the cellular anoxia in cyanide poisoning; the mechanism is uncertain, but it is reasonable to administer high-flow oxygen.

Carbon monoxide (CO) is a colourless, odourless gas formed by the incomplete combustion of hydrocarbons and poisoning results from its inhalation. The concentration (% saturation) of CO in the blood may confirm exposure (cigarette smoking alone may account for up to 10%) but is no guide to the severity of poisoning. CO binds reversibly to haemoglobin with about 250 times greater affinity than oxygen. Binding to one of the four oxygen binding sites on the haemoglobin molecule significantly increases the affinity of the other three binding sites for oxygen which further reduces the delivery of oxygen to hypoxic tissues. In addition, CO has an even higher affinity for cardiac myoglobin, further worsening cardiac output and tissue oxygenation. Poor correlation between carboxyhaemoglobin in the blood and observed toxicity suggests that other mechanisms are involved.

Symptoms commence at about 10% carboxyhaemoglobin with a characteristic headache. Death may occur from myocardial and neurological injury at levels of 50%–70%. Severe breathlessness is not a feature typical of severe intoxication. Delayed symptoms (2–4 weeks) include parkinsonism, cerebellar signs and psychiatric disturbances.

Investigations should include direct estimation of carboxyhaemoglobin in the blood. Consider the diagnosis even if the level is low and some time has passed since exposure or high flow oxygen has been given. Pao_2 levels should be normal. Oxygen saturation is accurate only if directly measured and not calculated from the Pao_2. Administer oxygen through a tight-fitting mask and continue for at least 12 h. Evidence for the efficacy of hyperbaric oxygen is conflicting and transport to hyperbaric chambers may present logistic problems, but it is advocated when the blood carboxyhaemoglobin concentration exceeds 40%, there is unconsciousness, neurological defect, ischaemic change on the ECG, pregnancy, or the clinical condition does not improve after 4 h of normobaric therapy.

Lead poisoning arises from a variety of occupational (house renovation and stripping old paint), and recreational sources. Environmental exposure has been a matter of great concern, as witnessed by the protective legislation introduced by many countries to reduce pollution, e.g. by removing lead from petrol. Lead in the body comprises a rapidly exchangeable component in blood (2%, biological $t_{1/2}$; 35 days) and a stable pool in dentine and the skeleton (95%, biological $t_{1/2}$; 25 years). Lead binds to sulfhydryl groups and interferes with haem production. Since haem-containing proteins play a vital role in cellular oxidation, lead poisoning has wide-ranging effects, particularly in young children. With mild poisoning there is lethargy and abdominal discomfort; severe abdominal symptoms and peripheral neuropathy and CNS disturbances indicate more serious toxicity. Serum lead values over 100 micrograms/mL are associated with impaired cognitive development in children; levels above 1 000 micrograms/mL are potentially fatal.

Mild lead poisoning (< 450 micrograms/mL) may be treated by removal from exposure and monitoring. Moderate poisoning requires oral chelation therapy such as *D*-penicillamine (unlicensed) or more recently with *succimer* (2,3-dimercaptosuccinic acid, DMSA), a water-soluble analogue of dimercaprol with a high affinity for lead. Severe lead poisoning calls for parenteral therapy to initiate excretion and *sodium calcium edetate* is commonly used to chelate lead from bone and the extracellular space; urinary lead excretion diminishes over 5 days as the extracellular store is exhausted. Redistribution of lead from bone to brain may account for subsequent worsening of symptoms (colic and encephalopathy).

Dimercaprol is more effective than sodium calcium edetate at chelating lead from the soft tissues such as brain, which is the rationale for *combined therapy with sodium calcium edetate*.

Methanol is widely available as a solvent and in paints and antifreezes, and constitutes a cheap substitute for ethanol. Methanol itself has low toxicity but its metabolites are highly toxic. As little as 10 mL may cause permanent blindness and 30 mL may kill. Methanol, like ethanol, is metabolised by zero-order processes that involve the hepatic alcohol and aldehyde dehydrogenases, but, whereas ethanol forms ethanal and ethanoic acid (partly responsible for the unpleasant effects of 'hangover'), methanol forms methanal and methanoic acid. Blindness may occur because aldehyde dehydrogenase present in the retina (for the interconversion of retinol and retinene) allows the local formation of methanal. Acidosis is due to the methanoic acid, which itself enhances pH-dependent hepatic lactate production, adding the problems of lactic acidosis.

The clinical features include severe malaise, vomiting, abdominal pain and tachypnoea (due to the acidosis). Loss of visual acuity and scotomata indicate ocular damage and, if the pupils are dilated and non-reactive, permanent loss of sight is probable. Coma and circulatory collapse may follow. The key laboratory finding is a high anion gap acidosis. Blood methanol can be measured but does not correlate closely with the clinical picture.

Therapy is directed at:
- *Correcting the metabolic acidosis*. Achieving this largely determines the outcome; sodium bicarbonate is given intravenously in doses up to 2 mol in a few hours, carrying an excess of sodium which must be managed. Methanol is metabolised slowly and relapse may accompany too early discontinuation of bicarbonate.
- *Inhibiting methanol metabolism*. Ethanol, which occupies the dehydrogenase enzymes in preference to methanol, competitively prevents metabolism of methanol to its toxic products. A single oral dose of ethanol 1 mL/kg (as a 50% solution or as the equivalent in gin or whisky) is followed by 0.25 mL/kg·h orally or intravenously, aiming to maintain the blood ethanol at about 100 mg/100 mL until no methanol is detectable in the blood. Fomepizole (4-methylpyrazole), another competitive inhibitor of alcohol dehydrogenase, is effective in severe methanol poisoning and is less likely to cause cerebral depression (it is available in the UK on a named-patient basis).
- *Eliminating methanol and its metabolites*. Haemodialysis is two to three times more effective than is peritoneal dialysis and is indicated in severe cases.

Folinic acid 30 mg intravenously 6-hourly may protect against retinal damage by enhancing formate metabolism.

Ethylene glycol. Ethylene glycol is readily accessible as a constituent of antifreezes for car radiators (available as a 95% concentration). Its use to give 'body' and sweetness to white table wines was criminal. Metabolism to glycolate and oxalate causes acidosis and renal damage, a situation that is further complicated by lactic acidosis. The lethal dose for an adult is around 100 mL.

In the first 12 h after ingestion the patient appears as though intoxicated with alcohol but without the characteristic odour. Subsequently there is increasing acidosis, pulmonary oedema and cardiac failure. In 2–3 days renal pain and tubular necrosis develop because calcium oxalate crystals form in the urine. Intravenous sodium bicarbonate corrects the acidosis, and with calcium gluconate, the hypocalcaemia. As with methanol (above), ethanol or fomepizole competitively inhibit the metabolism of ethylene glycol and haemodialysis eliminates the poison.

Hydrocarbons. Common hydrocarbons include paraffin oil (kerosene), petrol (gasoline) and benzene. The specific toxic effects depend upon the chemical structure of the hydrocarbon, the dose and route of administration. In general, they cause CNS depression and pulmonary damage from inhalation. It is vital to avoid aspiration into the lungs with spontaneous vomiting.

Volatile solvent abuse. Solvent abuse or 'glue sniffing' is common among teenagers, especially males, although the prevalence has probably declined over the last 35 years. Data from 2004 suggested that 6% of 15-year-olds had engaged in the practice in the previous year. The success of the modern chemical industry provides easy access to these substances as adhesives, dry cleaners, air fresheners, deodorants, aerosols and other products. Viscous products are taken from a plastic bag, liquids from a handkerchief or plastic bottle.

The immediate euphoriant and excitatory effects give way to confusion, hallucinations and delusions as the dose is increased. Chronic abusers, notably of toluene, develop peripheral neuropathy, cerebellar disease and dementia; damage to the kidney, liver, heart and lungs also occurs with solvents. Evidence from 2006 suggested that one person per week dies in the UK from this practice and in 60% of these cases there was no previous history of abuse, suggesting that death commonly occurs on the first use. Over 50% of deaths from the practice follow cardiac arrhythmia, probably caused by sensitisation of the myocardium to catecholamines and by vagal inhibition from laryngeal stimulation due to aerosol propellants sprayed into the throat. Most deaths have been related to butane lighter fuel inhalation due to its particular tendency to induce cardiac arrhythmias. Death may also occur from acute intoxication impairing judgment, leading to accidents.

Acute solvent poisoning requires immediate cardiorespiratory resuscitation and anti-arrhythmia

treatment. Toxicity from carbon tetrachloride and chloroform involves the generation of phosgene, a First World War gas, which is inactivated by cysteine and by glutathione, formed from cysteine. Recommended treatment is therefore with *N*-acetylcysteine, as for poisoning with paracetamol.

Herbicides and pesticides

Organophosphorus pesticides are anticholinesterases; an account of poisoning and its management is given later. Organic carbamates are similar.

Dinitro-compounds. Dinitro-ortho-cresol (DNOC) and dinitrobutylphenol (DNBP) are selective weedkillers and insecticides, and cases of poisoning occur accidentally, e.g. by ignoring safety precautions. These substances can be absorbed through the skin and the hands, resulting in yellow staining of face or hair. Symptoms and signs indicate a very high metabolic rate (due to uncoupling of oxidative phosphorylation); copious sweating and thirst proceed to dehydration and vomiting, weakness, restlessness, tachycardia and deep, rapid breathing, convulsions and coma. Treatment is urgent and consists of cooling the patient and attention to fluid and electrolyte balance. It is essential to differentiate this type of poisoning from that due to anticholinesterases, because atropine given to patients poisoned with dinitrocompound will stop sweating and may cause death from hyperthermia.

Phenoxy herbicides (2,4-D, mecoprop, dichlorprop) are used to control broad-leaved weeds. Ingestion causes nausea, vomiting, pyrexia (due to uncoupling of oxidative phosphorylation), hyperventilation, hypoxia and coma. Urine alkalinisation accelerates elimination. Organochlorine pesticides, e.g. dicophane (DDT), may cause convulsions in acute overdose. Treat as for status epilepticus.

Rodenticides include warfarin and thallium; for strychnine, which causes convulsions, give diazepam.

Paraquat is a widely used herbicide that is extremely toxic if ingested; a mouthful of the commercial solution taken and spat out may be sufficient to kill. It is highly corrosive and can be absorbed through the skin. A common sequence is: ulceration and sloughing of the oral and oesophageal mucosa, renal tubular necrosis (5–10 days later), pulmonary oedema and pulmonary fibrosis. Whether the patient lives or dies depends largely on the condition of the lung. Treatment is urgent and includes activated charcoal or aluminium silicate (Fuller's earth) by mouth as adsorbents. Haemodialysis may have a role in the first 24 h, the rationale being to reduce the plasma concentration and protect the kidney, failure of which allows the slow but relentless accumulation of paraquat in the lung.

Diquat is similar to paraquat but the late pulmonary changes may not occur.

Incapacitating agents

CS (chlorobenzylidene malononitrile, a tear 'gas'). It is possible that a physician will be called upon to treat individuals who have been exposed to incapacitating agents. Such agents are designed to cause a temporary disablement that lasts for little longer than the period of exposure. CS is a solid that is disseminated as an aerosol (particles of 1 micron in diameter) by including it in a pyrotechnic mixture. It is an aerosol or smoke, not a gas. The particles aggregate and settle to the ground in minutes, so that the risk of prolonged exposure out of doors is not great. The onset of symptoms occurs immediately on exposure and they disappear dramatically.

According to the concentration of CS to which a person is exposed, the effects vary from a slight pricking or peppery sensation in the eyes and nasal passages up to the maximal symptoms of streaming from the eyes and nose, spasm of the eyelids, profuse lachrymation and salivation, retching and sometimes vomiting, burning of the mouth and throat, cough and gripping pain in the chest. Exposed subjects absorb small amounts only, and the plasma $t_{1/2}$ is about 5 s. There appear to be no long-lasting sequelae but, plainly, it would be prudent to assume that patients with asthma or chronic bronchitis could suffer an exacerbation from high concentrations.

CN (chloroacetophenone, a tear gas) is generally used as a solid aerosol or smoke; solutions (Mace) are used at close quarters.

CR (dibenzoxazepine) entered production in 1973 after testing on army volunteers. In addition to the usual properties (above) it may induce a transient rise in intraocular pressure. Its solubility allows use in water 'cannons'.

POISONING BY BIOLOGICAL SUBSTANCES

Many plants form substances that are important for their survival either by enticing animals, which disperse their spores, or by repelling potential predators. Poisoning occurs when children eat berries or chew flowers, attracted by their colour; adults may mistake non-edible for edible varieties of salad plants and fungi (mushrooms) for they may resemble one another closely and some are greatly prized by epicures. Ingestion of plants is responsible for a significant number of calls to poison information services (10% in US and German surveys) but serious poisonings are rare. Deaths from plant poisoning are thus very rare in industrialised societies. A recent study from the USA covering the period 1983—2000 identified only 30 fatalities over this 18-year period. Plant poisoning is, however, a significant problem in the developing world. Such deaths are almost exclusively deliberate suicide or homicide.

In addition many plants may cause cutaneous irritation, e.g. directly with nettle (*Urtica*), or dermatitis following sensitisation with *Primula*. Gastrointestinal symptoms, nausea, vomiting, diarrhoea and abdominal pain occur with numerous plants.

The treatment of plant poisonings consists mainly of giving activated charcoal to adsorb toxin in the gastrointestinal tract, supportive measures to maintain cardiorespiratory function, and control of convulsions with diazepam.

Specific measures. In 'death cap' (*Amanita phalloides*) mushroom poisoning, high dose penicillin or silibinin (an extract of the milk thistle) may be used to inhibit amatoxin uptake by the liver and its enterohepatic circulation. Antitoxins, e.g. Digibind, are used for poisoning with plants that produce toxic cardiac glycosides.

SUMMARY

Deliberate overdose with drugs is a common clinical problem. Poisoning may also occur as a result of accidental ingestion, occupational exposure and in the context of recreational substance use. The effective management of poisoning is based upon the use of general supportive measures, reduction of drug absorption or increase in elimination and the use of specific pharmacological agents ('antidotes'). This chapter will examine: background, initial assessment, resuscitation, supportive treatment, prevention of further absorption of the poison, acceleration of elimination of the poison, specific antidotes, psychiatric and social assessment, poisoning by non-drug chemicals (heavy metals, cyanide, methanol, ethylene glycol, hydrocarbons, volatile solvents, heavy metals, herbicides and pesticides), poisoning by biological substances.

IMPORTANT TERMINOLOGY

antidotes　解毒药

resuscitation　复苏

supportive treatment　支持疗法

specific antidotes　特异性解毒药

toxidromes　中毒综合征

alkalinisation　碱化作用

acidification　酸化作用

haemodialysis　血液透析

peritoneal dialysis　腹膜透析

metabolic acidosis　代谢性酸中毒

CHALLENGE YOURSELF

1. It is important to obtain information on the poison that has been taken. What are the key pieces of information are?
2. What are the main methods used for accelerating elimination of the poison?
3. What drugs can be readily tested for and detected in urine in the emergency department?

Minjie Wei

Chapter 10

Neurological disorders

Part 1. Cholinergic mechanisms and drugs

These drugs act on post-synaptic acetylcholine receptors (cholinoceptors) at all sites in the body where acetylcholine is the effective neurotransmitter. They initially stimulate and usually later block transmission. In addition, like acetylcholine, they act on the non-innervated receptors that relax peripheral blood vessels.

Uses of cholinergic drugs

- For myasthenia gravis, both to diagnose (edrophonium) and to treat symptoms (neostigmine, pyridostigmine, distigmine).
- To lower intraocular pressure in chronic simple glaucoma (pilocarpine).
- To bronchodilate patients with airflow obstruction (ipratropium, tiotropium).
- To improve cognitive function in Alzheimer's disease (rivastigmine, donepezil).

CLASSIFICATION

Direct-acting (receptor agonists)

- Choline esters (bethanechol, carbachol), which act at all sites, like acetylcholine, but are resistant to degradation by acetylcholinesterases (AChE; see Fig. 10.1). Muscarinic effects are much more prominent than nicotinic.

- Alkaloids (pilocarpine, muscarine) act selectively on end-organs of postganglionic, cholinergic neurones. Effects are exclusively muscarinic.

Indirect-acting

Cholinesterase inhibitors, or anticholinesterases (physostigmine, neostigmine, pyridostigmine, distigmine, galantamine, rivastigmine, donepezil), block acetylcholinesterase (AChE), the enzyme that destroys acetylcholine, allowing endogenous acetylcholine to persist and produce intensified effects.

SITES OF ACTION (Fig. 10.1)

- Autonomic nervous system (Fig. 10.1, sites 1 and 2).
- Neuromuscular junction (Fig. 10.1, site 1).
- Central nervous system (CNS).
- Non-innervated sites: blood vessels, chiefly arterioles (Fig. 10.1, site 3).
- Acetylcholine is released from nerve terminals to activate a post-synaptic receptor, except on blood vessels, where the action of cholinergic drugs is unrelated to cholinergic 'vasodilator' nerves. It is also produced in tissues unrelated to nerve endings, e.g. placenta and ciliated epithelial cells, where it acts as a local hormone (autacoid) on local receptors.

A list of principal effects is given below. Not all occur with every drug and not all are noticeable at therapeutic doses. For example, CNS effects of cholinergic drugs are best seen in cases of anticholinesterase poisoning. Atropine antagonises all the effects of cholinergic drugs except nicotinic actions on autonomic ganglia and the neuromuscular junction, i.e. it has antimuscarinic but not antinicotinic effects.

Fig. 10.1 The different origins of acetylcholine (ACh) activating nicotinic (N) versus muscarinic (M) cholinergic receptors. The three sites (numbered 1–3) are referred to in the text.

PHARMACOLOGY

Autonomic nervous system

There are two distinct classes of receptor for acetylcholine, defined on the basis of their preferential activation by the alkaloids nicotine (from tobacco) and muscarine (from a toxic mushroom, *Amanita muscaria*).

It was Henry Dale who, in 1914, first made this functional division, which remains a robust and useful way of classifying cholinergic drug effects. He noted that the actions of acetylcholine and substances acting like it at autonomic ganglia and the neuromuscular junction mimic the stimulant effects of nicotine (hence nicotinic). In contrast, the actions at postganglionic cholinergic endings (parasympathetic endings plus the cholinergic sympathetic nerves to the sweat glands) and non-innervated

receptors on blood vessels resembled the alkaloid, muscarine (hence muscarinic).

Parasympathetic division. Stimulation of cholinoceptors in autonomic ganglia and at postganglionic endings affects chiefly the following organs:

- Eye: miosis and spasm of the ciliary muscle occur so that the eye is accommodated for near vision. Intraocular pressure falls.
- Exocrine glands: there is increased secretion most noticeably from salivary, lachrymal, bronchial and sweat glands. The last are cholinergic, but anatomically part of the sympathetic system; some sweat glands, e.g. axillary, may be adrenergic.
- Heart: bradycardia occurs with atrioventricular block, and eventually cardiac arrest.
- Bronchi: there is bronchoconstriction and mucosal hypersecretion that may be clinically serious in asthmatic subjects, in whom cholinergic drugs should be avoided if possible.
- Gut: motor activity is increased and may cause colicky pain. Exocrine secretion is also increased. Tone in sphincters falls, which may cause defaecation (anal sphincter) or acid reflux/regurgitation (oesophageal sphincter).
- Urinary bladder and ureters contract and the drugs promote micturition.

Sympathetic division. Only the ganglia are stimulated and cholinergic nerves to the adrenal medulla. These effects are overshadowed by effects on the parasympathetic system and are usually seen only if atropine has been given to block the latter, when tachycardia, vasoconstriction and hypertension occur.

Neuromuscular (voluntary) junction

The neuromuscular junction has cholinergic nerve endings and so is activated when anticholinesterases allow acetylcholine to persist, causing muscle fasciculation. Prolonged activation leads to a secondary depolarising neuromuscular block.

Central nervous system

There is usually stimulation followed by depression but considerable variation between drugs is observed, possibly due to differences in CNS penetration. In overdose, mental excitement occurs, with confusion and restlessness, insomnia (with nightmares during sleep), tremors and dysarthria, and sometimes even convulsions and coma. Nicotinic receptor activation in the CNS is also thought to be important for cognitive processing, which appears to be impaired in schizophrenic subjects.

Blood vessels

There is stimulation of cholinergic vasodilator nerve endings in addition to the more important dilating action on arterioles and capillaries mediated through non-innervated muscarinic receptors. Activation of these receptors stimulates nitric oxide production from the vascular endothelium that relaxes the underlying smooth muscle.

Choline esters

Acetylcholine

As acetylcholine has such importance in the body it is not surprising that attempts have been made to use it therapeutically. But a substance with such a huge variety of effects and rapid destruction in the body is unlikely to be useful when given systemically, as its use in psychiatry illustrates.

Acetylcholine was first injected intravenously as a therapeutic convulsant in 1939, in the reasonable expectation that the fits would be less liable to cause fractures than those following therapeutic leptazol (pentylenetetrazole) convulsions. Recovery rates of up to 80% were claimed in various psychotic conditions. Enthusiasm began to wane, however, when it was shown that the fits were due to anoxia resulting from cardiac arrest and not to pharmacological effects on the brain.

The following description is typical:

A few seconds after the injection (which was given as rapidly as possible, to avoid total destruction in the blood) the patient sat up 'with knees drawn up to the chest, the arms flexed and the head bent forward. There were repeated violent coughs, sometimes with flushing. Forced swallowing and loud peristaltic rumblings could be heard'. Respiration was laboured and irregular. 'The coughing abated as the patient sank back in the bed. Forty seconds after the injection the radial and apical pulse were zero and the patient became comatose.' The pupils dilated, and deep reflexes were hyperactive. In 45 seconds the patient went into opisthotonos with brief apnoea.

Lachrymation, sweating and borborygmi were prominent. The deep reflexes became diminished. The patient then relaxed and 'lay quietly in bed – cold moist and gray. In about 90 seconds, flushing of the face marked the return of the pulse'. The respiratory rate rose and consciousness returned in about 125 seconds. The patients sometimes micturated but did not defaecate. They 'tended to lie quietly in bed after the treatment'. 'Most of the patients were reluctant to be retreated.'

Other choline esters

Carbachol is not destroyed by cholinesterase; its actions are most pronounced on the bladder and gastrointestinal tract, so that the drug was used to stimulate these organs, e.g. after surgery. These uses are now virtually obsolete, e.g. catheterisation is preferred for bladder atony. It is occasionally applied topically (3% solution) to the eye as a miotic.

Bethanechol resembles carbachol in its actions but is some 10-fold less potent (it differs by a single b-methyl group) and has no significant nicotinic effects at clinical doses.

Alkaloids with cholinergic effects

Nicotine is a social drug that lends its medicinal use as an adjunct to stopping its own abuse as tobacco. It is available as gum to chew, dermal patches, a nasal spray or an inhalator. These deliver a lower dose of nicotine than cigarettes and appear to be safe in patients with ischaemic heart disease. The patches are slightly better tolerated than the gum, which releases nicotine in a more variable fashion depending on the rate at which it is chewed and the salivary pH, which is influenced by drinking coffee and carbonated drinks. Nicotine treatment is reported to be nearly twice as effective as placebo in achieving sustained withdrawal from smoking (18% versus 11% in one review). Treatment is much more likely to be successful if it is used as an aid to, not a substitute for, continued counselling. Bupropion is possibly more effective than the nicotine patch and the partial nicotinic agonist, varenicline, slightly more effective still. The efficacy of varenicline is tempered by its ability to cause suicidal ideation and behaviour.

Pilocarpine, from a South American plant (Pilocarpus spp.), acts directly on muscarinic receptors (see Fig. 10.1); it also stimulates and then depresses the CNS. The chief clinical use of pilocarpine is to lower intraocular pressure in primary open-angle glaucoma (also called chronic simple or wide-angle glaucoma), as an adjunct to a topical β-blocker; it produces miosis, opens drainage channels in the trabecular network and improves the outflow of aqueous humour. Oral pilocarpine is available for the treatment of xerostomia (dry mouth) in Sjö gren's syndrome, or following irradiation of head and neck tumours. The commonest adverse effect is sweating, an effect actually exploited in a diagnostic test for cystic fibrosis.

Anticholinesterases

At cholinergic nerve endings and in erythrocytes there is a specific enzyme that destroys acetylcholine, true cholinesterase or acetylcholinesterase. In various tissues, especially plasma, there are other esterases that are not specific for acetylcholine but that also destroy other esters, e.g. suxamethonium, procaine (and cocaine) and bambuterol (a prodrug that is hydrolysed to terbutaline). Hence, they are called pseudocholinesterases. Chemicals that inactivate these esterases (anticholinesterases) are used in medicine and in agriculture as pesticides. They act by allowing naturally synthesised acetylcholine to accumulate instead of being destroyed. Their effects are explained by this accumulation in the CNS, neuromuscular junction, autonomic ganglia, postganglionic cholinergic nerve endings (which are principally in the parasympathetic nervous system) and in the walls of blood vessels, where acetylcholine has a paracrine role not necessarily associated with nerve

endings. Some of these effects oppose one another, e.g. the effect of anticholinesterase on the heart will be the result of stimulation at sympathetic ganglia and the opposing effect of stimulation at parasympathetic (vagal) ganglia and at postganglionic nerve endings.

Physostigmine is an alkaloid, obtained from the seeds of the West African Calabar bean (spp. Physostigma), which has had long use both as a weapon and as an ordeal poison. It acts for a few hours. It has been shown to have some efficacy in improving cognitive function in Alzheimer-type dementia.

Neostigmine ($t_{1/2}$ 2 h) is a synthetic reversible anticholinesterase whose actions are more prominent on the neuromuscular junction and the alimentary tract than on the cardiovascular system and eye. It is therefore used principally in myasthenia gravis and as an antidote to competitive neuromuscular blocking agents; its use to stimulate the bowels or bladder after surgery is now obsolete. Neostigmine is effective orally, and by injection (usually subcutaneous). But higher doses may be used in myasthenia gravis, often combined with atropine to reduce the unwanted muscarinic effects.

Pyridostigmine is similar to neostigmine but has a less powerful action that is slower in onset and slightly longer in duration, and perhaps with fewer visceral effects. It is used in myasthenia gravis.

A more recent use of anticholinesterase drugs has been to improve cognitive function in patients with Alzheimer's disease, where both the degree of dementia and amyloid plaque density correlate with the impairment of brain cholinergic function. Donepezil, galantamine (which has additional nicotinic agonist properties) and rivastigmine are licensed in the UK for this indication. They are all reversible inhibitors that are orally active and cross the blood–brain barrier readily.

Anticholinesterase poisoning

The anticholinesterases used in therapeutics are generally of the carbamate type that reversibly inactivates cholinesterase only for a few hours. This contrasts markedly with the very long-lived inhibition caused by inhibitors of the organophosphate (OP) type. In practice, the inhibition is so long that clinical recovery from organophosphate exposure is usually dependent on synthesis of new enzyme. This process may take weeks to complete, although clinical recovery is usually evident in days. Cases of acute poisoning are usually met outside therapeutic practice, e.g. after agricultural, industrial or transport accidents.

Substances of this type have also been developed and used in war, especially the three G agents: GA (tabun), GB (sarin) and GD (soman). Although called nerve 'gas', they are actually volatile liquids, which facilitates their use. Where there is known risk of exposure, prior use of pyridostigmine, which occupies cholinesterases reversibly for a few hours (the lesser evil), competitively protects them from access by the irreversible warfare agent (the greater evil); soldiers during the Gulf Wars expecting attack were provided with preloaded syringes (of the same design as the Epipen) for delivering adrenaline/epinephrine as antidote therapy. Organophosphate agents are absorbed through the skin, the gastrointestinal tract and by inhalation. Diagnosis depends on observing a substantial part of the list of actions below.

Typical features of acute poisoning involve the gastrointestinal tract (salivation, vomiting, abdominal cramps, diarrhoea, involuntary defaecation), the respiratory system (bronchorrhoea, bronchoconstriction, cough, wheezing, dyspnoea), the cardiovascular system (bradycardia), the genitourinary system (involuntary micturition), the skin (sweating), the skeletal system (muscle weakness, twitching) and the nervous system (miosis, anxiety, headache, convulsions, respiratory failure). Death is due to a combination of the actions in the CNS, to paralysis of the respiratory muscles by peripheral depolarising neuromuscular block, and to excessive bronchial secretions and constriction causing respiratory failure. At autopsy, ileal intussusceptions are commonly found.

Quite frequently and typically 1–4 days after resolution of symptoms of acute exposure, the intermediate syndrome may develop, characterised by a proximal flaccid limb paralysis that may reflect

muscle necrosis. Even later, after a gap of 2–4 weeks, some exposed persons exhibit delayed polyneuropathy, with sensory and motor impairment usually of the lower limbs. Claims of chronic effects (subtle cognitive defects, peripheral neuropathy) following recurrent, low-dose exposure, as with organophosphate used as sheep dip, continue to be the subject of investigation but, as yet, there is no conclusive proof.

Treatment. As the most common circumstance of accidental poisoning is exposure to pesticide spray or spillage, contaminated clothing should be removed and the skinwashed. Attendants should take care to ensure that they themselves do not become contaminated.

- Atropine is the mainstay of treatment; 2 mg is given i.m. or i.v. as soon as possible and repeated every 15–60 min until dryness of the mouth and a heart rate exceeding 70 beats per minute indicate that its effect is adequate. A poisoned patient may require 100 mg or more for a single episode. Atropine antagonises the muscarinic parasympathomimetic effects of the poison, i.e. due to the accumulated acetylcholine stimulating postganglionic nerve endings (excessive secretion and vasodilatation), but has no effect on the neuromuscular block, which is nicotinic.

- Mechanical ventilation may therefore be needed to assist the respiratory muscles; special attention to the airway is vital because of bronchial constriction and excessive secretion.

- Diazepam may be needed for convulsions.

- Atropine eye drops may relieve the headache caused by miosis.

- Enzyme reactivation. The organophosphate (OP) pesticides inactivate cholinesterase by irreversibly phosphorylating the active centre of the enzyme. Substances that reactivate the enzyme hasten the destruction of the accumulated acetylcholine and, unlike atropine, they have both antinicotinic and antimuscarinic effects. The principal agent is pralidoxime, which should be given by slow intravenous injection (diluted) over 5–10 min, initially 30 mg/kg repeated every 4–6 h or by intravenous infusion, 8 mg/kg·h; usual maximum 12 g in 24 h.

Its efficacy is greatest if administered within 12 h of poisoning, then falls off steadily as the phosphorylated enzyme is further stabilised by 'ageing'. If significant reactivation occurs, muscle power improves within 30 min.

Poisoning with reversible anticholinesterases is appropriately treated by atropine and the necessary general support; it lasts only hours.

In poisoning with irreversible agents, erythrocyte or plasma cholinesterase content should be measured if possible, both for diagnosis and to determine when a poisoned worker may return to the task (should he or she be willing to do so). Return should not be allowed until the cholinesterase exceeds 70% of normal, which may take several weeks. Recovery from the intermediate syndrome and delayed polyneuropathy is slow and is dependent on muscle and nerve regeneration.

DISORDERS OF NEUROMUSCULAR TRANSMISSION

Myasthenia gravis

In myasthenia gravis synaptic transmission at the neuromuscular junction is impaired; most cases have an autoimmune basis and some 85% of patients have a raised titre of autoantibodies to the muscle acetylcholine receptor. The condition is probably heterogeneous, as about 15% do not have receptor antibodies, or have antibodies to another neuromuscular junction protein (muscle specific kinase, MuSK) and, rarely, it occurs with D-penicillamine used for rheumatoid arthritis.

Neostigmine was introduced in 1931 for its stimulant effects on intestinal activity. In 1934 it occurred to Dr Mary Walker that, as the paralysis of myasthenia had been (erroneously) attributed to a curare-like substance in the blood, physostigmine (eserine), an anticholinesterase drug known to antagonise curare, might be beneficial. It was, and she reported this important observation in a short letter. Soon after this she used neostigmine by mouth, with greater benefit.

Pathogenesis. The clinical features of myasthenia gravis are caused by specific autoantibodies to the nicotinic acetylcholine receptor. These antibodies accelerate receptor turnover, shortening their typical lifetime in the skeletal muscle membrane from around 7 days, to 1 day in a myasthenic. This process results in marked depletion of receptors from myasthenic skeletal muscle (about 90%), explaining its fatigability. The frequent finding of a specific human leucocyte antigen (HLA) haplotype (A1-B8-Dw3) in myasthenics and concurrent hyperplasia or tumours of the thymus support the autoimmune basis for the disease.

Diagnosis. Edrophonium dramatically and transiently (5 min) relieves myasthenic muscular weakness. A syringe is loaded with edrophonium 10 mg; 2 mg is given i.v. and if there is no improvement in weakness in 30 s the remaining 8 mg is injected. Adults without suitable veins may receive 10 mg by i.m. injection. Atropine should be at hand to block severe cholinergic autonomic (muscarinic) effects, e.g. bradycardia, should they occur. Titres of acetylcholine receptor antibodies should also be measured to confirm the diagnosis.

Treatment involves immunosuppression, thymectomy (unless contraindicated) and symptom relief with drugs:

- Immunosuppressive treatment is directed at eliminating the acetylcholine receptor autoantibody. Prednisolone induces improvement or remission in 80% of cases. The dose should be increased slowly using an alternate day regimen until the minimum effective amount is attained; an immunosuppressive improvement may take several weeks. Azathioprine may be used as a steroid-sparing agent. Prednisolone is effective for ocular myasthenia, which is fortunate, for this variant of the disease responds poorly to thymectomy or anticholinesterase drugs. Some acute and severe cases respond poorly to prednisolone with azathioprine and, for these, intermittent plasmapheresis or immunoglobulin i.v. (to remove circulating anti-receptor antibody) can provide dramatic short-term relief.

- Thymectomy should be offered to those with generalised myasthenia gravis under 40 years of age, once the clinical state allows and unless there are powerful contraindications to surgery. Most cases benefit and about 25% can discontinue drug treatment. Thymectomy should also be undertaken in all myasthenic patients who have a thymoma, but the main reason is to prevent local infiltration, as the procedure is less likely to relieve the myasthenia.

- Symptomatic drug treatment is decreasingly used. Its aim is to increase the concentration of acetylcholine at the neuromuscular junction with anticholinesterase drugs. The mainstay is usually pyridostigmine, starting with 60 mg by mouth 4-hourly. It is preferred because its action is smoother than that of neostigmine, but the latter is more rapid in onset and can with advantage be given in the mornings to get the patient mobile. Either drug can be given parenterally if bulbar paralysis makes swallowing difficult. An antimuscarinic drug, e.g. propantheline (15–30 mg t.i.d.), should be added if muscarinic effects are troublesome.

Excessive dosing with an anticholinesterase can actually worsen the muscle weakness in myasthenics if the accumulation of acetylcholine at the neuromuscular junction is sufficient to cause depolarising blockade (cholinergic crisis). It is important to distinguish this type of muscle weakness from an exacerbation of the disease itself (myasthenic crisis). The dilemma can be resolved with a test dose of edrophonium 2 mg i.v. (best before next dose of anticholinesterase), which relieves a myasthenic crisis but worsens a cholinergic one. The latter may be severe enough to precipitate respiratory failure and should be attempted only with full resuscitation facilities, including mechanical ventilation, at hand.

A cholinergic crisis should be treated by withdrawing all anticholinesterase medication, mechanical ventilation if required, and atropine i.v. for muscarinic effects of the overdose. The neuromuscular block is a nicotinic effect and will be unchanged by atropine. A resistant myasthenic crisis may be treated by withdrawal of drugs and mechanical ventilation for a few days. Plasmapheresis or immunoglobulin i.v. may be beneficial by removing anti-receptor antibodies.

Lambert–Eaton syndrome

Separate from myasthenia gravis is the Lambert–Eaton syndrome, in which symptoms similar to those of myasthenia gravis occur in association with a carcinoma; in 60% of patients this is a small-cell lung cancer. The defect here is pre-synaptic with a deficiency of acetylcholine release due to an autoantibody directed against L-type voltagegated calcium channels.

Patients with the Lambert–Eaton syndrome do not usually respond well to anticholinesterases. The drug 3,4-diaminopyridine (3,4-DAP) increases neurotransmitter release and also the action potential (by blocking potassium conductance), producing a nonspecific enhancement of cholinergic neurotransmission. It should be taken orally, four or five times a day. Adverse effects due to CNS excitation (insomnia, seizures) can occur. An example of an orphan drug without a product licence, 3,4-DAP is available in the UK on a 'named patient' basis.

Drug-induced disorders of neuromuscular transmission

Quite apart from the neuromuscular blocking agents used in anaesthesia, a number of drugs possess actions that impair neuromuscular transmission and, in appropriate circumstances, give rise to:

- Postoperative respiratory depression in people with otherwise normal neuromuscular transmission.

- Aggravation or unmasking of myasthenia gravis.

- A drug-induced myasthenic syndrome.

  These drugs include:

Antimicrobials. Aminoglycosides (neomycin, streptomycin, gentamicin), polypeptides (colistimethate sodium, polymyxin B) and perhaps the quinolones (e.g. ciprofloxacin) may cause postoperative breathing difficulty if they are instilled into the peritoneal or pleural cavity. It appears that the antibiotics both interfere with the release of acetylcholine and also have a competitive curare-like effect on the acetylcholine receptor.

Cardiovascular drugs. Those that possess local anaesthetic properties (quinidine, procainamide, lidocaine) and certain b-blockers (propranolol, oxprenolol) interfere with acetylcholine release and may aggravate or reveal myasthenia gravis.

Other drugs. Penicillamine causes some patients, especially those with rheumatoid arthritis, to form antibodies to the acetylcholine receptor and a syndrome indistinguishable from myasthenia gravis results. Spontaneous recovery occurs in about two-thirds of cases when penicillamine is withdrawn. Phenytoin may rarely induce or aggravate myasthenia gravis, or induce a myasthenic syndrome, possibly by depressing release of acetylcholine. Lithium may impair pre-synaptic neurotransmission by substituting for sodium ions in the nerve terminal.

Part 2. Drugs that oppose acetylcholine

These may be divided into:

- Antimuscarinic drugs, which act principally at postganglionic cholinergic (parasympathetic) nerve endings, i.e. atropine-related drugs. Muscarinic receptors can be subdivided according to their principal sites, namely in the brain (M1), heart (M2) and glandular, gastric parietal cells and smooth muscle cells (M3). As with many receptors, the molecular basis of the subtypes has been defined together with two further cloned subtypes M4 and M5, the precise functional roles of which remain to be clarified.
- Antinicotinic drugs:
  - ganglion-blocking drugs
  - neuromuscular blocking drugs

Antimuscarinic drugs

Atropine is the prototype drug of this group and will be described first. Other named agents will be mentioned only in so far as they differ from atropine. All act as non-selective and competitive antagonists of the various muscarinic receptor subtypes (above). Atropine is a simple tertiary amine; certain others are quaternary nitrogen compounds, a modification that increases antimuscarinic potency in the gut, imparts ganglion-blocking effects and reduces CNS penetration.

Atropine

Atropine is an alkaloid from the deadly nightshade, Atropa belladonna. It is a racemate (DL-hyoscyamine), and almost all of its antimuscarinic effects are attributable to the L-isomer alone. Atropine is more stable chemically as the racemate, which is the preferred formulation. In general, the effects of atropine are inhibitory but in large doses it stimulates the CNS. Atropine also blocks the muscarinic effects of injected cholinergic drugs, both peripherally and on the CNS. The clinically important actions of atropine at parasympathetic postganglionic nerve endings are listed below; they are mostly the opposite of the activating effects on the parasympathetic system produced by cholinergic drugs.

Exocrine glands. All secretions except milk are diminished. Dry mouth and dry eye are common. Gastric acid secretion is reduced but so also is the total volume of gastric secretion, so that pH may be little altered. Sweating is inhibited (sympathetic innervation but releasing acetylcholine). Bronchial secretions are reduced and may become viscid, which can be a disadvantage, as removal of secretion by cough and ciliary action is rendered less effective.

Smooth muscle is relaxed. In the gastrointestinal tract there is reduction of tone and peristalsis. Muscle spasm of the intestinal tract induced by morphine is reduced, but such spasm in the biliary tract is not significantly affected. Atropine relaxes bronchial muscle, an effect that is useful in some asthmatics. Micturition is slowed and urinary retention may be induced, especially when there is pre-existing prostatic enlargement.

Ocular effects. Mydriasis occurs with a rise in intraocular pressure due to the dilated iris blocking drainage of the intraocular fluid from the angle of the anterior chamber. An attack of glaucoma may be induced in eyes predisposed to primary angle (also called acute closed-angle or narrow angle) closure and is a medical emergency. There is no significant effect on pressure in normal eyes. The ciliary muscle is paralysed and so the eye is accommodated for distant vision. After atropinisation, normal pupillary reflexes may not be regained for 2 weeks. Atropine use is a cause of unequally sized and unresponsive pupils.

Cardiovascular system. Atropine reduces vagal tone, thus increasing the heart rate and enhancing conduction in the bundle of His. As efficacy depends on the level of vagal tone, full atropinisation may increase heart rate by 30 beats/min in a young subject, but has little effect in the elderly.

Atropine has no significant effect on peripheral blood vessels in therapeutic doses but in overdose there is marked vasodilatation.

Central nervous system. Atropine is effective against both the tremor and rigidity of parkinsonism. It prevents or abates motion sickness.

Antagonism to cholinergic drugs. Atropine opposes the effects of muscarinic agonists on the CNS, at postganglionic cholinergic nerve endings and on peripheral blood vessels. It does not block cholinergic effects at the neuromuscular junction or significantly at the autonomic ganglia, i.e. atropine opposes the muscarine-like but not the nicotine-like effects of acetylcholine.

Pharmacokinetics. Atropine is readily absorbed from the gastrointestinal tract and may also be injected by the usual routes, including intratracheal instillation in an emergency setting. The occasional cases of atropine poisoning following use of eye drops are due to the solution running down the lachrymal ducts into the nose and being swallowed. Atropine is in part destroyed in the liver and in part excreted unchanged by the kidney ($t_{1/2}$ 2 h).

Dose. 0.6–1.2 mg by mouth at night or 0.6 mg i.v., repeated as necessary to a maximum of 3 mg per day; for chronic use atropine has largely been replaced by other antimuscarinic drugs.

Poisoning with atropine (and other antimuscarinic drugs) presents with the more obvious periph-eral effects: dry mouth (with dysphagia), mydriasis, blurred vision, hot, flushed, dry skin, and, in addition, hyperthermia (CNS action plus absence of sweating), restlessness, anxiety, excitement, hallucinations, delirium, mania. The cerebral excitation is followed by depression and coma or, as it has been described with characteristic American verbal felicity, 'hot as a hare, blind as a bat, dry as a bone, red as a beet and mad as a hen'. Poisoning is typically seen (especially in children) following ingestion of the rather attractive berries of solanaceous plants, e.g. deadly nightshade and henbane. Treatment involves activated charcoal to adsorb the drug, sponging to cool the patient and diazepam for the central excitement.

Other antimuscarinic drugs

In the following accounts, the peripheral atropine-like effects of the drugs may be assumed; only differences from atropine are described.

Hyoscine (scopolamine) is structurally a close relative of atropine. It differs chiefly in being a CNS depressant, although it may sometimes cause excitement. Elderly patients are often confused by hyoscine and so it is avoided in their anaesthetic premedication. Mydriasis is also briefer than with atropine.

Hyoscine butylbromide (strictly N-butylhyoscine bromide; Buscopan) also blocks autonomic ganglia. If injected, it is an effective relaxant of smooth muscle, including the cardia in achalasia, the pyloric antral region and the colon, properties utilised by radiologists and endoscopists. It may sometimes be useful for colic.

Homatropine is used for its ocular effects (1%and 2% solutions as eye drops). Its action is shorter than that of atropine, and it is therefore less likely to cause serious increases in intraocular pressure; the effect wears off in a day or two. Complete cycloplegia cannot always be obtained unless repeated instillations are made every 15 min for 1–2 h. Its effects are especially unreliable in children, in whom cyclopentolate or atropine is preferred. The pupillary dilatation may be reversed by physostigmine eye drops.

Tropicamide (Mydriacyl) and cyclopentolate

(Mydrilate) are useful (as 0.5% or 1%solutions) for mydriasis and cycloplegia. They are quicker and shorter acting than homatropine. Both cause mydriasis in 10–20 min and cycloplegia shortly thereafter. The duration of action is 4–12 h.

Ipratropium (Atrovent) is used as an inhaled bronchodilator for both acute asthma and chronic obstructive pulmonary disease (COPD), and in chronic COPD. It has very limited efficacy in most chronic asthmatics.

Tiotropium (Spiriva) is a long-acting (>24 h) alternative to ipratropium, but only for patients with chronic COPD. It is not licensed for acute bronchoconstriction because of its slow onset of action.

Flavoxate (Urispas) is used for urinary frequency, tenesmus and urgency incontinence because it increases bladder capacity and reduces unstable detrusor contractions.

Oxybutynin is also used for detrusor instability, but antimuscarinic adverse effects may limit its value.

Propantheline (Pro-Banthine) also has ganglionblocking properties. It may be used as a smooth muscle relaxant, e.g. for irritable bowel syndrome and diagnostic procedures.

Dicyclomine (Merbentyl) is an alternative.

Benzhexol. (trihexyphenidyl) and orphenadrine: see parkinsonism.

Propiverine, tolterodine and trospium diminish unstable detrusor contractions and are used to reduce urinary frequency, urgency and incontinence.

Oral antimuscarinics have occasional use in the treatment of hyperhidrosis.

Uses of antimuscarinic drugs

- **For their central actions** – some (trihexyphenidyl (benzhexol) and orphenadrine) are used against the rigidity and tremor of parkinsonism, especially drug-induced parkinsonism, where doses higher than the usual therapeutic amounts are often needed and tolerated. They are used as antiemetics (principally hyoscine, promethazine). Their sedative action is used in anaesthetic premedication (hyoscine).

- **For their peripheral actions** – atropine, homatropine and cyclopentolate are used in ophthalmology to dilate the pupil and to paralyse ocular accommodation. Patients should be warned of a transient, but unpleasant, stinging sensation, and that they cannot read or drive (at least without dark glasses) for at least 3–4 h. Tropicamide is the shortest acting of the mydriatics. If it is desired to dilate the pupil and to spare accommodation, a sympathomimetic, e.g. phenylephrine, is useful.

  In anaesthesic premedication, atropine, and hyoscine* block the vagus and reduce mucosal secretions; hyoscine also has useful sedative effects. Glycopyrronium* is frequently used during anaesthetic recovery to block the muscarinic effects of neostigmine given to reverse a nondepolarising neuromuscular blockade.

  In the respiratory tract, ipratropium* is a useful bronchodilator in chronic obstructive pulmonary disease and acute asthma.

- **For their actions on the gut**, against muscle spasm and hypermotility, e.g. against colic (pain due to spasmof smooth muscle), and to reduce morphine-induced smooth muscle spasm when the analgesic is used against acute colic.

- **In the urinary tract**, flavoxate, oxybutynin, propiverine, tolterodine, trospium and propantheline* are used to relieve muscle spasm accompanying infection in cystitis, and for detrusor instability.

- **In disorders of the cardiovascular system**, atropine is useful in bradycardia following myocardial infarction.

- **In cholinergic poisoning**, atropine is an important antagonist of both central nervous, parasympathomimetic and vasodilator effects, though it has no effect at the neuromuscular junction and will not prevent voluntary muscle paralysis. It is also used to block muscarinic effects when cholinergic drugs, suchasneostigmine, are used for their effect on the neuromuscular junction in myasthenia gravis.

Disadvantages of the antimuscarinics include glaucoma and urinary retention, where there is prostatic hypertrophy.

---

*Quaternary ammonium compounds (see text).

Part 3. Adrenergic mechanisms and drugs

ADRENERGIC MECHANISMS

The discovery in 1895 of the hypertensive effect of adrenaline/epinephrine was initiated by Dr Oliver, a physician in practice, who conducted a series of experiments on his young son into whom he injected an extract of bovine suprarenal and detected a 'definite narrowing of the radial artery'. The effect was confirmed in animals and led eventually to the isolation and synthesis of adrenaline/epinephrine in the early 1900s. Many related compounds were examined and, in 1910, Barger and Dale invented the word sympathomimetic and also pointed out that noradrenaline/norepinephrine mimicked the action of the sympathetic nervous system more closely than did adrenaline/epinephrine.

Adrenaline/epinephrine, noradrenaline/norepinephrine and dopamine are synthesised in the body and are used in therapeutics. The pathway is: tyrosine→ dopa→dopamine→noradrenaline/norepinephrine→ adrenaline/epinephrine. The final step to adrenaline/ epinephrine only occurs in the adrenal medulla.

CLASSIFICATION OF SYMPATHOMI-METICS

By mode of action

Noradrenaline/norepinephrine is synthesised and stored in vesicles within adrenergic nerve terminals (Fig. 10.2). The vesicles can be released from these stores by stimulating the nerve or by drugs (ephedrine, amfetamine). The noradrenaline/norepinephrine stores can also be replenished by intravenous infusion of noradrenaline/norepinephrine, and abolished by reserpine or by cutting the sympathetic nerve. Sympathomimetics may be classified on the basis of their sites of action (Fig. 10.2) as acting:

1. **Directly:** adrenoceptor agonists, e.g. adrenaline/ epinephrine, noradrenaline/norepinephrine, isoprenaline (isoproterenol), methoxamine, xylometazoline, metaraminol (entirely); and dopamine and phenylephrine (mainly).

Fig 10.2 Noradrenergic nerve terminal releasing noradrenaline/norepinephrine (NA) to show the sites of action of drugs that impair or mimic adrenergic function. α and β refer to adrenergic receptor subtypes; MAO, monoamine oxidase.

2. **Indirectly:** by causing a release of preformed noradrenaline/norepinephrine from stores in nerve endings, e.g. amfetamines, tyramine; and ephedrine (largely).

3. **By both mechanisms** (1 and 2, though one usually predominates): other synthetic agents.

All of the above mechanisms operate in both the central and peripheral nervous systems, but discussion below will focus on agents that influence peripheral adrenergic mechanisms.

Tachyphylaxis (rapidly diminishing response to repeated administration) is a particular feature of group 2 drugs. It reflects depletion of the 'releasable' pool of noradrenaline/norepinephrine from adrenergic nerve terminals that makes these agents less suitable as, for example, pressor agents than drugs in group 1. Longer-term tolerance to the effects of direct sympathomimetics is much less of a clinical problem and reflects an alteration in adrenergic receptor density or coupling to second messenger systems.

Interactions of sympathomimetics with other vasoactive drugs are complex. Some drugs block the reuptake mechanism for noradrenaline/norepinephrine in adrenergic nerve terminals and potentiate the pressor effects of noradrenaline/norepinephrine, e.g. cocaine, tricyclic antidepressants or highly noradrenaline/norepinephrine-selective reuptake inhibitors (NSRIs) such as reboxetine (see Fig. 10.2). Others deplete or destroy the intracellular stores within adrenergic nerve terminals (e.g. reserpine and guanethidine) and thus block the action of indirect sympathomimetics.

Sympathomimetics are also generally optically active drugs, with only one stereoisomer conferring most of the clinical efficacy of the racemate (a 50:50 mixture of stereoisomers); for instance, L-noradrenaline/norepinephrine is at least 50 times as active as the D-form. Noradrenaline/norepinephrine, adrenaline/epinephrine and phenylephrine are all used clinically as their L-isomers.

Consequences of adrenoceptor activation

All adrenoceptors are members of the G-coupled family of receptor proteins, i.e. the receptor is coupled to its effector protein through special transduction proteins called G-proteins (themselves a large protein family). The effector protein differs among adrenoceptor subtypes. In the case of β-adrenoceptors, the effector is adenylyl cyclase and hence cyclic AMP is the second messenger molecule. For a-adrenoceptors, phospholipase C is the commonest effector protein and the second messenger here is inositol trisphosphate (IP3).

Selectivity for adrenoceptors

Selectivity is relative, not absolute; some agonists act on both α and β receptors, some are partial agonists and, if sufficient drug is administered, many will extend their range. The same applies to selective antagonists (receptor blockers), e.g. a $β_1$- selective-adrenoceptor blocker can cause severe exacerbation of asthma ($αβ_2$ effect), even at low dose.

Adrenoceptor agonists

α + β effects, non-selective: adrenaline/epinephrine is used as a vasoconstrictor (α) with local anaesthetics, as a mydriatic (α), and in the emergency treatment of anaphylactic shock.

$α_1$ effects: noradrenaline/norepinephrine (with slight β effect on the heart) is selectively released physiologically, but as a therapeutic agent it is used for hypotensive states, excepting septic shock where dopamine and dobutamine are preferred (for their cardiac inotropic effect). Other agents with predominantly $α_1$ effects are imidazolines (xylometazoline, oxymetazoline), metaraminol, phenylephrine, phenylpropanolamine, ephedrine and pseudoephedrine; some are used solely for topical vasoconstriction (nasal decongestants).

$α_2$ effects in the central nervous system: clonidine, moxonidine.

β effects, non-selective (i.e. $β_1$ + $β_2$): isoprenaline (isoproterenol). Used as a bronchodilator ($β_2$), positive cardiac inotrope and to enhance conduction in heart block ($β_1$, $β_2$), it has been largely superseded by more selective agents. Other non-selective β agonists (ephedrine and orciprenaline) are also obsolete.

β_1 **effects, with some α effects:** dopamine, used in cardiogenic shock.

β_1 **effects:** dobutamine, used for cardiac inotropic effect.

β_2 **effects**, used in asthma, or to relax the uterus, include: salbutamol, terbutaline, fenoterol, pirbuterol, reproterol, rimiterol, isoxsuprine, orciprenaline, ritodrine.

Adrenoceptor antagonists (blockers)

Effects of a sympathomimetic

The overall effect of a sympathomimetic depends on the site of action (receptor agonist or indirect action), on receptor specificity and on dose; for instance adrenaline/epinephrine ordinarily dilates muscle blood vessels (β_2; mainly arterioles, but veins also) but in very large doses constricts them (α). The end results are often complex and unpredictable, partly because of the variability of homeostatic reflex responses and partly because what is observed, e.g. a change in blood pressure, is the result of many factors, e.g. vasodilatation (β) in some areas, vasoconstriction (α) in others, and cardiac stimulation (β).

To block all the effects of adrenaline/epinephrine and noradrenaline/norepinephrine, antagonists for both α and β receptors must be used. This can be a matter of practical importance, e.g. in phaeochromocytoma.

Physiological note. The termination of action of noradrenaline/norepinephrine released at nerve endingsis by:

- reuptake into nerve endings by the noradrenaline/norepinephrine transporter where it is stored in vesicles or metabolised by monoamine oxidase (MAO) (Fig. 10.2)
- diffusion away from the area of the nerve ending and the receptor (junctional cleft)
- metabolism (by extraneuronal MAO and catechol-O-methyltransferase, COMT).

These processes are slower than the rapid destruction of acetylcholine at the neuromuscular junction by extracellular acetylcholinesterase seated alongside the receptors. This reflects the differing signalling

requirements: almost instantaneous (millisecond) responses for voluntary muscle movement versus the much more leisurely contraction of arteriolar muscle to control vascular resistance.

Synthetic non-catecholamines in clinical use have a $t_{\frac{1}{2}}$ of hours, e.g. salbutamol 4 h, because they resist enzymatic degradation by MAO and COMT. They may be given orally, although much higher doses are then required versus parenteral routes. They penetrate the central nervous system (CNS) and may have prominent effects, e.g. amfetamine. Substantial amounts appear in the urine.

Pharmacokinetics

Catecholamines (adrenaline/epinephrine, noradrenaline/norepinephrine, dopamine, dobutamine, isoprenaline) (plasma $t_{\frac{1}{2}}$ approx. 2 min) are metabolised by MAO and COMT. These enzymes are present in large amounts in the liver and kidney, and account for most of the metabolism of injected catecholamines. MAO is also present in the intestinal mucosa (and in peripheral and central nerve endings). COMT is present in the adrenal medulla and tumours arising from chromaffin tissue, but not in sympathetic nerves. This explains the recent discovery that the COMT product, metanephrines, is a more sensitive and specific marker of phaeochromocytoma than measurement of the parent catecholamines. Because of both enzymes catecholamines are ineffective when swallowed (they are not bioavailable), but non-catecholamines, e.g. salbutamol and amfetamine, are effective orally.

Adverse effects

These may be deduced from their actions (Fig. 10.3). Tissue necrosis due to intense vasoconstriction (α) around injection sites occurs as a result of leakage from intravenous infusions. The effects on the heart (β_1) include tachycardia, palpitations, cardiac arrhythmias including ventricular tachycardia and fibrillation, and muscle tremor (β_2). Sympathomimetic drugs should be used with great caution in patients with heart disease.

The effect of the sympathomimetic drugs on the

Fig. 10.3 Cardiovascular effects of noradrenaline/norepinephrine, adrenaline/epinephrine and isoprenaline (isoproterenol): pulse rate (beats/min), blood pressure in mmHg (dotted line is mean pressure), peripheral resistance in arbitrary units.

pregnant uterus is variable and difficult to predict, but serious fetal distress can occur, due to reduced placental blood flow as a result both of contraction of the uterine muscle (α) and arterial constriction (α). β₂ agonists are used to relax the uterus in premature labour, but unwanted cardiovascular actions (tachycardia in particular) can be troublesome for the mother. The oxytocin antagonist atosiban does not have these unwanted effects.

The differences are due to the differential a- and b-agonist selectivities of these agents.

Sympathomimetics and plasma potassium. Adrenergic mechanisms have a role in the physiological control of plasma potassium concentration. The Na/K pump that shifts potassium into cells is activated by β₂-adrenoceptor agonists (adrenaline/epinephrine, salbutamol, isoprenaline) and can cause hypokalaemia. β₂-adrenoceptor antagonists block the effect.

The hypokalaemic effect of administered (β₂) sympathomimetics may be clinically important, particularly in patients with pre-existing hypokalaemia, e.g. due to intense adrenergic activity such as occurs in myocardial infarction, in fright (admission to hospital is accompanied by transient hypokalaemia),

or with previous diuretic therapy, and patients taking digoxin. In such subjects the use of a sympathomimetic infusion or of an adrenaline/epinephrine-containing local anaesthetic may precipitate cardiac arrhythmia. Hypokalaemia may occur during treatment of severe asthma, particularly where the β₂-receptor agonist is combined with theophylline.

β-adrenoceptor blockers, as expected, enhance the hyperkalaemia of muscular exercise, and one of their benefits in preventing cardiac arrhythmias after myocardial infarction may be due to block of β₂-receptor-induced hypokalaemia.

Overdose of sympathomimetics is treated according to rational consideration of mode and site of action.

INDIVIDUAL SYMPATHOMIMETICS

The classic, mainly endogenous, substances will be described first despite their limited role in therapeutics, and then the more selective analogues that have largely replaced them.

Catecholamines

Traditionally catecholamines have had a dual nomenclature (as a consequence of a company patenting the name Adrenalin), broadly European and North American. The North American naming system has been chosen by the World Health Organization as recommended international nonproprietary names (rINNs), and the European Unionhas directed member states to use rINNs. Byexception, adrenaline and noradrenaline are the terms used in the titles of monographs in the European Pharmacopoeia and are thus the official names in the member states. Because uniformity has not yet been achieved, and because of the scientific literature, we use both names.

Adrenaline/epinephrine

Adrenaline/epinephrine (α- and β-adrenoceptor effects) is used:

- as a vasoconstrictor with local anaesthetics (1 in 80 000 or weaker) to prolong their effects (about two-fold)
- as a topical mydriatic (sparing accommodation; it also lowers intraocular pressure)
- for severe allergic reactions, i.e. anaphylactic shock, intramuscularly or intravenously. The route must be chosen with care. The subcutaneous route is not recommended as the intense vasoconstriction slows absorption.

Adrenaline/epinephrine is used in anaphylactic shock because of its mix of actions, cardiovascular and bronchial; it may also stabilise mast cell membranes and reduce release of vasoactive autacoids. Patients who are taking non-selectiveβ-blockers may not respond to adrenaline/epinephrine (use intravenous salbutamol) and indeed may develop severe hypertension.

Adrenaline/epinephrine (topical) decreases intraocular pressure in chronic open-angle glaucoma, as does dipivefrine, an adrenaline/epinephrine ester prodrug. These drugs are contraindicated in closed-angle glaucoma because they are mydriatics. Hyperthyroid patients are intolerant of adrenaline/epinephrine.

Accidental overdose with adrenaline/epinephrine occurs occasionally. It is rationally treated with propranolol to block the cardiac b effects (cardiac arrhythmia) and phentolamine or chlorpromazine to control the a effects on the peripheral circulation that will be prominent when theβ effects are abolished. Labetalol (α+β blockade) is a good alternative. β-adrenoceptor block alone is hazardous as the then unopposed α-receptor vasoconstriction causes (severe) hypertension. Use of other classes of antihypertensives is irrational and may even cause adrenaline/epinephrine release.

Noradrenaline/norepinephrine (chiefly α and β_1 effects)

The main effect of administered noradrenaline/norepinephrine is to raise the blood pressure by constricting the arterioles and so increasing the total peripheral resistance, with reduced blood flow (except in coronary arteries which have few a1 receptors). Though it does have some cardiac stimulant (β_1) effect, the resulting tachycardia is masked by the profound reflex bradycardia caused by the hypertension. Noradrenaline/norepinephrine is given by intravenous infusion to obtain a controlled and sustained response; the effect of a single intravenous injection is unpredictable and would last only a minute or so. It is used where peripheral vasoconstriction is specifically required, e.g. vasodilatation of septic shock. Adverse effects include peripheral gangrene and local necrosis following accidental extravasation from a vein; tachyphylaxis occurs and withdrawal must be gradual.

Isoprenaline (isoproterenol)

Isoprenaline (isopropylnoradrenaline) is a nonselective β-receptor agonist, i.e. it activates both β_1 and β_2 receptors. It relaxes smooth muscle, including that of the blood vessels and airways, and has negligible metabolic or vasoconstrictor effects. It causes a marked tachycardia, which is its main disadvantage in the treatment of bronchial asthma. It is still occasionally used in complete heart block, massive overdose of a β-blocker, and in cardiogenic shock (for hypotension).

Dopamine

Dopamine activates different receptors depending on the dose used. At the lowest effective dose it stimulates specific dopamine (D_1) receptors in the CNS and the renal and other vascular beds (dilator); it also activates presynaptic autoreceptors (D_2) which suppress release of noradrenaline/norepinephrine. As the dose is increased, dopamine acts asanagonist on β_1-adrenoceptors in the heart (increasing contractility and rate); at high doses it activates a-adrenoceptors (vasoconstrictor). It is given by continuous intravenous infusionbecause, like all catecholamines, its $t_{1/2}$ is short (2min). Anintravenous infusion (2–5micrograms/kg·min) increases renal blood flow (partly through an effect oncardiac output). As the dose rises the heart is stimulated, resulting in tachycardia and increased cardiac output. At these higher doses, dopamine is referred to as an 'inoconstrictor'.

Dopamine is stable for about 24 h in sodium chloride ordextrose. Subcutaneous leakage causes vasoconstriction and necrosis (compare with noradrenaline/norepinephrine), and should be treated by local injection of an α-adrenoceptor blocking agent (phentolamine 5 mg, diluted). It may be mixed with dobutamine.

Dobutamine

Dobutamine is a racemic mixture of D- and L-dobutamine. The racemate behaves primarily as aβ_1-adrenoceptor agonist with greater inotropic than chronotropic effects on the heart; it has some α-agonist effect, but less than dopamine. It is useful in shock (with dopamine) and in low-output heart failure (in the absence of severe hypertension).

Dopexamine

Dopexamine is a synthetic catecholamine whose principal action is as an agonist for the cardiac β_2-adrenoceptors (positive inotropic effect). It is also a weak dopamine agonist (thus causing renal vasodilatation) and inhibitor of noradrenaline/norepinephrine uptake, thereby enhancing stimulation of cardiacβ_1 receptors by noradrenaline/norepinephrine. It is used occasionally to optimise the cardiac output, particularly perioperatively.

Non-catecholamines

Salbutamol, fenoterol, rimiterol, reproterol, pirbuterol, salmeterol, ritodrine and terbutaline are β-adrenoceptor agonists that are relatively selective for β_2 receptors, so that cardiac (chiefly β_1-receptor) effects are less prominent. Tachycardia still occurs because of atrial (sinus node) β_2-receptor stimulation; the β_2-adrenoceptors are less numerous in the ventricle and there is probably less risk of serious ventricular arrhythmias than with the use of nonselective catecholamines. The synthetic agonists are also longer acting than isoprenaline because they are not substrates for COMT, which methylates catecholamines in the liver. They are used principally in asthma, and to reduce uterine contractions in premature labour.

Salbutamol

Salbutamol (Ventolin) ($t_{1/2}$ 4 h) is taken orally, 2–4 mg up to four times per day; it also acts quickly by inhalation and the effect can last for 4–6 h, which makes it suitable for both prevention and treatment of asthma. Of an inhaled dose less than 20% is absorbed and can cause cardiovascular effects. It can also be given by injection, e.g. in asthma, premature labour (β_2 receptor) and for cardiac inotropic (β_1) effect in heart failure (where the β_2-vasodilator action is also useful). Clinically important hypokalaemia can also occur (the shift of potassium into cells). The other drugs above are similar.

Salmeterol. (Serevent) is a variant of salbutamol that has an additional binding site adjacent to the β_2-adrenoceptor; this results in slow onset (15–30 min) and long duration of action (12–18 h). This behaviour is distinct from the other widely used long-acting β_2-agonist, formoterol, which has a rapid bronchodilator effect like salbutamol (within a few minutes).

Ephedrine

Ephedrine ($t_{1/2}$ approx. 6 h) is a plant alkaloid with

indirect sympathomimetic actions that resemble those of adrenaline/epinephrine peripherally and amfetamine centrally. Hence, (in adults) it produces increased alertness, anxiety, insomnia, tremor and nausea; children may be sleepy when taking it. In practice, central effects limit its use as a sympathomimetic in asthma.

Ephedrine is well absorbed when given orally and, unlike most other sympathomimetics, undergoes relatively little first-pass metabolism in the liver (it is not a substrate for MAO or COMT); it is excreted largely unchanged by the kidney. It differs from adrenaline/epinephrine principally in that its effects come on more slowly and last longer. Tachyphylaxis occurs on repeated dosing. It can be given by mouth for reversible airways obstruction, topically as a mydriatic and mucosal vasoconstrictor or by slow intravenous injection to reverse hypotension from spinal or epidural anaesthesia. Newer drugs that are better suited for these purposes have largely replaced it. It is sometimes useful in myasthenia gravis (adrenergic agents enhance cholinergic neuromuscular transmission). Pseudoephedrine is similar to ephedrine but much less active.

Phenylpropanolamine (norephedrine) is similar but with fewer CNS effects. Prolonged administration of phenylpropanolamine to women as an anorectic has been associated with pulmonary valve abnormalities and stroke, leading to its withdrawal in some countries.

Amfetamine (Benzedrine) and dexamfetamine (Dexedrine) act indirectly. They are seldom used for their peripheral effects, which are similar to those of ephedrine, but usually for their effects on the CNS (narcolepsy, attention deficit in children).

Phenylephrine has actions qualitatively similar to those of noradrenaline/norepinephrine but of longer duration, up to several hours. It can be used as a nasal decongestant (0.25%–0.5% solution), but sometimes irritates. In the doses usually given, the CNS effects are minimal, as are the direct effects on the heart. It is also used as a mydriatic and briefly lowers intraocular pressure.

SHOCK

Definition. Shock is a state of inadequate organ perfusion (oxygen deficiency) sufficient adversely to affect cellular metabolism, causing the release of enzymes and vasoactive substances, i.e. it is a low flow or hypoperfusion state.

Typically the blood pressure is low, reflecting reduced cardiac output. The exception is septic shock, where the cardiac output is typically high, but it is maldistributed (due to constriction, dilatation, shunting), leading to poor oxygen utilisation and tissue injury (warm shock).

The essential element, hypoperfusion of vital organs, is present whatever the cause, whether pump failure (myocardial infarction), maldistribution of blood (septic shock) or loss of intravascular volume (bleeding or increased permeability of vessels damaged by bacterial cell products, burns or anoxia). Functions of vital organs, such as the brain (consciousness), lungs (gas exchange) and kidney (urine formation) are clinical indicators of adequacy of perfusion of these organs.

Treatment may be summarised as follows:

- Treatment of the cause: bleeding, infection, adrenocortical deficiency.
- Replacement of any fluid lost from the circulation.
- Perfusion of vital organs (brain, heart, kidneys) and maintenance of the mean blood pressure.

Blood flow (oxygen delivery) rather than blood pressure is of the greatest immediate importance for the function of vital organs. A reasonable blood pressure is needed to ensure organ perfusion, but peripheral vasoconstriction may maintain a normal mean arterial pressure despite a very low cardiac output. Under these circumstances, blood flow to vital organs will be inadequate and multiple organ failure will ensue unless the patient is resuscitated adequately.

The decision on how to treat shock depends on assessment of the pathophysiology:

- whether cardiac output, and thus peripheral blood flow, is inadequate (low pulse volume, cold-constricted periphery)
- whether cardiac output is normal or high and

peripheral blood flow is adequate (good pulse volume and warm dilated periphery), but there is maldistribution of blood

- whether the patient is hypovolaemic or not, or needs a cardiac inotropic agent, a vasoconstrictor or a vasodilator

Types of shock

In poisoning by a cerebral depressant or after spinal cord trauma, the principal cause of hypotension is low peripheral resistance due to reduced vascular tone. The cardiac output can be restored by infusing fluid and/or giving vasoactive drugs (e.g. noradrenaline/norepinephrine, metaraminol).

In central circulatory failure (cardiogenic shock, e.g. after myocardial infarction) the cardiac output and blood pressure are low because of pump failure; myocardial perfusion is dependent on aortic pressure. Venous return (central venous pressure) is normal or high. The low blood pressure may trigger the sympathoadrenal mechanisms of peripheral circulatory failure summarised below.

Not surprisingly, the use of drugs in low-output failure caused by acute myocardial damage is disappointing. Vasoconstriction (by an α-adrenoceptor agonist) may raise the blood pressure by increasing peripheral resistance, but the additional burden on the damaged heart can further reduce the cardiac output. Cardiac stimulation with a β_1-adrenoceptor agonist may fail; it increases myocardial oxygen consumption and may cause an arrhythmia. Dobutamine or dopamine offers a reasonable choice if a drug is judged necessary; dobutamine is preferred as it tends to vasodilate, i.e. it is an 'inodilator'. If there is bradycardia (as sometimes complicates myocardial infarction), cardiac output can be increased by accelerating the heart rate by vagal block with atropine.

Septic shock is severe sepsis with hypotension that is not corrected by adequate intravascular volume replacement. It is caused by lipopolysaccharide (LPS) endotoxins from Gram-negative organisms and other cell products from Gram-positive organisms; these initiate host inflammatory and procoagulant responses through the release of cytokines, e.g. interleukins, and the resulting diffuse endothelial damage is responsible for many of the adverse manifestations of shock. The procoagulant state, in particular, predisposes to the development of microvascular thrombosis that leads to tissue ischaemia and organ hypoperfusion. Activation of nitric oxide production by LPS and cytokines worsens the hypoperfusion by decreasing arterial pressure. This initiates a vigorous sympathetic discharge that causes constriction of arterioles and venules; the cardiac output may be high or low according to the balance of these influences.

There is a progressive peripheral anoxia of vital organs and acidosis. The veins (venules) dilate and venous pooling occurs so that blood is sequestered in the periphery; effective circulatory volume decreases because of this and fluid is lost into the extravascular space from endothelial damage caused by bacterial products.

When septic shock is recognised, appropriate antimicrobials should be given in high dose immediately after taking blood for culture. Beyond that, the primary aim of treatment is to restore cardiac output and vital organ perfusion by increasing venous return to the heart, and to reverse the maldistribution of blood. Increasing intravascular volume will achieve this, guided by the central venous pressure to avoid overloading the heart. Oxygen is essential as there is often uneven pulmonary perfusion.

After adequate fluid resuscitation has been established, inotropic support is usually required. Noradrenaline/norepinephrine is the vasoactive drug of choice for septic shock: its potent a-adrenergic effect increases the mean arterial pressure and its modest b1 effect may raise cardiac output, or at least maintain it as the peripheral vascular resistance increases. Dobutamine may be added to augment cardiac output further. Some clinicians use adrenaline/epinephrine, in preference to noradrenaline/norepinephrine plus dobutamine, on the basis that its powerful α and β effects are appropriate in the setting of septic shock; it may exacerbate splanchnic ischaemia and lactic acidosis.

Hypotension in (atherosclerotic) occlusive vascular disease is particularly serious, for these patients are dependent on pressure to provide the necessary blood flow in vital organs whose supplying vessels are less able to dilate. It is important to maintain an adequate mean arterial pressure, whichever inotrope is selected.

Choice of drug in shock

On present knowledge the best drug would be one that both stimulates the myocardium and selectively modifies peripheral resistance to increase flow to vital organs.

- Dobutamine is used when cardiac inotropic effect is the primary requirement.
- Adrenaline/epinephrine is used when a more potent inotrope than dobutamine is required, e.g. when the vasodilating action of dobutamine compromises mean arterial pressure.
- Noradrenaline/norepinephrine is used when vasoconstriction is the first priority, plus some cardiac inotropic effect, e.g. septic shock.

Additionally, recombinant activated protein C (APC) drotrecogin α can be given to reverse the procoagulant state of septic shock. Inflammatory conditions such as septic shock inhibit the generation of endogenous APC, which normally inactivates factors Va and VIIIa, with the result that production of these procoagulant factors is unchecked. Recombinant human APC improved survival of patients with septic shock and multi-organ failure in a large randomised controlled trial.

Monitoring drug use

Modern monitoring by both invasive and non-invasive techniques is complex and is undertaken in units dedicated to, and equipped for, this activity. The present comment is an overview. Monitoring normally requires close attention to heart rate and rhythm, blood pressure, fluid balance and urine flow, pulmonary gas exchange and central venous pressure. The use of drugs in shock is secondary to accurate assessment of cardiovascular state (especially of peripheral flow) and to other essential management, treatment of infection and maintenance of intravascular volume.

Restoration of intravascular volume

In an emergency, speed of replacement is more important than its nature. Crystalloid solutions, e.g. isotonic saline, Hartmann's, Plasma-Lyte, are immediately effective, but they leave the circulation quickly. (Note that dextrose solutions are completely ineffective because they distribute across both the extracellular and intracellular compartments.) Macromolecules (colloids) remain in the circulation longer. The two classes (crystalloids and colloids) may be used together.

The choice of crystalloid or colloid for fluid resuscitation remains controversial. A Cochrane review of over 56 clinical trials with mortality data concluded that in critically ill patients there was no evidence that colloids offered superior survival over the use of crystalloids in patients following trauma, burns or surgery. Colloids are also much more expensive than crystalloids.

Artificial colloidal solutions include dextrans (glucose polymer), gelatin (hydrolysed collagen) and hydroxyethyl starch.

Dextran 70 (mol. wt. 70 000) has a plasma restoring effect lasting for 5–6 h. Dextran 40 is used to decrease blood sludging and so to improve peripheral blood flow.

Gelatin products (e.g. Haemaccel, Gelofusine) have a plasma restoring effect of 2–3 h (at best).

Etherified starch. Several hydroxyethyl starch solutions are available, with widely differing effects on plasma volume: high molecular weight (450 000) solutions restore volume for 6–12 h, whereas the effect of medium molecular weight (200 000) starches lasts for 4–6 h.

Adverse effects include anaphylactoid reactions; dextran and hydroxyethyl starch can impair haemostatic mechanisms.

Part 4. Epilepsy

Definitions

A seizure is a clinical symptom or sign caused by abnormal electrical discharges within the cerebral cortex. For example, a tonic–clonic seizure refers to a pattern by which a patient loses consciousness, becomes generally stiff (tonic), and subsequently jerks all limbs (clonus); whereas a complex partial seizure refers to a constellation of impaired consciousness, déjà vu sensations, epigastric rising sensation, olfactory hallucinations and motor automatisms, e.g. lip smacking. By contrast, epilepsy refers to the clinical syndrome of recurrent seizures, and implies a pathological state that predisposes to further future seizures. Hence having one, or even a single cluster of seizures (i.e. over a few days) does not in itself qualify as epilepsy, since these seizures may have been due to a febrile illness or drug intoxication that themselves later resolve. By contrast, having at least two seizures, separated by at least a few weeks, is usually sufficient to signify epilepsy. Only one-third of people having seizures develop chronic epilepsy.

Pathology and seizure types

Epilepsy affects 0.5%–1% of the general population, while the lifetime risk of having a seizure is 3–5 %. There are both multiple causes and multiple seizure types. Approximately half of adult epilepsy is believed to be due to genetic or early developmental causes, although the exact nature of these – e.g. sodium channel mutations or cerebral palsy – are determined in only a small minority. The other half of adult epilepsy is due to acquired causes, such as alcohol, stroke, traumatic head injury or brain tumours.

The cause of epilepsy determines the seizure type. Genetic causes (i.e. 'primary') predispose to generalised seizures characterised by tonic–clonic or absence seizures (lapses of consciousness lasting seconds), myoclonus (random limb jerk at other times), photosensitivity (seizures triggered by flashing lights), EEG showing a 3-Hz spikeand- wave pattern, and a normal MRI brain. Conversely, where focal brain injury has occurred, e.g. brain tumour or stroke, and the brain scan is abnormal, focal epileptic discharges occur within the brain leading to a partial seizure – i.e. when only a narrow set of brain functions are disturbed, e.g. causing single limb jerking (implying motor cortex involvement). Importantly, partial seizures can propagate very quickly to become a 'secondary generalised seizure'. Another common cause of adult-onset partial epilepsy is maldevelopment of the medial temporal lobes ('mesial temporal sclerosis') believed to be due to injury, e.g. hypoxia or infection, during fetal or early childhood life, and sometimes apparent as atrophic hippocampi and amygdala on high-resolution MRI.

PRINCIPLES OF MANAGEMENT

- Identification of underlying cause and treatment of this where possible, e.g. cerebral neoplasm or arteriovenous malformation.
- Educate the patient about the disease, duration of treatment and need for compliance.
- Counselling the patient about avoiding harm from seizures, e.g. driving regulations, swimming or bathing alone and climbing, as well as other dangerous pursuits, to be avoided.
- Avoid precipitating factors, e.g. alcohol, sleep deprivation, stroboscopic light.
- Anticipate natural variation, e.g. fits may occur particularly or exclusively around menstruation in women (catamenial epilepsy).
- For most cases with recurrent seizures, an antiepileptic drug is prescribed with subsequent monitoring and adjustment of dosage or drug type.
- Consider surgical therapies in patients with refractory seizures, e.g. vagal nerve stimulation, temporal lobectomy. For childhood refractory epilepsy, a ketogenic diet – i.e. high fat: carbohydrate ratio – is useful, as ketone bodies are antiepileptogenic.
- Acute treatment of generalised convulsive seizures consists of ensuring the patient lies on the floor away from danger, and is postictally manoeuvred into the recovery position. If a seizure continues for more than a few minutes, rectal or buccal diazepam or intranasal midazolam can be given. If convulsive seizures last for more than 5 min, patients should be transferred to hospital for consideration of intravenous benzodiazepine and phenytoin.

Practical guide to antiepilepsy drugs

When to initiate. Following a single seizure the chance of a further seizure is approximately 25% over the following 3 years. Furthermore, only 33% of single seizure patients develop chronic epilepsy. Hence the majority of first seizures are provoked by a reversible, and often recognisable, factor, e.g. infection, drug toxicity, surgery. For these reasons, following a single seizure anticonvulsants are not generally prescribed, whereas after two or more distinct seizure episodes (i.e. with more than a few weeks apart between episodes), they generally are prescribed. Immediate treatment of single or infrequent seizures does not affect long-term remission but introduces the potential for adverse effects. Patients need to be made aware that anticonvulsant therapy reduces harm caused by generalised seizures, and may also reduce the risk of sudden death in epilepsy (SUDEP), that usually occurs during sleep.

Monotherapy. Although the choice of anticonvulsants is large (approximately 20), first-line therapy is generally restricted to one of only a few drugs that have a good track record and are relatively safe and well-tolerated. Initial therapy is confined to a single drug (i.e. monotherapy) that is usually effective in stopping seizures or at least significantly decreasing their frequency. The majority of epilepsy patients (70%) can remain on monotherapy for adequate control, although sometimes the choice of monotherapy may need to be switched to allow for tolerance or optimisation of seizure control. As the number of single anticonvulsants tried increases, the incremental likelihood that any new one will offer a significant reduction in seizures decreases: from 50% response to a first drug, to an additional 30% to a second drug, to an extra 10% to a third drug, and less than 5% for any subsequent drug tried.

What drug to initiate. For older types of anticonvulsants, knowing the seizure type – i.e. whether partial or primary generalised – mattered, because in certain cases the spectrum of seizure efficacy is limited, and, moreover, certain seizure types can be worsened by ill-chosen drugs. For example, carbamazepine is an effective first-line therapy for partial seizures but may worsen primary generalised, absence or myoclonic seizures; similarly phenytoin can worsen absence and myoclonic seizures. Ethosuximide, by contrast, is only effective in primary generalised, and not partial, seizures.

More modern anticonvulsants, by contrast, are in general effective over a much broader range of seizure types allowing for more confidence of use even when seizure type is uncertain. Thus sodium valproate, lamotrigine and levetiracetam are active against both primary and secondary generalised epilepsy, and being relatively well tolerated, account for most first-line prescriptions. In one head-to-head study comparing popular first-line therapies for generalised and partial seizures, lamotrigine was generally tolerated better than other drugs, while valproate was the most efficacious; carbamazepine and topiramate were more likely to cause unwanted effects.[7]

Women of reproductive age and children. These categories of patients prompt selection of particular drugs and avoidance of others. **Polytherapy.** If a trial of three or so successive anticonvulsants (i.e. taken as monotherapy at adequate dosage for at least several months) does not control a patient's epilepsy, it may be worthwhile trying dual therapy. Polytherapy offers the theoretical advantage of controlling neuronal hyperexcitability by more than one mechanism, that can be synergistic. In reality, increasing polytherapy often adheres to the law of diminishing returns, viz. the proportion of uncontrolled patients who show a positive response decreases at each addition of drug number And at the same time, adverse effects become more likely.

Abrupt withdrawal. Effective therapy must never be stopped suddenly, as this is a well-recognised trigger for status epilepticus, which may be fatal. But if rapid withdrawal is required by the occurrence of toxicity, e.g. due to a severe rash or significant liver dysfunction, a new drug ought to be started simultaneously. The speed by which the dose of a new drug can be raised varies according to drug type and urgency.

Circumstantial seizures. In cases where fits are

liable to occur at a particular time, e.g. the menstrual period, adjust the dose to achieve maximal drug effect at this time or confine drug treatment to this time. For example, in catamenial epilepsy, clobazam can be useful given only at period time.

Once treatment is stable, patients should keep to a particular proprietary brand as different brands of the same generic agent (e.g. carbamazepine) may exhibit varying pharmacokinetics.

Dosage and administration

The manner in which drug dosing is initiated depends on: ① the drug type, and ② the frequency and severity of the patient's seizures (i.e. the relative urgency with which therapeutic levels are reached). Phenytoin and phenobarbital allow for a rapid loading (within 24 h); valproate, levetiracetam and oxcarbazepine allow for escalation over days or a few weeks, whilst lamotrigine and carbamazepine require gradual escalations over many weeks. If seizures are infrequent at the time of presentation, e.g. every few weeks, antiepileptics should generally be started at their lowest dose, with small increments made every 1–2 weeks. In this way, the risk of unwanted effects, especially dizziness or 'feeling drunk' are minimised. A slow introduction of lamotrigine is also essential to reduce the risk of rash or more severe hypersensitivity reactions, Most drugs have a generally recognised maintenance dose range; the lowest dose within this range that achieves a reasonable degree of seizure control should be established. Monitoring of blood concentrations is helpful in guiding dosage of carbamazepine, phenytoin and phenobarbital, but not other anticonvulsants.

Failure to respond

In patients who continue fitting in spite of the recommended maintenance dose range having been reached, there are numerous possible explanations:

- Non-compliance, diarrhoea and vomiting, patients instructed to be 'nil by mouth' (revealed by measuring blood concentrations of drug).
- Inadequate dosing, including the possibility of drug interaction, e.g. another drug reducing the effective dose of the anticonvulsant by hepatic enzyme induction.
- Pregnancy also causes hepatic induction, and reduces the effective dose of lamotrigine.
- Increase in the severity of an underlying disease, e.g. enlargement of a brain tumour, or new disease.
- Drug resistance, e.g. genetic polymorphisms in hepatic cytochromes (such as CYP 2 C9) that metabolise drugs, sodium channel subunit SCN1A, or the P glycoprotein drug transporter (ABCB1 gene) that expels drugs from neurones.

Drug withdrawal

If patients have remained seizure-free for more than a few years, it is reasonable to consider withdrawal of antiepilepsy drug therapy. The prognosis of a seizure disorder is determined by:

- Type of seizure disorder – benign rolandic epilepsy, solely petit mal or grand mal seizures confer a high chance of full remission, whereas juvenile myoclonic epilepsy, temporal or frontal lobe epilepsies often require lifelong treatment.
- Time to remission – early remission carries a better outlook.
- Number of drugs required to induce remission – rapid remission on a single drug is a favourable indicator for successful withdrawal.
- MRI brain scan findings – presence of an underlying lesion predicts difficult control.
- EEG findings – epileptogenic activity is a predictor of poor outcome for drug withdrawal.
- Associated neurological deficit or learning difficulty – control is often difficult.
- Length of time of seizure freedom on treatment – the longer the period, the better the outlook.

Discontinuing antiepilepsy medication is associated with about 20% relapse during withdrawal and a further 20% relapse over the following 5 years; after this period relapse is unusual. A general recommendation is to withdraw the antiepilepsy drug over a period of 6 months.

If a fit occurs during this time, full therapy must recommence until the patient has been free from seizures for several years.

Driving regulations and epilepsy

Multiple driving regulations exist that relate epilepsy (and neurological conditions predisposing to epilepsy, e.g. brain surgery) to stipulations regarding driving (according to the UK Driving Vehicle Licensing Authority). These rules are based upon statistical data relating specific diagnoses or clinically described events (e.g. blackouts without warning) with the risk of future blackout and/or car accidents. Epileptic patients who wish to continue driving therefore need to contact their national driving licensing body so that each case can be judged on its merits; while waiting for a decision, patients must not drive.

In general in the UK, patients suffering seizures, or blackouts of undetermined cause, are not permitted to drive a car for 1 year from their last attack. Exceptions include: patients who have had exclusively nocturnal seizures for at least 3 years, or patients in whom a single seizure has occurred more than 6 months earlier, providing they have a normal brain scan and EEG; these groups are usually permitted to drive.

Pregnancy and epilepsy

Pregnancy worsens epilepsy in about a third of patients, but also improves epilepsy in another third. One of the main concerns in this patient group is that all anticonvulsants increase the chance of teratogenicity slightly, with valproate, phenytoin and phenobarbital carrying most risk. The toxicological hazard must be weighed against the risk of seizures which themselves can be harmful to mother and unborn baby, and are likely to worsen if anticonvulsants are discontinued. For instance, the risk of major congenital anomalies in the fetus is 1% for healthy mothers, 2% in untreated epileptic mothers (in observational studies, so generally not severe epileptics), and 2%–3% in mothers on epilepsy monotherapy. Valproate, by contrast, has been associated with a malformation rate of approximately 10%, while 20–30% of children are subsequently found to have mild learning disabilities or require 'special needs' education. The UK maintains a national drug monitoring register of all pregnant women taking antiepileptic drugs.

Doctor–patient discussions about what antiepileptic drug, if any, and at what dose, are required preconception. Advance planning is preferred because:

- neural tube defects are related to deficiencies in folic acid stores before pregnancy, so that antiepileptic drugs that affect stores, e.g. valproate, can be avoided, and folic acid 5 mg per day given for several months in advance.
- adjustments in dose and type of drug can be avoided in the early stages of pregnancy as there is a higher risk of toxicity and seizure breakthrough during this critical phase of fetal development. In general, patients having seizures with blackouts should be on an effective dose of an anticonvulsant, because of the risks of anoxia, lactic acidosis and trauma.

During pregnancy, liver enzymes become induced, which has implications in epilepsy. Firstly, patients on lamotrigine before conception require a gradually increased dose during the pregnancy, to cope with enhanced catabolism (lowering lamotrigine plasma concentration). Secondly, enzyme-inducing drugs often aggravate a relative deficiency of vitamin K that occurs in final trimester women, predisposing to postpartum haemorrhage; vitamin K is therefore given by mouth during the last 2 weeks of pregnancy.

Breast feeding

Antiepilepsy drugs pass into breast milk: phenobarbital, primidone and ethosuximide in significant quantities, phenytoin and sodium valproate less so. There is a risk that the baby will become sedated or suckle poorly but provided there is awareness of these effects, the balance of advantage favours breast feeding while taking antiepilepsy drugs.

Epilepsy and oral contraceptives

Many antiepileptic drugs induce steroid-metabolising enzymes and so can cause hormonal contraception to fail. This applies to: carbamazepine, oxcarbazepine, phenytoin, barbiturates, and topiramate. Patients receiving any of these drugs and wishing to remain on the combined contraceptive pill need a higher dose of oestrogen (at least 50 micrograms/day), which they should take back-to-back for three cycles ('tri-cycling'), before stopping for 3 days, and then repeating the pattern. Even this method offers a suboptimal level of contraception, and a non-oestrogenic form of contraception is preferred. Lamotrigine is not an enzyme inducer but can decrease levonorgestrel plasma concentration through other mechanisms.

Epilepsy in children

Seizures in children tend to arise from different sets of causes (usually genetic or cerebral palsy) from those arising in adults, and can carry either very good long-term outcomes, e.g. spontaneous resolution, or, less commonly, bad outcomes, e.g. gradual deterioration. Treatments are similar to those used in adults, but certain seizure types necessitate drugs that are rarely used in adults, e.g. ethosuximide for absence seizures, or vigabatrin for refractory partial seizures (partly because children may become irritable or more cognitively impaired with drugs such as valproate and phenobarbital).

Febrile convulsions. Seizures triggered by fever due to any cause (typically viral infection) are common in young children (3 months – 5 years old). Two-thirds of such children will have only one attack, and in total only 2% will progress to adult epilepsy. For this reason, continuous prophylaxis is seldom given, except for those cases where atypical febrile seizures occur, e.g. lasting for more than 15 min, have focal features or recur within the same febrile illness. Long-term antiepileptic therapy is avoided where possible in children due to recognised adverse effects of most such drugs on learning and social development. Febrile convulsions may be treated on an ad hoc basis by issuing parents with a specially formulated solution of diazepam for rectal administration (absorption from a suppository is too slow) that allow for easy and early administration. Febrile convulsions may be prevented by treating febrile children with paracetamol and cooling with sponge soaks.

Status epilepticus

Status epilepticus refers to continuous or repeated epileptic seizures for more than 30 min. It often arises in patients already known to have epilepsy, in whom antiepileptic drug therapy has been inappropriately withdrawn or not taken. It can be the first presentation of epilepsy, due to an acquired brain insult, e.g. viral encephalitis.

Status epilepticus is a medical emergency. In the first instance, general resuscitation (airway control, oxygen, intravenous saline, etc.) is required. Treatment of seizures is initially with the intravenous benzodiazepine lorazepam (0.5–4 mg). Lorazepam is preferred to diazepam because it has a longer effective t½ and is less lipophilic and so accumulates less in fat, causing less delayed toxicity (hypotension and respiratory depression). The speed of action of lorazepam and diazepam are both rapid. Phenytoin i.v. may be started simultaneously to suppress further seizures, given as a loading dose (15–20 mg/kg bodyweight) over 1 h, while monitoring ECG and blood pressure for arrhythmias and hypotension. Subsequently a maintenance dose of approximately 300 mg/day is given and adjusted according to plasma levels (corrected for albumin). Phenobarbital maybe given i.v. as a third-line drug when seizures continue. At this point, the level of sedation (due both to seizures and drugs) is usually sufficiently great to warrant general anaesthesia, e.g. with propofol or thiopental, combined with intubation, mechanical ventilation and intensive care management. Pharmacologically induced sedation is removed periodically to allow for assessment of seizure activity (both from clinical observations and using EEG).

If resuscitation facilities are not immediately available, diazepam by rectal solution is a useful option. In some cases, midazolam (nasally) may be preferred, e.g. in children or those with severe learning disability. Intravenous benzodiazepines should not be used if resuscitation facilities are unavailable as there is risk of respiratory arrest.

Always investigate and treat the cause of a generalised seizure. Give aciclovir i.v. if viral encephalitis is suspected or, if status is triggered by removing an antiepileptic drug, it must be re-instituted. Magnesium sulphate is the treatment of choice for seizures related to eclampsia.

PHARMACOLOGY OF INDIVIDUAL DRUGS

Modes of action

Antiepilepsy (anticonvulsant) drugs aim to inhibit epileptogenic neuronal discharges and their propagation, while not interfering significantly with physiological neural activity. They act by one of five different mechanisms given below. It is generally recommended that when more than one drug is needed to control seizures, then drugs chosen should be selected from different classes of action, both to target epileptogenesis at more than one control point (resulting in synergistic effects) and to reduce unwanted effects.

Decreases electrical excitability. Examples: phenytoin, carbamazepine, lamotrigine, lacosamide. These drugs reduce cell membrane permeability to ions, particularly fast, voltage-dependent sodium channels which are responsible for the inward current that generates an action potential. Receptor blockage is typically use-dependent, meaning that only cells firing repetitively at high frequency are blocked, which permits discrimination between epileptic and physiological activity. A further potential avenue for reducing neuronal depolarisation is to use a potassium channel opener, e.g. retigabine.

Decreases synaptic vesicle release. Examples: calcium channel blockers: e.g. gabapentin; levetiracetam. Calcium channel activation is required for synaptic vesicle release and so calcium channel blockers may act by decreasing synaptic transmission, and therefore activity propagation, especially during periods of high burst activity. Calcium channel blockade may also reduce excitoxicity – a pathological process by which repetitive neuronal depolarisation leads to calcium entry into neurones, with resultant cell death. Gabapentin and pregabalin are specific for high voltage-gated P/Q type calcium channels, whereas ethosuximide is specific for low-voltage-gated T-type calcium channels. Other drugs such as lamotrigine, valproate and topiramate block calcium channels as just one of many cellular actions.

Levetiracetam uniquely inhibits synaptic vesicle protein 2A (SV2A), thereby reducing synaptic vesicle recycling.

Enhancement of gamma-aminobutyric acid (GABA) transmission. Examples: enzodiazepines, phenobarbital, valproate, vigabatrin, tiagabine. By enhancing GABA, the principal inhibitory transmitter of the brain, neuronal membrane permeability to chloride ions is increased, which secondarily reduces cell excitability. Benzodiazepines and barbiturates activate the GABA receptor via specific benzodiazepine and barbiturate binding sites.

Inhibition of excitatory neurotransmitters, e.g. glutamate. Examples: topiramate, felbamate. Glutamate inhibition both stops neuronal excitation in the short term, and excitotoxicity and cell death in the long term.

Other actions. Example: lacosamide, which as well as inhibiting sodium channel conductance, also targets a neuronal protein called 'collapsin-response mediator protein 2' (CRMP2).

Sodium channel blockers

Carbamazepine

Carbamazepine (Tegretol) acts predominantly as a voltage dependent sodium channel blocker, thereby reducing membrane excitability.

Pharmacokinetics. Carbamazepine is metabolised to an epoxide; both compounds possess antiepileptic activity but the epoxide may cause more adverse effects. The $t_{1/2}$ of carbamazepine falls from 35 h to 20 h over the first few weeks of therapy due to autoinduction of hepatic enzymes. For this reason, the dose of carbamazepine is gradually increased, over many weeks, with the expectation that plasma-levels will remain within a therapeutic range over this time. Other drugs relying on hepatic metabolism may also have their effective plasma level decreased due to induction secondary to carbamazepine, e.g. glucocorticosteroids, contraceptive pill, theophylline, warfarin, as well as other anticonvulsants, e.g. phenytoin. The metabolism of carbamazepine itself may be inhibited by valproate and to a lesser extent, by lamotrigine and levetiracetam (thereby raising carbamazepine plasma levels).

Uses. Carbamazepine is effective for partial seizures with or without secondary generalisation. It is also first-line treatment for trigeminal neuralgia. It is not recommended for primary generalised seizures (especially myoclonic epilepsy), which can be worsened by it.

Adverse effects follow from the fact that it depresses electrical excitability. In the central nervous system (CNS) this results in cerebellar and brainstem dysfunction (causing dizziness, diplopia, ataxia, nausea and reversible blurring of vision), as well as drowsiness; in the heart this can result in depression of cardiac atrioventricular (AV) conduction. Rashes, including serious reactions such as Stevens–Johnson syndrome, tend to be more of a problem for this drug than other anticonvulsants. A further set of issues arise from the hepatic induction property of carbamazepine: both osteomalacia and folic acid deficiency may occur due to enhanced metabolism of vitamin D and folic acid, respectively. Elderly patients receiving any enzyme-inducing drug should be screened for osteoporosis with bone-density scanning, and treated with bisphosphonates if necessary. Other unwanted effects can include gastrointestinal symptoms, headache, blood disorders, e.g. leucopenia, syndrome of inappropriate antidiuretic hormone (causing hyponatraemia), liver and thyroid dysfunction. Carbamazepine impairs cognitive function less than phenytoin.

Oxcarbazepine

Oxcarbazepine, like its analogue carbamazepine, acts by blocking voltage-sensitive sodium channels. It is rapidly and extensively metabolised in the liver; the t½ of the parent drug is 2 h, but that of its principal metabolite (which also has therapeutic activity) is 11 h. Unlike carbamazepine, it does not form an epoxide, which may explain its lower frequency of unwanted effects; these include dizziness, headache and hyponatraemia, and selective cytochrome enzyme induction (potentially causing failure of oestrogen contraception). Monitoring of plasma sodium may be necessary in the elderly and patients on diuretics. Oxcarbazepine is used either as monotherapy or as addon therapy for partial seizures. The speed with which the dose can be escalated is generally quicker than that for carbamazepine.

Phenytoin

Phenytoin (diphenylhydantoin, Epanutin, Dilantin) acts principally by blocking neuronal voltage-dependent sodium ion channels; this action is described as membrane stabilising, and discourages the spread (rather than the initiation) of seizure discharges.

Pharmacokinetics. Phenytoin provides a good example of the application of pharmacokinetics for successful prescribing.

Saturation kinetics. Phenytoin is hydroxylated extensively in the liver, a process that becomes saturated at about the doses needed for therapeutic effect. Thus phenytoin at low doses exhibits first-order kinetics but saturation or zero-order kinetics develop as the therapeutic plasma concentration range (10–20 mg/L) is approached, i.e. dose increments of equal size produce a disproportional rise in steady-state plasma concentration. Thus dose increments should become smaller as the dose increases (which is why there is a 25 mg capsule), and plasma concentration monitoring is advisable. Phenytoin given orally is well absorbed, allowing for achievement of therapeutic range concentrations within 24 h (as may be required in patients with frequent seizures).

Enzyme induction and inhibition. Phenytoin is a potent inducer of hepatic enzymes that metabolise other drugs (carbamazepine, warfarin), dietary and endogenous substances (including vitamin D and folate), and phenytoin itself. This latter causes a slight fall in steady-state phenytoin concentration over the first few weeks of therapy, though this may not be noticeable with progressive dose increments. Drugs that inhibit phenytoin metabolism (causing its plasma concentration to rise) include sodium valproate, isoniazid and certain non-steroidal anti-inflammatory drugs.

Uses. The main role of phenytoin in modern practice is in the emergency control of seizures, including status epilepticus, because of its reliable antiepileptic effect, and because an effective treatment dose can be loaded rapidly. It may also be used to prevent partial seizures with or without secondary generalisation, but is not generally used first line in this regard because of its adverse effect profile. It may worsen primary generalised epilepsies, such as absence or myoclonic seizures, and so is not used for these conditions unless status epilepticus occurs.

Other uses. The membrane-stabilising effect of phenytoin finds use in cardiac arrhythmias, trigeminal neuralgia and myotonic dystrophy (an inherited disorder in which skeletal muscle becomes overexcitable).

Adverse effects of phenytoin are multitudinous, especially with years of therapy, which fact, together with its narrow therapeutic range, is why phenytoin is not favoured for long-term therapy. Unwanted effects related to the nervous system include cognitive impairment, cerebellar ataxia, dyskinesias, tremor and peripheral neuropathy. Cutaneous reactions include rashes (dose related), coarsening of facial features, hirsutism, lupus-like syndrome, gum hyperplasia (due to inhibition of collagen catabolism), and Dupuytren's contracture (caused by free-radical formation). Haematological effects include: macrocytic anaemia due to increased folate metabolism (treatable with folate supplementation), IgA hypergammaglobulinaemia, lymphadenopathy and pseudolymphoma. Osteomalacia due to increased metabolism of vitamin D occurs after years of therapy and calls for bone-density scanning.

Intravenous phenytoin is associated with cardiac depression, distal ischemia ('purple-glove syndrome') and, if drug extravasation occurs, local but severe ulceration.

Overdose causes cerebellar symptoms and signs, coma, apnoea or even paradoxically, seizures. The patient may remain unconscious for a long time because of saturation kinetics, but will recover with standard care.

Lamotrigine

Lamotrigine (Lamictal) stabilises pre-synaptic neuronal membranes by blocking voltage-dependent sodium and calcium channels, and reduces the release of excitatory amino acids, such as glutamate and aspartate. The $t_{1/2}$ of 24 h allows for a single daily dose.

Lamotrigine is a favoured first-line drug for partial and generalised epilepsy, being both effective and well tolerated. It is also used in bipolar disorder as a mood stabiliser. It has few cognitive or sedating effects relative to other antiepileptic drugs.

It causes rash in about 10% of patients, including, rarely, serious reactions such as Stevens–Johnson syndrome and toxic epidermal necrolysis (potentially fatal). The risk of rash lessens if treatment begins with a low dose and escalates slowly, whereas concomitant use of valproate, which inhibits lamotrigine metabolism, adds to the hazard. Carbamazepine, phenytoin and barbiturates accelerate the metabolic breakdown of lamotrigine, thereby prompting an increase in the prescribed lamotrigine dose. Other specific unwanted effects of lamotrigine include insomnia and headache, the latter effect distinguishing it from valproate and topiramate that are used for migraine prevention. Insomnia may respond to lamotrigine taken once daily in the morning.

Lacosamide

Lacosamide (Vimpat) selectively facilitates a 'slow-inactivating' component of the voltage-gated sodium channel, which predominates under high-frequency neural activity (e.g. seizures), without affecting 'fast-inactivating' sodium channel states that characterise more standard patterns of neural firing frequency. This offers seizure control while reducing common antiepileptic unwanted effects such as sedation or cognitive impairment. Lacosamide also targets a neuronal protein called 'collapsin-response mediator protein 2' that is involved in neuronal differentiation, axonal outgrowth and gene expression. Whether this property confers additional disease-modifying properties to lacosamide (as distinct from its antiseizure property) is unknown.

Lacosamide is effective in refractory partial epilepsy, and has the advantage of being available as a syrup and i.v. formulation. The $t_{1/2}$ is 13 h, and unwanted effects include dizziness, nausea, headache and prolongation of the PR interval on the ECG.

GABA-potentiators

Sodium valproate

Sodium valproate (valproic acid, Epilim) acts on sodium and calcium channels, as well as GABAA receptors, the latter action by virtue of inhibiting GABA transaminase (thereby increasing GABA levels, and hence neuronal inhibition).

Sodium valproate is metabolised extensively in the liver ($t_{1/2}$ 13 h). It is a non-specific metabolic inhibitor, both of its own metabolism, and that of other anticonvulsants including lamotrigine, phenytoin and carbamazepine. To avoid toxicity, patients taking valproate and starting such drugs as second-line therapy should receive lower does of the second anticonvulsant. By contrast, the metabolism of valproate is accelerated by enzyme-inducing drugs, e.g.carbamazepine.

Sodium valproate is effective for both generalised and partial epilepsies, as well as for migraine prevention and mania (for which it acts as a mood stabiliser).

Adverse effects. The main concerns, particularly to women, are weight gain, impaired glucose tolerance, teratogenicity, polycystic ovary syndrome and loss of hair, which grows back curly. Nausea and dyspepsia may be a more general problem, ameliorated by using an enteric-coated formulation. Some patients exhibit a rise in liver enzymes, which is usually transient and without sinister import, but patients should be closely monitored until the biochemical tests return to normal as, rarely, liver failure occurs (risk maximal at 2–12 weeks); this is often indicated by anorexia, malaise and a recurrence of seizures. Other reactions include pancreatitis, coagulation disorder due to inhibition of platelet aggregation or thrombocytopenia, and hyperammonaemia that can present with acute confusion.

Barbiturates

Some of the earliest effective antiepileptic drugs came from the barbiturate family: namely, phenobarbital ($t_{1/2}$ 100 h), and primidone (Mysoline), the latter being metabolised largely to phenobarbital, i.e. it is a prodrug. The main use of phenobarbital is for status epilepticus because of its potent antiepileptic effect and the ability to give it intravenously. It is also used as an adjunct for long-term control of refractory partial seizures, but suffers from a high level of unwanted effects (especially sedation), including cardiac or respiratory arrest if overdosed, and dependency/addiction, and interactions (enzyme induction). Withdrawal from barbiturates must be performed very slowly (typically over months) because of a high risk of inducing seizures.

Benzodiazepines

Lorazepam and diazepam are first-line drugs for rapid control of acute seizures, but are not recommended for longterm prophylaxis due to unwanted effects: mainly sedation, tolerance and addiction. Clonazepam (Rivotril) ($t_{1/2}$ 25 h) is used mainly as an adjunct in myoclonic epilepsy due to its additional effects as a muscle relaxant. Clobazam finds use as an oral method for establishing rapid seizure control, e.g. in patients with a first presentation of frequent symptomatic seizures, and may be effective for drug-resistant partial seizures. Its effectiveness may wane after a few months due to tolerance. Both clonazepam and clobazam should be avoided in patients with anxiety or a history of drug addiction, due to risk of addiction or misuse.

Calcium channel blockers

Gabapentin

Gabapentin (Neurontin) is an analogue of GABA that is sufficiently lipid soluble to cross the blood–brain barrier. Its main action may be through inhibition of voltage-gated calcium channels, especially via interactions with the $\alpha_2\delta$ subunit. It also facilitates GABAergic transmission, as its name suggests. It is excreted unchanged and, has the advantage of not inducing or inhibiting hepatic metabolism of other drugs.

Gabapentin is effective only for partial seizures and secondary generalised epilepsy. It is also beneficial for neuropathic pain, and anxiety.

Gabapentin may cause somnolence, unsteadiness, dizziness and fatigue, although the likelihood of these decreases if dosing is started very low (e.g. 100 mg three times per day) and increased gradually (e.g. to 900 mg three times per day).

Pregabalin

Pregabalin (Lyrica) acts similarly to gabapentin, and is sometimes used in place of gabapentin when the latter has been ineffective for refractory partial seizures. Its main adverse effects are confusion, dizziness and weight gain. As well as being an antiepileptic it is commonly used against neuropathic pain, and it possesses anxiolytic properties.

Ethosuximide

Ethosuximide (Zarontin) ($t_{1/2}$ 55 h) is a member of the succinimide family that differs from other antiepilepsy drugs in that it blocks a particular type of calcium channel that is active in primary generalised epilepsies – especially absence seizures (petit mal) and myoclonic epilepsy. For this reason its main use is among children. Adverse effects include gastric upset, CNS effects, and allergic reactions including eosinophilia and other blood disorders, and lupus erythematosus.

Carbonic anhydrase inhibitors

Carbonic anhydrase inhibition reduces central nervous excitability, and is a property shared by topiramate, zonisamide and acetazolamide. Acetazolamide is rarely used now as an antiepileptic, but the other two find roles as adjuncts in partial epilepsy, as well as migraine. They also share common unwanted effects, namely weakness, anorexia, weight loss, depression, paraesthesia and renal stones (due to alkalosis).

Topiramate

Topiramate (Topamax), acts via various mechanisms, including carbonic anhydrase inhibition, voltage-gated sodium channel blockade, glutamate receptor blockade and enhancement of GABA activity The $t_{1/2}$ of 21 h allows once-daily dosing; it is excreted in the urine, mainly as unchanged drug.

Topiramate is used for partial seizures, as well as for migraine prevention (a property it shares with valproate). Unlike valproate, which causes weight gain, topiramate causes weight loss (considered an advantage by many women). Other unwanted effects include cognitive impairment, e.g. naming difficulty, acute myopia and raised intraocular pressure.

Levetiracetam

Levetiracetam (Keppra) is unique in inhibiting synaptic vesicle protein 2A (SV2A), which secondarily reduces synaptic vesicle recycling. It is effective for both partial and generalised seizures, is relatively well tolerated, and appears not to interact with other drugs. It is also rapidly and completely absorbed after oral administration, and can reach maintenance dose relatively quickly. For these reasons, it has become increasingly popular as a first-line agent for many seizure types. Its therapeutic index appears to be high, with the commonest adverse effects being weakness, dizziness and drowsiness. Relatively specific unwanted effects of levetiracetam are emotional lability, behavioural disturbance and psychosis, and it should be used with caution in patients with prior mood disturbance, learning disability or head injury. It is metabolised predominantly in the kidney, making it a drug of choice in liver disease, but use at lower dose in renal impairment.

Part 5. Parkinson's disease and parkinsonism

Definitions

Parkinson's disease refers to a specific neurodegenerative disease characterised pathologically by intracellular accumulation of Lewy bodies and subsequent neuronal loss, predominantly within the substantia nigra pars compacta (SNpc). This midbrain nucleus normally provides dopaminergic input to the neo-striatum (caudate and putamen), a critical aspect to motor control; one cardinal feature of Parkinson's disease is that motor symptoms are reversible by administration of dopaminergic drugs. By contrast, parkinsonism refers to the clinical symptoms and signs of Parkinson's disease (tremor, rigidity, brady-kinesia and postural imbalance) that may arise either from Parkinson's disease or one of its mimics; the latter include extensive small-vessel cerebral isch-emia due to hypertension, neuroleptic drugs or other neurodegenerative disease such as multiple-systems atrophy (MSA) or Huntington's disease. Note that parkinsonism due to conditions other than Parkin-son's disease generally responds poorly to dopami-nergic therapies. Another distinguishing feature is that symptoms and signs of Parkinson's disease, but not other causes, are often asymmetric.

Pathophysiology of Parkinson's disease

Parkinson's disease is the second commonest neuro-degenerative disease after Alzheimer's disease. Both diseases show an exponentially increasing risk with age, with the risk of Parkinson's disease rising from approximately 0.2% under the age of 60 to 1% over the age of 60 and 4% of people over 85 years old. At the time that a clinical diagnosis first becomes appar-ent, radioactive dopamine uptake scans (sensitive to dopaminergic neurones) reveal that approximately 70% of the patient's nigrostriatal dopaminergic neurones have already been lost. The implication of this finding is that treatments which might actually halt neuronal death ('disease-modifying drugs' as opposed to 'symptomatic treatments') should ideally be used in presymptomatic cases, e.g. as identified by dopamine scanning of the elderly, or relatives of affected individuals. In only about 15% of Parkinson's cases is there a clear family history, and not more than 10% of cases are caused by a recognised gene mutation. Furthermore, no current treatment strate-gies have been shown to prevent disease progression,

with the possible exception of rasagiline. Rather, existing drug therapies primarily serve to enhance dopaminergic neurotransmission, whose deficiency underlies the main symptoms of Parkinson's disease.

The pathophysiology of Parkinson's disease, and its critical dependency upon dopamine, arises from an imbalance between two striatal–thalamic–cerebral cortical circuits (Fig. 10.4). To understand this, it is useful to remember that under normal circumstances the globus pallidus INternus (GPi) INhibits thalamic communication with the frontal cortex, thereby braking voluntary movements. Since dopaminergic input to the striatum itself suppresses GPi (via a 'direct' pathway), loss of dopaminergic input allows

Fig. 10.4 Schematic diagram of principal 'volitional' motor pathways, and their interaction with dopaminer-gic input in health (A) and in Parkinson's disease (B). In A, normal dopaminergic tone favours the direct path-way which involves two sequential inhibitions, and so overall motor activation (i.e. a '_' and '_' making a 't'). In B, inadequate dopaminergic input favours the indirect pathway which involves three sequential inhibitions, and so overall motor inhibition (i.e. a '_' and '_' and '_', making a '_').

the GPi to be overactive, thereby favouring inhibition of motor cortex, and so causing slowness of movement (bradykinesia) or freezing. Loss of dopamine also encourages an indirect pathway between striatum, subthalamic nucleus and GPi, which has the net effect of increasing GPi braking of movement. Therefore replacing dopamine can increase the relative contribution of the 'direct' relative to 'indirect' pathway. Furthermore, inducing neurosurgical stereotactic against the globus pallidus or subthalamus can offer a reduction in bradykinesia.

OBJECTIVES OF THERAPY

The main goal of treatment in Parkinson's disease is to manage symptoms for as long as possible while minimising treatment-associated complications. The following principles motivate pharmacological strategies:

Enhancement of dopaminergic neurotransmission. This can be achieved by:

- Administering the dopamine precursor levodopa.
- Decreasing endogenous clearance and breakdown of dopamine by inhibiting monoamine oxidase (selegiline, rasagiline) or catechol-O-methyltransferase (entacapone, tolcapone).
- Stimulating dopamine receptors with agonists (ropinirole, pramipexole, cabergoline, rotigotine, apomorphine).
- Increasing pre-synaptic dopamine release (amantadine–this mechanism being only one of many by which this drug may be effective).
- Avoiding dopamine antagonists (especially traditional neuroleptics such as haloperidol, and antiemetics such as prochlorperazine).

Note that the most seemingly obvious treatment strategy–ingesting or infusing dopamine – is ineffective because dopamine is rapidly metabolised in the gut, blood and liver by monoamine oxidase and catechol-O-methyltransferase. Furthermore, intravenously administered dopamine, or dopamine formed in peripheral tissues, is insufficiently lipid soluble to penetrate the CNS.

Pre-empting and treating levodopa-induced motor complications. Although levodopa is the most effective symptomatic treatment at all stages of the disease, its main drawback is that it usually results in treatment-induced fluctuations in motor control ('on–off' phenomena) and dyskinesias (i.e. excessive purposeless movements appearing as restlessness or rocking) by about 5–10 years from treatment initiation. One of the main factors associated with this complication is the total previous exposure to levodopa. Hence, in patients under approximately 70 years old, it is preferable to begin therapy with drugs other than levodopa, typically dopamine agonists or an MAO inhibitor. As the disease progresses, and symptoms become more severe in spite of non-levodopa therapies, levodopa is introduced, albeit in small doses, and increasing only very gradually so that only the smallest dose providing reasonable symptom relief is used. In patients over 70 years old, long-term dyskinesias are not so relevant, and moreover alternatives to levodopa, namely dopamine agonists, anticholinergics and amantadine, are more prone to cause confusion in this age group.

One of the theories for why motor fluctuations occur is related to the pulsatile nature by which levodopa is traditionally administered, which results in brain concentrations of levodopa (and dopamine) that rise and fall several times over a typical day. This is in contrast to the 'physiological mode' of dopamine release that is to a large extent tonic. Pulsatile, rather than smooth, administration of levodopa or dopamine agonists has been found in animal models to result in a gradual shortening of treatment response and dyskinesias. Consequently, methods which 'smooth' circulating levodopa concentrations may protect against eventual development of motor complications. Furthermore, a more sustained and steady supply of levodopa compared to conventional levodopa preparations can be achieved by using catechol-O-methyltransferase (COMT) inhibitors (entacapone or tolcapone) taken at the same time as levodopa, which has the effect of inhibiting dopamine catabolism, and so increasing dopamine availability. Using this strategy from the outset of Parkinson's disease is controversial, with one study[21] showing that levodopa-COMT inhibitors started as first-line therapy result in the sooner development of dyskinesias relative to standard levodopa therapy, possibly due to the fact that patients are exposed to higher effective concentrations of levodopa from early on.

Use of cholinergic drugs. One model of Parkinson's disease conceptualises its pharmacology in terms of a relative imbalance between dopamine levels (too low) and acetylcholine levels (too high). This model explains the fact that cholinergic (muscarinic-type receptor) antagonists are also effective for tremor andrigidity (but not bradykinesia). Morerecently, cholinesterase inhibitors (especially rivastigmine) that increase acetylcholine levels have been used successfully for psychosis and dementia in Parkinson's disease, without generally worsening the patient's motor symptoms. This observation challenges any simplistic relationship between acetylcholine excess and Parkinson's disease symptomatology.

Treatment of non-motor symptoms of Parkinson's disease. Consultations with patients should include enquiry into non-motor symptoms that are associated with Parkinson's disease, and, if present, treatments prescribed appropriately. These include: antidepressants for depression; laxatives for constipation; NSAIDs for pain (especially frozen shoulder); benzodiazepines for REM-sleep disorder; fludrocortisone for postural hypotension; cholinesterase inhibitors for psychosis or dementia; and salivary gland injections of botulinum toxin for sialorrhoea.

Recognition of conservative, surgical and co-morbidity therapies. Patients should be encouraged to keep mobile and exercise within their capabilities. Patients may need to be offered physiotherapy, speech therapy and occupational therapy, the latter of which will involve evaluation of potential risks in the environment, e.g. loose carpet, stairs. Patients with advanced disease who are not demented but suffer severe fluctuations may benefit from functional neurosurgery, the commonest procedure of which is bilateral deep brain electrical stimulation (DBS) of the subthalamic nucleus. Finally, coexisting morbidities, such as hypertension, diabetes and stroke, should be treated optimally, e.g. with antihypertensives, aspirin and statins, so as to reduce cerebral vascular injury, itself a cause of parkinsonism and dementia.

DRUGS FOR PARKINSON'S DISEASE

Dopaminergic drugs

Levodopa and dopa decarboxylase inhibitors

Levodopa ('dopa' stands for dihydroxyphenylalanine) is the natural amino acid precursor of dopamine. It is readily absorbed from the upper small intestine by active amino acid transport, and traverses the blood–brain barrier by a similar active transport mechanism. Within the brain levodopa is decarboxylated (by dopa decarboxylase) to dopamine.

A major disadvantage is that levodopa is also extensively decarboxylated to dopamine in peripheral tissues, such that only 1%–5% of an oral dose of levodopa reaches the brain. This means that large quantities of administered levodopa would be required for a meaningful antiparkinsonian effect. Such high doses cause a high rate of adverse effects caused by peripheral actions of levodopa and dopamine, notably nausea, cardiac arrhythmia and postural hypotension. Furthermore, high-dose levodopa inhibits gastric emptying and results in erratic delivery to the absorption site and fluctuations in plasma concentration. This problem has been largely circumvented by the development of peripheral decarboxylase inhibitors, which do not enter the CNS, and so selectively prevent peripheral conversion of levodopa to dopamine. Thus by combining levodopa with a peripheral decarboxylase inhibitor, unwanted effects due to peripheral dopamine production are minimised, while the proportion of ingested levodopa available for export into the CNS is maximised. Decarboxylase inhibitors are given in combination with levodopa in one of several formulations:

- Co-careldopa (carbidopa + levodopa in respective proportions 12.5/50, 25/100 and 50 mg/200 mg) (Sinemet).

- Co-beneldopa (benserazide+levodopa in proportions 12.5/50, 25/100, 50 mg/200 mg) (Madopar).
- Co-careldopa with entacapone (carbidopa + levodopa + entacapone in same proportions as co-careldopa plus entacapone 200 mg with each tablet) (Stalevo).

These combinations produce similar brain concentrations of dopamine as achievable by levodopa alone, but with only 25% of the levodopa dose given.

The half-life of levodopa given with a decarboxylase inhibitor is 90 min, but its acute motor benefit lasts for 6 h or so, while there is also a lesser effect that lasts for approximately 2 weeks. The acute motor response to levodopa gradually reduces with long-term therapy, which may be related to a progressively diminishing reserve of healthy dopaminergic neurones which store levodopa and allow gradual conversion to dopamine.

Dose management. Levodopa preparations are introduced gradually and titrated according to individual response. Compliance is important. Abrupt discontinuation of therapy can lead to relapse, that when extreme can resemble the neuroleptic malignant syndrome. A controlled-release preparation of levodopa/carbidopa is occasionally used for patients with nocturnal symptoms or akinesia on awakening, when it is prescribed for use before bedtime. This preparation has not proven to be useful for daytime fluctuations, as it increases levodopa levels slowly, and so either controls symptoms too slowly to be useful, or increases the likelihood of end-of-dose dyskinesias. A soluble form of co-beneldopa is also available which can help provide rapid relief of akinesia, e.g. on awakening, and may be more appropriate in patients with dysphagia.

Adverse effects. As mentioned above, the main drawback to levodopa use is the eventual development of motor complications, with about 50% of treated patients developing them within 5 years (although they can occur after only a few months with high doses, especially in young patients), and nearly all patients developing some by 10 years. These take the form of motor fluctuations, e.g. 'wearing off', when the duration of clinical response shortens with chronicity of treatment, or 'on–off fluctuations', when the patient's response to each levodopa dose consists of swinging abruptly between violent dyskinesias (during which the patient can move to a degree voluntarily, and so is 'on') and freezing (i.e. 'off'). Dyskinesias typically take the form of continual writhing, rocking or fidgeting movements (also termed 'chorea') of the limb, trunk, neck, lips or tongue. These are believed to arise from both pre-synaptic (e.g. diminution of dopa decarboxylase reserves) and post-synaptic (e.g. receptor down-regulation) mechanisms. Dyskinesias can occur coincident with both the peak levodopa blood concentration (e.g. mid-dose), or at the onset and offset of each dose's clinical effect (i.e. biphasic pattern).

Levodopa-induced dyskinesias are dose-related, so that in general the lowest dose of levodopa is used that achieves a reasonable degree of symptom relief. Further strategies that can be used against motor fluctuations/dyskinesias include: avoiding taking levodopa with meals; using small doses more often; slow-release levodopa preparations taken before sleep, and use of adjunctive medications such as dopamine agonists; amantadine, and COMT inhibitors (taken together with levodopa). In advanced cases, a nasoduodenal feeding tube can be placed that allows for continuous enteric infusion of levodopa gel (Duodopa), or patients can be offered deep brain stimulation. All these methods, in enhancing the effectiveness of dopamine or providing alternative antiparkinsonian methods, enable a reduction in levodopa dose, and so provide strategies in cases where dyskinesias are prominent.

In the short term, the main unwanted effect is nausea, which can be minimised by increasing dosage gradually, and offering patients a safe antiemetic such as domperidone (a peripherally confined dopamine antagonist) or cyclizine (an antihistamine), taken half an hour before levodopa. This is usually only required for the first few weeks. Postural hypotension may occur, although this can develop as a feature of advanced Parkinson's disease due to degeneration of noradrenergic nuclei within the brainstem and cord. Agitation and confusion, including visual hallucinations, may occur but it may be difficult to decide whether these are due to drug or to disease. Mental changes are particularly likely in the elderly, especially when there is pre-existing dementia. If acute confusion occurs, other Parkinson's drugs that cause confusion – antimuscarinics, amantadine or dopamine agonists should be progressively withdrawn before levodopa. Alternatively, the anticholinesterase rivastigmine, or atypical neuroleptics such as quetiapine or clozapine, may be of benefit.

Interactions. With non-selective monoamine oxidase inhibitors (MAOIs), the monoamine dopamine formed from levodopa is protected from destruction; it accumulates and also follows the normal path of conversion to noradrenaline/norepinephrine, by dopamine b-hydroxylase; severe hypertension results. This is not generally seen with the selective MAO-B inhibitors, selegiline or rasagiline, used as adjuncts in Parkinson's disease.

Levodopa antagonises the effects of antipsychotics (dopamine receptor blockers). Tricyclic antidepressants are safe.

Dopamine agonists

These mimic the effects of dopamine, the endogenous agonist, which stimulates both of the main types of dopamine receptor, D_1 and D_2 (coupled respectively to adenylyl cyclase stimulation and inhibition). The D_2 receptor is the principal target in Parkinson's disease, although chronic D_1-receptor stimulation potentiates response to the D_2 receptor. The main advantage of dopamine agonists relative to levodopa is that they do not result in significant motor fluctuations or dyskinesias, which may relate to their longer $t_{1/2}$, and to the fact that they are not dependent upon pre-synaptic conversion. Whether they also protect dopaminergic neurones by sparing the levodopa dose, and therefore reducing levodopa-induced oxidative damage, has been theorised but not proven. Conversely, dopamine agonists are not as effective as levodopa, and are limited by a higher rate of confusion and psychosis in the elderly. On the other hand, the problems of developing synthetic alternatives are:

- Reproducing the right balance of D_1 and D_2 stimulation (dopamine itself is slightly D_1 selective, in test systems, but its net effect in vivo is determined also by the relative amounts and locations of receptors – which differ in parkinsonian patients from normal).
- Avoiding the undesired effects of peripheral, mainly gastric, D_2 receptors.
- Synthesising a full, not partial, agonist.

Ergot derivatives (cabergoline, pergolide, lisuride, bromocriptine). These first-generation dopamine agonists are now not preferred because of their high rate of unwanted effects. In particular, the ergotamine component can cause fibrosis of internal organs after chronic exposure, leading to serious complications (below).

Cabergoline and pergolide are the best known drugs of this class; the former has the advantage of being very long acting (a $t_{1/2}$ of more than 80 h), allowing a once-daily (or even twice-weekly) administration. The $t_{1/2}$ of pergolide is 6 h, longer than that of levodopa. Both drugs therefore allow for a more enduring 'on' phase, and can relieve parkinsonian symptoms through the night and on awakening. The ergotamine property of these drugs can cause Raynaud's phenomenon (painful cold extremities due to vasospasm), while their additional properties as 5-hydroxytryptamine (5-HT) type 2 receptor agonists can cause pleural effusions, pulmonary or retroperitoneal fibrosis (the latter causing renal failure due to ureteric obstruction). Additionally, cardiac valve fibrosis may result in valvular incompetency, e.g. aortic regurgitation or pulmonary valve regurgitation (the latter a very rare valvular abnormality otherwise). These effects are also seen with chronic amfetamine use, e.g. dexfenfluramine (antiobesity drugs), possibly through effects on similar receptors. Consequently, patients who previously received ergot derivatives are now treated with non-ergot derivatives. In those patients who require ergotamine dopamine agonists (because non-ergotamine equivalents may be less effective), screening for potential complications is required, e.g. by measuring plasma creatinine and performing echocardiograms 6-monthly.

Bromocriptine is a D_2-receptor agonist and a weak a-adrenoceptor antagonist. It is commonly used to suppress the production of prolactin in patients with prolactinomas (pituitary tumours) but now only rarely for Parkinson's disease because nausea, vomiting and postural hypotension are more prominent than with more modern dopamine agonists. Pleural effusions and retroperitoneal fibrosis may also occur with prolonged use.

Non-ergot dopamine agonists (ropinirole, pramipexole, rotigotine). These drugs are currently preferred as first-line therapy in newly diagnosed patients under the age of 70 years old. Beyond this age group, the long-term complications of levodopa are not felt to be so relevant (and are milder in older-onset Parkinson's patients) allowing for levodopa use from the outset. Furthermore, psychosis or confusion (unwanted effects of all dopamine agonists) are more likely in elderly patients taking these drugs.

Both ropinirole and pramipexole are relatively selective dopamine 2 receptor agonists, and are generally more effective against tremor than other symptoms. Both drugs are started at low dose and increased over weeks or months, to a maintenance dose (e.g. ropinirole starts at 0.75 mg/day and typically is increased to 9 mg/day over 9 weeks). The relatively short $t\frac{1}{2}$ of these drugs necessitates thrice daily administration but formulations that allow oncedaily administration are available. The dopamine agonist rotigotine can be used daily as a transdermal patch, and is particularly convenient in Parkinson's patients with dysphagia.

Apart from psychosis in elderly patients, the other notable unwanted effects of the non-ergot dopamine agonists are: postural hypotension, ankle oedema, daytime somnolence (including sudden sleep attacks in a minority of patients), and impulse-control disorders in about 15%, including punding, hypersexuality, gambling, eating binges and compulsive shopping. Some of these behaviours may be more likely in Parkinson's disease patients, independent of a treatment effect, due to a dysregulated dopamine-prefrontal reward system. Where obsessionality develops on dopamine agonist therapy, this usually occurs in patients already taking a high daily levodopa dose,

and indeed can lead to addiction and patient-initiated escalation of drug doses. The approach in these cases is gradually to withdraw the dopamine agonist.

Inhibition of dopamine metabolism: MAO-inhibitorsand COMT inhibitors

Monoamine oxidase (MAO) enzymes have an important function in modulating the intraneuronal content of neurotransmitters. The enzymes exist in two principal forms, A and B, defined by specific substrates, some of which cannot be metabolised by the other form. The therapeutic importance of recognising these two forms arises because they are to some extent present in different tissues, and the enzyme at these different locations can be selectively inhibited by the individual inhibitors: moclobemide for MAO-A and selegiline or rasagiline for MAO-B.

Selegiline. is a selective, irreversible inhibitor of MAO type B. The problem with non-selective MAO inhibitors is that they prevent degradation of dietary amines, especially tyramine, which may then act systemically as sympathomimetics (causing the so-called hypertensive 'cheese reaction'). Selegiline does not cause the cheese reaction, because MAO-A in the liver and sympathetic nerve endings is unaffected, allowing tyramine to be metabolised. In the CNS, selegiline reduces intraneuronal degradation of dopamine, but has no effect on synaptic cleft concentrations of other neuromodulatory amines, such as serotonin and noradrenaline/ norepinephrine. The effects of these amines can be enhanced by MAO-A inhibitors used as antidepressants.

Rasagiline is another MAO type B inhibitor, but has an advantage over selegiline in not producing amfetamine metabolites, which are believed to be part of the reason for confusion in susceptible patients. Furthermore, two trials of rasagiline have suggested that patients who take this early in their disease course show an enduring benefit (of up to 6 years), relative both to patients on placebo, and to those who are treated with rasagiline only after a delay of 9 months. While potentially evidence for a 'disease modifying', rather than merely a symptomatic treatment effect, longer-term follow-up of these patients, and further independent trials will be required to confirm this.

Entacapone inhibits catechol-O-methyltransferase (COMT), one of the principal enzymes responsible for the metabolism of dopamine, and so prolongs the action of levodopa. It is most effective for patients who experience only short-lived 'on' periods with levodopa, and in whom frequent levodopa doses are used (typically at 3–4-hourly intervals), by providing a more predictable and stable response. It is taken at the same time as levodopa, usually as part of the same drug formulation (Stalevo). Entacapone is preferred to long-acting preparations of levodopa, whose main disadvantage is their slow onset of action. The adverse effects of entacapone include increased dyskinesias (by increasing the effective brain levodopa concentration), bodily fluids e.g. urine, turning orange, and diarrhoea.

Tolcapone is a COMT inhibitor that can be more effective than entacapone; it is taken three times per day, not necessarily at the same time as levodopa. Its main drawback is hepatotoxicity, resulting in liver failure in approximately 1 in 13 000 cases, thereby necessitating fortnightly screening blood tests.

Antimuscarinic (anticholinergic) drugs

Antimuscarinic drugs benefit parkinsonism by blocking acetylcholine receptors in the CNS, thereby partially redressing the imbalance created by decreased dopaminergic activity. Their use originated when hyoscine was given to parkinsonian patients in an attempt to reduce sialorrhoea by peripheral effect, and it then became apparent that they had other beneficial effects in this disease. Synthetic derivatives are now used orally. These include benzhexol (trihexyphenidyl), orphenadrine, benzatropine, procyclidine, biperiden. There is little to choose between these. Antimuscarinics produce modest improvements in tremor, rigidity, sialorrhoea, muscular stiffness and leg cramps, but do not generally help with bradykinesia. They are also effective intramuscularly or intravenously in acute drug-induced dystonias.

Unwanted effects include dry mouth, blurred vision, constipation, urine retention, acute glaucoma, hallucinations, memory defects and acute confusional states (which, once again, are more likely in elderly patients).

Amantadine

Amantadine antedates the discovery of dopamine receptor subtypes, and its discovery as an antiparkinsonian drug was an example of serendipity. It is an antiviral drug which, given for influenza to a parkinsonian patient, was noticed to be beneficial. The two effects are probably unrelated. It appears to act by increasing synthesis and release of dopamine, and by diminishing neuronal reuptake. It also has a slight antimuscarinic effect. The drug is much less effective than levodopa, whose action it enhances slightly, but it has the advantage of reducing levodopa- induced dyskinesias. It is more effective than the standard antimuscarinic drugs, with which it has an additive effect. Amantadine is relatively free from adverse effects but there do occur ankle oedema (probably a local effect on blood vessels), postural hypotension, livedo reticularis and CNS disturbances, e.g. insomnia, hallucinations and, rarely, fits. It is more likely to cause confusion in the elderly and so is preferred for younger patients.

Drug-induced parkinsonism

The classical antipsychotic drugs block dopamine receptors, and their antipsychotic activity relates closely to this action, which notably involves the D_2 receptor, the principal target in Parkinson's disease. It comes as no surprise, therefore, that these drugs, as well as certain calcium antagonists, e.g. flunarizine (used for migraine) and valproate, can induce a state with clinical features very similar to those of idiopathic Parkinson's disease. An important distinguishing measure between drug-induced parkinsonism and Parkinson's disease is that the former shows a normal dopamine-transporter binding using a DAT scan, since the nigrostriatal terminals (on which the transporter is located) are intact; in Parkinson's disease there is typically a (asymmetric) reduction in transporter binding. The piperazine phenothiazines, e.g. trifluoperazine, and the butyrophenones, e.g. haloperidol, are most commonly involved, whereas neuroleptics with high antimuscarinic blocking activity, e.g. thioridazine, are less likely to cause this.

Treatment of drug-induced parkinsonism firstly involves consideration of whether the offending drug can be withdrawn, or replaced, e.g. by an atypical antipsychotic such as quetiapine, lanzapine or clozapine, that provokes fewer extrapyramidal effects. After withdrawal of the offending drug, most cases resolve completely within 7 weeks. When drug-induced parkinsonism is troublesome, an antimuscarinic drug, e.g. trihexyphenidyl, is beneficial, while levodopa and dopamine agonists are not (and risk provoking psychosis).

Tardive dyskinesias, such as repetitive orofacial or lingual movements, that come on after neuroleptics have been withdrawn, are distinct from drug-induced parkinsonism, can be worsened by anticholinergics, and so are instead treated with reinstatement of the offending drug if appropriate, switching to an atypical neuroleptic, e.g. quetiapine, and addition of either tetrabenazine (which depletes pre-synaptic dopamine) or clonazepam.

Part 6. Multiple sclerosis

Multiple sclerosis (MS) is the archetypal neuroinflammatory disease and the commonest cause of neurodisability in young adults. In recent years there has been a rapid expansion in the number of available disease-modifying immunomodulatory therapies, all of which are normally given by a specialist MS centre. It is important to distinguish the inflammatory component of MS, which usually manifests itself as self-terminating relapses, from a more insidious neurodegenerative component that is the cause of long-term 'progressive' disability. Most drug therapies target the former process without appearing to have significant impact on the latter.

First-line injectable disease-modifying drugs

Interferon (IFN) β was the first treatment consistently to show a reduction in the number of symptomatic relapses, and demyelinating lesions observable on MRI. IFNβ also delays disability by 12–18 months in relapsing/remitting disease, probably by reducing relapses (rather than because of an effect on progression). Clinical trials show that in ambulant MS patients with relapsing/remitting disease, IFNβ produces a relative reduction in risk of relapse of approximately one-third. Furthermore, in previously healthy patients who present with a 'clinically isolated syndrome', i.e. a single episode of neurological disturbance associated with MRI white matter lesions, IFNβ delays the occurrence of a second episode. Thus the drug may suppress the onset of multiple sclerosis (taken as the point at which more than one neurological episode has occurred).

IFNβ is a polypeptide, normally produced by fibroblasts, whose natural purpose is probably as an effector of an antiviral response. It has multiple immunological effects, including suppression of antibody production, cytokine modulation (e.g. increasing interleukin-10 while decreasing tumour necrosis factor-a and interleukin-1), and inhibition of antigen presentation, T-cell proliferation, differentiation and migration into the brain. As a therapy it is produced as a human recombinant product within either mammalian cells (type 1a; Avonex or Rebif) or modified E. coli bacteria (type 1b: Betaferon or Betaseron) formulations, with only the Rebif formulation available in more than one dose. It is not indicated for patients with purely progressive forms of disease, although it may still be effective at reducing relapses in patients who have entered a relapsing, progressive phase (i.e. continuous disability progression with superimposed temporary exacerbations).

IFNβ is usually self-injected either subcutaneously three times per week, or i.m. once per week. Unwanted effects of IFNβ are usually minor, with some patients experiencing 'flu-like symptoms, nausea, mildly deranged liver or thyroid function tests, mood disturbance (it is thus relatively contraindicated in patients with a history of depression or suicidal thoughts) and less commonly, seizures. With IFNβ, especially type 1b preparations, some patients develop neutralising antibodies, resulting in a clear decrease in therapeutic efficacy in approximately one-third of patients. The finding of raised antibody levels may prompt change in therapy.

Glatiramer acetate (co-polymer) is an oligopeptide that suppresses various components of the MS-immune response. Like IFNβ, it is self-administered, albeit in daily subcutaneous injections, and has the advantage of not inducing neutralising antibodies. The range of patients in which it is effective, and its level of efficacy, matches that of IFNβ.

Oral disease-modifying drugs

The development of oral disease-modifying therapies for multiple sclerosis promises to transform patient experience by offering patients a considerably more practical and painless therapy compared to the previous mainstay of treatment – IFNβ. Furthermore, preliminary trials suggest that the effectiveness of these therapies is superior to that of IFNβ, with relative reductions in relapse rate approaching 50% and relative reductions in new MRI lesions of 50%–80%.

Sphingolipid (also called fingolimod) is high-affinity agonist at the sphingosine-1-phosphate receptor, causing receptor down-regulation. This receptor is normally required to allow lymphocyte egress from lymph nodes, and so the drug suppresses trafficking of autoreactive T cells into the blood. ECG monitoring is required as it can cause heart block. Laquinimod shifts the immunophenotype of T-helper lymphocytes to a Th2 pattern (characterised by IL-4 secretion), and away from a Th1 pattern (characterised by interferon-g secretion), the latter of which is believed to be contributory to ongoing relapses. Fumarate is a citric acid cycle intermediate that acts in a similar way to laquinimod, but may also act to up-regulate antioxidant enzymes via the Nrf2 signalling pathway. It can cause flushing, pruritus and abdominal pain. Cladribine acts as a purine nucleotide antagonist that suppresses DNA replication necessary for lymphocyte and monocyte division (indeed its original use was for the treatment of leukaemia). It has the advantage that only two 5-day courses per year need be taken to produce a significant MS-treatment effect. Thus adverse effects seen with high doses of this drug used for cancer, e.g. nephrotoxicity and neuropathy, can mostly be avoided in MS treatment. A small excess of bone marrow suppression and opportunistic infection is still observed. Finally, teriflunomide is the active metabolite of leflunomide (used in rheumatoid arthritis) that blocks pyrimidine, and consequently, DNA synthesis. Similar to cladribine, it is associated with mild myelosuppression and upper respiratory tract infection.

Intravenous therapies

Monoclonal antibodies targeted against critical steps of the cell-mediated immune reactions that underlie MS are among the most effective immunomodulatory therapies in MS. But these drugs also carry the potential for serious unwanted effects (notably opportunistic infections) and are therefore reserved for patients with rapid deterioration who have failed to respond to less intensive immunomodulatory therapies such as IFNβ.

Natalizumab (Tysabri) targets the alpha4-beta1-integrin receptor VCAM-1 (vascular cell adhesion molecule) that is required for T lymphocytes to enter the central nervous system from the blood. Typically administered every 4 weeks, it decreases relapse rate by up to 70%. A real concern is that approximately 1 in 1 000 treated patients (predominantly those taking additional immunosuppressants) develop progressive multifocal leukoencephalopathy (PML). This is an aggressive cerebral white-matter disease caused by reactivation of the Jakob–Creutzfeldt virus, previously seen only in diseases characterised by immunocompromise, such as advanced HIV infection or lymphoma. Unlike PML in these diseases which are nearly always fatal, PML associated with natalizumab can be reversed if therapy discontinues soon after its development (MRI scans are necessary every few months while on treatment).

Alemtuzumab (MabCampath or Campath) comprises monoclonal antibodies against CD52 – a marker of mature lymphocytes. In certain patients with frequent relapses it has been able to completely suppress their future occurrence. This occurs at the risk of provoking new organ-based autoimmune diseases, especially thyroid disease (in 40%), immune thrombocytopenic purpura (ITP) and Goodpasture's disease (that can cause life-threatening bleeding and renal failure, respectively).

Other intravenous therapies used in advanced cases of MS include mitoxantrone, a cytotoxic drug that decreases interleukin-10 production, but which can cause infertility, cardiomyopathy and promyelocytic leukaemia, rituximab (anti-CD20 monoclonal antibody), i.v. immunoglobulin, cyclophosphamide and bone-marrow ablation with subsequent autologous stem-cell transplantation.

Symptomatic therapies

Corticosteroid therapy is often used for acute, disabling attacks of MS. The drugs decrease the length of an attack but do not reduce the number of recurrent attacks or the final disability. Methylprednisolone (0.5–1 g) is given i.v. or by mouth over a 3–5-day period. Intravenous treatment appears to benefit relapses of optic neuritis more than do oral steroids but usually requires hospital admission.

Urinary frequency and urgency (spastic bladder) is common, for which the antimuscarinics propantheline or oxybutynin can be useful by acting as a detrusor relaxant. Constipation is treated with laxatives, while impotence may respond to sildenafil. In progressive disease, muscle spasticity can be severe and disabling. Oral baclofen or tizanidine, or locally injected botulinum toxin can reduce spasticity, but over-treatment may lead to flaccid weakness. Intranasal cannabinoid is a more recent treatment for spasticity. Very occasionally, baclofen given intrathecally by an implanted pump can relieve severe spas-

ticity. Fatigue is common in MS and may respond to amantadine or modafinil. Depression or psychosis, features of MS, require specific treatments. Finally, the role of general supportive measures, such as ramps, wheelchairs, stairlifts, prevention of bedsores, cannot be overstated.

IMPORTANT TERMINOLOGY

cholinergic drugs   胆碱能药物

anticholinergic drugs   抗胆碱能药物

anticholinesterases   抗胆碱酯酶

adrenergic mechanisms   肾上腺素能机制

aympathomimetics   拟交感神经药

neurological disorders   神经系统疾病

epilepsy   癫痫

Parkinson's disease   帕金森病

multiple sclerosis   多发性硬化

seizure   惊厥

calcium channel blockers   钙通道阻滞剂

monoamine oxidase   单胺氧化酶

substrate   底物

inhibitors   抑制剂

inducer   诱导剂

CHALLENGE YOURSELF

1. Please describe the classification and pharmacology of Cholinergic drugs.
2. Please describe the clinical application of anticholinergic drugs.
3. Please detail the classification of adrenergic drugs by mode of action and selectivity for adrenoceptors.
4. Please detail the management principles of epilepsy.
5. Please detail the treatment drugs of Parkinson's disease.

Zhi Dong

Chapter 11

Psychotropic drugs

Psychiatric disorders, including depression, schizophrenia, anxiety, sleep disorders, dementia, and attention deficit/hyperactivity disorder, affect millions of people around the world. Without intervention, they can have devastating effects and interfere with daily life. Decades of research led to a variety of therapeutic options for people with psychiatric disorders, but how well they work varies greatly from person to person. Researchers in neuroscience and related disciplines are studying genes and brain areas affected by psychiatric disorders in animals and humans in an effort to develop better therapies alongside more traditional treatments. Scientists hope to create new paths to treatments that offer faster relief with fewer side effects, and diagnostic tests that identify psychiatric disorders earlier. This chapter considers the drugs for the psychiatric disorders, as well as the drugs for sleep disorders and dementia.

Diagnostic issues

Older classifications of psychiatric disorder divided diseases into 'psychoses' and 'neuroses'. The term 'psychosis' is still widely used to describe a severe mental illness with hallucinations, delusions, extreme abnormalities of behavior including marked overactivity, retardation and catatonia, usually with lack of insight. Psychotic disorders include schizophrenia, severe depression and mania. Psychosis may also be due to illicit substances or organic conditions. Clinical features of schizophrenia are subdivided into 'positive symptoms', which include hallucinations, delusions and thought disorder, and 'negative symptoms' such as apathy, flattening of affect and poverty of speech.

Disorders formerly grouped under 'neuroses' include anxiety disorders (e.g. panic disorder, generalized anxiety disorder, obsessive–compulsive disorder, phobias and post-traumatic stress disorder), eating disorders (e.g. anorexia nervosa and bulimia nervosa), depression (provided there are no 'psychotic' symptoms) and sleep disorders.

Also falling within the scope of modern psychiatric diagnostic systems are organic mental disorders (e.g. dementia in Alzheimer's disease), disorders due to substance misuse, personality disorders, disorders of childhood and adolescence, and mental retardation.

Drug therapy in relation to psychological treatment

No account of drug treatment strategies for psychiatric illness is complete without considering psychological therapies. Psychotherapies range widely, from simple counseling (supportive psychotherapy) through psychoanalysis to newer techniques such as cognitive behavioural therapy.

As a general rule, psychotic illnesses require drugs as first-line treatment, with psychotherapy being adjunctive, for instance in promoting drug compliance, improving family relationships and helping individuals cope with distressing symptoms. By contrast, for depression and anxiety disorders, such as panic disorder and obsessive–compulsive disorder, forms of psychotherapy are available that provide alternative first-line treatment to medication. The choice between drugs and psychotherapy depends on treatment availability, previous history of response, patient preference and the ability of the patient to work appropriately with the chosen therapy. In many cases there is scope and sometimes advantage to the use of drugs and psychotherapy in combination.

All doctors who prescribe drugs engage in a 'therapeutic relationship' with their patients. A depressed person whose doctor is empathic, supportive and appears to believe in the efficacy of the drug prescribed is more likely to take the medication and to adopt a hopeful mindset than if the doctor seemed aloof and ambivalent about the value of psychotropic drugs. Remembering that placebo response rates of 30–40% are common in double-blind trials of antidepressants, we should never underestimate the importance of our relationship with the patient in enhancing the pharmacological efficacy of the drugs we use.

Part 1. Antidepressant drugs

Antidepressants can be broadly divided into four main classes, tricyclics (TCA, named after their three-ringed structure), selective serotonin reuptake inhibitors (SSRIs), monoamine oxidase inhibitors (MAOIs) and novel compounds, some of which are related to TCAs or SSRIs. Clinicians who wish to have a working knowledge of antidepressants would be advised to be familiar with the use of at least one drug from each of the four main categories tabulated. A more thorough knowledge-base would demand awareness of the distinct characteristics of the subgroups of novel compounds (e.g. serotonin and noradrenaline/norepinephrine reuptake inhibitors (SNRIs), mirtazapine, reboxetine and agomelatine) and differences between individual SSRIs and TCAs. As antidepressants are largely similar in their therapeutic efficacy, awareness of profiles of unwanted effects is of particular importance.

An alternative categorisation of antidepressants is based solely on mechanism of action (Fig. 11.1). The majority of antidepressants, including SSRIs, TCAs and related compounds, are reuptake inhibitors. Certain novel agents, including trazodone and mirtazapine, are receptor blockers, whereas MAOIs are enzyme inhibitors.

Mechanism of action

The monoamine hypothesis proposes that, in depression, there is deficiency of the neurotransmitters noradrenaline/norepinephrine and serotonin in the brain which can be restored by antidepressants. Drugs that alleviate depression also enhance monoamine availability and release (Fig. 11.2), increasing activity at postsynaptic receptors. It is relevant that (older) antihypertensive agents, e.g. reserpine, which reduced the availability of noradrenaline/norepinephrine, caused depression.

SSRIs act, as their name indicates, predominantly by preventing serotonin reuptake by blocking the cell-surface serotonin transporter; with little effect on noradrenaline/norepinephrine reuptake. Tricyclic antidepressants and reboxetine inhibit noradrenaline/norepinephrine reuptake, but tricyclic effects on serotonin reuptake vary widely; desipramine and protriptyline have no effect, whereas clomipramine is about five times more potent at blocking serotonin than noradrenaline/norepinephrine reuptake. SNRIs are capable of inhibiting reuptake of both transmitters. However, for venlafaxine a dose of at least 150 mg/day is required for noradrenaline/norepinephrine uptake blockade to be exerted. Mirtazapine also achieves an increase in noradrenergic and serotonergic neurotransmission, but through antagonism of presynaptic α_2-autoreceptors (receptors that mediate negative feedback for transmitter release). Other novel antidepressants include trazodone, which blocks several types of serotonin receptor (including the 5HT2A and 5HT2C receptors) as well as α-adrenoceptors and histaminergic receptors and acts as a partial agonist at the 5HT1A receptor, and agomelatine which acts both as an agonist of melatonin receptors and a blocker of the serotonin 5HT2C

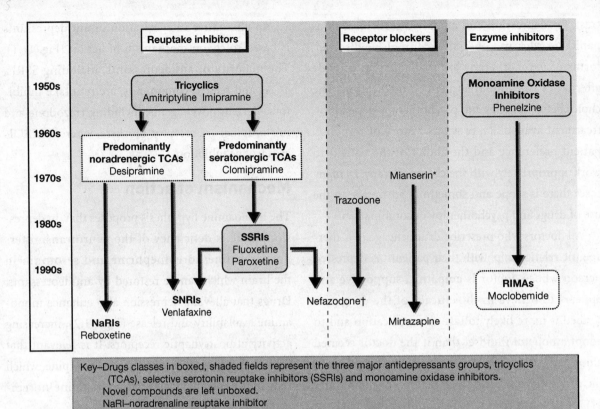

Key–Drugs classes in boxed, shaded fields represent the three major antidepressants groups, tricyclics (TCAs), selective serotonin reuptake inhibitors (SSRIs) and monoamine oxidase inhibitors.
Novel compounds are left unboxed.
NaRI–noradrenaline reuptake inhibitor
SNRI–serotonin, and noradrenaline reuptake inhibitor
RIMA–reversible inhibitor of monoamine oxidase
*–Mianserin is rarely used due to associations with aplastic anaemia
†–Nefazodone is both a reuptake inhibitor and receptor blocker no longer available in UK

Fig. 11.1 Flow chart of the evolution of antidepressant drugs, and classification by mechanism of action.

Physiological processes at the synapse:
1. When an electrical signal reaches the presynaptic terminal, presynaptic amine vesicles fuse with the neuronal membrane and release their contents into the synaptic cleft.
2. Amines in the synaptic cleft bind to postsynaptic receptors to produce a postsynaptic response.
3. Amines may be removed from the synaptic cleft by reuptake into the presynaptic neuron.
4. The monoamine oxidase enzyme breaks down presynaptic amines.

Effects of antidepressants:
A. Tricyclics prevent presynaptic reuptake of the amines noradrenaline and serotonin
B. SSRIs predominantly block reuptake of serotonin.
C. MAOIs reduce the activity of monoamine oxidase in breaking down presynaptic amines (leaving more available for release into the presynaptic cleft).
D. Some antidepressants (e.g. nefazodone) block postsynaptic receptors directly.

Fig. 11.2 Mechanism of action of antidepressant drugs at the synapse.

receptor, the combined effects of these actions leading to a rise in frontal cortex dopamine availability.

MAOIs increase the availability of noradrenaline/norepinephrine and serotonin by preventing their destruction by the monoamine oxidase type A enzyme in the presynaptic terminal. The older MAOIs, phenelzine, tranylcypromine and isocarboxazid, bind irreversibly to monamine oxidase by forming strong (covalent) bonds. The enzyme is thus rendered permanently ineffective such that amine metabolising activity can be restored only by production of fresh enzyme, which takes weeks. These MAOIs are thus called 'hit and run' drugs as their effects greatly outlast their detectable presence in the blood.

Although the monoamine hypothesis of depression is conceptually straightforward, it is in reality an oversimplification of a complicated picture. Other systems that are implicated in the aetiology of depression (and which provide potential targets for drug therapy) include the hypothalamic–pituitary–thyroid axis and the hypothalamic–pituitary–adrenal (HPA) axis. The finding that 50% of depressed patients have raised plasma cortisol concentrations constitutes evidence that depression may be associated with increased HPA drive.

Drugs with similar modes of action to antidepressants are found other uses in medicine. Bupropion (amfebutamone) inhibits reuptake of both dopamine and noradrenaline/norepinephrine. It was originally developed and used as an antidepressant but is now more frequently used to assist smoking cessation. It is also prescribed in attention deficit hyperactivity disorder. Sibutramine, licensed as an anorectic agent, is a serotonin and noradrenaline/norepinephrine reuptake inhibitor (SNRI).

Therapeutic efficacy

Provided antidepressant drugs are prescribed at an adequate dose and taken regularly, 60%–70% of patients with depression should respond within 3–4 weeks. Conventional meta-analysis have shown little evidence that any particular drug or class of antidepressant is more efficacious than others, but there are some possible exceptions to this general statement:

- Venlafaxine, in high dose (>150 mg/day) and Escitalopram may have greater efficacy than other antidepressants.
- Amitriptyline appears to be slightly more effective than other TCAs and also SSRIs for severe depression, but this advantage is compromised by its poor tolerability and lack of safety in overdose relative to more modern agents.
- The older MAOIs (e.g. phenelzine) may be more effective than other classes in 'atypical' depression, a form of depressive illness where mood reactivity is preserved, lack of energy may be extreme and biological features are the opposite of the normal syndrome, i.e. excess sleep and appetite with weight gain.

Selection

An antidepressant should be selected to match individual patients' requirements, such as the need or otherwise for a sedative effect, or the avoidance of antimuscarinic effects (especially in the elderly). In the absence of special factors, the choice rests on the weight of evidence of efficacy, the tolerability, the safety in overdose and the likelihood of an effective dose being reached. SSRIs and other newer drugs (e.g. mirtazapine and venlafaxine) are highlighted as best meeting these needs.

Mode of use

Antidepressants usually require 3–4 weeks for the full therapeutic effect to be achieved. When a minimal response is seen, an antidepressant can usefully be extended to 6 weeks to see whether further benefit is achieved. By contrast, patients may experience unwanted effects, especially 'jitteriness' or 'activation' symptoms such as increased anxiety and irritability, soon after starting treatment (they should be warned about this possibility), but such symptoms usually diminish with time. Some drugs have the advantage that they can be started at a dose which would be considered adequate for the therapeutic effect (e.g. most SSRIs) but in contrast many others, including all tricylic antidepressants, need to be started at a low and generally tolerable starting dose to the therapeutic dose. For example, imipramine should be started at 25–50 mg/day, with gradual increments to a recognised 'minimum therapeutic' dose, around 125 mg/day (140 mg/day for lofepramine). Low starting doses are particularly important for elderly patients. Only when the drug has reached the minimum therapeutic dose and been taken for at least 4 weeks can response or non-response be adequately established. However, some patients do achieve response or remission at subtherapeutic doses, for reasons of drug kinetics and limited capacity to metabolise, the self-limiting nature of depression, or by a placebo effect.

For SSRIs dose titration is often unnecessary as the minimum therapeutic dose can usually be tolerated as a starting dose. Divided doses are not usually required, and administration is by a single morning or evening dose. Evidence suggests that patients commencing treatment on SSRIs are more likely to reach an effective dose than those starting on TCAs. Of the novel compounds, trazodone usually requires titration to a minimum therapeutic dose of at least 200 mg/day. Response to reboxetine, venlafaxine and mirtazapine may occur at the starting dose, but some dose titration is commonly required. Venlafaxine is licensed for treatment-resistant depression by gradual titration from 75 to 375 mg/day. There is some need for dose titration when using MAOIs. Unlike other drug classes, reduction to a lower maintenance dose is recommended after a response is achieved if unwanted effects are problematical.

Changing and stopping antidepressants

When an antidepressant fails through lack of efficacy despite an adequate trial or due to unacceptable adverse effects, a change to a drug of a different class is generally advisable. For a patient who has not responded to an SSRI it is logical to try a novel compound such as venlafaxine, mirtazapine or reboxetine, or sometimes a tricyclic antidepressant. Any of these options may offer a greater increase in synaptic noradrenaline/norepinephrine than the ineffective SSRI.

Evidence also suggests that patients failing on one SSRI may respond to a different drug within the class, an approach that is particularly useful where other antidepressant classes have been unsuccessful previously, are contraindicated, or have characteristics that the patient or doctor feels are undesirable. Awareness of biological differences between drugs within a class may also be helpful when patients cannot tolerate other drug classes. For instance, among SSRIs, paroxetine has the most affinity for the serotonin transporter and fluoxetine the least, while among TCAs, clomipramine has more important serotonergic enhancing effects than the others.

When changing between antidepressant doses, a conservative approach would be to reduce the first antidepressant progressively over 2 or more weeks before starting the new drug. The gradual reduction is particularly important with paroxetine and venlafaxine which are known to cause 'discontinuation syndromes' if stopped abruptly, and less important with fluoxetine due to its long half-life active metabolite which offers 'built-in' protection against withdrawal problems. A more proactive approach would involve 'cross-tapering' the second antidepressant – i.e. starting it while the first antidepressant is being reduced and gradually titrating the dose up. However, an important exception concerns changes to or from MAOIs, which must be handled with great caution due to the dangers of interactions between antidepressants (see below). Therefore MAOIs cannot safely be introduced within 2 weeks of stopping most antidepressants (3 weeks for imipramine and clomipramine; combination of the latter with tranylcypromine is particularly dangerous), and not until 5 weeks after stopping fluoxetine, due to its long half-life active metabolite. Similarly, other antidepressants should not be introduced until 2–3 weeks have elapsed from discontinuation of MAOI. No washout period is required when using the reversible MAOI, moclobemide.

When a patient achieves remission, the antidepressant should be continued for at least 9 months at the dose that returned mood to normal. Premature dose reduction or withdrawal is associated with increased risk of relapse. In cases where three or more depressive episodes have occurred, evidence suggests that long-term continuation of an antidepressant offers protection, as further relapse is almost inevitable in the next 3 years. When ceasing use of an antidepressant, the dose should be reduced gradually to avoid discontinuation syndromes (symptoms include anxiety, agitation, nausea and mood swings). Discontinuation of SSRIs and venlafaxine are associated additionally with dizziness, electric shock-like sensations and paraesthesia. Short $t_{1/2}$ drugs that do not produce active metabolites (e.g. paroxetine, venlafaxine) and TCAs are most likely to cause such problems.

Augmentation

The development of many new antidepressants in recent years has reduced the need to use augmentation strategies. Nevertheless augmentation, i.e. the addition of a second drug to an existing antidepressant, can be used when two or more standard antidepressants have successively failed to alleviate depressive symptoms despite treatment at an adequate dose for an adequate time. Some of the augmentations discussed may even be used earlier than this if there is an indication or justification for the augmenting drug specific to the individual patient.

One strategy which has come to prominence is to augment (or combine) an SSRI or SNRI antidepressant with the novel antidepressant mirtazapine. The initial justification for this combination stems from mirtazapine's unorthodox mechanism of action – the idea being that the presynaptic adjustments effected by mirtazapine could act additively or even synergistically with the monoamine reuptake inhibition of SSRIs and SNRIs. A second justification is more practical – mirtazapine is known to improve the quality of sleep and serotonin reuptake inhibitors may initially disrupt this, thus mirtazapine can be added both to boost the antidepressant effect and to address an unresolved problem with sleep. An evidence base does exist both for mirtazapine–venlafaxine and mirtazapine–fluoxetine co-prescription in depression, with both combinations reported as providing significantly higher remission rates than fluoxetine alone. Ease of initiation of these combinations, along with the evidence of enhanced effectiveness, means that these are currently the most commonly used augmentation strategies for treatment of depression in psychiatry inpatients in the UK.

Another important augmentation strategy employs the mood stabiliser lithium carbonate. Controlled trials suggest that up to 50% of patients who have not responded to standard antidepressants can respond after lithium augmentation but the evidence is stronger for augmenting tricyclics than for augmenting SSRIs. Addition of lithium requires careful titration of the plasma concentration up to the therapeutic range, with periodic checks thereafter and monitoring for toxicity.

More recently, augmentation of SSRIs with atypical antipsychotics has been effective in clinical trials. Trial evidence is strongest using olanzapine, and also exists for quetiapine, risperidone and aripiprazole. Antipsychotics also have important potential for side-effects which must be taken into account before their introduction.

Tri-iodothyronine (T3) also aids antidepressant action, and most evidence points to added benefit with TCAs. When co-prescribing TCAs with thyroid hormone derivatives, be aware that the combination of lofepramine with the levo-isomer of thyroxine is contraindicated. The amino acid L-tryptophan and the β-adrenoceptor blocker pindolol may also be used to augment. Tryptophan increases 5-hydroxytryptamine (5HT) production, and pindolol may act by blocking negative feedback of 5HT on to 5HT1A-autoreceptors.

Other indications for antidepressants

Antidepressants may benefit most forms of anxiety disorder, including panic disorder, generalized anxiety disorder, post-traumatic stress disorder, obsessive–compulsive disorder and social phobia. SSRIs are recognised as first-line drug treatment for all five of these anxiety disorders.

Fluoxetine is effective in milder cases of the eating disorder bulimia nervosa, in higher doses (60 mg/day) than are required for depression. This effect is independent of that on depression (which may coexist), and may therefore involve a different mode of action. Antidepressants appear to be ineffective in anorexia nervosa. Antidepressants also have a role in pain control. The SNRI drug duloxetine is licensed for diabetic neuropathy while considerable trial evidence exists for use of the original tricyclic antidepressants imipramine and amitriptyline for the control of chronic pain.

Adverse effects

As most antidepressants have similar therapeutic efficacy, the decision regarding which drug to select often rests on adverse effect profiles and potential to cause toxicity. Selective serotonin reuptake inhibitors SSRIs have a range of unwanted effects including nausea, anorexia, dizziness, gastrointestinal disturbance, agitation, akathisia (motor restlessness) and anorgasmia (failure to experience an orgasm). They lack direct sedative effect, an advantage over older drugs in patients who need to drive motor vehicles or need to work or study. SSRIs can disrupt the pattern of sleep with increased awakenings, transient reduction in the amount of rapid eye movement (REM) and increased REM latency, but eventually sleep improves due to improved mood. SSRIs lack the side-effects of postural hypotension, antimuscarinic and antihistaminergic effects seen with TCAs. In contrast to both TCAs and mirtazapine, SSRIs may induce weight loss through their anorectic effects, at least in the short term. SSRIs are relatively safe in overdose.

The serotonin syndrome is a rare but dangerous complication of SSRI use and features restlessness, tremor, shivering and myoclonus, possibly leading on to hyperpyrexia, convulsions and delirium. The risk is increased by co-administration with drugs that enhance serotonin transmission, especially MAOIs, the antimigraine triptan drugs and St John's wort. The combination of fluoxetine or paroxetine with tramadol can also cause serotonin syndrome. These SSRIs inhibit the metabolism of tramadol to its active metabolite (which is responsible for the pain relief), leaving a build-up of unmetabolised tramadol which has sufficient serotonergic activity itself to interact with the SSRIs and enhance the risk of serotonin syndrome.

Novel compounds

Following the marketing success of SSRIs, many newer generation antidepressants have gained approval as treatments for MDD, including but not limited to serotonin and noradrenaline reuptake inhibitors (e.g. venlafaxine, desvenlafaxine and duloxetine), bupropion (a noradrenaline and dopamine reuptake Inhibitor), mirtazapine (noradrenaline and selective serotonin antagonist) and trazodone (serotonin antagonist and reuptake inhibitor). With the exception of agomelatine (melatonin receptor agonist with 5-HT$_{2C}$ receptor antagonist properties), all other agents primarily act through the modulation of monoaminergic neurotransmission. The aforementioned drugs along with SSRIs are so-called newer generation antidepressants. More recently, over the past 4 years, the US Food and Drugs Administration (FDA) has approved three additional antidepressants for the treatment of MDD, namely vilazodone, levomilnacipran and vortioxetine.

Venlafaxine produces unwanted effects that resemble those of SSRIs with a higher incidence of nausea. Sustained hypertension (due to blockade of noradrenaline/norepinephrine reuptake) is a problem in a small proportion of patients at high dose, and blood pressure should be monitored when more than 200 mg/day is taken. Venlafaxine appears to have some association with cardiac arrhythmias but whether this is to a degree that is clinically significant is unclear.

Duloxetine may cause early nausea, which tends to subside quickly. Other unwanted effects are somnolence, dizziness and constipation.

Mirtazapine has benefits in rarely being associated with sexual dysfunction and in improving sleep independent of mood but it may cause unwanted sedation and weight gain.

Trazodone is an option for depressed patients where heavy sedation is required. It also has the advantages of lacking antimuscarinic effects and of being relatively safe in overdose. Males should be warned of the possibility of priapism (painful penile erections), attributable to the drug's blockade of α_1-adrenoceptors.

Agomelatine is given at night when it appears to resynchronize circadian rhythms and therefore promotes improved sleep. Like mirtazapine it is rarely associated with sexual dysfunction, but its use necessitates early liver function tests.

Vilazodone is a novel antidepressant having a selective 5-HT reuptake inhibitor and 5-HT_{1A} receptor partial agonist profile, so it has been regarded as a serotonin partial agonist-reuptake inhibitor. Vilazodone is an effective and safe treatment option having novel mechanisms of action in patients with MDD. Relapse prevention effects and long-term efficacy of vilazodone should be established in adequately powered, large RCTs in the near future. More importantly, vilazodone's efficacy and tolerability should be compared with SSRI + buspirone in well controlled clinical trials.

Levomilnacipran, a dual serotonin-norepinephrine reuptake inhibitor, is one of the antidepressant drugs that clinicians use for routine depression care. Currently, there is inadequate evidence to conclude whether milnacipran is superior, inferior or the same as other antidepressive agents in terms of efficacy, acceptability and tolerability in the acute phase treatment of major depression. However, there is some evidence in favour of milnacipran over TCAs in terms of dropouts due to adverse events (acceptability) and the rates of experiencing adverse events (tolerability).

Vortioxetine is a multimodal antidepressant that acts as 5-HT transporter inhibitor as well as 5-HT_{3A} and 5-HT_7 receptors antagonist, 5-HT_{1A} and 5-HT_{1B} receptors partial agonist. It was recently approved in the US and the EU for the treatment of adult patients with MDD. Placebo -controlled and active- treatment trials support that VRX is effective and well -tolerated in MDD. Its combined serotonin reuptake inhibition with agonism, partial agonism and antagonism of a number of receptors might provide a broader spectrum of antidepressant activity than currently available agents.

Tricyclic antidepressants

The commonest unwanted effects are those of antimuscarinic action, i.e. dry mouth, constipation, blurred vision and difficulty with accommodation, raised intraocular pressure (glaucoma may be precipitated) and bladder neck obstruction (may lead to urinary retention in older males).

Patients may also experience: postural hypotension (through inhibition of α-adrenoceptors), which is often a limiting factor in the elderly; interference with sexual function; weight gain (through blockade of histamine H_1 receptors); prolongation of the QTc interval of the ECG, which predisposes to cardiac arrhythmias especially in overdose (use after myocardial infarction is contraindicated). Some TCAs (especially trimipramine and amitriptyline) are heavily sedating through a combination of antihistaminergic and α_1-adrenergic blocking actions, and this presents special problems to those whose lives involve driving vehicles or performing skilled tasks. In selected patients, sedation may be beneficial, e.g. a severely depressed person who has a disrupted sleep pattern or marked agitation.

There is great heterogeneity in adverse-effect profiles between TCAs. Imipramine and lofepramine cause relatively little sedation, and lofepramine is associated with milder antimuscarinic effects (but is contraindicated in patients with severe liver disease). When comparing SSRIs and TCAs for dropouts (a surrogate endpoint for tolerability), most meta-analyses show a small benefit in favour of SSRIs, although the older tricyclics imipramine and amitripyline are overrepresented in these meta-analyses.

Overdose. Depression is a risk factor for both parasuicide and completed suicide, and TCAs are commonly taken by those who deliberately self-harm. Dosulepin and amitriptyline are particularly toxic in overdose. Lofepramine is at least 15 times less likely to cause death from over dose; clomipramine and imipramine occupy intermediate positions.

Clinical features of overdose reflect the pharmacology of TCAs. Antimuscarinic effects result in warm, dry skin from vasodilatation and inhibition of sweating, blurred vision from paralysis of accommodation, papillary dilatation and urinary retention.

Consciousness is commonly dulled, and respiration depression and hypothermia may develop. Neurological signs including hyperreflexia, myoclonus, divergent strabismus and extensor plantar responses may accompany lesser degrees of impaired consciousness and provide scope for diagnostic confusion, e.g. with structural brain damage. Convulsions occur in a proportion of patients. Hallucinations and delirium occur during recovery of consciousness, often accompanied by a characteristic plucking at bedclothes.

Sinus tachycardia (due to vagal blockade) is a common feature but abnormalities of cardiac conduction accompany moderate to severe intoxication and may proceed to dangerous tachyarrhythmias or bradyarrhythmias. Hypotension may result from a combination of cardiac arrhythmia, reduced myocardial contractility and dilatation of venous capacitance vessels.

Supportive treatment suffices for the majority of cases. Activated charcoal by mouth is indicated to prevent further absorption from the alimentary tract and may be given to the conscious patient in the home prior to transfer to hospital. Convulsions are less likely if unnecessary stimuli are avoided, but severe or frequent seizures often precede cardiac arrhythmias and arrest, and their suppression with diazepam is important. Cardiac arrhythmias do not need intervention if cardiac output and tissue perfusion are adequate. Correction of hypoxia with oxygen, and acidosis by intravenous infusion of sodium bicarbonate are reasonable first measures and usually suffice.

Reboxetine is not structurally related to tricyclic agents but like lofepramine and desipramine acts predominantly by noradrenergic reuptake inhibition. Pseudo-antimuscarinic effects, particularly urinary hesistancy and dry mouth, trouble a minority of patients, postural hypotension may occur, as may impotence in males. It is relatively safe in overdose.

Monoamine oxidase inhibitors

Adverse effects include postural hypotension (especially in the elderly) and dizziness. Less common are headache, irritability, apathy, insomnia, fatigue, ataxia, gastrointestinal disturbances including dry mouth and constipation, sexual dysfunction (especially anorgasmia), blurred vision, difficult micturition, sweating, peripheral oedema, tremulousness, restlessness and hyperthermia. Appetite may increase inappropriately, causing weight gain.

Part 2. Antipsychotics

Classification

Originally tested as an antihistamine, chlorpromazine serendipitously emerged as an effective treatment for psychotic illness in the 1950s. Chlorpromazine-like drugs were originally termed 'neuroleptics' or 'major tranquillisers', but the preferred usage now is 'antipsychotics'. Classification is by chemical structure, e.g. phenothiazines, butyrophenones. Within the large phenothiazine group, compounds are divided into three types on the basis of the side-chain, as this tends to predict adverse effect profiles. The continuing search for greater efficacy and better tolerability led researchers and clinicians to reinvestigate clozapine, a drug that was originally licensed in the 1960s but subsequently withdrawn because of toxic haematological effects. Clozapine appeared to offer greater effectiveness in treatment-resistant schizophrenia, to have efficacy against 'negative' in addition to 'positive' psychiatric symptoms, and to be less likely to cause extrapyramidal motor symptoms. It regained its license in the early 1990s with strict requirements on dose titration and haematological monitoring. The renewed interest in clozapine and its unusual efficacy and tolerability stimulated researchers to examine other 'atypical' antipsychotic drugs.

Thus the most important distinction in modern-day classification of antipsychotic drugs is between the classical (typical) agents, such as chlorpromazine, haloperidol and zuclopenthixol, and the so-called atypical antipsychotics, which include clozapine and now risperidone, olanzapine, quetiapine, amisulpride, aripiprazole and others. These latter are 'atypical' in their mode of action, their lack of extrapyramidal motor symptoms and adverse effect profiles. Categorisation of atypical agents by their chemical structure is of limited value clinically as they are very heterogeneous. Similarly classification through a shared affinity for a particular receptor system has not been possible; as discussed below, the atypical antipsychotics are very heterogeneous in their receptor-binding profiles.

Indications

Antipsychotic drugs are used for the prophylaxis and acute treatment of psychotic illnesses including schizophrenia and psychoses associated with depression and mania. They also have an important role as an alternative or adjunct to benzodiazepines in the management of the acutely disturbed patient, for both tranquillisation and sedation. There is some evidence that atypical antipsychotics may be used for treatment resistant anxiety disorders after other treatments (e.g. SSRIs, SNRIs, pregabalin) have failed to produce an adequate response. Certain antipsychotics have an antidepressant effect that is distinct from their ability to alleviate the psychosis associated with depression, and as such can be used to augment the effect of antidepressants. Antipsychotics have also proved useful in the tic disorder Tourette's syndrome, and for recurrent self-harming behaviour.

Mechanism of action

The common action of conventional antipsychotics is to decrease brain dopamine function by blocking the dopamine D_2 receptors (Fig. 11.3). However, the atypical drugs act on numerous receptors and modulate several interacting transmitter systems. All atypicals (except amisulpride) exhibit greater affinity for 5HT2 receptors than D_2 receptors, unlike the classical agents. Atypical drugs that do antagonize dopamine D_2 receptors appear to have some selectivity of effect for those in the mesolimbic system (producing antipsychotic effect) rather than the nigrostriatal system

(associated with unwanted motor effects). Clozapine and risperidone exert substantial antagonism of α_2-adrenoceptors, a property that may explain their benefits against negative symptoms. Blockade of muscarinic acetylcholine receptors as with chlorpromazine and clozapine reduces the occurrence of extrapyramidal effects. Aripiprazole is a unique drug because it is a partial dopamine D_2-receptor agonist that acts conversely as an antagonist in regions where dopamine is overactive, such as the limbic system. It increases dopamine function where this is low (such as in the frontal cortex) and has little motor effect.

Fig. 11.3 Sagittal brain section illustrating dopaminergic pathways. ① Mesolimbic pathway (thought to be overactive in psychotic illness according to the dopamine hypothesis of schizophrenia); ② nigrostriatal pathway (involved in motor control, underactive in Parkinson's disease and associated with extrapyramidal motor symptoms); ③ tuberoinfundibular pathway (moderates prolactin release from the hypothalamus). VTA, ventrotegmental area.

Pharmacokinetics

Antipsychotics are well absorbed after oral administration and distribute widely. They are metabolised mainly by hepatic cytochrome P450 isoenzymes, e.g. CYP 2D6 (risperidone, perphenazine), CYP 3A4 (sertindole), CYP 1A2 (olanzapine, clozapine). Metabolism of some compounds is complex, e.g. zuclopenthixol and haloperidol are metabolised by both CYP 2D6 and CYP 3A4, which means that coprescription of inhibitors of either enzyme can cause raised plasma concentrations of these antipsychotics. Amisulpride is an exception to the general rule as it is mainly eliminated unchanged by the kidneys with little hepatic metabolism. Elimination $t_{1/2}$ values range from quetiapine 7 h, clozapine 12 h, haloperidol 18 h to olazapine 33 h. Depot preparations usefully release drug over 2–4 weeks after intramuscular injection (see below).

Efficacy

Symptoms in schizophrenia are defined as positive and negative. Although a classical antipsychotic drug should provide adequate treatment of positive symptoms including hallucinations and delusions, at least 60% of patients may have unresolved negative symptoms such as apathy, flattening of affect and alogia. Evidence suggests that clozapine may have a significant advantage against negative symptoms. This drug has a further advantage over all other antipsychotics, whether classical or atypical, in that it is the most effective agent for 'resistant' schizophrenia, i.e. where other antipsychotics prescribed at adequate doses fail to produce improvement or are not tolerated. Schizophrenia often runs a chronic relapsing and remitting course. Less than a quarter of patients avoid further episodes, with the most common reason for relapse being the stopping of medication against medical advice.

Mode of use

Atypical antipsychotics are all licensed for use in schizophrenia and are now recommended as the first-line treatment for newly diagnosed cases. Some also have licenses for psychosis in mania and for control of agitated or disturbed behaviour in the context of a psychotic illness.

The longer a psychosis is left untreated, the less favourable is the outcome, and drug treatment should be instigated as soon as an adequate period of assessment has allowed a provisional diagnosis to be established. Patients, who have never previously taken any antipsychotic agent, should start at the lowest available dose. For most atypical agents a period of dose titration by protocol from the starting dose up to a stated lowest therapeutic dose is usual, e.g. risperidone 4 mg/day, quetiapine 300 mg/day. Dose increases are indicated when there is no response until the desired effect on psychotic symptoms or calming of disturbed behaviour is achieved, the urgency of the situation determining the interval between increments until the maximum licensed dose is achieved. Conservative dose titration is advisable for the elderly and patients with learning disabilities (who may require antipsychotics for psychosis or severe behavioural disturbance).

Prescription of conventional antipsychotics follows similar rules to those for atypical drugs, starting at low doses in neuroleptic- naïve patients, e.g. haloperidol 0.5 mg/day in case the patient is particularly susceptible to adverse, especially extrapyramidal, motor side-effects. There is a wide range of effective doses for many classical agents (e.g. chlorpromazine, once the most prescribed antipsychotic but now rarely used, has a dose range from 25 to 1 000 mg/day). As the potency (therapeutic efficacy in relation to dose) of antipsychotic agents varies markedly between compounds, it is useful to think of the effective antipsychotic dose of classical agents in terms of 'chlorpromazine equivalents'. For example, haloperidol has a relatively high antipsychotic potency, such that 2–3 mg is equivalent to chlorpromazine 100 mg, whereas 200 mg sulpiride (low potency) is required for equivalent antipsychotic effect. Prescribing in excess of this requires specialist involvement. With co-prescribed antipsychotics, their total maximum antipsychotic dose should not exceed 1000 mg chlorpromazine equivalents per day, except under specialist supervision.

Clozapine may be initiated only under specialist supervision and usually after at least one other antipsychotic has failed through lack of efficacy or unacceptable adverse effects. Additionally, monitoring of leucocyte count is mandatory (danger of agranulocytosis) and blood pressure checking is required (for hypotensive effect). Patients are most vulnerable to agranulocytosis on initiation of therapy, with 75% of cases occurring in the first 18 weeks. The dose titration schedule must be followed strictly, starting with clozapine 12.5 mg at night and working up over a period of 4 weeks to a target therapeutic dose of 450 mg/day.

Alternative administration strategies in acute antipsychotic use

Preparations of antipsychotics for intramuscular injection are advantageous in patients who are unable or unwilling to swallow tablets, a common situation in psychosis or severe behavioural disturbance. Intramuscular preparations of the atypical antipsychotics olanzapine and aripiprazole are suitable for acute behavioural disturbance in schizophrenia but the conventional agent haloperidol is widely used. Formulations of risperidone and olanzapine that dissolve rapidly on contact with the tongue are available. These can be rapidly absorbed even by a disturbed and uncooperative patient.

Long-acting depot injections

Haloperidol, zuclopenthixol, fluphenazine, flupentixol, risperidone and pipothiazine are available as long-acting (2–4 weeks) depot intramuscular injections for maintenance treatment of patients with schizophrenia and other chronic psychotic disorders. Compliance is improved and there is less risk of relapse from ceasing to take medication. In view of the prolonged effect, it is prudent to administer a small initial test dose and review 5–10 days later for unwanted effects.

Rapid tranquillisation

Rapid tranquillisation protocols address the problem of severely disturbed and violent patients who have not responded to non-pharmacological approaches. The risks of administering psychotropic drugs (notably cardiac arrhythmia with high-dose antipsychotics) then greatly outweigh those of non-treatment.

A first step is to offer oral medication, usually haloperidol, olanzapine or risperidone with or without the benzodiazepine, lorazepam. If this is not accepted or fails to achieve control despite repeated doses, the intramuscular route is used to administer a benzodiazepine (e.g. lorazepam or midazolam) or an antipsychotic (e.g. haloperidol or olanzapine), or both (but intramuscular olanzapine should not be given with a benzodiazepine as excess sedation may

ensue). After emergency use of an intramuscular antipsychotic or benzodiazepine, pulse, blood pressure, temperature and respiration are monitored, and pulse oximetry (for oxygen saturation) if consciousness is lost.

Zuclopenthixol acetate i.m. was previously used for patients who do not respond to two doses of haloperidol i.m. This usually induces a calming effect within 2 h, persisting for 2–3 days. Clinicians are now becoming reluctant to use this heavily sedating preparation other than for patients who have previously responded well to it, and never use it for neuroleptic-naïve patients. Patients must be observed with care following administration.

Amobarbital and paraldehyde have a role in emergencies only when antipsychotic and benzodiazepine options have been exhausted.

Opinion statement for treating negative symptoms

Interest in the negative symptoms of schizophrenia has increased rapidly over the last several decades, paralleling a growing interest in functional, in addition to clinical, recovery, and evidence underscoring the importance negative symptoms play in the former. Efforts continue to better define and measure negative symptoms, distinguish their impact from that of other symptom domains, and establish effective treatments as well as trials to assess these. Multiple interventions have been the subject of investigation, to date, including numerous pharmacological strategies, brain stimulation, and nonsomatic approaches. Level and quality of evidence vary considerably, but to this point, no specific treatment can be recommended. This is particularly problematic for individuals burdened with negative symptoms in the face of mild or absent positive symptoms. Presently, clinicians will sometimes turn to interventions that are seen as more benign and in line with routine clinical practice. Strategies include use of atypical antipsychotics, ensuring the lowest possible antipsychotic dose that maintains control of positive symptoms (this can involve a shift from antipsychotic polypharmacy to monotherapy), possibly an antidepressant trial (given diagnostic uncertainty and the frequent use of these drugs in schizophrenia), and non-somatic interventions (e.g., cognitive behavioral therapy, CBT). The array and diversity of strategies currently under investigation highlight the lack of evidence-based treatments and our limited understanding regarding negative symptoms underlying etiology and pathophysiology. Their onset, which can precede the first psychotic break, also means that treatments are delayed. From this perspective, identification of biomarkers and/or endophenotypes permitting earlier diagnosis and intervention may serve to improve treatment efficacy as well as outcomes.

Adverse effects

Active psychotic illnesses often cause patients to have poor insight into their condition. Adverse drug effects can be the final straw in compromising already fragile compliance, leading to relapse. When atypical antipsychotics first came to prominence in the mid-1990s much was made of their lower propensity to cause several of the most troublesome side-effects of classical antipsychotics, especially extrapyramidal motor effects. However, while these problems are encountered less frequently, atypical drugs have a range of troublesome metabolic side-effects which had not been reported in the previous era of classic antipsychotics. Thus, to understand the current position relating to the pros and cons of atypical antipsychotics, it is necessary first to describe the side-effect profile of classical antipsychotic drugs.

Classical antipsychotics

It is rare for any patient taking classical antipsychotic agents to escape their adverse effects completely. Thus it is essential to discuss with patients the possibility of unwanted effects and regularly to review this aspect of their care.

Extrapyramidal symptoms. All classical antipsychotics produce these effects because they act by blocking dopamine receptors in the nigrostriatal pathway. Consequently some 75% of patients experience extrapyramidal symptoms shortly after starting the drug or increasing its dose (acute effects), or

sometime after a particular dose level has been established (tardive effects).

Acute extrapyramidal symptoms. Dystonias are manifest as abnormal movements of the tongue and facial muscles with fixed postures and spasm, including torticollis and bizarre eye movements. Parkinsonian symptoms result in the classical triad of bradykinesia, rigidity and tremor. Both dystonias and parkinsonian symptoms are believed to result from a shift in favour of cholinergic rather than dopaminergic neurotransmission in the nigrostriatal pathway. Anticholinergic (antimuscarinic) agents, e.g. procyclidine, orphenadrine or benztropine, act to restore the balance in favour of dopaminergic transmission but are liable to provoke antimuscarinic effects (dry mouth, urinary retention, constipation, exacerbation of glaucoma and confusion) and they offer no relief for tardive dyskinesia, which may even worsen. They should be used only to treat established symptoms and not for prophylaxis. Benzodiazepines are an alternative.

Akathisia is a state of motor and psychological restlessness, in which patients exhibit persistent foot tapping, moving of legs repetitively and being unable to settle or relax. A strong association has been noted between its presence in treated schizophrenics and subsequent suicide. A β-adrenoceptor blocker is the best treatment, although anticholinergic agents may be effective where akathisia coexists with dystonias and parkinsonian symptoms. Differentiating symptoms of psychotic illness from adverse drug effects is often difficult: drug induced akathisia may be mistaken for agitation induced by psychosis.

Tardive dyskinesia affects about 25% of patients taking classical antipsychotic drugs, the risk increasing with length of exposure. It was originally thought to be a consequence of up-regulation or supersensitivity of dopamine receptors, but a more recent view is that oxidative damage leads to increases in glutamate transmission. Patients display a spectrum of abnormal movements from minor tongue protrusion, lip-smacking, rotational tongue movements and facial grimacing, choreoathetoid movements of the head and neck, and even to twisting and gyrating of the whole body. Remission on discontinuing the causative agent is less likely than are simple dystonias and parkinsonian symptoms. Any anticholinergic agent should be withdrawn immediately. Reduction of the dose of classical antipsychotic is an option, but psychotic symptoms may then worsen or be 'unmasked'. Alternatively, an atypical antipsychotic can provide rapid improvement while retaining control of psychotic symptoms. Atypicals, particularly at high doses, can cause extrapyramidal effects, so this strategy is not always helpful. Clozapine, which does not appear to cause tardive dyskinesia, may be used in severe cases where continuing antipsychotic treatment is required and symptoms have not responded to other medication strategies.

If the classical antipsychotic is continued, tardive dyskinesia remits spontaneously in around 30% of patients within 1 year, but the condition is difficult to tolerate and patients may be keen to try other medications even where evidence suggests that the success rates for remission are limited. These include vitamin E, benzodiazepines, β-blockers, bromocriptine and tetrabenazine.

Cardiovascular effects. Postural hypotension may result from blockade of α_1-adrenoceptors; it is dose related. Prolongation of the QTc interval in the cardiac cycle may rarely lead to ventricular arrhythmias and sudden death. This observation led to the withdrawal from the market of thioridazine and droperidol, restrictions on the use of pimozide and general warnings regarding the use of several other antipsychotics including haloperidol.

Prolactin increase. Classical antipsychotics raise plasma prolactin concentration by blocking dopamine receptors in the tuberoinfundibular pathway, causing gynaecomastia and galactorrhoea in both sexes, and menstrual disturbances in women. A change to an atypical agent such as aripiprazole, quetiapine or olanzapine (but not risperidone or amisulpride) should minimize the effects. If continuation of the existing classical antipsychotic is obligatory, dopamine agonists such as bromocriptine and amantadine that reduce prolactin secretion may help.

Sedation. In the acute treatment of psychotic ill-ness this may be a highly desirable property, but it may be undesirable as the patient seeks to resume work, study or relationships.

Classical antipsychotics may also be associated with:

- Weight gain (a problem with almost all classical antipsychotics with the exception of loxapine; most pronounced with fluphenazine and flupentixol).
- Seizures (chlorpromazine is especially likely to lower the convulsion threshold).
- Interference with temperature regulation (hypothermia or hyperthermia, especially in the elderly).
- Skin problems (phenothiazines, particularly chlorpromazine, may provoke photosensitivity necessitating advice about limiting exposure to sunlight); rashes and urticaria may also occur.
- Sexual dysfunction (ejaculatory problems through α-adrenoceptor blockade).
- Retinal pigmentation (chlorpromazine can cause visual impairment if the dose is prolonged and high).
- Corneal and lens opacities.
- Blood dyscrasias (agranulocytosis and leucopenia).
- Osteoporosis (associated with increased prolactin levels).
- Jaundice (including cholestatic).

Atypical antipsychotics

Having considered the side-effect profile of classical antipsychotic agents, the adverse effects of atypical antipsychotics can be viewed as those shared with classical agents and those unique to one or more atypical agents.

Extrapyramidal effects occur less frequently than with classical agents (there is less blockade of dopamine D_2 receptors in the nigrostriatal pathway) but do occur with high doses of risperidone and olanzapine. Tardive dyskinesia is much less common with all of the atypical agents than with classical drugs. Anticholinergic (antimuscarinic) effects are most likely with clozapine and olanzapine. Sexual dysfunction and skin problems are rare with atypical antipsychotics. Adverse effects relating to prolactin stimulation are also rare, with the exception of risperidone and amisulpride (for which galactorrhea is as common as with classical drugs).

One of the most problematic side-effects with atypical antipsychotics, especially with olanzapine and clozapine, is these drugs' propensity to cause weight gain. The effect appears to be dose dependent for olanzapine but is often greater than 10 kg after 1 year's treatment with the 15 mg/day dose. Atypicals have also been implicated as causing metabolic disorders especially diabetes mellitus and hyperlipidaemia. Olanzapine, clozapine and quetiapine appear to be the most problematic. Obesity, impaired glucose tolerance and hyperlipidaemia, along with hypertension, are all features of metabolic syndrome. Hypertension can occur gradually with antipsychotics, most frequently as a consequence of weight gain. In a small number of cases hypertension may result from α_2-adrenoceptor blockade. However, hypertension is less commonly an antipsychotic side-effect than the other manifestations of metabolic syndrome and some atypical antipsychotics (notably clozapine and sertindole) are associated with postural hypotension. Atypical antipsychotics are associated with other important cardiovascualr effects. QTc prolongation is most likely to occur with sertindole (which is restricted for this reason), with quetiapine and zotepine associated with a lower level of risk (below that of the conventional antipsychotics haloperidol and pimozide). Olanzapine and risperidone are also associated with a greater risk of stroke in elderly patients with dementia.

Atypicals can also cause sedation. Clozapine is the most sedative followed by zotepine, quetiapine and olanzapine.

Clozapine warrants separate mention, given its value for patients with treatment-resistant schizophrenia or severe treatment-related extrapyramidal symptoms. Most important is the risk of agranulocytosis in up to 2% of patients (compared with 0.2% for classical antipsychotics). When clozapine was first licensed without requirement for regular blood counts, this problem caused appreciable mortality. With the introduction of strict monitoring, there have been no recorded deaths in the UK from agranulocytosis since clozapine was reintroduced, and internationally the death rate from agranulocytosis is now considerably less than 1 in 1 000. In addition to postural hypotension clozapine may cause tachycardia and provoke seizures in 3%–5% of patients at doses above 600 mg/day. Finally there are reported associations between clozapine use and cardiomyopathy and myocarditis, although both are very rare outcomes.

Lithium

Lithium salts were known anecdotally to have beneficial psychotropic effects as long ago as the middle of the 19th century, but scientific evidence of their efficacy was not obtained until 1949, when lithium carbonate was tried in manic patients; it was found to be effective in the acute state and, later, to prevent recurrent attacks.

The mode of action is not fully understood. Its main effect is probably to inhibit hydrolysis of inositol phosphate, so reducing the recycling of free inositol for synthesis of phosphatidylinositides, which if present in excess may interfere with cell homeostasis by promoting uncontrolled cell signalling. Other putative mechanisms involve the cyclic AMP 'second messenger' system, and monoaminergic and cholinergic neurotransmitters.

Indications and use. Lithium carbonate is effective treatment in more than 75% of episodes of acute mania or hypomania. Because its therapeutic action takes 2–3 weeks to develop, lithium is generally used in combination with a benzodiazepine such as lorazepam or diazepam (or with an antipsychotic agent where there are also psychotic features).

For prophylaxis, lithium is indicated when there have been two episodes of mood disturbance in 2 years, although in severe cases prophylactic use is indicated after one episode. When an adequate dose of lithium is taken consistently, around 65% of patients achieve improved mood control.

Patients who start lithium only to discontinue it within 2 years have a significantly poorer outcome than matched patients who are not given any pharmacological prophylaxis. The existence of a 'rebound effect' (recurrence of manic symptoms) during withdrawal dictates that long-term treatment with the drug is of great importance.

Lithium salts are ineffective for prophylaxis of bipolar affective disorder in around 35% of patients. The search for alternatives has centred on anticonvulsants, notably carbamazepine and sodium valproate and lamotrigine, and more recently the atypical antipsychotics.

Lithium is also used to augment the action of antidepressants in treatment-resistant depression.

Pharmaceutics. The dose of lithium ions (Li^+) delivered varies with the pharmaceutical preparation; thus it is vital for patients to adhere to the same pharmaceutical brand. For example, Camcolit 250-mg tablets each contain 6.8 mmol Li^+, Liskonum 450-mg tablets contain 12.2 mmol Li^+ and Priadel 200-mg tablets contain 5.4 mmol Li^+. The proprietary name must be stated on the prescription.

Monitoring. Dose is guided by monitoring the plasma concentration once steady state has been reached. Increments are made at weekly intervals until the concentration lies within the range 0.4 –1 mmol/L (maintenance at the lower level is preferred for elderly patients). The timing of blood sampling is important, and by convention a blood sample is taken prior to the morning dose, as close as possible to 12 h after the evening dose. Once the plasma concentration is at steady state and in the therapeutic range, it should be measured every 3 months. For toxicity monitoring, thyroid function (especially in women) and renal function (plasma creatinine and electrolytes) should be measured before initiation and every 3–6 months during therapy.

Patient education about the role of lithium in the prophylaxis of bipolar affective disorder is particularly important to achieve compliance with therapy; treatment cards, information leaflets and, where appropriate, video materials are used.

Adverse effects are encountered in three general categories:

- Those occurring at plasma concentrations within the therapeutic range (0.4–1 mmol/L), which include fine tremor (especially involving the fingers; a β-blocker may benefit), constipation, polyuria, polydipsia, metallic taste in the mouth, weight gain, oedema, goitre, hypothyroidism, acne, rash, diabetes insipidus and cardiac arrhythmias. Mild cognitive and memory impairment also occur.

- Signs of intoxication, associated with plasma concentrations greater than 1.5 mmol/L, are mainly gastrointestinal (diarrhoea, anorexia, vomiting) and neurological (blurred vision, muscle weakness, drowsiness, sluggishness and coarse tremor, leading on to giddiness, ataxia and dysarthria).

- Frank toxicity, due to severe overdosage or rapid reduction in renal clearance, usually associated with plasma concentrations over 2 mmol/L, constitutes a medical emergency. Hyperreflexia, hyperextension of limbs, convulsions, hyperthermia, toxic psychoses, syncope, oliguria, coma and even death may result if treatment is not instigated urgently.

Overdose. Acute overdose may present without signs of toxicity but with plasma concentrations well exceeding 2 mmol/L. This requires only measures to increase urine production, e.g. by ensuring adequate intravenous and oral fluid intake while avoiding sodium depletion (and a diuretic is contraindicated; see above). Treatment is otherwise supportive, with special attention to electrolyte balance, renal function and control of convulsions. Where toxicity is chronic, haemodialysis may be needed, especially if renal function is impaired. Plasma concentration may rise again after acute reduction, because lithium leaves cells slowly, and also due to continued absorption from sustained-release formulations. Whole bowel irrigation may be an option for significant ingestion, but specialist advice should be sought.

CLASSIFICATION OF ANXIETY DISORDERS

The diagnostic criteria of DSM-IV (Diagnostic and Statistical Manual) or ICD-10 (International Classification of Disease) are generally used. Both divide anxiety into a series of subsyndromes with clear operational criteria to assist in distinguishing them. At any one time many patients may have symptoms of more than one syndrome, but making the primary diagnosis is important as this can markedly influence the choice of treatment.

The key features of each anxiety disorder follow, with a practical description of the preferred choice of medication, its dose and duration.

Panic disorder (PD)

The main feature is recurrent, unexpected panic attacks. These are discrete periods of intense fear accompanied by characteristic physical symptoms such as skipping or pounding heart, sweating, hot flushes or chills, trembling/shaking, breathing difficulties, chest pain, nausea, diarrhea and other gastrointestinal symptoms, dizziness or light-headedness. The first panic attack often occurs without warning but may subsequently become associated with specific situations, e.g. in a crowded shop, driving. Anticipatory anxiety and avoidance behaviour develop in response to this chain of events. The condition must be distinguished from alcohol withdrawal, caffeinism, hyperthyroidism and (rarely) phaeochromocytoma.

Patients experiencing panic attacks often do not know what is happening to them, and because the symptoms are similar to those of cardiovascular, respiratory or neurological conditions, often present to non-psychiatric services, e.g. casualty departments, family doctors, medical specialists, where they may either be extensively investigated or given reassurance that there is nothing wrong. A carefully taken history reduces the likelihood of this occurrence.

Treatment. The choice lies between a fast-acting benzodiazepine, such as lorazepam or alprazolam, and one with delayed efficacy but fewer problems of withdrawal, such as a tricyclic antidepressant (TCA) or an SSRI. The different time course of these two classes of agent in panic disorder is depicted in Figure 11.4.

Benzodiazepines rapidly reduce panic frequency and severity and continue to be effective for months; significant tolerance to the therapeutic action is uncommon. On withdrawal of the benzodiazepine,

Fig. 11.4 Schematic representation of the time course of panic treatments.

even when it is gradual, increased symptoms of anxiety and panic attacks may occur, reaching a maximum when the final dose is stopped. Indeed, some patients find they are unable to withdraw and remain long-term on a benzodiazepine.

Antidepressants (both SSRIs and TCAs) have a slower onset of action and may cause an initial increase in both anxiety and panic frequency, such that a patient may discontinue medication, even after a single dose. This provoking reaction usually lasts for no more than 2–3 weeks after which panic frequency and severity improve quickly, but patients need help to stay on treatment in the first weeks. The doctor needs to give a clear explanation of the likely course of events and the antidepressant should be started at half the usual initial dose to reduce the likelihood of exacerbation. The dose of antidepressant required to treat panic disorder is generally as high as, or higher than, that for depression and maximal benefit may not emerge for 8–12 weeks. Patients should therefore receive as large a dose as can be tolerated for this length of time.

General comments about treating anxiety disorders

- There is need to discuss the benefits and risks of specific treatments with patients before treatment and take account of their clinical features, needs, preferences and availability of local services when choosing treatments.
- SSRIs are usually effective in anxiety disorders and are generally suitable for first-line treatment.
- Benzodiazepines are effective in many anxiety

disorders but their use should be short term except in treatment-resistant cases.

- SNRIs, TCAs, MAOIs, pregabalin and antipsychotics need to be considered in relation to their evidence base for specific conditions and their individual risks and benefits.

- With all antidepressants, especially SSRIs and SNRIs, there should be specific discussion and monitoring of possible adverse effects early in treatment, and also on stopping the drugs after a week of treatment; this latter also applies to benzodiazepines.

- SSRI/SNRI treatment is often slow to produce the therapeutic effect, and it is advisable to wait 12 weeks to assess efficacy.

- in a first episode, patients may need medication for at least 6 months, withdrawing over a further 4–8 weeks if they are well. Those with recurrent illness may need treatment for 1–2 years to enable them to learn and put into place psychological approaches to their problems. In many cases the illness is life-long and chronic maintenance treatment is justified if it significantly improves their well-being and function.

- Specific psychological treatments are also effective in treatment.

- When initial treatments fail, consider switching to another evidence-based treatment, combining evidence-based treatments (only when there are no contraindications), and referring to regional or national specialist services in refractory patients.

SLEEP DISORDERS

Types of sleep disorder

Several types of sleep disorder are recognised, and their differentiation is important; a simplified summary is given below but reference to DSM-IV, ICD-10 and ICSD4 will clarify the exact diagnostic criteria:

- Insomnia: not enough sleep or sleep of poor quality; problems of falling asleep (initial insomnia) or staying asleep (maintenance insomnia), or waking too early.

- Hypersomnia: excessive daytime sleepiness.
- Parasomnia: unusual happenings in the night, including nightmares, night terrors, sleep walking, and REM behaviour disorder.
- Other: sleep scheduling disorders (circadian rhythm disorder), restless legs syndrome, periodic leg movements of sleep.

Drugs for insomnia

Chronic insomnia is a prevalent (10%) medical disorder defined by difficulty falling or staying asleep or non-restorative sleep combined with impaired daytime functioning. Current research suggests that arousal and wakefulness are promoted by parallel neurotransmitter systems whose cell bodies are located in brainstem or midbrain centres, with projections to the thalamus and forebrain. These activating neurotransmitters are noradrenaline/norepinephrine, serotonin, acetylcholine, dopamine and histamine. In addition the newly discovered orexin system with cell bodies in the hypothalamus promotes wakefulness through regulating arousal 'pathways' (and inhibiting sedative ones).

The promotion of sleep is regulated by a number of other neurotransmitters; primary among these is gaminobutyric acid (GABA), the major inhibitory neurotransmitter in the brain. The majority of brain cells are inhibited by GABA so increasing its function reduces arousal and produces sleep, and eventually anaesthesia. There are many subsets of GABA neurons distributed throughout the brain but a particular cluster in the hypothalamus (ventrolateral preoptic nucleus) can be considered to be the sleep 'switch'. These neurons switch off brain arousal systems at the level of the cell bodies and therefore promote sleep. GABA receptors in the cortex can also promote sedation and sleep by inhibiting the target neurons of the arousal system. Most drugs used in insomnia act by increasing the effects of GABA at the $GABA_A$ receptor.

The GABAA-benzodiazepine receptor complex

GABAergic neurons are distributed widely in the CNS and GABA controls the state of neuronal excitability in all brain areas. The balance between excitatory inputs (mostly glutamatergic) and inhibitory GABAergic activity determines neuronal activity. If the balance swings in favour of GABA, then sedation, amnesia, muscle relaxation and ataxia appear and nervousness and anxiety are reduced. The mildest reduction of GABAergic activity (or increase in glutamate) elicits arousal, anxiety, restlessness, insomnia and exaggerated reactivity.

When GABA binds with the $GABA_A$ receptor, the permeability of the central pore of the receptor complex opens, so allowing more chloride ions into the neuron and decreasing excitability. Classical benzodiazepines (BZDs) in clinical use bind to another receptor on the complex (the benzodiazepine receptor) and enhance the effectiveness of GABA, producing a larger inhibitory effect (Fig. 11.5). These drugs are agonists at the receptor and an antagonist, flumazenil, prevents agonists from binding at the receptor site; it is used clinically to reverse benzodiazepine actions.

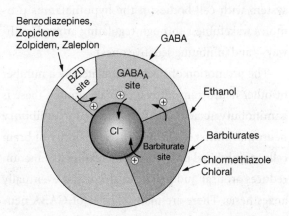

Fig. 11.5 Schematic representation of the binding sites on the $GABA_A$–benzodiazepine receptor complex. Note that drugs binding to the benzodiazepine (BZD) receptor site do not open the chloride channel directly, but rather augment the capacity of GABA to do so. Conversely agents such as the barbiturates both potentiate GABA and at higher concentrations have a direct effect on the chloride channel. This explains why barbiturates and alcohols are more toxic in overdose than the benzodiazepines.

Benzodiazepines

A general account of the benzodiazepines is appropriate here, although their indications extend beyond use as hypnotics. All benzodiazepines, and newer benzodiazepine-like drugs such as zopiclone and

zolpidem, are safe and effective for insomnia if the substance with the right timing of onset of action and elimination is chosen. They should not be used for patients with sleep-related breathing disorders such as obstructive sleep apnoea (see below) which is exacerbated by benzodiazepines. Objective measures of sleep show that they decrease time to sleep onset and waking during the night. They also improve subjective sleep. Other changes in sleep architecture are to some extent dependent on duration of action, with the very short-acting compounds having the least effect. Most commonly very light (stage 1) sleep is decreased, and stage 2 sleep is increased. Higher doses of longer-acting benzodiazepines partially suppress slow wave sleep.

Pharmacokinetics. Benzodiazepines are effective after administration by mouth but enter the circulation at very different rates that are reflected in the speed of onset of action, e.g. alprazolam is rapid, and oxazepam is slow. Hepatic breakdown produces metabolites, some with long $t_{\frac{1}{2}}$ which greatly extend drug action, e.g. chlordiazepoxide, clorazepate and diazepam all form demethyldiazepam ($t_{\frac{1}{2}}$ 80 h).

Uses. Oral benzodiazepines are used for: insomnia, anxiety, alcohol withdrawal states, muscle spasm due to a variety of causes, including tetanus and cerebral spasticity. Injectable preparations are used for rapid tranquillisation in psychosis, anaesthesia and sedation for minor surgery and invasive investigations. The choice of drug as hypnotic and anxiolytic is determined by pharmacokinetic properties.

Doses. Tolerance to the anxiolytic effects does not seem to be a problem. In sleep disorders the situation is not so clear; studies of subjective sleep quality show enduring efficacy, and the necessity for dose escalation in sleep disorders is rare, but the objective sleep effects have not been studied systematically over weeks and months.

Dependence. Both animal and human research has shown that brain $GABA_A$ receptors do change in function during chronic treatment with benzodiazepines, and therefore will take time to return to premedication status after cessation. Features of withdrawal and dependence vary. Commonly there is a kind of psychological dependence based on the fact that the treatment works to reduce patients' anxiety or sleep disturbance, and therefore they are unwilling to stop. If they do stop, there can be relapse, where original symptoms return. There can also be a rebound of symptoms, particularly after stopping hypnotics, with a worsening of sleep disturbance for one or two nights, longer sleep onset latency and increased waking during sleep – this is common. In anxiety disorders there may be a few days of increased anxiety and edginess which then resolves, probably in 10%–20% of patients. More rarely, there is a longer withdrawal syndrome that is characterized by the emergence of symptoms not previously experienced, e.g. agitation, headache, dizziness, dysphoria, irritability, fatigue, depersonalisation, hypersensitivity to noise and visual stimuli. Physical symptoms include nausea, vomiting, muscle cramps, sweating, weakness, muscle pain or twitching and ataxia. After prolonged high doses abrupt withdrawal may cause confusion, delirium, psychosis and convulsions. The syndrome is ameliorated by resuming medication but resolves in weeks; in a very few patients it persists, and these people have been the subject of much research, mainly focusing on their personality and cognitive factors.

Withdrawal of benzodiazepines should be gradual after as little as 3 weeks' use, but for long-term users it should be very slow, e.g. about of the dose every 2 weeks, aiming to complete it in 6–12 weeks. Withdrawal should be slowed if marked symptoms occur and it may be useful to substitute a long $t_{\frac{1}{2}}$ drug (diazepam) to minimize rapid fluctuations in plasma concentrations. Abandonment of the final dose may be particularly distressing. In difficult cases withdrawal may be assisted by concomitant use of an antidepressant.

Adverse effects. In addition to the above, benzodiazepines affect memory and balance. Hazards with car driving or operating machinery can arise from sedation, amnesia and impaired psychomotor function. Amnesia for events subsequent to administration occurs with high doses given i.v., e.g. for endoscopy, dental surgery (with local anaesthetic),

cardioversion, and in these situations it can be regarded as a blessing. Paradoxical behaviour effects and perceptual disorders, e.g. hallucinations occur occasionally. Headache, giddiness, alimentary tract upsets, skin rashes and reduced libido can occur.

Benzodiazepines in pregnancy. Benzodiazepines should be avoided in early pregnancy as far as possible as their safety is not established with certainty. Safety in pregnancy is not only a matter of avoiding prescription during an established pregnancy, for individuals may become pregnant on long-term therapy. Benzodiazepines cross the placenta and can cause fetal cardiac arrhythmia, muscular hypotonia, poor suckling, hypothermia and respiratory depression in the newborn.

Non-benzodiazepine hypnotics that act at the GABAA-benzodiazepine receptor

Although structurally unrelated to the benzodiazepines, these drugs act on the same receptor, so their effects can be blocked by flumazenil, the receptor antagonist. Those described below are all effective in insomnia, have low propensity for tolerance, rebound insomnia, withdrawal symptoms and abuse potential. Data from long-term studies suggests these agents are safe and effective over at least 12 months. Withdrawal effects similar to the benzodiazepines hypnotics occur but to a lesser extent.

Zopiclone has an onset of action that is relatively rapid (about 1 h) and that lasts for 6–8 h, making it suitable for both initial and maintenance treatment of insomnia. It may cause fewer problems on withdrawal than benzodiazepines. The duration of action is prolonged in the elderly, and in hepatic insufficiency. About 40% of patients experience a metallic aftertaste (genetically determined). People who take zopiclone have been shown to be at increased risk of road traffic accidents. Care should be taken with concomitant medication that affects its metabolic pathway.

Zolpidem is an imidazopyridine, and has a faster onset (30–60 min) and shorter duration of action. In patients over 80 years clearance is slower and action longer lasting.

199

Zaleplon, a pyrazolopyrimidine, has a fast onset and short duration of action. In volunteers, it appeared to have no effect on psychomotor (including driving) skills when taken at least 5 h before testing. It may be taken during the night when the patient has awoken and cannot get back to sleep, as long as this is at least 5 h before having to drive.

Other drugs that act on the GABAA benzodiazepine receptor

Chloral hydrate, clomethiazole and barbiturates also enhance GABA function, but at high doses have the additional capacity directly to open the membrane chloride channel; this may lead to potentially lethal respiratory depression and explains their low therapeutic ratio. These drugs also have a propensity for abuse/misuse and thus are very much second-line treatments.

Chloral hydrate has a fast (30–60 min) onset of action and 6–8 h duration of action. Chloral hydrate, a prodrug, is rapidly metabolised by alcohol dehydrogenase into the active hypnotic trichloroethanol ($t_{1/2}$ 8 h). Chloral hydrate is dangerous in serious hepatic or renal impairment, and aggravates peptic ulcer. Interaction with ethanol is to be expected since both are metabolised by alcohol dehydrogenase. Alcohol (ethanol) also appears to induce the formation of trichloroethanol which attains higher concentrations if alcohol is taken, increasing sedation. Triclofos and chloral betaine are related compounds.

Clomethiazole is structurally related to vitamin B_1 and is a hypnotic, sedative and anticonvulsant. When taken orally, it is subject to extensive hepatic first pass metabolism (which is defective in the old and in liver-damaged alcoholics who exhibit higher peak plasma concentrations); the $t_{1/2}$ is 4 h. It may also be given i.v. It is comparatively free from hangover but it can cause nasal irritation and sneezing. Dependence occurs and use should always be brief.

Other drugs used in insomnia

Antihistamines. Most proprietary (over-the-counter) sleep remedies contain H_1-receptor antihistamines with sedative action. Promethazine has a slow (1–2 h) onset and long duration of action ($t_{1/2}$ 12 h). It reduces sleep onset latency and awakenings during the night after a single dose, but there have been no studies showing enduring action. It is sometimes used as a hypnotic in children. There are no controlled studies showing improvements in sleep after other antihistamines. Alimemazine is used for short-term sedation in children. Most antihistamine sedatives have a relatively long action and may cause daytime sedation.

Antidepressants. In the depressed patient, improvement in mood is almost always accompanied by improvement in subjective sleep, and therefore choice of antidepressant should not usually involve additional consideration of sleep effects. Nevertheless, some patients are more likely to continue with medication if there is a short-term improvement, in which case mirtazapine or trazodone may provide effective antidepressant together with sleep promoting effects. Antidepressant drugs, particularly those with $5HT_2$-blocking effects, may occasionally be effective in long-term insomnia. Antipsychotics have been used to promote sleep in resistant insomnia occurring as part of another psychiatric disorder, probably because of the combination of $5HT_2$-antagonism, $\alpha1$-adrenoceptor antagonism and histamine H_1-receptor antihistamine effects in addition to their primary dopamine antagonist effects. Their long action leads to daytime sedation, and extrapyramidal movement disorders may result from their blockade of dopamine receptors. They therefore should be used with great care in the context of insomnia. Nevertheless, modern antipsychotics, e.g. quetiapine, are being used for intractable insomnia, usually at a dose well below the one required to treat psychosis, e.g. 25–50 mg/day.

Melatonin, the hormone produced by the pineal gland during darkness, has been investigated for insomnia. A prolonged release formulation is licensed for insomnia characterized by poor quality of sleep in people over 55 years, whose melatonin rhythm may be supposed to be reduced. Melatonin may also be used therapeutically to reset circadian rhythm to prevent jet-lag on long-haul flights, and for blind or partially sighted people who cannot use daylight to synchronize their natural rhythm.

Melatonin is metabolised mainly by CYP 1A enzymes and may interact with other active substances that affect these enzymes. For this reason it should not be taken with fluvoxamine, 5- or 8-methoxypsoralen, or cimetidine, and caution should be exercised in patients on oestrogens (e.g. contraceptive or hormone replacement therapy).

Suvorexant, the first orexin receptor antagonist (for orexin 1 and orexin 2 receptor) was approved by FDA in 2014 for the treatment of insomnia with sleep onset and/or sleep maintenance difficulties.

Hypersomnia

Sleep-related breathing disorders causing excessive daytime sleepiness are rarely treated with drugs. Sleepiness caused by the night-time disruption of sleep apnoea syndrome is sometimes not completely abolished by the standard treatment of continuous positive airway pressure overnight, and wake-promoting drugs, e.g. modafinil, may have a role in these patients.

Narcolepsy is a chronic neurological disorder, characterized by excessive daytime sleepiness (EDS) and sleep attacks, usually accompanied by cataplexy (attacks of muscle weakness on emotional arousal). These symptoms are often associated with the intrusion into wakefulness of other elements of rapid eye movement (REM) sleep, such as sleep paralysis and hypnagogic hallucinations, i.e. in a transient state preceding sleep.

Stimulants are effective in the treatment of EDS due to narcolepsy. Modafinil is usually preferred as it is not a controlled drug, failing which methylphenidate or dexamfetamine are added or substituted. In narcolepsy, patients usually need a stimulant for their hypersomnia and an antidepressant for their cataplexy. Combining an SSRI antidepressant with modafinil has been shown to be safe, but dexamfetamine and methylphenidate must not be given with MAOIs. Cataplexy is most effectively treated with 5HT uptake-blocking drugs such as clomipramine or fluoxetine, or other antidepressant drugs, e.g. reboxetine, or the MAOI selegiline.

Modafinil is a wake-promoting agent whose specific mechanism of action is not properly known; it does not appear to be overtly stimulant like the amfetamines. Its onset of action is slow and lasts 8–12 h. Potential for abuse is low. Modafinil is used in narcolepsy and other hypersomnias (e.g. that with sleep apnoea), and also promotes wakefulness in normal people who need to stay awake for long periods, e.g. military personnel. Its use is associated with a wide variety of gastrointestinal, CNS and other unwanted effects; contraindications to its use include moderate to severe hypertension, a history of left ventricular hypertrophy. Modafinil accelerates the metabolism of oral contraceptives, reducing their efficacy.

Amfetamines release dopamine and noradrenaline/ norepinephrine in the brain. This causes a behavioural excitation, with increased alertness, elevation of mood, increase in physical activity and suppression of appetite. Dexamfetamine, the dextrorotatory isomer of amfetamine, is about twice as active in humans as the laevo- isomer and is the main prescribed amfetamine. It is rapidly absorbed orally and acts for 3–24 h; most people with narcolepsy find twice a day dosing optimal to maintain alertness during the day. About 40% of narcoleptic patients find it necessary to increase their dose, suggesting some tolerance. Although physical dependence does not occur, mental and physical depression may develop following withdrawal.

Unwanted effects include edginess, restlessness, insomnia and appetite suppression, weight loss, and increase in blood pressure and heart rate. Amfetamines are commonly abused because of their stimulant effect but this is rare in narcolepsy. Contraindications to its use include moderate to severe hypertension, hyperthyroidism, and a history of drug or alcohol abuse.

Methylphenidate also promotes dopamine release but its principal action is to inhibit uptake of central neurotransmitters. Its effects and adverse effects resemble those of the amfetamines. Methylphenidate has a low systemic availability and slow onset of action, making it less liable to abuse. Its short duration of effect (3–4 h) requires that patients with narcolepsy need to plan the timing of tablet-taking to fit with daily activities. It is also used in attention deficit/hyperactivity disorder.

Unwanted effects include anxiety, anorexia and difficulty sleeping; these usually subside. Methylphenidate reduces expected weight gain and has been associated with slight growth retardation. Monitoring of therapy should include height and weight, also blood pressure and blood counts (thrombocytopenia and leucopenia occur). It should not be used in patients with hyperthyroidism, severe angina, or cardiac arrhythmias.

Parasomnias

Nightmares arise out of REM sleep and are reported by the patient as structured, often stereotyped dreams that are very distressing. Usually the patient wakes up fully and remembers the dream. Psychological methods of treatment may be appropriate, e.g. a program of rehearsing the dream and inventing a different pleasant ending. Nightmares of a particularly distressing kind are a feature of posttraumatic stress disorder. Case reports indicate benefit from various pharmacological agents, but no particular drug emerges as superior.

Night terrors and sleep-walking arise from slow wave sleep, and they are often coexistent. There is usually a history dating from childhood, and often a family history. Exacerbations commonly coincide with periods of stress, and alcohol increases their likelihood. In a night terror, patients usually sit or jump up from deep sleep (mostly in the first few hours of sleep) with a loud cry, look terrified and move violently, sometimes injuring themselves or others. They appear asleep and uncommunicative, often returning to sleep without being aware of the event. These terrors are thought to be a welling up of anxiety from deep centres in the brain which is normally inhibited by cortical mechanisms. If the disorder is sufficiently frequent or disabling, night terrors respond to the SSRI paroxetine (also effective in sleepwalkers) or the benzodiazepine clonazepam.

REM behaviour disorder, first described in 1986, consists of lack of paralysis during REM sleep which results in brief acting out of dreams, often vigorously with injury to self or others. Rarely, it can occur acutely as a result of drug or alcohol withdrawal, or in patients taking high doses of antidepressants such as clomipramine, venlafaxine or mirtazapine. More commonly it is chronic and either idiopathic or associated with neurological disorder.

Part 3. Drugs for Alzheimer's disease (dementia)

Alzheimer's and vascular (multi-infarct) disease are the two most common forms of dementia, accounting for about 80% of presentations. Alzheimer's disease is associated with deposition of β-amyloid in brain tissue and abnormal phosphorylation of the intracellular tau (τ) proteins causing abnormalities of microtubule assembly and collapse of the cytoskeleton. Pyramidal cells of the cortex and subcortex are particularly affected.

Evidence indicates that cholinergic transmission is diminished in Alzheimer's disease. The first three drugs available for use in Alzheimer's each act to enhance acetylcholine activity by inhibiting the enzyme acetylcholinesterase which metabolises and inactivates synaptically released acetylcholine. Consequently acetylcholine remains usable for longer. Individual drugs are categorised by the type of enzyme inhibition they cause. Donepezil is classed as a reversible' agent, as binding to the acetylcholinesterase enzymes lasts only minutes, whereas rivastigmine is considered 'pseudo-irreversible' as inhibition lasts for several hours. Galantamine is associated both with reversible inhibition and with enhanced acetylcholine action on nicotinic receptors. Clinical trials show that these agents produce an initial increase in patients' cognitive ability. There also may be associated global benefits, including improvements in non-cognitive aspects such as depressive symptoms. But the drugs do not alter the underlying process, and the relentless progress of the disease is paralleled by a reduction in acetylcholine production with a decline in cognition.

A fourth drug licensed for use in Alzheimer's disease is memantine. Overactive glutamate signalling has been linked to cell death and this drug is known to be a glutamine modulator through antagonism of NMDA receptors. Initially thought to have an entirely novel mode of action related to its effects on dampening excess glutamate neurotransmission, subsequent work suggests that memantine does have additional activity as an acetylcholine stimulant.

The beneficial effects of drugs are therefore to:

- stabilise the condition initially and sometimes improve cognitive function
- delay the overall pace of decline (and therefore the escalating levels of support required)
- postpone the onset of severe dementia.

The severity of cognitive deficits in patients suffering from dementia can be quantified by a simple 30-point schedule, the mini mental state examination (MMSE) of Folstein. A score of 21–26 denotes mild, 10–20 moderate and less than 10 severe Alzheimer's disease. The MMSE can also be used to monitor progress.

In 2001 the view of the UK National Institute for Health and Clinical Excellence (NICE) was that, subject to certain conditions, the drugs available at that time should be available as adjuvant therapy for those with a MMSE score above 12 points. Subsequent guidelines first suggested that the cost/benefit ratio for the three anticholinesterase inhibitor drugs was favourable only in those with moderate dementia (MMSE score between 10 and 20 points), only for this limitation to be subsequently removed. Guidelines for prescribing anticholinesterase inhibitors also advise the following:

- Alzheimer's disease must be diagnosed and assessed in a specialist clinic; the clinic should also assess cognitive, global and behavioural functioning, activities of daily living, and the likelihood of compliance with treatment.
- Treatment should be initiated by specialists but may be continued by family practitioners under a shared-care protocol.
- The carers' views of the condition should be sought before and during drug treatment.
- The patient should be assessed every 6 months and drug treatment should continue only if the MMSE score remains at or above 10 points and if treatment has had a worthwhile effect on global, behavioural and functional parameters.

Use of memantine in dementia is now supported by good quality evidence and it has been widely prescribed in the UK and many other countries. It enabled a reduction in the co-prescription of antipsychotic medication previously used for behavioural symptoms such as agitation and aggression. A small evidence base also suggests that the combination of memantine with an acetylcholinesterase inhibitor may be more effective than the acetylcholinesterase inhibitor alone.

Doses are:

- Donepezil 5–10 mg nocte increasing to 10 mg nocte after 1 month.
- Galantamine 4 mg twice daily increasing to 8–12 mg twice daily at 4-week intervals.
- Rivastigmine 1.5 mg twice daily increasing to 3–6 mg twice daily at 2-week intervals.
- Memantine 5 mg daily increasing weekly by 5 mg to a maximum of 20 mg daily.

Adverse effects of the three anticholinesterse inhibitors inevitably include cholinergic symptoms, with nausea, diarrhoea and abdominal cramps appearing commonly.

There may also be bradycardia, sinoatrial or atrioventricular block. Additionally, urinary incontinence, syncope, convulsions and psychiatric disturbances occur. Rapid dose increase appears to make symptoms more pronounced. Hepatotoxicity is a rare association with donepezil.

Memantine has a different side-effect profile with constipation, hypertension, headache, dizziness and drowsiness being highlighted as the most common adverse effects. Memantine has been reported as having an association with seizures, which may be a consideration in patients who have had previous fits.

The deterioration of function in dementia of Alzheimer's disease is often accompanied by acute behavioural disturbance. Memantine and the acetylcholinesterase inhibitors may be helpful in controlling this but in severe cases or where psychotic symptoms are present treatment with antipsychotics may be required. Be aware that if a person with dementia has Lewy body disease rather than Alzheimer's, antipsychotics may worsen the presentation.

Part 4. Drugs in attention deficit/hyperactivity disorder

Attention deficit hyperactivity disorder (ADHD) affects 5% of children and between 2% and 3% of adults in the UK (NICE 2008). ADHD is characterized by inattention, impulsivity and motor overactivity. Treatment of ADHD should be initiated only by a specialist and form part of a comprehensive treatment program of psychological, educational and social measures. Stimulant drugs are the first-choice treatment for ADHD in both children and adults. Methylphenidate and dexamfetamine increase synaptic dopamine and noradrenaline/norepinephrine; dexamfetamine also blocks the reuptake of both neurotransmitters. Methylphenidate is the first-line treatment in the UK for ADHD; it is available both in conventional and extended release formulations which can be combined to obtain maximum therapeutic effect. Treatment in children is frequently restricted to school terms, giving the child a 'drug holiday' when out of school. Drug holidays are necessary to determine efficacy of treatment, adjust or change dosage and avoid tolerance effects. Treatment in adults is more complex as attentional requirements are often continuous, so drug holidays may not be possible. Dosage tends to be slightly higher and combinations of different psychotropic drugs are more common. Dexamfetamine is an alternative that has similar efficacy to methylphenidate in ADHD and is the preferred drug in children with epilepsy. It has a greater potential for abuse than methylphenidate.

Unwanted effects of stimulants include some slowing of growth, loss of appetite and sleep, irritability, increased blood pressure and occasionally other cardiovascular problems. Weight, blood pressure and pulse should be monitored in both adults and children. In children height should also be monitored to assess growth. Stimulants in instant release formulations can be abused and some have been diverted to intravenous injection; prodrug and retarded release formulations have recently been introduced to combat this problem. Both methylphenidate and dexamfetamine are controlled drugs in the UK (class B schedule 2 of the Misuse of Drugs Act), so prescribing restrictions apply.

Atomoxetine, a noradrenaline/norepinephrine reuptake inhibitor (like reboxetine), is now licensed for ADHD. It is thought to act by increasing noradrenaline/norepinephrine and dopamine availability in the frontal cortex (where dopamine is taken up into noradrenergic nerve terminals). It has no known abuse liability and is not a controlled drug. The α-adrenoceptor blocker clonidine, tricyclic antidepressants (TCAs), bupropion and the stimulant modafinil may have a role in ADHD where methylphenidate, dexamfetamine and atomoxetine are contraindicated or have failed to produce benefit.

Part 5. Drugs for psychiatric illness in childhood

Children do suffer psychiatric illnesses. Many drugs used in childhood psychiatric illness are not properly tested in young people. Now there are regulatory pressures for drugs (in general) to have safety tests in children subsequent to their licensing in adults. Some drugs are deemed not to have adequate risk/benefit ratios in children, e.g. in depression most SSRI drugs are not recommended (an exception is fluoxetine for which evidence of efficacy and safety in children does exist). Similar caveats apply to the use of TCAs in childhood. By contrast, there are good efficacy data for several SSRIs in obsessive–compulsive disorder and social anxiety disorder, and for benefit of risperidone for aggression in children with autism.

SUMMARY

Psychiatric illnesses are often associated with co-morbid conditions, and may share the common mechanisms in the central nervous system. Thus, the drugs are sometime required for the treatment of different emotional disorders. These also indicated that mechanisms of many psychiatric illnesses are still unclear. Different psychiatric illnesses may share some similar symptoms, while same illness may show opposite behavioral changes at different times. Antidepressants are used for the treatment of clinical depression, as well as often for anxiety and a range of other disorders. Anxiolytics (including sedatives) are used for anxiety disorders and related problems such as insomnia. Mood stabilizers are used primarily in bipolar disorder. Antipsychotics are used for psychotic disorders, notably for positive symptoms in schizophrenia, and also increasingly for a range of other disorders. Stimulants are commonly used, notably for ADHD.

IMPORTANT TERMINOLOGY

psychiatric disorder　精神疾病

selective serotonin reuptake inhibitors (SSRIs)　选择性 5- 羟色胺再摄取抑制剂

monoamine oxidase inhibitors (MAOIs)　单胺氧化酶抑制剂

tricylic antidepressants　三环类抗抑郁药

extrapyramidal symptoms　锥体外系症状

post-traumatic stress disorder (PTSD)　创伤后应激障碍

generalized anxiety disorder (GAD)　广泛性焦虑症

obsessive–compulsive disorder　强迫症

classical benzodiazepines (BZDs)　苯二氮䓬类

attention deficit hyperactivity disorder (ADHD)　注意缺陷多动障碍力不足过动症

CHALLENGE YOURSELF

1. Based on the major classification of antidepressants and the mechanism of action, review the clinic usage of antidepressants.
2. How to distinguish the depression and anxiety, and the treatments between them.
3. The category of the drugs for Alzheimer's disease and the clinic evaluation.

Minggao Zhao

Chapter 12

Pain and analgesics

INTRODUCTION

Definition of pain

The International Association for the Study of Pain defines pain as 'an unpleasant sensory and emotional experience associated with actual or potential tissue damage, or described in terms of such damage'. This implies that the degree of pain experienced by the patient may be unrelated to the extent of underlying tissue damage, and that emotional or spiritual distress can add to the patient's experience of pain (Fig. 12.1).

This chapter focuses on the use of drugs for pain relief and illustrates the use of many analgesics that may be encountered in clinical practice. However, cli-nicians should recognise that the experience of pain is influenced by physical, emotional and psychological factors. While drug therapy is an expedient (and familiar) form of treatment, successful management of pain requires a more holistic approach that addresses all the components of pain. For instance, a patient's pain may not result from his/her disorders but loneliness or hopelessness.

Nociception

Pain alerts us to ongoing or potential tissue damage and the ability to sense pain is vital to our survival. The physiological process by which pain is perceived is known as *nociception*. While the neurobiology of nociception is complex, its appreciation provides a useful framework for understanding the way analgesics work (Fig. 12.2).

Our nervous system is alerted to actual or potential tissue injury by the activation of the peripheral terminals of highly specialised primary sensory neurones called *nociceptors*. Nociceptors have unmyelinated (C-fibre) or thinly myelinated (Aδ-fibre) axons. Their cell bodies lie in the dorsal root ganglia of the spinal cord or in the trigeminal ganglia. Different nociceptors encode discrete intensities and modalities of pain, depending upon their expression of ion-channel receptors. These receptors are *transducers*. They convert noxious stimuli into action potentials. Some of these transducers have been identified, including those that respond to heat (>46℃), cold (<10℃) and direct chemical irritants such as capsaicin.

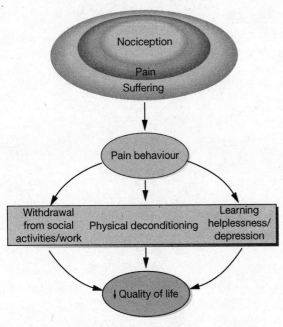

Fig. 12.1 A model of pain perception.

Fig. 12.2 Schematic representation of nociceptive pathways. Noxious stimuli such as protons (H⁺), temperature (temp) etc. applied to end-organs activate nociceptors. Injury leads to the release of prostaglandins such as prostaglandin E_2 (PGE₂), serotonin (5-HT), nerve growth factor (NGF) etc. from damaged cells, bradykinin (BK) from blood vessels and substance P (sP) from nociceptors. These agents either activate nociceptors directly or sensitise them to subsequent stimuli by parallel activation of intracellular kinases by G-protein-coupled receptors and tyrosine kinase receptors. Primary nociceptive afferents (C-fibres, Ad-fibres) of dorsal root ganglion (DRG) neurones synapse on second order neurones (S) in the spinal dorsal horn (magnified in inset). Here, glutamate (Glu) and sP released from primary afferent terminals (A) activate glutamate receptors (NMDA R, AMPA R, mGluRs) and neurokinin-1 (NK-1) receptors, respectively, located postsynaptically on spinal neurones. These synapses are negatively modulated by spinal inhibitory interneurones (I), which employ enkephalins (Enk) or γ-aminobutyric acid (GABA) as neurotransmitters. Spinal neurones convey nociceptive information to the brain and brainstem. Activation of descending noradrenergic/norepinergic and/or serotonergic systems, which originate in the brain and brainstem, leads to the activation of spinal inhibitory interneurones (I) thereby resulting in antinociception.

Action potentials that result from the transduction of noxious stimuli are conducted along the axon of the sensory neurone into the spinal cord. Conduction of the action potentials in sensory neurones depends on voltage-gated sodium channels, including two that are predominately expressed in nociceptors; $Na_v1.7$ and $Na_v1.8$.

The central terminal of the nociceptor makes synaptic contact with *dorsal horn neurones* within the spinal cord. Glutamate, an amino acid, is the main excitatory neurotransmitter released at these synapses. Its release can be inhibited by ligands that act to activate receptors found on the central terminal of the nociceptors (pre-synaptic inhibition). These include the opioids, cannabinoids, γ-aminobutyric acid (GABA)-receptor ligands and the anticonvulsants, gabapentin and pregabalin. Opioids and GABA also influence the action of glutamate on the dorsal horn neurones. They act on post-synaptic receptors to open potassium or chloride channels. This results in hyperpolarisation of the neurone, which inhibits its activity.

Other neurotransmitters may also be released by the central terminal of the nociceptors. For example, substance P is released during high-intensity and repetitive noxious stimulation. It mediates slow excitatory post-synaptic potentials and results in a localised depolarisation that facilitates the activation of N-methyl-D-aspartate (NMDA) receptors by glutamate. The end-result is a progressive increase in the output from dorsal horn neurones. This amplified output is thought to be responsible for the escalation of pain when the skin is repeatedly stimulated by noxious heat – a phenomenon known as wind-up.

Nociceptive output from the spinal cord is further modulated by descending inhibitory neurones that originate from supraspinal sites such as the periaqueductal gray or the rostral ventromedial medulla and terminate on nociceptive neurones in the spinal cord as well as on spinal inhibitory interneurones that store and release opioids. Stimulation of these brain regions, either electrically or chemically (e.g. opioids), produces analgesia in humans. Transmission through these inhibitory pathways is facilitated by monoamine neurotransmitters such as noradrenaline/norepinephrine and serotonin.

Finally, dorsal horn neurones send projections to supraspinal areas in the brainstem, hypothalamus, and thalamus and then, through relay neurones, to the cortex where the sensation of pain is perceived. The mechanism by which the cortex produces the conscious appreciation of pain is the focus of much research.

Classification of clinical pain

Rational pharmacological treatment of clinical pain depends on a number of factors, including the underlying cause and duration of pain, the patient's general medical condition and prognosis. Clinical pain is generally divided into three broad categories: acute, chronic, and cancer-related.

Acute pain, such as that experienced after trauma or surgery, typically resolves with healing of the injured tissue, and can usually be effectively managed with the appropriate use of pharmacotherapy. Poorly controlled post-surgical pain is associated with the development of complications such as pneumonia, myocardial ischaemia, paralytic ileus and thromboembolism, as well as an increased risk of the patient developing chronic pain. Effective analgesia in this setting not only reduces patient anxiety and provides subjective comfort, but also helps to blunt autonomic and somatic reflex responses. Effective analgesia can promote early mobilisation and increased appetite, and this, in turn, can improve postoperative outcome. Moreover, research suggests that analgesia given before surgical incision may reduce subsequent postoperative pain. Clinicians have attempted to exploit the concept of pre-emptive analgesia with varying success.

Chronic pain is commonly defined as pain that persists beyond the period expected for healing, or pain that is associated with progressive, non-malignant disease. Chronic pain may be due to the persistent stimulation of nociceptors in areas of ongoing tissue damage (e.g. chronic pain due to rheumatoid arthritis). In many instances, chronic pain can persist long after the healing of damaged tissue. In some patients, chronic pain presents without any identified ongoing tissue damage or antecedent injury.

Neuropathic pain is defined as a chronic pain resulting from damage to the nervous system. Neuropathic pain can be due to damage to the peripheral nervous system, such as patients with diabetic or AIDS polyneuropathy, post-herpetic neuralgia, or lumbar radiculopathy, or to the central nervous system, such as patients with spinal cord injury, multiple sclerosis, or stroke. The mechanisms of neuropathic pain remain the subject of much research.

Cancer-related pain refers to pain that is the result of primary tumour growth, metastatic disease, or the toxic effects of chemotherapy and radiation, such as neuropathies due to neurotoxic antineoplastic drugs.

Evaluation of pain

Achieving optimal pharmacological management of the patient's pain will depend on the type and cause of pain, as well as the psychological and physical condition of the patient. A comprehensive evaluation of the pain is, therefore, essential if we are to treat the patient successfully and safely. Underlying organic pathology must be excluded unless an obvious cause of pain is apparent (e.g. after recent surgery or trauma). The presence of organic pathology should also be suspected if the patient's pain presents in an unusual way, or is of a much greater magnitude than would normally be expected from the assumed pathology.

Once an organic explanation has been eliminated, additional tests are unhelpful. The illusory sense of progress such tests provide for both physician and patient may perpetuate maladaptive behaviour and impede the return to more normal function.

The evaluation of persistent pain should include pain location, quality, severity, duration, course, timing (including frequency of remissions and degree of fluctuation), exacerbating and relieving factors, and co-morbidities associated with the pain (with emphasis on psychological issues, depression, and anxiety). The efficacy and adverse effects of currently or previously used drugs and other treatments should also be determined.

If appropriate, the patient should be asked if litigation is ongoing or whether financial compensation for injury will be sought. A personal or family history of chronic pain can often give insight into the current problem. The patient's level of function should be assessed in detail, focusing on family relationships (including sexual), social network, and employment or vocation. The interviewer should elicit how the patient's pain affects the activities of normal living.

It is also important to determine what the pain means to the patient. In some patients, reporting pain may be more socially acceptable than reporting feelings of depression or anxiety. Pain and suffering should also be distinguished. In cancer patients, in particular, suffering may be due as much to loss of function and fear of impending death as to pain. The patient's expression of pain represents more than the pathology intrinsic to the disease.

Thorough physical examination is essential, and can often help to identify underlying causes and to evaluate, further, the degree of functional impairment. A basic neurological examination may identify features associated with neuropathic pain including:

- *Allodynia* – pain due to a stimulus which does not normally provoke pain.
- *Hyperalgesia* – an increased response to a stimulus which is normally painful.
- *Paraesthesia* – abnormal sensation, e.g. 'pins and needles'.
- *Dyaesthesia* – a painful paraesthesia, e.g. burning foot pain in diabetic neuropathy.

PHARMACOTHERAPY

An *analgesic* is defined as a drug that relieves pain. Analgesics are classified as *opioids* and *non-opioids* (e.g. NSAIDs). Co-analgesics or adjuvants are drugs that have a primary indication other than pain but are analgesic in some conditions. For example, antidepressants and anticonvulsants also act to reduce nociceptive transmission in neuropathic pain.

The efficacy and effectiveness of any given analgesic varies widely between individuals. Analgesics also have a relatively narrow therapeutic window, and drug dosages are often limited by the onset of adverse side-effects. For these reasons, an analgesic should be titrated for an individual patient until an acceptable balance is achieved between subjective pain relief and adverse drug effects.

NON-OPIOID ANALGESICS

NSAIDs (non-steroidal anti-inflammatory drugs)

Mechanism of analgesia

Endothelial damage produces an inflammatory response in tissues. Damaged cells release intracellular contents, such as adenosine triphosphate, hydrogen and potassium ions. Inflammatory cells recruited to the site of damage produce cytokines, chemokines and growth factors. A profound change to the chemical environment of the peripheral terminal of nociceptors occurs. Some factors act directly on the nociceptor terminal to activate it and produce pain, and others sensitise the terminal so that it becomes hypersensitive to subsequent stimuli. This process is known as peripheral sensitisation.

Prostanoid is a major sensitiser that is produced at the site of tissue injury. NSAIDs act by inhibiting cyclo-oxygenase, an enzyme involved in the production of prostanoid, as well as other prostaglandins. This enzyme has a number of isoforms, the most studied being cyclo-oxgenase-1 (COX-1) and cyclo-oxygenase-2 (COX-2). Their actions are inhibited by NSAIDs. Increased COX-2 production is induced by tissue injury and accounts for the efficacy of COX-2-specific inhibitor drugs (COXIBs). The inhibitory effect of NSAIDs on the production of other prostaglandins is responsible for the common side-effects of these drugs. Among other functions, the prostaglandins produced by cyclo-oxygenase act to protect the gastric mucosa, maintain normal blood flow in the kidney and preserve normal platelet function. Inhibition of prostaglandin production, therefore, can cause gastric irritation, damage to the kidney and an increased risk of bleeding.

Clinical use

NSAIDs are among the most commonly prescribed analgesics and, unless contraindicated, are effective and appropriate analgesics for use in acute inflammatory pain. There is much evidence to suggest that NSAIDs are effective in cancer-related pain. The benefit of NSAIDs in chronic non-cancer-related pain is less certain, with efficacy only proven in chronic inflammatory musculoskeletal pain, mainly from studies in rheumatoid arthritis. NSAIDs are generally ineffective in neuropathic pain conditions, and a careful risk–benefit assessment should be made prior to use in view of the side-effects associated with long-term use.

Choice of NSAID and route of administration

There is little difference in the clinical benefit conferred by any particular NSAID. However, NSAIDs differ in their pharmacokinetic properties and side-effects. This should be taken into account when choosing a non-steroidal agent for long-term use. For example, the oxicams (e.g. piroxicam, tenoxi-

cam) are metabolised slowly and have a high degree of enteropathic circulation. These NSAIDs have long elimination half-lives (but also higher incidences of gastrointestinal and renal side-effects).

NSAIDs should be given orally when possible. The same dose of NSAID is equally effective whether injected or taken orally. Topical application of NSAIDs for musculoskeletal pain is an exception as it is effective and is associated with a lower incidence of side-effects.

Side-effects

All NSAIDs are associated with dose-dependent side-effects. In particular, there is a risk of gastrointestinal bleed, renal toxicity and a possibility of cardiac-related complications. The morbidity related to gastrointestinal adverse effects is considerable (~5 per 1 000 patients per year of treatment) and catastrophic bleeding can occur without any preceding warning symptoms. For this reason, it is recommended that, when used in the longer term, NSAIDs should be prescribed along with an appropriate gastro-protective agent.

COX-2-specific NSAIDs provide analgesia with a reduced risk of GI bleed (but have a similar risk of renal toxicity). Trials have shown a slightly increased risk of cardiac complications in at-risk patients. Subsequent trials, however, have indicated that increased cardiac risk may also be associated with the use of non-selective NSAIDs (possibly as a result of hypertension secondary to fluid retention). Current guidelines suggest that all cyclo–oxygenase-inhibiting drugs should be used with caution in patients with known cardiovascular or cerebrovascular disease, i.e. at the lowest effective dose, and for the shortest possible time.

Paracetamol (acetaminophen)

The major advantage of paracetamol over the NSAIDs is its relative lack of adverse effects; this justifies its use as a first-line analgesic. It can be used on its own, or synergistically with non-steroidal drugs or opioids. Paracetamol is also an antipyretic with very weak anti-inflammatory properties. There is increasing evidence that its analgesic effect is central and results from the activation of descending serotonergic pain-inhibiting pathways, but its primary site of action may still be inhibition of prostaglandin synthesis (via COX-3 inhibition). Its major drawback is the liver toxicity seen in acute overdose due to the accumulation in the liver of benzoquinones.

Nefopam

Nefopam is chemically distinct and pharmacologically unrelated to any presently known analgesic and has been used in Europe for intravenous and oral administration since 1976. It is a racemic mixture of its two enantiomers. Although its mechanism of action remains largely unknown, nefopam is thought to increase the inhibiting tone of serotonergic and noradrenergic/norepinephrinergic descending pathways by inhibiting the synaptic uptake of dopamine, noradrenaline/norepinephrine and serotonin. Compared to NSAIDs and opioids, nefopam has the advantages of minimal effects on platelet aggregation and not depressing the central nervous system. There have been rare fatal overdoses with the oral form of the drug, characterised by convulsions and arrhythmia. Its sympathomimetic action precludes its use in patients with limited coronary reserve, prostatitis and glaucoma. Minor side-effects (nausea, dizziness and sweating) are observed in 15%–30% of treated patients. Nefopam has been abused primarily for its psychostimulant effects, which are probably linked to its dopamine-reuptake inhibition properties.

OPIOID ANALGESICS

Opium (the dried juice of the seed head of the opium poppy) was used in prehistoric times. Modern medical practice still benefits from the use of its alkaloids, employing them as analgesics, tranquillisers, antitussives and in the treatment of diarrhea.

The principal active ingredient in crude opium was isolated in 1806 by Friedrich Sertürner, who tested pure morphine on himself and three young men. He observed that the drug caused cerebral depression and relieved toothache, and named it

after Morpheus, the Greek god of dreams. Opium contains many alkaloids, but the only important opiates (drugs derived from opium) are morphine (10%) and codeine. Papaverine is occasionally used as a vasodilator.

Opioid is a generic term for natural or synthetic substances that bind to specific opioid receptors in the CNS, producing an agonist action.

Mechanism of action of opioids

Opioids produce their effects by activating specific G protein-coupled receptors in the brain, spinal cord and peripheral nervous system. There are three major classes of opioid receptor: δ-opioid (OP1, DOR), κ-opioid (OP2, KOR) and μ-opioid (OP3, MOR), that correspond respectively to their endogenous ligands, enkephalin, dynorphin and β-endorphin. Although studies suggest the existence of subtypes of all three major opioid receptor classes, the evidence is controversial and the sub-classification is of little practical value except, perhaps, to explain the change in side-effect profile sometimes seen during opioid rotation in long-term opioid use or cancer-related pain.

Agonist activity at opioid receptors acts to open potassium channels and prevent the opening of voltage-gated calcium channels. This reduces neuronal excitability and inhibits the release of pain neurotransmitters.

Classification of opioid drugs

Opioids have been traditionally classified as *strong*, *intermediate* and *weak*, according to their perceived analgesic properties and propensity for addiction. This approach can be misleading, as it implies that weak opioids such as codeine are less effective but safe. Codeine may be less potent than morphine but can cause respiratory depression if given insufficient quantities. Codeine-like drugs are also frequently abused. Opioids may also be classified according to their structure. As described later, the properties of opioids may be predicted on the basis of activity on opioid and other receptor systems. The functional classification is probably of most clinical use (Table 12.1).

Table 12.1 Classification of opioids

Traditional		
Strong	**Intermediate**	**Weak**
Morphine Diamorphine Fentanyl	Partial agonists Mixed agonist–antagonist	Codeine
Structural		
Morphinans	**Phenylperidines**	**Diphenylprophylamines**	**Esters**
Morphine Codeine	Meriperidine Fentanyl	Methadone, Dextropropoxyphene	Remifentanil
Functional		
Pure agonists	**Partial agonists**	**Mixed action**	**Antagonists**
Morphine Codeine	Buprenorphine	Pentazocine Nalbupine Butorphanol	Naxolone

Opioid pharmacodynamics

Opioids act to reduce the intensity and unpleasantness of pain. The common side-effects are due to their action on different opioid receptors. They include sedation, euphoria, dysphoria, respiratory depression, constipation, pruritis, and nausea and vomiting. It is important to note, however, that many of these side-effects tend to diminish with time as tolerance to the opioid develops. Constipation and dry mouth (leading to increased risk of dental caries) are more resistant to the development of tolerance and remain problems with long-term use. Impairment of hypothalamic function also occurs with long-term opioid use and may result in loss of libido, impotence and infertility. Adverse effects associated with the use of opioids in acute pain (and occasionally in chronic non-malignant pain) can often be managed simply by reducing the opioid dose or switching to a different opioid. In palliative medicine, unwanted effects related to long-term opioid use are often treated proactively, laxatives for constipation, excessive sedation by methylphenidate or dextroamphetamine. Rotating to another opioid, or using more frequent but smaller doses of opioids may also help.

Systemic effects of opioid analgesics

Central nervous system

Opioids reduce the intensity and unpleasantness of pain. Patients taking opioid analgesics often report less distress, even when they can still perceive pain. Sedation occurs frequently, particularly in the early stages of treatment, but often resolves although it can remain a problem, especially at higher doses, and is a common cause of drug discontinuation in the chronic pain population.

The sensitivity of the respiratory centre to hypercarbia and hypoxaemia is reduced by opioids. Hypoventilation, due to a reduction in respiratory rate and tidal volume, ensues. Cough is inhibited by a central action. Prolonged apnoea and respiratory obstruction can occur during sleep. These effects are more pronounced when the respiratory drive is impaired by disease, for example in chronic obstructive pulmonary disease, obstructive sleep apnoea and raised intracranial pressure.

Opioid-related respiratory depression is more common in patients being treated for acute pain than in patients established on long-term opioids. Respiratory depression in use relates to high blood opioid concentrations, for example with an inappropriately large dose that fails to account for differences in patient physiology (e.g. in hypovolaemic trauma or the elderly), or because the patient is unable to excrete the drug efficiently (as a consequence of renal impairment). Respiratory depression is unusual in patients established on long-term opioids due to the development of tolerance. Sudden changes to the patient's physiological state (e.g. the development of acute renal failure) may produce increases in blood opioid concentration and precipitate toxic effects.

Nausea and vomiting commonly accompany opioids used for acute pain. The mechanism may be activation of opioid receptors within the chemoreceptor trigger zone within the medulla, although opioid effects on the gastrointestinal tract and vestibular function probably play a role. Antiemetics are effective.

Miosis occurs due to an excitatory effect on the

parasympathetic nerve innervating the pupil. Pinpoint pupils are characteristic of acute poisoning; at therapeutic doses the pupils are merely smaller than normal.

Cardiovascular system

Opioids cause peripheral vasodilatation and impair sympathetic vascular reflexes. Postural hypotension may occur, but this is seldom troublesome in the reasonably fit patient and is rare with long-term use. Intravenous administration of opioids to patients who are hypovolaemic or have poor cardiac reserve can result in marked hypotension. Intravenous morphine titrated carefully may benefit patients with acute myocardial infarct and left ventricular failure as morphine reduces sympathetic drive (from pain and anxiety) and preload (by venodilatation), thereby reducing the work of the heart.

Gastrointestinal tract

Opioids cause a tonic increase of smooth muscle tone along the gastrointestinal tract. Reduced peristalsis and delayed gastric emptying results in constipation, greater absorption of water and increased viscosity of feces, and exacerbation of the constipation (but the effect is useful in diarrhea). Opioid-induced constipation in palliative care can be managed by increasing the fibre content of the diet to>10 g/day (unless bowel obstruction exists) and prescribing a stool softener (e.g. docusate sodium 100 mg twice or three times daily), usually with a stimulant laxative (e.g. senna or bisacodyl). Stimulant laxatives should be started at a low dose (e.g. Senna 15 mg daily) and increased as necessary. Persistent constipation can be managed with an osmotic laxative (e.g., magnesium citrate) given for 2 or 3 days or with lactulose daily (e.g.15 mL twice daily).

Pressure within the biliary tree due to spasm of the sphincter of Oddi is increased after opioid administration and gives rise to colicky pain with morphine which can be both diagnosed and relieved by a small dose of the opioid antagonist naloxone. Pethidine (meperidine) is held to produce less spasm in the sphincter of Oddi than other opioids due to its atropine-like effects and is preferred for biliary tree and pancreatic pain. At higher equi-analgesic doses, the effect of pethidine on the sphincter is similar to other opioids, and confers no advantage.

Urogenital tract

Increased tone in the detrusor muscle and contraction of the external sphincter, together with inhibition of the voiding reflexes may aggravate urinary retention.

Others

Opioid administration is often associated with cutaneous vasodilatation that results in the flushing of the face, neck and thorax. This may, in part, be due to histamine release. Pruritus is common with epidural or intrathecal administration of opioids and appears to be mediated by opioid receptor activation, as it is reversed by naloxone.

Pharmacokinetics

Bio-availability varies between opioids after oral administration but is generally poor. Methadone is an exception (80%) (Table 12.2).

Table 12.2 Approximate oral bio-availability of opioids	
Opioid	Approximate oral bio-availability %
Hydromorphone	20
Morphine	30
Diamorphine	30
Meperidine	30
Codeine	60
Oxycodone	60
Levorphanol	70
Tramadol	80
Methadone	80

Most opioids have a large volume of distribution (i.e exceeding total body water) and most have an elimination half-life in the range (3–10 h). Notable exceptions are alfentanil ($t_{\frac{1}{2}}$ 1.6 h) and remifentanil ($t_{\frac{1}{2}}$ 0.06 h) and methadone ($t_{\frac{1}{2}}$ 20–45 h; see section on methadone). Controlled-release opioids typically require days to approach steady-state plasma levels.

Duration of analgesia usually correlates with half-life unless the parent drug has active metabolites (morphine) or if the drug has a high affinity for opioid receptors (buprenorphine). Opioid sensitivity is increased in the neonate and in the elderly. Variation in response and the narrow therapeutic index of opioids make it essential to titrate effects for individual patients. For opioid-naïve patients with acute pain, frequent monitoring of pain relief, sedation, respiratory rate and blood pressure is necessary to guide dosage adjustment.

Route of administration

The oral route is preferred as it is simple, non-invasive and relatively affordable. It requires little in the form of direct medical supervision or complex delivery equipment. The slower onset of action renders this route less convenient for use in acute pain. The oral route is also unsuitable when patients suffer from emesis, dysphagia, gastrointestinal obstruction or malabsorption or in acute trauma where the patient may have delayed gastric emptying.

If parenteral administration is necessary, the intravenous route is preferable to intramuscular injection for repeated boluses because it is less painful. Also, intramuscular or subcutaneous routes of administration should not be used if the patient is peripherally vasoconstricted (e.g. in the acute trauma patient), as the establishment of normal peripheral blood flow, as the patient is resuscitated, may result in a sudden redistribution of the drug to the central circulation. Continuous intravenous or subcutaneous infusion should be considered if repeated parenteral doses pro-duce a prominent bolus effect (i.e. toxicity) at peak levels early in the dosing interval or break-through pain at trough levels. Patient-controlled analgesia (PCA) systems (in which the patient can trigger additional drug delivery) can be added to an infusion to provide supplementary doses. These systems are safe for both home and hospitalised patients, but are contraindicated for sedated and confused patients.

Epidural and intrathecal administration of opioids requires special expertise. The dorsal horn of the spinal cord is rich in opioid receptors, and equivalent analgesia can be provided using a lower dose of opioid, resulting in fewer systemic side-effects. However, rostral spread of the drug can result in delayed toxicity (e.g. respiratory depression) during acute administration, and the cost of infusion systems, staffing and monitoring must also be taken into account. The use of intraventricular morphine appears to be beneficial in treating recalcitrant pain due to head and neck malignancies and tumours (e.g., superior sulcus tumours, breast carcinoma) that affect the brachial plexus.

PHARMACOLOGY OF INDIVIDUAL OPIOIDS

Opioid agonist drugs

Morphine

Morphine remains the most widely used opioid analgesic for the treatment of severe pain. It is the gold standard against which other opioids are compared. Commonly given intramuscularly, intravenously, or orally, it can also be administered per rectum and into the epidural space or cerebrospinal fluid. Unlike most opioids, it is relatively water soluble. Metabolism is by hepatic conjugation and its half life is about 2–4 h. The duration of useful analgesia provided by morphine is about 3–6 h, but varies greatly with different drug preparations and routes of administrations.

Morphine 6-glucuronide (M6G), one of its major metabolites, is an agonist at the μ receptor and also at the distinct M6G receptor. It is more potent than morphine. As it is excreted in the urine, it accumulates if renal function is impaired. With repeated use of morphine, morphine 6-glucuronide is responsible for a significant amount of pharmacological activity.

Diamorphine

Diamorphine (3,6-diacetyl morphine), or heroin, is a semi-synthetic drug that was first made from morphine at St Mary's Hospital, London, in 1874. In almost every country, except the UK, the manufacture of diamorphine, even for use in medicine, is now illegal.

Diamorphine has no direct activity at the μ receptor. It is rapidly converted within minutes to morphine and 6-monoacetylmorphine. The effects of diamorphine are principally due to the actions of morphine and 6-monoacetylmorphine on the μ and, to a lesser extent, the κ receptors.

Diamorphine given parenterally has a $t_{1/2}$ of 3 min. When given orally, it is subject to complete presystemic or first-pass metabolism and only morphine ($t_{1/2}$ 3 h) and other metabolites reach the systemic circulation. Thus oral diamorphine is essentially a prodrug. It is likely that there are no significant differences in the pharmacodynamics of diamorphine when compared to morphine when used for acute pain, de-spite the common belief that diamorphine is associated with more euphoria and less nausea and vomiting. Its greater potency (greater efficacy in relation to weight and, therefore, requiring a smaller volume) and lipid-solubility make diamorphine suitable for delivery by subcutaneous infusion through a syringe driver when continuous pain control is required in palliative care that can no longer be achieved by the enteral route (oral, buccal, rectal).

Codeine

Codeine is obtained naturally or by methylation of morphine. It has a low affinity for opioid receptors and most of its analgesic effect results from its metabolism (about 10%) to morphine. The polymorphic CYP2D6 enzyme is responsible for this transformation and it is absent in some individuals (e.g. 7% of the Caucasian population whilst very low in Chinese and Japanese), suggesting that these patients will derive little benefit from codeine.

Codeine alone is a relatively poor analgesic but can be effective for mild to moderate pain, especially when combined with paracetamol. It can also be useful for the short-term symptomatic control of persistent cough or mild diarrhoea. Prolonged use is often associated with chronic constipation, especially at higher doses (more than30 mg four times daily).

Dihydrocodeine

Dihydrocodeine (DF118) is a low-efficacy opioid with an analgesic potency similar to that of codeine. It is used to relieve moderate acute and chronic pain on its own or as a compound tablet (co-dydramol; dihydrocodeine 10 mg plus paracetamol 500 mg). Although active metabolites (dihydromorphine and dihydromorphine-6-O-glucuronide) account for some of its pharmacological effects, dihydrocodeine itself has analgesic activity and may be a more reliable analgesic when compared to codeine.

Oxycodone

Oxycodone is a semi-synthetic opioid that has been in clinical use since 1917. Its potency is approximately twice that of morphine. Oxycodone is currently used as a controlled-release preparation for cancer and chronic non-malignant pain. The immediate-release solution and tablets are available for acute or breakthrough pain. Parental oxycodone is an alternative when opioids cannot be given orally. Both oxycodone and morphine provide effective analgesia in acute and chronic pain. Oxycodone may have a more favourable pharmacokinetic profile. Its oral bio-availability, at about 80%, is significantly higher. This results in reduced inter-individual variation in plasma concentrations after oral administration. It has a similar adverse-effect profile to morphine, with a slightly reduced incidence of psychotropic effects.

A fixed-dose oral formulation (Targinact) of oxycodone combined with naloxone has been shown to be effective in patients who derive benefit from opioid therapy, but where use of the opioid is limited because of intractable constipation. Naloxone provides competitive antagonism of the opioid-receptor mediated effects of oxycodone in the gut, thus reducing constipation. Since the bio-availability of naloxone after oral administration is less than 3%, systemic effects from the antagonist drug are unlikely. The recommended maximum daily dose of Targinact is 80 mg oxycodone hydrochloride and 40 mg naloxone hydrochloride.

Hydromorphone

Hydromorphone is a semi-synthetic opioid used primarily for the treatment of cancer-related pain. It can be administered intravenously, orally, and rectally. Hydromorphone is five times as potent as morphine when given by the oral route and eight to nine times as potent when given intravenously, with a similar duration of action. The liver is its principal site of metabolism. In contrast to morphine, the 6-glucuronide metabolite is not produced in any significant amount, the main metabolite being hydromorphone-3-glucuronide. Some metabolites are active but they are present in such small amounts that they are unlikely to have a significant effect except perhaps in renal failure.

Methadone

Methadone is a synthetic opioid used commonly as a maintenance drug in opioid addicts and increasingly used in cancer and chronic non-malignant pain. It is rapidly absorbed after oral administration and is extensively metabolised to products that are excreted in the urine. The principal feature of methadone is its long duration of action, due to high protein binding and slow liver metabolism. The elimination half-life of methadone is 20–45 h, making it suitable for use in long-term therapy, but less useful for acute pain. Steady state concentration is only reached after several days with regular administration and dosages must be carefully titrated.

When used in cancer-related pain or chronic non-malignant pain, an opioid of short half-life should be provided for breakthrough pain, rather than an extra dose of methadone. The long duration of action also favours its use for the treatment of opioid withdrawal.

Fentanyl

Fentanyl is one of the first short-acting opioids developed for use in anaesthesia. It is approximately 100 times more potent than morphine but undergoes hepatic metabolism to produce inactive metabolites. At low doses, it has a short duration of action due to redistribution of the drug. Its terminal half-life is relatively long (1.5–6 h) and, at higher doses, when tissue sites are saturated, its duration of action is much higher. The long $t_{1/2}$ and high lipid solubility make fentanyl ideal for use as a transdermal patch. These preparations are used commonly in cancer-related pain and chronic non-malignant pain.

Oral transmucosal fentanyl citrate offers a unique way of treating breakthrough and incident pain. The transmucosal route offers rapid onset of action in 5–15 min, with peak plasma concentrations at 22 min. Absorption takes place at the buccal and sublingual mucosa, first-pass effect is avoided and overall bio-availability is 50%.

Alfentanil

Alfentanil is less potent and has a shorter half-life than fentanyl. Despite its lower lipid solubility, it has a more rapid onset of action. This is because a greater proportion of the unbound drug is un-ionised and able to diffuse freely across the blood–brain barrier. Like fentanyl, it accumulates with prolonged infusion and the plasma $t_{1/2}$ increases with the duration of infusion.

Remifentanil

Remifentanil is a μ-opioid receptor agonist with an analgesic potency similar to fentanyl and a speed of onset similar to alfentanil. It is broken down by blood and tissue esterases and has a short and predictable $t_{1/2}$ (approximately 5 min) which is not affected by renal or hepatic function or plasma cholinesterase deficiency.

Its main metabolite is a carboxylic acid derivative which is excreted by the kidneys. Although this accumulates in renal failure, significant pharmacological effects are unlikely as its potency relative to remifentanil is only 0.1%–0.3%.

Remifentanil is unique in that its plasma half-life re-mains constant even after prolonged infusion. This property favours its use during anaesthesia, when a rapid wake-up time is desirable (e.g. after neurosurgery).

Papaveretum

Papaveretum is a mixture of opium alkaloids, the

principal constituents being morphine (50%), codeine, papaverine and noscapine. Noscapine may be teratogenic, and is no longer a component of commercially available papaveretum in the UK.

Partial agonist opioid analgesics

Buprenorphine

Buprenorphine is a partial agonist at the μ receptor. The partial agonist activity, however, is thought to occur at a higher dose than would be normally used therapeutically and is, therefore, rarely clinically significant. It is 30 times more potent than morphine and its receptor affinity (tenacity of binding) is high. This means that it dissociates from the receptor very slowly. Thus, its peak effect may occur up to 3 h after administration, and its duration of action as long as 10 h. In theory, a partial agonist has less potential for respiratory depression and abuse. Respiratory depression can occur with buprenorphine overdose and, because of its affinity with the μ receptor, may only be partially reversed by naloxone. A respiratory stimulant (doxapram) may be needed in overdose or, occasionally, mechanical ventilation.

Because of extensive first-pass metabolism when swallowed, buprenorphine is normally given by the buccal (sublingual) route or by i.m. or slow i.v. injection. It is a useful analgesic in acute pain because administration by injection can be avoided (for children, or for patients with a bleeding disorder or needle phobia). Its low incidence of drug dependency has led to its increased use in withdrawing opioid addicts and in chronic non-malignant pain. Its prolonged half-life and high lipid-solubility make it suitable for use as a transdermal patch preparation.

Meptazinol

Meptazinol is a high-efficacy partial agonist opioid with central cholinergic activity that is thought to add to its analgesic effect. It is used to relieve acute or chronic pain of moderate intensity. It is thought to have a low incidence of confusion and a low potential for abuse. Its poor oral bio-availability and partial agonist activity make it less useful in severe pain.

Mixed agonist–antagonist opioid analgesics

Drugs in this class include pentazocine, butorphanol, and nalbuphine. They act as partial agonists at the κ receptor and weak antagonist at the μ receptor. Consequently, they may cause withdrawal symptoms in patients dependent on other opioids. As analgesics, mixed agonist–antagonist opioids are not as efficacious as pure μ agonists. Compared to morphine, they produce less dependence (but this definitely occurs), more psychotomimetic effects (κ receptor), and less sedation and respiratory depression (naloxone can reverse the respiratory depression in overdose). They are given to relieve moderate to severe pain, but dysphoric adverse effects often limit their usefulness.

Pentazocine is one sixth as potent as morphine, nalbuphine is slightly less potent than morphine and butorphanol is five to nine times as potent. Adverse effects include nausea, vomiting, dizziness, sweating, hypertension, palpitations, tachycardia and central nervous system disturbance (euphoria, dysphoria, psychotomimesis). Pentazocine has effects on the cardiovascular system, raising systolic blood pressure and pulmonary artery pressure, and should be avoided in myocardial infarction.

Opioids with action on other systems

Pethidine (meperidine)

Pethidine (meperidine) was discovered in 1939 during a search for atropine-like compounds. Its use as a treatment for asthma was abandoned when its opioid agonist properties were appreciated.

Pethidine is primarily a μ-receptor agonist. Despite its structural dissimilarity to morphine, pethidine shares many similar properties, including antagonism by naloxone. It is extensively metabolised in the liver and the parent drug and metabolites are excreted in the urine. Normeperidine is a pharmacologically active metabolite. It can cause central excitation and, eventually, convulsions, if it accumulates after prolonged intravenous administration or in renal impairment.

Pethidine has atropine-like effects, including dry mouth and blurred vision (cycloplegia and sometimes mydriasis, though usually miosis). It can produce euphoria and is associated with a high incidence of dependence. Its use as an analgesia in obstetric practice was based on early clinical research which showed that, unlike morphine, pethidine did not appear to delay labour. However, the doses of pethidine used in these early studies were low and it is now established that pethidine confers no added advantage over other opioids at higher equi-analgesic doses.

Pethidine is eight to ten times less potent than morphine, has poor and variable oral absorption, with a short duration of action in the range of 2–3 h. For all these reasons, it is recommended that pethidine should be avoided if alternatives are available.

Tramadol

Tramadol is presented as a mixture of two stereoisomers. It is a centrally acting analgesic with relatively weak μ-opioid receptor activity. However, it also inhibits neuronal reuptake of noradrenaline/norepinephrine and enhances serotonin release, and this is thought to account for some of its analgesic action.

It is rapidly absorbed from the gastrointestinal tract. Roughly 20% of an oral dose undergoes first-pass metabolism and less than 30% of a dose is excreted unchanged in the urine. Production of the O-desmethyl-tramadol metabolite is dependent on the cytochrome CYP2D6 enzyme. This metabolite is an active μ agonist with a greater receptor affinity than tramadol. Tramadol is approximately as effective as pethidine for postoperative pain.

Tramadol is less likely to depress respiration and has a lower incidence of constipation compared to opioids, but has a high incidence of nausea and dizziness. It can cause seizures (rare) and should be used with caution insusceptible patients.

Opioid antagonists

Naloxone

Naloxone is a competitive antagonist at μ-, δ-, κ-, and σ-opioid receptors and acts to reverse the effects of most opioid analgesics. It acts within minutes when given intravenously and slightly less rapidly when given intramuscularly. However, the duration of antagonism (approximately 20 min) is usually shorter than that of opioid-induced respiratory depression. Close monitoring of the patient and repeated doses of naloxone may therefore be necessary.

A common starting dosage in an opioid-naïve patient with acute opioid over dosage is 0.4 mg i.v. every 2–3 min until effect. For patients receiving long-term opioid therapy, it should be used only to reverse respiratory depression and must be administered more cautiously to avoid precipitating withdrawal or severe pain. A reasonable starting dose is 0.04 mg (dilute a 0.4 mg ampoule in 10 mL saline) i.v. every2–3 min until the respiratory rate improves.

Choice of opioid analgesic

An opioid may be preferred because of favourable experience, lower cost (methadone is least expensive), availability, route of administration or duration of action. Opioids with a short half-life (morphine and diamorphine) should be used as first-line agents for acute pain but may be replaced with longer-acting drugs if pain persists.

Knowledge of equi-analgesic doses of opioids is essential when changing drugs or routes of administration (Table 12.3 and 12.4). Cross-tolerance between drugs is in-complete, so when one drug is substituted for another, the equi-analgesic dose should be reduced by 50%. The only exception is methadone,

Table 12.3	Relative potency of opioids	
Drug	Oral: parenteral potency ratio*	Parenteral potency relative to morphine**
Morphine	1:6	1.0
Codeine	2:3	0.1
Hydromorphone	1:5	6.0
Meperidine	1:4	0.15
Oxycodone	1:2	1.0
Methadone	1:2	1.0

* Oral–parenteral ratio: for example, morphine is six times more potent parenterally than orally.
** Potency relative to morphine: for example, hydromorphone is six times more potent than an equal dose of morphine when given parenterally.

which should be reduced by 75%–90%. Opioid rotation is commonly used in cancer-related and chronic non-malignant pain as a means of reducing side-effects and limiting the development of tolerance.

Table 12.4	Opioid oral analgesic equivalents	
Analgesic	Single dose	Equi-analgesic dose Oral morphine
Codeine	60 mg	5 mg
Dihydrocodeine	60 mg	8 mg
Tramadol	50 mg	10 mg
Meptazinol	200 mg	8 mg
Buprenorphine sublingual	200 micrograms	10 mg
Hydromorphone	1.3 mg	10 mg
Methadone	1 mg	10 mg
Oxycodone	5 mg	10 mg

TOLERANCE, DEPENDENCE AND ADDICTION

Although the use of strong opioid analgesics in cancer-related pain is well established, physicians are often reluctant to prescribe opioids in acute, and especially in chronic, non-malignant pain. Patients (and their families, friends and employers) are, likewise, wary about the long-term use of opioids. The reasons for this reluctance may stem from previous experiences of the genuine problems associated with long-term opioid use in patients or, more often, due to the perception of opioids as dangerous and addictive drugs. Patients and physicians also frequently confuse tolerance and dependence with drug addiction.

Tolerance indicates the need to increase the dose of a drug with time to achieve the same analgesic effect. It is due to physiological adaptation to the drug. In practice, tolerance can be managed by increasing the dose of the opioid drug over time. Tolerance to the adverse effects of opioids (e.g. constipation) is often less predictable, and the development of side-effects may prevent further escalation of the drug.

It is important to distinguish a gradual reduction in efficacy of an analgesic that is due to the development of tolerance from the onset of pain due to progression of the underlying disease process or new pathology.

Dependence is the physical manifestation of tolerance and its effects are observed soon after abrupt withdrawal of a long-term opioid. The severity of withdrawal symptoms varies depending on the patient, the drug and the length of treatment, and includes symptoms such as coryza, tremor, sweating, abdominal cramps, myalgia, vomiting and diarrhoea. Acute withdrawal can usually be avoided by reducing the drug dose gradually at the end of treatment by about 50% every 2 days (but may require a slower rate of withdrawal in some long-term patients). Patients on long-term opioid therapy should not be given mixed agonist/antagonist drugs, as they can precipitate withdrawal.

Addiction is a behavioural problem characterised by drug-seeking activity in the individual in order to experience its psychotropic effects. This drug-seeking behaviour may persist despite the knowledge that continued use of the drug will result in considerable physical, emotional, social or economic harm. The incidence of addiction in patients taking opioid medications for acute pain is negligible, and is low even in patients on long-term opioids for chronic non-malignant pain (<10%), provided that the patients are carefully screened for drug misuse potential and adequately monitored. The risk of iatrogenic addiction in patients prescribed opioids for cancer-related pain is believed to be extremely low.

Pain relief in opioid addicts

Drug addicts can suffer from pain. Physicians, particularly in hospitals, are often guilty of withholding or under-prescribing opioids for drug-addicted patients in acute pain. This stems from unfounded fears of 'worsening' the addiction, distrust of the patient's motives or misguided attempts to 'cure' the patient of his addiction.

Before treating opioid addicts with acute pain, physicians should attempt to establish the patient's daily opioid intake prior to hospital admission. The patient should then be maintained with an equivalent daily dose of opioid medication throughout their admission. Physicians should be aware that the strength of street drugs is highly variable. The addicted patient may also have an acute medical condition that alters opioid pharmacokinetics unpredictably. It is safer, therefore, to first prescribe an appropriate dose of an opioid with a short duration of action on an 'as required' basis, in order to assess opioid requirements, before conversion to longer-acting opioids for maintenance.

The opioid-addicted patient with acute pain will require appropriate analgesia in addition to the calculated maintenance dose. Non-opioid analgesics are useful adjuncts, but should not be used as a substitute for opioid analgesia. The use of opioid agonist-antagonist compounds in known or suspected active opioid addicts is absolutely contraindicated as these drugs may precipitate withdrawal.

CO-ANALGESICS

Co-analgesics (adjuvant analgesics) are important for the treatment of cancer-related and chronic non-malignant pain. These agents provide an 'opioid-sparing' effect and are effective for the treatment of neuropathic pain associated with many cancers. In chronic non-malignant pain, co-analgesics are frequently used as 'first-line' drugs, and form the mainstay of treatment for chronic neuropathic pain. As co-analgesics are generally used in other medical conditions (e.g. as anticonvulsants or antidepressants), their basic pharmacology will be covered in the relevant chapters elsewhere. This chapter highlights the use of co-analgesics in the context of pain management.

Multipurpose adjuvant analgesics

Corticosteroids

Corticosteroids are among the most widely used adjuvant analgesics in palliative care. They improve quality of life in cancer patients by virtue of their analgesic effects and other beneficial effects on appetite, nausea, mood and malaise. Corticosteroids may also reduce oedema around metastases or damaged nerve plexuses. Patients with advanced cancer who experience pain and other symptoms often respond favourably to a relatively small dose of corticosteroid (e.g. dexamethasone 1–2 mg twice daily).

Neuroleptics

Methotrimeprazine has proven very useful in bedridden patients with advanced cancer who experience pain associated with anxiety, restlessness or nausea. In this setting, the sedative, anxiolytic and antiemetic effects of this drug can be useful, and side-effects, such as orthostatic hypotension, are less clinically significant. Treatment can be started at 6–25 mg/day in three divided doses at mealtimes and increased until optimum effect. Alternatively, as a sedative, a single night-time dose of 10–25 mg can be given.

Benzodiazepines

Benzodiazepines have limited analgesic effects but are often used as a short-term treatment for painful muscle spasm. Their use, however, must be balanced by the potential for side-effects, including sedation and confusion. With the important exception of clonazepam, which is widely accepted for use in the management of neuropathic pain, these drugs are generally prescribed only if another indication exists, such as anxiety or insomnia.

Adjuvant analgesics used in neuropathic pain

Antidepressants

At present, the evidence for analgesic efficacy is greatest for the tertiary amine tricyclic drugs, such as amitriptyline, doxepin and imipramine. The secondary aminetricyclic antidepressants (such as desipramine and nortriptyline) have fewer side-effects and are preferred when there are serious concerns about sedation, anticholinergic effects or cardiovascular toxicity. Dual-reuptake inhibitors (venlafaxine, duloxetine) may be beneficial for patients who obtain relief from tricyclics but find the adverse effects a problem. Duloxetine is currently licensed for the treatment of pain from diabetic neuropathy and fibromyalgia and has been shown to be effective in clinical trials. There is little evidence, however, to suggest that duloxetine is more efficacious compared to tricyclic antidepressant drugs for the treatment of neuropathic pain.

The dose of duloxetine required to treat pain is 60–120 mg, which also has clinically relevant antidepressant effects. This is in contrast to other antidepressant drugs used in neuropathic pain where the analgesic effect of the drugs occurs at a smaller dose and within a shorter time from onset (1–2 weeks) than any antidepressant effect. The drugs should be started at a low dose to minimise initial side-effects (e.g. amitriptyline 10 mg daily in the elderly and 10–25 mg daily in younger patients). Education of the patient is essential. They should be informed that the analgesic effect of the antidepressant medication can take days or weeks to develop, and that the drug must be taken on a regular basis for effect. It is common for patients to report taking the medication intermittently as a supplement to simple analgesics 'when the pain is bad'. Patient compliance is often improved when physicians emphasis that the drugs are being prescribed for their analgesic effects and not for their antidepressant properties.

Abrupt withdrawal of the antidepressant drugs should be avoided as it can cause a variety of unpleasant symptoms, thought to be related to rebound cholinergic activity. These include vivid dreams, restlessness and gastrointestinal hyperactivity. These symptoms can be minimised if the drug dose is reduced gradually at intervals of 5–10 days.

Anticonvulsants

In 1853, Alfred Trousseau, then director of the medical clinic at the Hôtel-Dieu in Paris, suggested that painful paroxysms seen in trigeminal neuralgia were due to discharges in the trigeminal system that were similar to the neuronal discharges seen in epilepsy. Trousseau's hypothesis was tested by Bergouigan who successfully used phenytoin to treat trigeminal neuralgia. Carbamazepine was studied in the same condition during a placebo-controlled double-blind design that was among the first of its kind in pain medicine. Since then, anticonvulsants have been extensively used in a wide variety of neuropathic pain syndromes, particularly those associated with 'lancinating' or 'shooting' pain. Animal studies have shown that peripheral nerve fibres in persistent pain syndromes have altered expression of certain ion channels, particularly novel sodium channels, and N-type calcium channels.

Carbamazepine, phenytoin and sodium valproate have been used for many years to treat neuropathic pain. However, carbamazepine remains the only anticonvulsant licensed within the UK for the treatment of trigeminal neuralgia. All anticonvulsants produce side-effects such as dizziness and drowsiness. Carbamazepine, in particular, may suppress bone marrow function and cause hyponatraemia. Its use requires regular blood monitoring.

Gabapentin and pregabalin are newer anticonvulsant agents that show good efficacy in clinical trials of neuropathic pain. These drugs bind to the $\alpha_2\delta$-1 subunit of voltage-dependent calcium channels and may work by preventing the formation of excitatory synapses within the central nervous system. Gabapentin is generally better tolerated than the older anticonvulsants and has a licence in the UK for the treatment of neuropathic pain. It is not metabolised by the liver and has few clinically significant drug interactions. It should be started at a dose of 300 mg at night (100 mg in the elderly) and titrated upwards as tolerated or to a dose of 600–1 200 mg three times daily. A saturable gut transport mechanism limits bio-availability at high oral doses (but also protects against overdosage). Pregabalin shares a similar mode of action to gabapentin, but has the advantage of more linear pharmacokinetics and can be given as a twice daily preparation (normal maintenance dose up to 300 mg twice daily).

Local anaesthetics

Local anaesthetic agents are specifically developed to provide local and regional anaesthesia. The use of systemic local anaesthetics in neuropathic pain was first suggested in the 1950s, and was popularised by subsequent studies that showed effectiveness in the treatment of painful diabetic neuropathy. Parenteral administration is, however, impractical for long-term treatment. Lidocaine infusions are mostly used to identify the subgroup of patients with neuropathic pain who respond to sodium channel blockade. Patients who respond favourably to lidocaine infusion may proceed to a trial of its oral analogue, mexiletine.

A topical lidocaine patch preparation, consisting of an adhesive dressing infused with a preparation containing 5% lidocaine may be useful for the treatment of post-herpetic neuralgia and other peripheral neuropathic pain conditions. Lidocaine 5% transdermal patches show reasonable efficacy in clinical trials with minimal systemic absorption of the local anaesthetic agent. Their ease of use and lack of side-effects may encourage use for the treatment of post-herpetic neuralgia and other neuropathic pain disorders.

Capsaicin

Capsaicin (derived from chili peppers) activates specific vanilloid receptors found in C-nociceptors. Initial topical application causes a transient burning sensation. With repeated applications, however, desensitisation of the nociceptors occurs. This is the basis for its use in chronic pain conditions.

Clinical trials using topically applied 0.025%–0.075% capsaicin cream (applied four times daily) show good results for pain due to diabetic neuropathy and post-herpetic neuralgia. However, repeated applications for several weeks are required and compliance is often poor.

A topical patch preparation containing 8% capsaicin is available for use in peripheral neuropathic pain conditions. This preparation has been shown to provide longer-lasting pain relief (-3 months) with a single 30–60 minute application. Application of the patch requires preparation of the skin beforehand with local anaesthetic.

Clonidine

Clonidine has agonist activity at α_2 and imidazoline receptors and is an effective analgesic when given intravenously or via the epidural or intrathecal routes. Oral preparations also exist and are well-absorbed, with 75%–95% bio-availability. Its greater potency when given centrally means that analgesic efficacy can be obtained with smaller doses and a reduced incidence of side-effects. Clonidine has been shown to augment the analgesic potency of epidural local anaesthetic agents and opioids, and has proven efficacy in chronic pain disorders, including cancer pain. The major side-effects are sedation and hypotension. The latter is caused primarily by central sympatholysis, and may be compounded by concomitant bradycardia. Chronic administration leads to a risk of rebound hypertension if withdrawn suddenly.

Cannabinoids

Delta-9-tetrahydrocannabinol (THC) is the only constituent of cannabis with clinically significant analgesic properties. THC is a partial agonist at the cannbinoid-1 receptor (CB-1r), which mediates its analgesic effects. The CB-1r is widely expressed throughout the CNS (including the brain), which accounts for the psychotrophic effects of THC. Clinical trials continue to suggest that THC is useful for the treatment of refractory chronic pain, particularly in multiple sclerosis, cancer or HIV. Additionally, the cannabinoid is an antiemetic and stimulates the appetite.

THC and related cannabinoids are formulated for the oral and oromucosal routes. The oral preparations are pure and synthetically derived. The oromucosal preparation Sativex® is plant-derived and comprises THC and cannabidiol (CBD) in equal proportions. Cannabidiol does not possess analgesic properties but may attenuate the psycho-activity of THC via an anxiolytic effect. Sativex® is currently licensed in Canada for the symptomatic relief of neuropathic pain in multiple sclerosis and pain from cancer.

The oral bio-availability of THC is poor and varies highly between individuals. Peak plasma concentration improves with fasting and occurs 2–4 h after drug ingestion. The oromucosal route avoids the hepatic first pass effect and consequently has a quicker onset and greater bio-availability. Consequently, patients may themselves adjust the dose of Sativex until pain relief is achieved with tolerable side-effects.

Ziconotide

Ziconotide (previously called SNX-111) is the synthetic form of the hydrophilic conopeptide ω-MVIIA, which is found in the venom of the Pacific fish-hunting snail, Conus magus. Notably, ziconotide is the only truly novel analgesic that has emerged from decades of pharmaceutical research and development.

Ziconotide binds reversibly and tightly to a subset of voltage-sensitive calcium channels (N-type channels) which are found in the dorsal horn of the spinal cord and localised to the pre-synaptic central terminals of primary afferent neurones. The binding of ziconotide inhibits these channels, which reduces nociceptive transmission at the spinal level. N-type calcium channels are found throughout the CNS and account for the adverse effects of ziconotide. Common adverse effects are dizziness, nausea, confusion, and headache. More severe, but rare side-effects are hallucinations, thoughts of suicide, new or worsening depression. Consequently, the drug is contraindicated in patients with a history of psychosis, schizophrenia, clinical depression or bipolar disorder.

Ziconotide is only administered intrathecally to minimise adverse effects. The optimal dose is achieved by slow titration over weeks as an infusion via an intrathecal pump. The method of delivery is complex, costly and invasive. Consequently, ziconotide is only approved for the management of severe chronic pain in patients for whom intrathecal therapy is warranted and who have been shown to be intolerant of, or refractory to, other treatment, such as systemic analgesics, adjunctive therapies or intrathecal morphine. Drug tolerance does not occur and there are minimal withdrawal effects after prolonged infusion.

Ketamine

Ketamine is a non-competitive NMDA antagonist that acts at the phencyclidine (PCP) binding site in the NMDA receptor. Controlled studies show good analgesic efficacy in peripheral and central neuropathic pain, fibromyalgia and chronic ischaemic pain. The drug can be given using various routes of administration but trials most frequently report the use of intravenous boluses of 0.1–0.45 mg/kg, followed in some studies by infusions of around 5–7micrograms/kg·min. Oral bio-availability is poor and impaired by poor taste, but the drug is now available as a more tolerably flavoured oral ketamine solution. The drug is often associated with adverse effects, including unpleasant dreams, hallucinations, and visual and auditory disturbances. Ketamine may have a synergistic effect when combined with opioids.

Adjuvants used for bone pain

Bisphosphonates

Bisphosphonates (previously known as diphosphonates) are analogues of inorganic pyrophosphate that inhibit osteoclast activity and, consequently, reduce bone resorption in a variety of illnesses. This effect, presumably, underlines the putative analgesic efficacy of these compounds in bone pain. Currently the evidence for analgesic effects is best for pamidronate. Potential differences in the analgesia produced by the various drugs in this class require additional study, and neither dose-dependent effects nor long-term risks or benefits in cancer patients are established. The use of any bisphosphonate requires monitoring of serum calcium, phosphate, magnesium and potassium.

PHARMACOTHERAPY OF ACUTE MIGRAINE HEADACHES

Migraine is characterised by episodic attacks of moderate-severe throbbing headache with a number of associated symptoms that include nausea, vomiting, photophobia and phonophobia. In around one third of patients with migraine, the headache can be accompanied by focal neurological symptoms (aura). In Europe and the USA, about18% of women and 6% of men suffered at least one migraine attack in the past year. Migraine has been ranked among the world's most disabling medical illnesses. Its socio-economic impact is substantial, with an estimated annual cost of $17 billion for treatment costs alone.

The pathophysiology of migraine is complex but a likely causative factor is the release of vasoactive peptides from the sensory nerve terminals that innervate meningeal blood vessels, causing dilatation of the arteries in the meninges, perivascular inflammation and amplification of the nociceptive afferent nerve supply. Sensory input from dural and cerebrovascular sensory fibres is amplified and perceived as pain (allodynia). Activation of the sympathetic nervous system is the likely cause of autonomic symptoms such as nausea and vomiting. Sensory symptoms (aura) are produced by a transient, spreading disturbance in cortical function. Migraine possesses features of inflammatory and functional pain, as well as objective neurologic dysfunction. Diagnosis is based on the headache's characteristics and associated symptoms.

Management of migraine

Migraine is best thought of, and managed as, a chronic pain syndrome. Non-pharmacological management of migraine involves helping patients to identify and avoid triggering factors such as stress, foods containing vasoactive amines (e.g. chocolate, cheese), bright lights, loud noises, hormonal changes and hypoglycaemia. Other behavioural and psychological interventions used for prevention include relaxation training, thermal biofeedback combined with relaxation training, electromyography biofeedback and cognitive behavioural therapy.

Pharmacotherapy of migraine is either abortive or preventive.

Abortive treatment of migraine

Drugs used to abort an acute attack of migraine are either non-specific (analgesics) or specific (triptans and ergots).

Simple analgesics such as acetylsalicylic acid (900 mg) or paracetamol (1 000 mg), with or without the addition of caffeine, can often be effective for mild to moderate headaches. The addition of domperidone

(10 mg by mouth) or metoclopramide (10 mg by mouth) may help reduce nausea. NSAIDs, such as naproxen (500–1000 mg by mouth or rectally, with an antiemetic), ibuprofen (400–800 mg by mouth), or tolfenamic acid (200 mg by mouth) can also be very useful, when tolerated. All tend to be most effective when given early during the headache.

With frequent use, these medications tend to increase headache frequency and may cause a state of refractory daily or near-daily headache; so-called 'analgesic-associated chronic daily headache' (CDH). Codeine-containing compound analgesics are notorious and their use requires careful monitoring for worsening symptoms. Patients who require regular analgesics may be more easily treated with standard preventatives.

When simple measures fail, or more aggressive treatment is required, more specific drugs are required.

Selective 5-HT$_1$ agonists (triptans)

Triptans are serotonin (5-hydroxytryptamine or 5-HT) antagonists with high affinity for 5-HT$_{1B}$ or 5-HT$_{1D}$ receptors. Action at the 5-HT$_{1B}$ receptors on blood vessels produces cranial vasoconstriction. Action at presynaptic 5-HT$_{1D}$ receptors inhibits the release of vasoactive peptides and nociceptive neurotransmitters. Recent comparative randomised trials of triptans show efficacy rates similar to those of simple analgesics and NSAIDs. In patients without cardiovascular contraindications, triptans are safe, effective and appropriate first-line treatments for patients who have a moderate to severe headache and in patients where simple or combination analgesics have failed to provide adequate relief. Triptan therapy is most effective when used early when the headache is mild, but it is uncertain if they are best used after the resolution of the aura and the optimal timing is probably patient-dependent.

The choice of triptan also depends upon patient preference, as well as the character, duration and severity of the headache, convenience and cost. Non-oral administration may be beneficial in cases when the headache intensifies rapidly, or severe nausea and emesis are early features of the headache. Only sumatriptan is available for parenteral administration.

The onset of action of most triptans is 20–60 min (10 min for sumatriptan). If necessary, patients can take another dose after 2 or 4 h. If the appropriate dose of triptan is ineffective or has unacceptable side-effects, consider a switch to an alternative triptan formulation. The drugs can be used in combination with other simple analgesics, NSAIDs and antiemetics. There is a risk of developing serotonin syndrome) if given in combination with other serotonin-reuptake inhibitor drugs (e.g. SSRI or MAOI antidepressants). While the risk of causing birth defects is probably low, triptans should not be used routinely during pregnancy.

Minor adverse effects such as flushing and neck or chest tightness are very common. In most cases, this is not caused by coronary vasoconstriction. There are reported cases of serious cardiovascular events and triptans should be avoided in patients who have, or are at high risk of developing, coronary heart disease.

Frequent use of triptans is also associated with the development of analgesic-associated chronic daily headache and, in general, the use of the drugs should be limited to an average of 2 days per week.

Sumatriptan

Sumatriptan (Imigran) is rapidly absorbed after oral administration and undergoes extensive (84%) presystemic metabolism. Its elimination half-life is 2.5 h. The oral dose is 50–100 mg, and should not exceed 200 mg in a 24-hour period. The oral route may be avoided by giving sumatriptan 20 mg intranasally (disagreeable taste). This can be repeated once after 2 h, but no more than 40 mg should be given in 24 h. When a rapid response is required, sumatriptan 6 mg can be given subcutaneously (bio-availability by the subcutaneous route is 96%) and, again, can be repeated once in a 24-hour period.

Sumatriptan is generally well tolerated. As well as the commonly reported symptoms of neck and chest tightness, sumatriptan is also associated with malaise, fatigue, dizziness, vertigo and sedation. Nausea and vomiting may follow oral or subcutaneous administration.

Other triptans include zolmitriptan, naratriptan, rizatriptan, almotriptan, frovatriptan and eletriptan. All have similar safety profiles, but varying duration of action. The therapeutic response and adverse effects of different triptans are often idiosyncratic, and several drugs may have to be tried before one is found that offers relief with minimal adverse events.

Ergotamine

Although ergotamine is a useful antimigraine compound, it is no longer considered a first-line drug for migraine because of its adverse effects. Ergots have much greater receptor affinity at serotonergic (5-HT_{1A}, 5-HT_2), adrenergic, and dopaminergic receptors compared to triptans. Peripheral vasoconstriction that results from ergotamine administration can persist for as long as 24 h, and repeated doses lead to cumulative effects long outlasting the migraine attack. It may precipitate angina pectoris, probably by increasing cardiac pre- and afterload. Ergotamine should never be used for prophylaxis of migraine.

Preventive treatment for migraine

For patients who are unable to achieve adequate pain relief with the use of the standard analgesic medications and triptans, the use of medications to reduce the frequency and intensity of migraine attacks may be appropriate. Other indications for preventative medications include troublesome adverse events from standard drug therapies, acute drug overuse, very frequent headaches (more than two per week), special circumstances such as hemiplegic migraine, or attacks with a risk of permanent neurological injury.

Medications used for prophylaxis include β-adrenergic blockers, non-steroidal anti-inflammatory drugs, and antineuropathic medications such as the antidepressants, calcium-channel antagonists and anticonvulsants. Those with the best documented effectiveness are β-adrenergic blockers, pizotifen, and the anticonvulsant drugs, sodium valproate and topiramate.

Choice of migraine prophylactic agent is based on effectiveness, adverse events, and coexistent and co-morbid conditions. Women of childbearing potential should be educated about the risk of drugs in pregnancy and encouraged to consider contraception. Because of the risks of adverse effects, especially drowsiness, on commencing treatment, all the migraine prophylactic drugs should be started at a low dose and increased slowly until therapeutic effects develop or the maximum dose is reached. A full therapeutic trial may take 2–6 months. Patients should try to avoid overusing drugs for acute attacks during the trial period. If headaches are well controlled, treatment can be tapered down and may be discontinued if the patient remains symptom-free.

Pizotifen

Pizotifen is an antihistamine drug with serotonin-antagonist activity. It is structurally related to the tricyclic antidepressant drugs and shares their potential for antimuscarinic adverse effects such as dry mouth, urinary retention and constipation. Its antihistamine action produces drowsiness, and the drug also causes weight gain. Treatment is usually started at 500 micrograms at night and titrated upwards to effect. It is rare to exceed a dose of 1 mg three times daily (or as a single 3 mg dose at night).

Topiramate

The introduction of topiramate is arguably the most important recent advance in migraine prophylaxis. Topiramate is an anticonvulsant with a number of actions that include enhanced GABA activity, voltage-gated Na^+ and Ca^{2+} channel inhibition, reduced activity of glutamate at AMPA/kainite post-synaptic receptors, and inhibition of the presynaptic release of calcitonin gene-related protein (CGRP). The net result is a reduction in excitatory transmission and an increase in inhibitory neurotransmission.

Topiramate reduces the frequency of migraine attacks, starting with 25 mg at night and increasing gradually as tolerated. The optimal effect occurs at 100 mg daily, with little effect at 50 mg, and an increased incidence of unwanted effects at higher doses. Positive effects were usually seen within the first month of treatment and continued with longer-term use.

Adverse effects include paraesthesia, fatigue and dizziness. Unlike many of the antineuropathic medications, topiramate is not associated with weight gain.

SUMMARY

Pain is an unpleasant sensory and emotional experience associated with actual or potential tissue damage, or described in terms of such damage. The physiological process by which pain is perceived is known as nociception. Clinical pain is generally divided into three broad categories: acute, chronic, and cancer-related. Acute pain usually results from trauma or surgery, typically resolves with healing of the injured tissue, and can usually be effectively managed with the appropriate use of pharmacotherapy. Chronic pain is commonly defined as pain that persists beyond the period expected for healing, or pain that is associated with progressive, non-malignant disease. Neuropathic pain is a chronic pain resulting from damage to the nervous system. Cancer-related pain refers to pain that is the result of primary tumour growth, metastatic disease, or the toxic effects of chemotherapy and radiation, such as neuropathies due to neurotoxic antineoplastic drugs.

An analgesic is defined as a drug that relieves pain. Analgesics are classified as opioids and non-opioids (e.g. non-steroidal anti-inflammatory drugs, NSAIDs). NSAIDs act by inhibiting cyclo-oxygenase, an enzyme involved in the production of prostanoid, as well as other prostaglandins. NSAIDs are among the most commonly prescribed analgesics and, unless contraindicated, are effective and appropriate analgesics for use in acute inflammatory pain. The side-effects of NSAIDs are the risks of gastro-intestinal bleed, renal toxicity and a possibility of cardiac-related complications. The drugs include paracetamol, nefopam, *etc.*

Opioid analgesics refer to drugs that are derived from natural opiates or their synthetic analogues. Opioids produce their effects by activating specific G protein-coupled receptors in the brain, spinal cord and peripheral nervous system. Opioids have been traditionally classified as strong, intermediate and weak, according to their perceived analgesic properties and propensity for addiction. The systemic effects include reducing the intensity and unpleasantness of pain via influencing center nervous system, causing peripheral vasodilatation and impairing sympathetic vascular reflexes, increasing of smooth muscle tone along the gastrointestinal tract and increasing tone in the detrusor muscle and contraction of the external sphincter, together with inhibition of the voiding reflexes may aggravate urinary retention. The opioids include morphine, diamorphine, codeine, dihydrocodeine, oxycodone, hydromorphone, methadone, fentanyl, alfentanil, remifentanil, papaveretum, buprenorphine and meptazinol, *etc.* The side-effects of opioids include sedation, euphoria, dysphoria, respiratory depression, constipation, pruritis, and nausea and vomiting. Naloxone is a competitive antagonist at μ-, δ-, κ-, and σ-opioid receptors and acts to reverse the effects of most opioid analgesics. Multipurpose adjuvant analgesics include corticosteroids, neuroleptics and benzodiazepines.

IMPORTANT TERMINOLOGY

analgesics　止痛药

pain　疼痛

acute pain　急性疼痛

chronic pain　慢性疼痛

neuropathic pain　神经性疼痛

cancer-related pain　癌痛

nociception　痛感

nociceptors　痛觉感受器

non-opioid analgesics　非阿片类止痛药

NSAIDs (non-steroidal anti-inflammatory drugs)　非甾体抗炎药

opioid analgesics　阿片类止痛药

co-analgesics (adjuvant analgesics)　止痛辅助用药

acute migraine　急性偏头痛

cannabinoids　大麻素类

anticonvulsants　抗惊厥药

selective 5-HT$_1$ agonists　选择性 5-羟色胺激动剂

triptans　曲坦类药物

CHALLENGE YOURSELF

Why does a doctor prescribe morphine for those who suffer from both cancer pain and diarrhea? Please give your reason.

Xuanbin Wang

Chapter | **13** |

Anaesthesia and neuromuscular block

The administration of general anaesthetics and neuromuscular blocking drugs is generally confined to trained specialists. Nevertheless, non-specialists are involved in perioperative care and will benefit from an understanding of how these drugs act. Doctors from a variety of specialties use local anaesthetics and the pharmacology of these drugs is discussed in detail.

GENERAL ANAESTHESIA

With the introduction of general anaesthesia in the 1840s, surgeons could operate with careful deliberation. The problem of inducing quick, safe and easily reversible unconsciousness for any desired length of time in humans began to be solved. The next important developments in anaesthesia were in the 20th century when the appearance of new drugs, both as primary general anaesthetics and as adjuvants (muscle relaxants), new apparatus and clinical expertise in rendering prolonged anaesthesia safe enabled surgeons to increase their range. No longer was the duration and type of surgery determined by patients' capacity to endure pain

Phases of general anaesthesia

Balanced surgical anaesthesia (hypnosis, analgesia and muscle relaxation) with a single drug would require high doses that would cause adverse effects such as slow and unpleasant recovery, and depression of cardiovascular and respiratory function. In modern practice, different drugs are used to attain each objective so that adverse effects are minimised.

The perioperative period may be divided into three phases, and several factors determine the choice of drugs given in each of these.

Before surgery (premedication)

Anxiolysis and amnesia. A patient who is going to have a surgical operation is naturally apprehensive; this anxiety is reduced by reassurance and a clear explanation of what to expect. Very anxious patients will secrete a lot of adrenaline/epinephrine from the suprarenal medulla and this may make them more liable to cardiac arrhythmias with some anaesthetics. In the past, sedative premedication was given to virtually all patients undergoing surgery. This practice has changed dramatically because of the increasing proportion of operations undertaken as 'day cases' and the recognition that sedative premedication prolongs recovery. Sedative premedication is now reserved for those who are particularly anxious or those undergoing major surgery. Benzodiazepines, such as temazepam (10–30 mg for an adult), provide anxiolysis and amnesia for the immediate presurgical period.

Analgesia is indicated if the patient is in pain before surgery, or the analgesia can be given preemptively to prevent postoperative pain. Severe preoperative pain is treated with a parenteral opioid such as morphine. Non-steroidal anti-inflammatory drugs (NSAIDs) and paracetamol are commonly given orally before operation to prevent postoperative pain after minor surgery. For moderate or major surgery, these drugs are supplemented with an opioid towards the end of the procedure.

Timing. Premedication is given about an hour before surgery.

Gastric contents. Pulmonary aspiration of gastric contents can cause severe pneumonitis. Patients at risk of aspiration are those with full stomachs, in the third trimester of pregnancy or with an incompetent gastro-oesophageal sphincter. A single dose of an antacid, e.g. sodium citrate, may be given before a general anaesthetic to neutralise gastric acid in high-risk patients. Alternatively or additionally, a histamine H_2-receptor blocker, e.g. ranitidine, or proton pump inhibitor, e.g. omeprazole, will reduce gastric secretion volume as well as acidity. Metoclopramide usefully hastens gastric emptying, increases the tone of the lower oesophageal sphincter and is an antiemetic.

The aim is to induce unconsciousness, analgesia and muscle relaxation – the anaesthetic triad. Total muscular relaxation (paralysis) is required for some surgical procedures, e.g. intra-abdominal surgery, but most surgery can be under- taken without neuromuscular blockade.

During surgery general anaesthetic

Induction

1. Usually intravenous: pre-oxygenation followed by a small dose of an opioid, e.g. fentanyl or alfentanil to provide analgesia and sedation, followed by propofol or, less commonly, thiopental, etomidate or ketamine to induce anaesthesia. Airway patency is maintained with a supraglottic airway device (e.g. laryngeal mask airway (LMA)), a tracheal tube or, for very short procedures, an oral airway and facemask. Insertion of a tracheal tube usually requires paralysis with a neuromuscular blocker and is undertaken if there is a risk of pulmonary aspiration from regurgitated gastric contents or from blood.

2. Inhalational induction, usually with sevoflurane, is undertaken less commonly. It is used in children, particularly if intravenous access is difficult, and in patients at risk from upper airway obstruction.

Maintenance

1. Most commonly with oxygen and air, or nitrous oxide and oxygen, plus a volatile agent, e.g. sevoflurane, desflurane or isoflurane. Additional doses of a neuromuscular blocker or opioid are given as required.

2. A continuous intravenous infusion of propofol can be used to maintain anaesthesia. This technique of total intravenous anaesthesia is relatively common because the quality of recovery may be better than after inhalational anaesthesia. The propofol infusion is often combined with an infusion of remifentanil, an ultra-short-acting opioid. When appropriate, peripheral nerve block with a local anaesthetic, or neural axis block, e.g. spinal or epidural, provides intraoperative analgesia and muscle relaxation. These local anaesthetic techniques provide excellent postoperative analgesia.

After surgery

The anaesthetist ensures that the effects of neuromuscular blocking drugs and opioid-induced respiratory depression have either worn off or have been adequately reversed by an antagonist; the patient is not left alone until conscious, with protective reflexes restored, and with a stable circulation.

Relief of pain after surgery can be achieved with several techniques. An epidural infusion of a mixture of local anaesthetic and opioid provides excellent pain relief after major surgery such as laparotomy. Parenteral morphine, given intermittently by a nurse or a patient-controlled system, will also relieve moderate or severe pain but has the attendant risk of nausea, vomiting, sedation and respiratory depression. The addition of regular paracetamol and a NSAID, given orally or parenterally (the rectal route is used much less commonly now), will provide additional pain relief and reduce the requirement for morphine.

Postoperative nausea and vomiting (PONV) is common after laparotomy and major gynaecological surgery, e.g. abdominal hysterectomy. The use of propofol, particularly when given to maintain anaesthesia, has reduced the incidence of PONV. Antiemetics, such as cyclizine, metoclopramide and ondansetron, may be helpful. Dexamethasone also reduces the incidence of PONV. Many anaesthetists use a combination of two or three of these drugs, a strategy which has been shown to be particularly effective.

Some special techniques

Dissociative anaesthesia is a state of profound analgesia and anterograde amnesia with minimal hypnosis during which the eyes may remain open; it can be produced by ketamine. It is particularly useful where modern equipment is lacking or where access to the patient is limited, e.g. in prehospital or military settings.

Sedation and amnesia without analgesia is provided by intravenous midazolam or, less commonly nowadays, by diazepam. These drugs can be used alone for procedures causing mild discomfort, e.g. endoscopy, and with a local anaesthetic where more pain is expected, e.g. removal of impacted wisdom teeth. Benzodiazepines produce anterograde, but not retrograde, amnesia. By definition, the sedated patient remains responsive and cooperative.

Benzodiazepines can cause respiratory depression and apnoea, especially in the elderly and in patients with respiratory insufficiency. The combination of an opioid and a benzodiazepine is particularly dangerous. Benzodiazepines depress laryngeal reflexes and place the patient at risk of inhalation of oral secretions or dental debris. A continuous infusion of low-dose propofol provides very effective sedation that can be rapidly titrated to produce the desired effect. Use of propofol in this way should be undertaken only by those with advanced airway skills, such as anaesthetists and some emergency physicians.

Entonox, a 50:50 mixture of nitrous oxide and oxygen, is breathed by the patient using a demand valve. It is particularly useful in the prehospital environment and for brief procedures, such as splinting limbs.

PHARMACOLOGY OF ANAESTHETICS

All successful general anaesthetics are given intravenously or by inhalation because these routes enable closest control over blood concentrations and thus of effect on the brain.

Mode of action

General anaesthetics act on the brain, primarily on the midbrain reticular activating system, and the spinal cord. Many anaesthetics are lipid soluble and there is good correlation between this and anaesthetic effectiveness (the Overton–Meyer hypothesis); the more lipid soluble tend to be the more potent anaesthetics, but such a correlation is not invariable. Some anaesthetic agents are not lipid soluble and many lipid-soluble substances are not anaesthetics.

Until recently it was thought that the principal site of action of general anaesthetics was relatively non-specific action in the neuronal lipid bilayer membrane. The current view is that anaesthetic agents interact with proteins to alter the activity of specific neuronal ion channels, particularly the fast neurotransmitter receptors such as nicotinic acetylcholine, γ-aminobutyric acid (GABA) and glutamate receptors. The suppression of motor responses to painful stimuli by anaesthetics is mediated mainly by the spinal cord, whereas hypnosis and amnesia are mediated within the brain.

Comparison of the efficacy of inhalational anaesthetics is made by measuring the minimum alveolar concentration (MAC) in oxygen required to prevent movement in response to a standard surgical skin incision in 50% of subjects. The MAC of the volatile agent is reduced by the co-administration of nitrous oxide.

INHALATION ANAESTHETICS

The preferred inhalation anaesthetics are those that are minimally irritant and non-flammable, and comprise nitrous oxide and the fluorinated hydrocarbons, e.g. sevoflurane.

Pharmacokinetics (volatile liquids, gases)

The depth of anaesthesia is correlated with the tension (partial pressure) of anaesthetic drug in brain tissue. This is driven by the development of a series of tension gradients from the high partial pressure delivered to the alveoli and decreasing through the blood to the brain and other tissues. The gradients are dependent on the blood/gas and tissue/ gas solubility coefficients, as well as on alveolar ventilation and organ blood flow.

An anaesthetic that has high solubility in blood, i.e. a high blood/gas partition coefficient, will provide a slow induction and adjustment of the depth of anaesthesia. Here, the blood acts as a reservoir (store) for the drug so that it does not enter the brain readily until the blood reservoir is filled. A rapid induction can be obtained by increasing the concentration of drug inhaled initially and by hyper- ventilating the patient.

Anaesthetics with low solubility in blood, i.e. a low blood/gas partition coefficient (nitrous oxide, desflurane, sevoflurane), provide rapid induction of anaesthesia because the blood reservoir is small and anaesthetic is available to pass into the brain.

During induction of anaesthesia the blood is taking up anaesthetic selectively and rapidly, and the resulting loss of volume in the alveoli leads to a flow of anaesthetic into the lungs that is independent of respiratory activity. When the anaesthetic is discontinued the reverse occurs and it moves from the blood into the alveoli. In the case of nitrous oxide, this can account for as much as 10% of the expired volume and so can significantly lower the alveolar oxygen concentration. Mild hypoxia occurs and lasts for as long as 10 min. Oxygen is given to these patients during the last few minutes of anaesthesia and the early post-anaesthetic period. This phenomenon, diffusion hypoxia, occurs with all gaseous anaesthetics, but is most prominent with gases that are relatively insoluble in blood, for they will diffuse out most rapidly when the drug is no longer inhaled, i.e. just as induction is faster, so is elimination.

Nitrous oxide is especially powerful in this respect because it is used at concentrations of up to 70%.

Nitrous oxide

Nitrous oxide is a gas with a slightly sweetish smell that is neither flammable nor explosive. It produces light anaesthesia without demonstrably depressing the respiratory or vasomotor centre provided that normal oxygen tension is maintained.

Advantages. Nitrous oxide reduces the requirement for other more potent and intrinsically more toxic anaesthetics. It has a strong analgesic action; inhalation of 50% nitrous oxide in oxygen (Entonox) may have similar effects to standard doses of morphine. Induction is rapid and not unpleasant, although transient excitement may occur, as with all anaesthetics. Recovery time rarely exceeds 4 min even after prolonged administration.

Disadvantages. Nitrous oxide is expensive to buy and to transport. It must be used in conjunction with more potent anaesthetics to produce full surgical anaesthesia.

Uses. Nitrous oxide is used to maintain surgical anaesthesia in combination with other anaesthetic agents, e.g. isoflurane or propofol, and, if required, muscle relaxants. Entonox provides analgesia for obstetric practice and for emergency treatment of injuries.

Dosage and administration. For the maintenance of anaesthesia, nitrous oxide must always be mixed with at least 30% oxygen. For analgesia, a concentration of 50% nitrous oxide with 50% oxygen usually suffices.

Contraindications. Any closed, distensible, air-filled space expands during administration of nitrous oxide, which moves into it from the blood. It is therefore contraindicated in patients with: demonstrable collections of air in the pleural, pericardial or peritoneal spaces; intestinal obstruction; arterial air embolism; decompression sickness; severe chronic obstructive airway disease; emphysema. Nitrous oxide will cause pressure changes in closed, non-compliant spaces such as the middle ear, nasal sinuses and the eye.

Precautions. Continued administration of oxygen may be necessary during recovery, especially in elderly patients.

Adverse effects. The incidence of nausea and vomiting increases with the duration of anaesthesia. Exposure to nitrous oxide for more than 4 h can cause megaloblastic changes in the bone marrow. Because prolonged and repeated exposure of staff, as well as of patients, may be associated with bone marrow depression and teratogenic risk, scavenging systems are used to minimise ambient concentrations in operating theatres.

Halogenated anaesthetics

Halothane was the first halogenated agent to be used widely, but in the developed world it has been largely superseded by isoflurane, sevoflurane and desflurane. A description of isoflurane is provided, and of the others in so far as they differ. The MAC in oxygen of some volatile anaesthetics is: isoflurane 1.2%, enflurane 1.7%, sevoflurane 2.0%, desflurane 6.0%, halothane 0.74%.

Isoflurane

Isoflurane is a volatile colourless liquid that is not flammable at normal anaesthetic concentrations. It is relatively insoluble and has a lower blood/gas coefficient than halothane or enflurane, which enables rapid adjustment of the depth of anaesthesia. It has a pungent odour and can cause bronchial irritation, making inhalational induction unpleasant. Isoflurane is minimally metabolised (0.2%), and none of the breakdown products has been related to anaesthetic toxicity.

Respiratory effects. Isoflurane causes respiratory depression and diminishes the ventilatory response to carbon dioxide. Although it irritates the upper airway, it is a bronchodilator.

Cardiovascular effects. Anaesthetic concentrations of isoflurane, i.e. 1–1.5 MAC, cause only slight impairment of myocardial contractility. Isoflurane causes peripheral vasodilation and reduces blood pressure. It does not sensitise the heart to catecholamines. In low concentrations (< 1 MAC), cerebral blood flow, intracranial pressure and cerebral autoregulation are maintained. Isoflurane is a potent coronary vasodilator and in the presence of a coronary artery stenosis it may cause redistribution of blood away from an area of inadequate perfusion to one of normal perfusion. This phenomenon of 'coronary steal' may cause regional myocardial ischaemia.

Other effects. Isoflurane relaxes voluntary muscles and potentiates the effects of non-depolarising muscle relaxants. Isoflurane depresses cortical EEG activity and does not induce abnormal electrical activity or convulsions.

Sevoflurane

Sevoflurane is less chemically stable than the other volatile anaesthetics in current use. About 2.5% is metabolised in the body and it is degraded by contact with carbon dioxide absorbents, such as soda lime. The reaction with soda lime causes the formation of a vinyl ether (compound A), which may be nephrotoxic. Sevoflurane is less soluble than isoflurane and is very pleasant to breathe, which makes it an excellent choice for inhalational induction of anaesthesia, particularly in children. The respiratory and cardiovascular effects of sevoflurane are very similar to isoflurane, but sevoflurane does not cause 'coronary steal'. In many hospitals, despite its higher cost, sevoflurane is displacing isoflurane as the most commonly used volatile anaesthetic.

Desflurane

Desflurane has the lowest blood/gas partition coefficient of any inhaled anaesthetic agent and thus gives particularly rapid onset and offset of effect. As it undergoes negligible metabolism (0.03%), any release of free inorganic fluoride is minimised; this characteristic favours its use for prolonged anaesthesia. Desflurane is extremely volatile and cannot be administered with conventional vaporisers. It has a very pungent odour and causes airway irritation to an extent that limits its rate of induction of anaesthesia. Despite this limitation, its very rapid recovery characteristics, even after very prolonged anaesthesia, make it an increasingly popular choice for major surgery.

Halothane

Halothane has the highest blood/gas partition coefficient of the volatile anaesthetic agents and recovery from halo- thane anaesthesia is comparatively slow. It is pleasant to breathe. Halothane reduces cardiac output more than any of the other volatile anaesthetics. It sensitises the heart to the arrhythmic effects of catecholamines and hypercapnia; arrhythmias are common, in particular atrioventricular dissociation, nodal rhythm and ventricular extrasystoles. Halothane can trigger malignant hyperthermia in those who are genetically predisposed.

About 20% of halothane is metabolised and it induces hepatic enzymes, including those of anaesthetists and operating theatre staff. Hepatic damage occurs in a small proportion of exposed patients. Typically fever develops 2–3 days after anaesthesia, accompanied by anorexia, nausea and vomiting. In more severe cases this is followed by transient jaundice or, very rarely, fatal hepatic necrosis. Severe hepatitis is a complication of repeatedly administered halothane anaesthesia (incidence of 1 in 50 000) and follows immune sensitisation to an oxidative metabolite of halothane in susceptible individuals. This serious complication, along with the other disadvantages of halothane and the popularity of sevoflurane for inhalational induction, has almost eliminated its use in the developed world. It remains in common use in other parts of the world because it is comparatively inexpensive.

Oxygen in anaesthesia

Supplemental oxygen is always used with inhalational anaesthetics to prevent hypoxia, even when air is used as the carrier gas. The concentration of oxygen in inspired anaesthetic gases is usually at least 30%, but oxygen should not be used for prolonged periods at a greater concentration than is necessary to prevent hypoxaemia. After prolonged administration, concentrations greater than 80% have a toxic effect on the lungs, which presents initially as a mild substernal irritation, progressing to pulmonary exudation and atelectasis. Use of unnecessarily high concentrations of oxygen in incubators causes retrolental fibroplasia and permanent blindness in premature infants.

INTRAVENOUS ANAESTHETICS

Intravenous anaesthetics should be given only by those fully trained in their use and who are experienced with a full range of techniques of managing the airway, including tracheal intubation.

Pharmacokinetics

Intravenous anaesthetics enable an extremely rapid induction because the blood concentration can be raised quickly, establishing a steep concentration gradient and expediting diffusion into the brain. The rate of transfer depends on the lipid solubility and arterial concentration of the unbound, non-ionised fraction of the drug. After a single induction dose of an intravenous anaesthetic, recovery occurs quite rapidly as the drug is redistributed around the body and the plasma concentration reduces. Recovery from a single dose of intravenous anaesthetic is thus dependent on redistribution rather than rate of metabolic breakdown. With the exception of propofol, repeated doses or infusions of intravenous anaesthetics will cause considerable accumulation and prolong recovery. Attempts to use thiopental as the sole anaesthetic in war casualties led to it being described as an ideal form of euthanasia.

It is common practice to induce anaesthesia intravenously and then to use a volatile anaesthetic for maintenance. When administration of a volatile anaesthetic is stopped, it is eliminated quickly through the lungs and the patient regains consciousness. The recovery from propofol is rapid, even after repeated doses or an infusion. This advantage, and others, has resulted in propofol displacing thiopental as the most popular intravenous anaesthetic.

Propofol

Induction of anaesthesia with 1.5–2.5 mg/kg occurs within 30 s and is smooth and pleasant with a low incidence of excitatory movements. Some preparations of propofol cause pain on injection, but adding lidocaine 20 mg to the induction dose eliminates this. The recovery from propofol is rapid, and the incidence of nausea and vomiting is extremely low, particularly when propofol is used as the sole anaesthetic. Recovery from a continuous infusion of propofol is relatively rapid as the plasma concentration decreases by both redistribution and metabolic clearance (predominantly as the glucuronide). Special syringe pumps incorporating pharmacokinetic algorithms enable the anaesthetist to select a target plasma propofol concentration (e.g. 4 micrograms/mL for induction of anaesthesia) once details of the patient's age and weight have been entered. This technique of target-controlled infusion (TCI) provides a convenient method for giving a continuous infusion of propofol.

Central nervous system. Propofol causes dose-dependent cortical depression and is an anticonvulsant. It depresses laryngeal reflexes more than barbiturates, which is an advantage when

Cardiovascular system. Propofol reduces vascular tone, which lowers systemic vascular resistance and central venous pressure. The heart rate remains unchanged and the result is a fall in blood pressure to about 70%–80% of the preinduction level and a small reduction in cardiac output.

Respiratory system. Unless it is undertaken very slowly, induction with propofol causes transient apnoea. On resumption of respiration there is a reduction in tidal volume and increase in rate.

Thiopental

Thiopental is a very short-acting barbiturate that induces anaesthesia smoothly, within one arm-to-brain circulation time. The typical induction dose is 3–5 mg/kg. Rapid distribution (initial $t_{1/2}$ 4 min) allows swift recovery after a single dose. The terminal $t_{1/2}$ of thiopental is 11 h and repeated doses or continuous infusion lead to significant accumulation in fat and very prolonged recovery. Thiopental is metabolised in the liver. The incidence of nausea and vomiting after thiopental is slightly higher than that after propofol. The pH of thiopental is 11 and extravasa-

tion causes considerable local damage. Accidental intraarterial injection will also cause serious injury distal to the injection site.

Central nervous system. Thiopental has no analgesic activity and may be antanalgesic. It is a potent anticonvulsant. Cerebral metabolic rate for oxygen consumption ($CMRO_2$) is reduced, causing cerebral vasoconstriction, reduction in cerebral blood flow and intracranial pressure.

Cardiovascular system. Thiopental reduces vascular tone, causing hypotension and a slight compensatory increase in heart rate. Antihypertensives or diuretics may augment the hypotensive effect.

Respiratory system. Thiopental reduces respiratory rate and tidal volume.

Methohexitone

Methohexitone is a barbiturate similar to thiopental but its terminal $t_{1/2}$ is considerably shorter. Since the introduction of propofol, its use is confined almost entirely to inducing anaesthesia for electroconvulsive therapy (ECT). Propofol shortens seizure duration and may reduce the efficacy of ECT.

Etomidate

Etomidate is a carboxylated imidazole. It causes pain on injection and excitatory muscle movements are common on induction of anaesthesia. There is a 20%–50% incidence of nausea and vomiting associated with its use. Etomidate causes adrenocortical suppression by inhibiting 11β- and 17β-hydroxylase, and for this reason is not used for prolonged infusion. Even after a single dose of etomidate, adrenocortical suppression can last for as long as 72 h and in septic patients is associated with an increased incidence of organ failure. Despite all of these disadvantages it remains in common (although decreasing) use, particularly for emergency anaesthesia, because it causes less cardiovascular depression and hypotension than thiopental or propofol. It should not be used in patients with sepsis.

Ketamine

Ketamine is a phencyclidine (hallucinogen) derivative and an antagonist of the NMDA receptor. In anaesthetic doses it produces a trance-like state known as dissociative anaesthesia (sedation, amnesia, dissociation, analgesia).

Advantages. Anaesthesia persists for up to 15 min after a single intravenous injection and is characterised by profound analgesia. Ketamine may be used as the sole analgesic for diagnostic and minor surgical interventions. In contrast to most other anaesthetic drugs, ketamine usually causes a tachycardia and increases blood pressure and cardiac output, making it an increasingly popular choice for inducing anaesthesia in shocked patients. Because pharyngeal and laryngeal reflexes are only slightly impaired, the airway may be less at risk than with other general anaesthetic techniques. It is a potent bronchodilator and is sometimes used to treat severe bronchospasm in asthmatics requiring mechanical ventilation.

Disadvantages. Ketamine produces no muscular relaxation. It increases intracranial and intraocular pressure. Hallucinations with delirium can occur during recovery (the emergence reaction), but are minimised if ketamine is used solely as an induction drug and followed by a conventional inhalational anaesthetic. Their incidence is reduced by giving a benzodiazepine both as a premedication and after the procedure.

Uses. Subanaesthetic doses of ketamine can be used to provide analgesia for painful procedures of short duration such as the dressing of burns, radiotherapeutic procedures, marrow sampling and minor orthopaedic procedures. Ketamine can be used for induction of anaesthesia before giving inhalational anaesthetics, or for both induction and maintenance of anaesthesia for short-lasting diagnostic and surgical interventions that do not require skeletal muscle relaxation. It is of particular value for children requiring frequent, repeated anaesthetics. It is increasingly popular for inducing anaesthesia in critically ill patients.

Recovery of consciousness is gradual. Emergence reactions are lessened by benzodiazepine premedication and by avoiding unnecessary disturbance of the patient during recovery.

Contraindications include: moderate to severe hypertension, cerebral trauma (although this is controversial), intracerebral mass or haemorrhage, or other causes of raised intracranial pressure; eye injury and increased intraocular pressure; psychiatric disorders such as a schizophrenia and acute psychoses.

Use in pregnancy. Ketamine is contraindicated in pregnancy before term, as it has oxytocic activity. It is also contraindicated in patients with eclampsia or preeclampsia. It may be used for assisted vaginal delivery by an experienced anaesthetist. Ketamine is better suited for use during caesarean section; it causes less fetal and neonatal depression than other anaesthetics.

MUSCLE RELAXANTS

Neuromuscular blocking drugs

A lot of surgery, especially of the abdomen, requires that voluntary muscle tone and reflex contraction be inhibited. This could be attained by deep general anaesthesia (but with risk of cardiovascular depression, respiratory complications and slow recovery) or by regional nerve blockade (which may be difficult to do or contraindicated, e.g. if there is a haemostatic defect).

Selective relaxation of voluntary muscle with neuromuscular blocking drugs enables surgery under light general anaesthesia with analgesia; it also facilitates tracheal intubation, quick induction and quick recovery. However, mechanical ventilation and technical skill are required. Neuromuscular blocking drugs should be given only after induction of anaesthesia.

Drugs acting at the myoneural junction produce complete paralysis of all voluntary muscle so that movement is impossible and mechanical ventilation is needed. It is plainly important that a paralysed patient should be unconscious during surgery.

Mechanisms

When an impulse passes down a motor nerve to voluntary muscle it causes release of acetylcholine from the nerve endings into the synaptic cleft. This activates receptors on the membrane of the motor endplate, a specialised area on the muscle fibre, opening ion channels for momentary passage of sodium, which depolarises the endplate and initiates muscle contraction.

Neuromuscular blocking drugs used in clinical practice interfere with this process. Natural substances that prevent the release of acetylcholine at nerve endings exist, e.g. Clostridium botulinum toxin and some venoms.

There are two principal mechanisms by which drugs used clinically interfere with neuromuscular transmission:

1. By competition with acetylcholine (atracurium, cisatracurium, mivacurium, pancuronium, rocuronium, vecuronium). These drugs are competitive antagonists of acetylcholine. They do not cause depolarisation themselves but protect the endplate from depolarisation by acetylcholine. The result is a flaccid paralysis. Reversal of this type of neuromuscular block can be achieved with anticholinesterase drugs, such as neostigmine, which prevent the destruction by cholinesterase of acetylcholine released at nerve endings, enable the concentration to build up and so reduce the competitive effect of a blocking agent. Rocuronium and vecuronium can also be reversed with the modified γ-cyclodextrin, sugammadex.

2. By depolarisation of the motor endplate (suxamethonium). Such agonist drugs activate the acetylcholine receptor on the motor endplate; at their first application voluntary muscle contracts but, as they are not destroyed immediately, like acetylcholine, the depolarisation persists. It might be expected that this prolonged depolarisation would cause muscles to remain contracted, but this is not so (except in chickens). With prolonged administration, a depolarisation block changes to a competitive block (dual block). Because of the uncertainty of this situation, a competitive blocking drug is preferred for anything other than short procedures.

Competitive antagonists

Atracurium is unique in that it is altered spontaneously in the body to an inactive form ($t_{1/2}$ 30 min) by a passive chemical process (Hofmann elimination). The duration of action (15–35 min) is thus uninfluenced by the state of the circulation, the liver or the kidneys, a significant advantage in patients with hepatic or renal disease and in the aged. It has very little direct effect on the cardiovascular system but at doses of greater than 0.5–0.6 mg/kg histamine release may cause hypotension and bronchospasm.

Cisatracurium is a stereoisomer of atracurium; it is less prone to cause histamine release.

Vecuronium is a synthetic steroid derivative that produces full neuromuscular blockade about 3 min after a dose of 0.1 mg/kg, lasting for 30 min. It has no cardiovascular side effects and does not cause histamine release.

Rocuronium is another steroid derivative that has the advantage of a rapid onset of action, such that 0.6 mg/kg allows tracheal intubation to be achieved after 60 s. It has negligible cardiovascular effects and a similar duration of action to vecuronium.

Mivacurium belongs to the same chemical family as atracurium and is the only nondepolarising neuromuscular blocker that is metabolised by plasma cholinesterase. It is comparatively short acting (10–15 min), depending on the initial dose. Mivacurium can cause some hypotension because of histamine release.

Pancuronium was the first steroid-derived neuromuscular blocker in clinical use. It is longer acting than vecuronium and causes a slight tachycardia.

Antagonism of competitive neuromuscular block

Neostigmine

The action of competitive acetylcholine blockers is antagonised by anticholinesterase drugs, which enable accumulation of acetylcholine. Neostigmine is given intravenously, mixed with glycopyrronium to prevent bradycardia caused by the parasympathetic autonomic effects of the neostigmine. It acts in 4 min and its effects last for about 30 min. Too much neostigmine can cause neuromuscular block by depolarisation, which will cause confusion unless there have been some signs of recovery before neostigmine is given. Progress can be monitored with a nerve stimulator.

Sugammadex

Sugammadex comprises a ring-like structure of low molecular weight sugars. This γ-cyclodextrin was designed specifically to encapsulate rocuronium: the negatively charged hydrophilic outer core attracts the positively charged rocuronium and pulls the drug into its lipophilic core. The result is an inactive water-soluble complex that is excreted by the kidneys. A full neuromuscular block from rocuronium can be reversed with sugammadex in less than 3 min. Neostigmine can be used only when the block from rocuronium has started to recover spontaneously (perhaps 30 min after initial injection) and it has many unwanted effects that are not a feature of sugammadex. Vecuronium can also be reversed by sugammadex. The relatively high cost of sugammadex is currently prohibiting its widespread adoption.

Depolarising neuromuscular blocker

Suxamethonium (succinylcholine)

Paralysis is preceded by muscle fasciculation, and this may be the cause of the muscle pain experienced commonly after its use. The pain may last for 1–3 days and can be minimised by preceding the suxamethonium with a small dose of a competitive blocking agent.

Suxamethonium is the neuromuscular blocker with the most rapid onset and the shortest duration of action (although the onset of rocuronium is almost as fast and with sugammadex the recovery is faster than that of suxamethonium). Tracheal intubation is possible in less than 60 s and total paralysis lasts for up to 4 min with 50% recovery in about 10 min ($t_{1/2}$ for effect). It is indicated particularly for rapid sequence induction of anaesthesia in patients who are at risk of aspiration – the ability to secure

the air- way rapidly with a tracheal tube is of the utmost importance. If intubation proves impossible, recovery from suxamethonium and resumption of spontaneous respiration is relatively rapid. Unfortunately, if it is impossible to ventilate the paralysed patient's lungs, recovery may not be rapid enough to prevent the onset of hypoxia.

Suxamethonium is destroyed by plasma pseudocholinesterase and so its persistence in the body is increased by neostigmine, which inactivates that enzyme, and in patients with hepatic disease or severe malnutrition whose plasma enzyme concentrations are lower than normal. Approximately 1 in 3 000 of the European population have hereditary defects in amount or kind of enzyme, and cannot destroy the drug as rapidly as normal individuals. Paralysis can then last for hours and the individual requires ventilatory support and sedation until recovery occurs spontaneously. Repeated injections of suxamethonium can cause bradycardia, extrasystoles and even ventricular arrest. These are probably due to activation of cholinoceptors in the heart and are prevented by atropine. It can be used in Caesarean section as it does not cross the placenta readily. Suxamethonium depolarisation causes a release of potassium from muscle, which in normal patients will increase the plasma potassium by 0.5 mmol/L. This is a problem only if the patient's plasma potassium concentration was already high, for example in acute renal failure. In patients with spinal cord injuries and those with major burns, suxamethonium may cause a grossly exaggerated release of potassium from muscle, sufficient to cause cardiac arrest.

Uses of neuromuscular blocking drugs

Only those who are competent at tracheal intubation and ventilation of the patient's lungs should use these drugs. The drugs are used:
- to provide muscular relaxation during surgery, to enable intubation in the emergency department, and occasionally to assist mechanical ventilation in intensive therapy units; and
- during electroconvulsive therapy to prevent

injury to the patient from excessive muscular contraction.

Other muscle relaxants

Drugs that reduce spasm of the voluntary muscles without impairing voluntary movement can be useful in spastic states, low back syndrome and rheumatism with muscle spasm. Baclofen is structurally related to γ-aminobutyric acid (GABA), an inhibitory central nervous system (CNS) transmitter; it inhibits reflex activity mainly in the spinal cord. Baclofen reduces spasticity and flexor spasms, but, as it has no action on voluntary muscle power, function is commonly not improved. Ambulant patients may need their leg spasticity to provide support, and reduction of spasticity may expose the weakness of the limb. It benefits some cases of trigeminal neuralgia. Baclofen is given orally ($t_{1/2}$ 3 h).

Dantrolene acts directly on muscle and prevents the re- lease of calcium from sarcoplasm stores.

Anaphylaxis

Anaphylactic reactions are caused by the interaction of antigens with specific immunoglobulin (Ig) E antibodies, which have been formed by previous exposure to the antigen. Anaphylactoid reactions are clinically indistinguishable from anaphylaxis but are not caused by previous exposure to a triggering agent and do not involve IgE. Intravenous anaesthetics and muscle relaxants can cause anaphylactic or anaphylactoid reactions; rarely, they are fatal. Muscle relaxants are responsible for 70% of anaphylactic reactions during anaesthesia, and suxamethonium accounts for almost half of these.

LOCAL ANAESTHETICS

Mode of action

Local anaesthetics prevent the initiation and propagation of the nerve impulse (action potential). By reducing the passage of sodium through voltage-gated sodium ion channels they raise the threshold of excitability; in consequence, conduction is blocked

at afferent nerve endings, and by sensory and motor nerve fibres. The fibres in nerve trunks are affected in order of size, the smallest (autonomic, sensory) first, probably because they have a proportionately greater surface area, and then the larger (motor) fibres. Paradoxically the effect in the CNS is stimulation.

Pharmacokinetics

The distribution rate of a single dose of a local anaesthetic is determined by diffusion into tissues with concentrations approximately in relation to blood flow (plasma $t_{1/2}$ of only a few minutes). By injection or infiltration, local anaesthetics are usually effective within 5 min and have a useful duration of effect of 1–1.5 h, which in some cases may be doubled by adding a vasoconstrictor.

Most local anaesthetics are used in the form of the acid salts, as these are both soluble and stable. The acid salt (usually the hydrochloride) dissociates in the tissues to liberate the free base, which is biologically active. This dissociation is delayed in abnormally acid, e.g. inflamed, tissues, but the risk of spreading infection makes local anaesthesia undesirable in infected areas.

Absorption from mucous membranes on topical application varies according to the compound. Those that are well absorbed are used as surface anaesthetics (cocaine, lidocaine, prilocaine). Absorption of topically applied local anaesthetic can be extremely rapid and give plasma concentrations comparable to those obtained by injection. This has led to deaths from overdosage, especially via the urethra.

For topical effect on intact skin for needling procedures, a eutectic mixture of bases of prilocaine or lidocaine is used (EMLA – eutectic mixture of local anaesthetics). Absorption is very slow and a cream is applied under an occlusive dressing for at least 1 h. Tetracaine gel 4% (Ametop) is more effective than EMLA cream and enables pain-free venepuncture 30 min after application.

Ester compounds (cocaine, procaine, tetracaine, benzocaine) are hydrolysed by liver and plasma esterases, and their effects may be prolonged where there is a genetic enzyme deficiency.

Amide compounds (lidocaine, prilocaine, bupivacaine, levobupivacaine, ropivacaine) are dealkylated in the liver.

Impaired liver function, whether caused by primary cellular insufficiency or low liver blood flow as in cardiac failure, may both delay elimination and cause higher peak plasma concentrations of both types of local anaesthetic. This is likely to be important only with large or repeated doses or infusions.

Prolongation of action by vasoconstrictors

The effect of a local anaesthetic is terminated by its removal from the site of application. Anything that delays its absorption into the circulation will prolong its local action and can reduce its systemic toxicity when large doses are used. Most local anaesthetics, with the exception of cocaine, cause vascular dilation. The addition of a vasoconstrictor such as adrenaline/epinephrine reduces local blood flow, slows the rate of absorption of the local anaesthetic, and prolongs its effect; the duration of action of lidocaine is doubled from 1 h to 2 h. Normally, the final concentration of adrenaline/epinephrine should be 1 in 200 000, although dentists use up to 1 in 80 000.

Do not use a vasoconstrictor for nerve block of an extremity (finger, toe, nose, penis). For obvious anatomical reasons, the whole blood supply may be cut off by intense vasoconstriction so that the organ may be damaged or even lost. Enough adrenaline/epinephrine can be absorbed to affect the heart and circulation, and reduce the plasma potassium concentration.

This can be dangerous in cardiovascular disease, and with co-administered tricyclic antidepressants and potassium- losing diuretics. An alternative vasoconstrictor is felypressin (synthetic vasopressin), which, in the concentrations used, does not affect the heart rate or blood pressure and may be preferable in patients with cardiovascular disease.

Other effects

Local anaesthetics also have the following clinically important effects in varying degree: Excitation of parts of the CNS, which may manifest as anxiety, restlessness, tremors, euphoria, agitation and even convulsions, which are followed by depression, an quinidine-like actions on the heart.

Uses

Local anaesthesia is generally used when loss of consciousness is neither necessary nor desirable, and also as an adjunct to major surgery to avoid high-dose general anaesthesia and to provide postoperative analgesia. It can be used for major surgery, with sedation, although many patients prefer to be unconscious. It is invaluable when the operator must also be the anaesthetist, which is often the case in some parts of the developing world.

Local anaesthetics may be used in several ways: surface anaesthesia, as solution, jelly, cream or lozenge; infiltration anaesthesia; block the sensory nerve endings and small cutaneous nerves; Regional anaesthesia.

Regional anaesthesia requires considerable knowledge of anatomy and attention to detail for both success and safety.

Nerve block means the anaesthetising of a region, small or large, by injecting the drug around, not into, the appropriate nerves, usually either a peripheral nerve or a plexus. The routine use of peripheral nerve stimulating needles and/or ultra- sound guidance has increased significantly the success rate of peripheral nerve or plexus blocks. Nerve block provides its own muscular relaxation as motor fibres are blocked as well as sensory fibres, although with care differential block, affecting sensory more than motor fibres, can be achieved. There are various specialised forms: brachial plexus, paravertebral, paracervical block. Sympathetic nerve blocks may be used in vascular disease to induce vasodilation.

Intravenous. A double cuff is applied to the arm, inflated above arterial pressure after elevating the limb to drain the venous system, and the veins filled with local anaesthetics e.g. 0.5%–1% lidocaine without adrenaline/epinephrine. The arm is anaesthetised in 6–8 min, and the effect lasts for up to 40 min if the cuff remains inflated. The cuff must not be deflated for at least 20 min. The technique is useful in providing anaesthesia for the treatment of injuries speedily and conveniently, and many patients can leave hospital soon after the procedure. The technique must be meticulously conducted, for sudden release of the full dose of local anaesthetic accidentally into the general circulation may cause severe toxicity and even cardiac arrest. Bupivacaine is no longer used for intravenous regional anaesthesia as cardiac arrest caused by it is particularly resistant to treatment.

Extradural (epidural) anaesthesia is used in the thoracic, lumbar and sacral (caudal) regions. Lumbar epidurals are used widely in obstetrics and low thoracic epidurals provide excellent analgesia after laparotomy. The drug is injected into the where it acts on the nerve roots. This technique is less likely to cause hypotension than spinal anaesthesia. Continuous analgesia is achieved if a local anaesthetic, often mixed with an opioid, is infused through an epidural catheter.

Subarachnoid (intrathecal) block (spinal anaesthesia). The drug is injected into the cerebrospinal fluid (CSF) and, by using a solution of appropriate specific gravity and tilting the patient, it can be kept at an appropriate level. Sympathetic nerve blockade causes hypotension. Headache due to CSF leakage is virtually eliminated by using very narrow atraumatic 'pencil point' needles.

Serious local neurological complications, e.g. infection and nerve injury, are extremely rare.

Opioid analgesics are used intrathecally and extradurally. They diffuse into the spinal cord and act on its opioid receptors; they are highly effective in skilled hands for post-surgical and intractable pain. Respiratory depression may occur. The effect begins in 20 min and lasts for up to 12 h. Diamorphine or other more lipid-soluble opioids, such as fentanyl, may be used.

Adverse reactions

Excessive absorption causes paraesthesiae (face and tongue), anxiety, tremors and even convulsions. The latter are very dangerous, are followed by respiratory depression, and may require diazepam or thiopental for control. Cardiovascular collapse and respiratory failure occur with higher plasma concentrations of the local anaesthetic; the cause is direct myocardial depression compounded by hypoxia associated with convulsions. Cardiopulmonary resuscitation must be started immediately. Intravenous lipid may improve resuscitation success after cardiac arrest caused by local anaesthetics.

Anaphylactoid reactions are very rare with amide local anaesthetics and some of those reported have been due to preservatives. Most reported reactions to amide local anaesthetics are due to co-administration of adrenaline/ epinephrine, intravascular injection or psychological effects (vasovagal episodes). Reactions with ester local anaesthetics are more common.

Individual local anaesthetics

Amides

Lidocaine is a first choice drug for surface use as well as for injection, combining efficacy with comparative lack of toxicity; the $t_{1/2}$ is 1.5 h. It is also useful in cardiac arrhythmias although it has been largely replaced by amiodarone for this purpose.

Prilocaine is used similarly to lidocaine ($t_{1/2}$ 1.5 h), but it is slightly less toxic. It used to be the preferred drug for intravenous regional anaesthesia but it is no longer available as a preservative-free solution and most clinicians now use lidocaine instead. Crystals of prilocaine and lidocaine base, when mixed, dissolve in one another to form a eutectic emulsion that penetrates skin and is used for dermal anaesthesia (EMLA; e.g. before venepuncture in children).

Bupivacaine is long acting ($t_{1/2}$ 3 h) and is used for peripheral nerve blocks, and for epidural and spinal anaesthesia. Although onset of effect is comparable to that of lidocaine, peak effect occurs later (30 min).

Levobupivacaine is the S-enantiomer of racemic bupivacaine. The relative therapeutic ratio (levobupivacaine: racemic bupivacaine) for CNS toxicity is indicating that levobupivacaine is marginally less toxic.

Ropivacaine may provide better separation of motor and sensory nerve blockade; effective sensory blockade can be achieved without causing motor weakness (although this fact is controversial). The rate of onset of ropivacaine is similar to that of bupivacaine, but its absolute potency and duration of effect are slightly lower. The indications for ropivacaine are similar to those of bupivacaine.

Esters

Cocaine (alkaloid) is used medicinally solely as a surface anaesthetic usually as a 4% solution, because adverse effects are both common and dangerous when it is injected. Even as a surface anaesthetic, sufficient absorption may take place to cause serious adverse effects and cases continue to be reported; only specialists should use it and the dose must be checked and restricted. Cocaine prevents the uptake of catecholamines (adrenaline/epinephrine, noradrenaline/norepinephrine) into sympathetic nerve endings, thus increasing their concentration at receptor sites, so that cocaine has a built in vasoconstrictor action, which is why it retains a (declining) place as a surface anaesthetic for surgery involving mucous membranes, e.g. nose. Other local anaesthetics do not have this action; indeed, most are vasodilators and added adrenaline/epinepehrine is not so efficient.

OBSTETRIC ANALGESIA AND ANAESTHESIA

The ideal drug must relieve labour pain without making the patient confused or uncooperative. It must not interfere with uterine activity nor must it influence the fetus, e.g. to cause respiratory depression by a direct action, by prolonging labour or by reducing uterine blood supply. It should also be suitable for use by a midwife without supervision.

Pethidine is used widely. There is little difference between the effects of equipotent doses of morphine and pethidine on analgesia, respiratory depression, and nausea and vomiting. All opioids have the potential to cause respiratory depression of the newborn but this can be reversed with naloxone if necessary. The popular choice of pethidine for analgesia during labour is not because of any clear pharmacological advantage, but because it remains the only opioid licensed for use by midwives.

Nitrous oxide and oxygen (50% of each: Entonox) may be administered for each contraction from a machine the patient works herself or supervised by a midwife (about 10 good breaths are needed for maximal analgesia).

Epidural local anaesthesia provides the most effective pain relief, but the technique should be undertaken only after adequate training. only anaesthetists insert epidural anaesthetics.

Spinal anaesthesia is now used much more commonly than epidural anaesthesia for Caesarean section. The vast majority of caesarean sections are now undertaken with regional rather than general anaesthesia.

General anaesthesia during labour presents special problems. Gastric regurgitation and aspiration are a particular risk. The safety of the fetus must be considered; all anaesthetics and analgesics in general use cross the placenta in varying amounts and, apart from respiratory depression, produce no important effects except that high doses interfere with uterine contraction and may be followed by uterine haemorrhage. Neuromuscular blocking agents can be used safely.

ANAESTHESIA IN PATIENTS ALREADY TAKING MEDICATION

Anaesthetists are in an unenviable position. They are expected to provide safe service to patients in any condition, taking any drugs. Sometimes there is opportunity to modify drug therapy before surgery, but often there is not. Anaesthetists require a particularly detailed drug history from the patient.

Drugs that affect anaesthesia

Adrenal steroids. Chronic corticosteroid therapy with the equivalent of prednisolone 10 mg daily within the previous 3 months suppresses the hypothalamic–pituitary–adrenal (HPA) system. Without corticosteroid supplementation perioperatively the patient may fail to respond appropriately to the stress of surgery and become hypotensive.

Antibiotics. Aminoglycosides, e.g. neomycin, gentamicin, potentiate neuromuscular blocking drugs.

Anticholinesterases can potentiate suxamethonium.

Antiepilepsy drugs. Continued medication is essential to avoid status epilepticus. Drugs must be given parenterally (e.g. phenytoin, sodium valproate) or rectally (e.g. carbamazepine) until the patient can absorb enterally.

Antihypertensives of all kinds; hypotension may complicate anaesthesia, but it is best to continue therapy. Hypertensive patients are particularly liable to excessive increase in blood pressure and heart rate during intubation, which can be dangerous if there is ischaemic heart disease. After surgery, parenteral therapy may be needed for a time.

β-Adrenoceptor blocking drugs can prevent the homeostatic sympathetic cardiac response to cardiac depressant anaesthetics and to blood loss.

Diuretics. Hypokalaemia, if present, will potentiate neuromuscular blocking agents and perhaps general anaesthetics.

Oral contraceptives containing oestrogen, and post-menopausal hormone replacement therapy predispose to thromboembolism. **Psychotropic drugs.** Neuroleptics potentiate or synergise with opioids, hypnotics and general anaesthetics.

Antidepressants. Monoamine oxidase inhibitors can cause hypertension when combined with certain catecholamines and some other adrenergic drugs.

ANAESTHESIA IN THE DISEASED, AND IN PARTICULAR PATIENT GROUPS

The normal response to anaesthesia may be greatly modified by disease. Some of the more important aspects include:

Respiratory disease and smoking predispose the patient to postoperative pulmonary complications, principally infective. The site of operation, e.g. upper abdomen, chest, and the severity of pain influence the impairment to ventilation and coughing.

Cardiac disease. The aim is to avoid the circulatory stress (with increased cardiac work, which can compromise the myocardial oxygen supply) caused by hypertension and tachycardia. Intravenous drugs are normally given slowly to reduce the risk of overdosage and hypotension.

Patients with fixed cardiac output, e.g. with aortic stenosis or constrictive pericarditis, are at special risk from reduced cardiac output with drugs that depress the myocardium and vasomotor centre, for they cannot compensate. Induction with propofol or thiopental is particularly liable to cause hypotension in these patients. Hypoxia is obviously harmful. Skilled technique rather than choice of drugs on pharmacological grounds is the important factor.

Hepatic or renal disease is generally liable to increase drug effects and should be taken into account when selecting drugs and their doses.

Malignant hyperthermia (MH) is a rare pharmacogenetic syndrome with an incidence of between 1 in 15 000 and 1 in 150 000 in North America, exhibiting autosomal dominant inheritance with variable penetrance. The condition occurs during or immediately after anaesthesia and may be precipitated by potent inhalation agents (halothane, isoflurane, sevoflurane) or suxamethonium. The patient may have experienced an uncomplicated general anaesthetic previously. The mechanism involves an abnormally in- creased release of calcium from the sarcoplasmic reticulum, often caused by an inherited mutation in the gene for the ryanodine receptor, which resides in the sarcoplasmic reticulum membrane. High calcium concentrations stimulate muscle contraction, rhabdomyolysis and a hypermetabolic state. Malignant hyperthermia is a life-threatening medical emergency. Oxygen consumption increases by up to three times the normal value, and body temperature may increase as fast as $1\,^{\circ}\text{C}$ every 5 min, reaching as high as $43\,^{\circ}\text{C}$. Rigidity of voluntary muscles may not be evident at the outset or in mild cases.

Dantrolene 1 mg/kg i.v. is given immediately. Further doses are given at 10 min intervals until the patient responds, to a cumulative maximum dose of 10mg/kg. Dantrolene ($t_{\frac{1}{2}}$ 9 h) probably acts by preventing the release of calcium from the sarcoplasm store that ordinarily follows depolarisation of the muscle membrane.

Non-specific treatment is needed for the hyperthermia (cooling, oxygen), and insulin and dextrose are given for hyperkalaemia caused by potassium release from contracted muscle. Hyperkalaemia and acidosis may trigger severe cardiac arrhythmias.

Once the immediate crisis has resolved, the patient and all immediate relatives should undergo investigation for MH. This involves a muscle biopsy, which is tested for sensitivity to triggering agents.

Anaesthesia in MH-susceptible patients is achieved safely with total intravenous anaesthesia using propofol and opioids. Dantrolene for intravenous use must be available immediately in every location where general anaesthesia is given. The relation of malignant hyperthermia syndrome with neuroleptic malignant syndrome (for which dantrolene may be used as adjunctive treatment) is uncertain.

Muscle diseases. Patients with myasthenia gravis are very sensitive to (intolerant of) competitive, but not to depolarising, neuromuscular blocking drugs.

Those with myotonic dystrophy may recover less rapidly than normal from central respiratory depression and neuromuscular block; they may fail to relax with suxamethonium.

Sickle cell disease. Hypoxia and dehydration can precipitate a crisis.

Atypical (deficient) pseudocholinesterase. There is delay in the metabolism of suxamethonium and mivacurium. The duration of neuromuscular block depends on the level of pseudocholinesterase activity.

Raised intracranial pressure will be made worse by high expired concentration inhalation agents, by hypoxia or hypercapnia, and in response to intubation if anaesthesia is inadequate. Without support from a mechanical ventilator, excessive doses of opioids will cause hypercapnia and increase intracranial pressure.

The elderly are liable to become confused by cerebral depressants, especially by hyoscine. Atropine also crosses the blood–brain barrier and can cause confusion in the elderly; glycopyrronium is prefer-

able. In general, elderly patients require smaller doses of all drugs than the young. The elderly tolerate hypotension poorly; they are prone to cerebral and coronary ischaemia.

Children. The problems with children are more technical, physiological and psychological than pharmacological.

Sedation in critical care units is used to reduce patient anxiety and improve tolerance to tracheal tubes and mechanical ventilation. Whenever possible, patients are sedated only to a level that enables them to open their eyes to verbal command; oversedation is harmful. Commonly used drugs include propofol and midazolam, and opioids such as fentanyl, alfentanil, morphine or remifentanil, and the centrally-acting alpha-2 agonists clonidine and dexmedetomidone.

Neuromuscular blockers are required only rarely to assist mechanical ventilation. If pain is treated properly and patient-triggered modes of ventilation are used, many patients in the critical care unit will not require sedation.

Reassurance from sympathetic nursing staff is extremely important and far more effective than drugs.

SUMMARY

This chapter described the drugs used in general anaesthesia, inhalation anaesthetics, intravenous anaesthetics, muscle relaxants including neuromuscular blocking drugs, local anaesthetics. The pharmacokinetics of some anaesthetics ware suggested. The uses of anesthetics under special conditions and the drug interactions between anaesthetics and other medicines ware described.

IMPORTANT TERMINOLOGY

nitrous oxide 氧化亚氮
isoflurane 异氟醚
halothane 氟烷
enflurane 恩氟烷
sevoflurane 七氟烷
desflurane 地氟烷

propofol　丙泊酚

thiopental　硫喷妥钠

etomidate　依托咪酯

ketamine　氯胺酮

methohexitone　美索比妥

atracurium　阿曲库铵

cisatracurium　顺阿曲库铵

pancuronium　泮库铵

vecuronium　维库铵

suxamethonium　琥珀胆碱

lidocaine　利多卡因

prilocaine　丙铵卡因

bupivacaine　布比卡因

levobupivacaine　左布比卡因

ropivacaine　罗哌卡因

cocaine　可卡因

CHALLENGE YOURSELF

1. What are the advantages and disadvantages of thiopental, ketamine, and propofol?

2. What are the main characteristics of common local anesthesia? What are their clinical application and adverse effects?

3. What are effects of the blood/gas partition coefficients on inhalation anesthetics?

4. What is local anaesthesia now used for Caesarean section?

5. What are differences between competition and depolarization types of muscle relaxants?

Jingshan Shi

Chapter | **14** |

Pharmacotherapy of Cardiovascular Diseases

Part 1. Arterial hypertension, angina pectoris, myocardial infarction and heart failure

DRUGS USED IN HYPERTENSION AND ANGINA

Two groups of drugs, β-adrenergic blockers and calcium channel blockers, are used in both hypertension and angina. Several drugs for hypertension are also used in the treatment of heart failure.

DIURETICS

Diuretics, particularly the thiazides, are useful antihypertensives. They cause an initial loss of sodium with a parallel contraction of the blood and extracellular fluid volume. The effect may reach 10% of total body sodium, but it is not maintained. After several months of treatment, the main blood pressure-lowering effect appears to reflect a reduced responsiveness of resistance vessels to endogenous vasoconstrictors, principally noradrenaline/norepinephrine. Although this hyposensitivity may be a consequence of the sodium depletion, thiazides are generally more effective antihypertensive agents than loop diuretics, despite causing less salt loss, and evidence suggests an independent action of thiazides on an unidentified ion channel on vascular smooth muscle cell membranes. Maximal effect on blood pressure is delayed for several weeks and other drugs are best

added after this time.

Adverse metabolic effects of thiazides on serum potassium, blood lipids, glucose tolerance and uric acid metabolism led to suggestions that they should be replaced by newer agents without these effects. It is now recognised that unnecessarily high doses of thiazides were used in the past and that with low doses, e.g. bendroflumethiazide 1.25–0.5 mg/day or less (or hydrochlorothiazide 12.5–25 mg), thiazides are both effective and well tolerated. Moreover, they are by far the least costly antihypertensive agents available worldwide and have proved to be the most effective in several outcome trials in preventing the major complications of hypertension, myocardial infarction and stroke.

The characteristic reduction in renal calcium excretion induced by thiazides may, in long-term therapy, also reduce the occurrence of hip fractures in older patients and benefit women with postmenopausal osteoporosis.

VASODILATORS

Organic nitrates

Organic nitrates (and nitrite) were introduced into medicine in the 19th century. De-nitration in the smooth muscle cell releases nitric oxide (NO), which is the main physiological vasodilator, normally produced by endothelial cells. Nitrodilators (a generic term for drugs that release or mimic the action of

NO) activate the soluble guanylate cyclase in vascular smooth muscle cells and cause an increase in intracellular cyclic guanosine monophosphate (GMP) concentrations. This is the second messenger which alters calcium fluxes in the cell, decreases stored calcium and induces relaxation. The result is a generalised dilatation of venules (capacitance vessels) and to a lesser extent of arterioles (resistance vessels), causing a fall of blood pressure that is postural at first; the larger coronary arteries especially dilate. Whereas some vasodilators can 'steal' blood away from atheromatous arteries, with their fixed stenoses, to other, healthier arteries, nitrates probably have the reverse effect as a result of their supplementing the endogenous NO. Atheroma is associated with impaired endothelial function, resulting in reduced release of NO and, possibly, its accelerated destruction by the oxidised low-density lipoprotein (LDL) in atheroma.

The venous dilatation causes a reduction in venous return and a fall in left ventricular filling pressure with reduced stroke volume, but cardiac output is sustained by the reflex tachycardia induced by the fall in blood pressure.

Pharmacokinetics. The nitrates are generally well absorbed across skin and the mucosal surface of the mouth or gut wall. Nitrates absorbed from the gut are subject to extensive first-pass metabolism in the liver, as shown by the substantially higher doses required by that route compared with sublingual application (and explains why swallowing a sublingual tablet of glyceryl trinitrate terminates its effect). They are first de-nitrated and then conjugated with glucuronic acid. The $t_{1/2}$ periods vary (see below), but for glyceryl trinitrate (GTN) it is 1–4 min. The denitration of GTN is in fact genetically determined as the enzyme responsible, a mitochondrial alcohol dehydrogenase, ALDH2, is polymorphic and in subjects carrying a common coding variant (E504K) sublingual GTN has reduced efficacy.

Tolerance to the characteristic vasodilator headache comes and goes quickly (hours). Ensuring that a continuous steady-state plasma concentration is avoided prevents tolerance. This is easy with occasional use of GTN, but with nitrates having longer $t_{1/2}$ (see below) and sustained-release formulations it is necessary to plan the dosing to allow a low plasma concentration for 4–8 h, e.g. overnight; alternatively, transdermal patches may be removed for a few hours if tolerance is suspected.

Uses. Nitrates are chiefly used to relieve angina pectoris and sometimes left ventricular failure. An excessive fall in blood pressure will reduce coronary flow as well as cause fainting due to reduced cerebral blood flow, so it is important to avoid accidental overdosing. Patients with angina should be instructed on the signs of overdose-palpitations, dizziness, blurred vision, headache and flushing followed by pallor – and what to do about it (see below).

The discovery that coronary artery occlusion by thrombosis is itself 'stuttering'–developing gradually over hours–and associated with vasospasm in other parts of the coronary tree has made the use of isosorbide dinitrate (Isoket) by continuous intravenous infusion adjusted to the degree of pain, a logical, and effective, form of analgesia for unstable angina.

Transient relief of pain due to spasm of other smooth muscle (colic) can sometimes be obtained, so that relief of chest pain by nitrates does not prove the diagnosis of angina pectoris.

Nitrates are contraindicated in angina due to anaemia.

Adverse effects. Collapse due to fall in blood pressure resulting from overdose is the commonest side-effect. The patient should remain supine with the legs raised above the head to restore venous return to the heart. The patient should also spit out or swallow the remainder of the tablet.

Nitrate headache, which may be severe, is probably due to the stretching of pain-sensitive tissues around the meningeal arteries resulting from the increased pulsation that accompanies the local vasodilatation. If headache is severe the dose should be halved. Methaemoglobinaemia can occur with heavy dosage.

Interactions. An important footnote to the use of nitrates (and NO dilators generally) has been the marked potentiation of their vasodilator effects observed in patients taking phosphodiesterase (PDE) inhibitors, such as sildenafil (Viagra) and tadalafil (Cialis). These agents target an isoform of PDE (PDE-5) expressed in the blood vessel wall. Other methylaxanthine PDE inhibitors, such as theophylline, do not cause a similar interaction because they are rather weak inhibitors of PDE-5, even at the doses effective in asthma. A number of pericoital deaths reported in patients taking sildenafil have been attributed to the substantial fall in blood pressure that occurs when used with a nitrate. This is an ironic twist for an agent in first-line use in erectile dysfunction that was originally developed as a drug to treat angina.

Glyceryl trinitrate (see also above)

Glyceryl trinitrate (1879) (trinitrin, nitroglycerin, GTN) ($t_{1/2}$ 3 min) is an oily, non-flammable liquid that explodes on concussion with a force greater than that of gunpowder. Physicians meet it mixed with inert substances and made into a tablet, in which form it is both innocuous and fairly stable. But tablets more than 8 weeks old or exposed to heat or air will have lost potency by evaporation and should be discarded. Patients should also be warned to expect the tablet to cause a burning sensation under the tongue if it still contains active GTN. An alternative is to use a nitroglycerin spray (see below), which, formulated as a pressurised liquid GTN, has a shelf-life of at least 3 years.

GTN is the drug of choice in the treatment of an attack of angina pectoris. The tablets should be chewed and dissolved under the tongue, or placed in the buccal sulcus, where absorption is rapid and reliable. Time spent ensuring that patients understand the way to take the tablets, and that the feeling of fullness in the head is harmless, is time well spent. The action begins in 2 min and lasts for up to 30 min. The dose in the standard tablet is 300 mg, and 500- or 600-mg strengths are also available; patients may use up to 6 mg daily in total, but those who require more than two or three tablets per week should take a long-acting nitrate preparation. GTN is taken at the onset of pain and as a prophylactic immediately before any exertion likely to precipitate the pain. Sustained-release buccal tablets are available (Suscard), 1–5 mg. Absorption from the gastrointestinal tract is good, but extensive hepatic first-pass metabolism renders the sublingual or buccal route preferable; an oral metered aerosol that is sprayed under the tongue (nitrolingual spray) is an alternative.

For prophylaxis. GTN can be given as an oral (buccal, or to swallow, Sustac) sustained-release formulation or via the skin as a patch (ointment); these formulations can be useful for sufferers from nocturnal angina.

Venepuncture. The ointment can assist difficult venepuncture and a transdermal patch adjacent to an intravenous infusion site can prevent extravasation and phlebitis, and prolong infusion survival.

Isosorbide dinitrate (Cedocard) ($t_{1/2}$ 20 min) is used for prophylaxis of angina pectoris and for congestive heart failure (tablets sublingual, and to swallow). An intravenous formulation, 500 mg/mL (Isoket), is available for use in left ventricular failure and unstable angina.

Isosorbide mononitrate (Elantan) ($t_{1/2}$ 4 h) is used for prophylaxis of angina (tablets to swallow). Hepatic first-pass metabolism is much less than for the dinitrate so that systemic bio-availability is more reliable.

Pentaerithrityl tetranitrate (Peritrate) ($t_{1/2}$ 8 h) is less efficacious than its metabolite pentaerithrityl trinitrate ($t_{1/2}$ 11 h).

Calcium channel blockers

Calcium is involved in the initiation of smooth muscle and cardiac cell contraction, and in the propagation of the cardiac impulse.

Vascular smooth muscle cells. Contraction of these cells requires an influx of calcium across the cell membrane. This occurs through voltage-operated ion channels (VOCs) and this influx is able to trigger further release of calcium from intracellular stores in the sarcoplasmic reticulum. The VOCs have relatively long opening times and carry large fluxes; hence they are usually referred to as L- type channels. The rise in intracellular free calcium results in activation of the contractile proteins, myosin and actin, with shortening of the myofibril and contraction of smooth muscle. During relaxation calcium is released from the myofibril and either pumped back into the sarcoplasm or lost through Na/Ca exchange at the cell surface.

There are three structurally distinct classes of calcium channel blocker:

- Dihydropyridines (the most numerous).
- Phenylalkylamines (principally verapamil).
- Benzothiazepine (diltiazem).

The differences between their clinical effects can be explained in part by their binding to different parts of the L-type calcium channel. All members of the group are vasodilators, and some have negative inotropic and negative chronotropic effects on the heart via effects on pacemaker cells in the conducting tissue. The attributes of individual drugs are described below.

The therapeutic benefit of the calcium blockers in hypertension and angina is due mainly to their action as vasodilators. Their action on the heart gives non-dihydropyridines an additional role as class 4 antiarrhythmics.

Pharmacokinetics. Calcium channel blockers in general are well absorbed from the gastrointestinal tract and their systemic bio-availability depends on the extent of first-pass metabolism in the gut wall and liver, which varies between the drugs. All undergo metabolism to less active products, predominantly by cytochrome P450 CYP3A4, which is the source of interactions with other drugs by enzyme induction and inhibition. As their action is terminated by metabolism, dose adjustments for patients with impaired renal function are therefore either minor or unnecessary.

Indications for use

- Hypertension: amlodipine, isradipine, nicardipine, nifedipine, verapamil.
- Angina: amlodipine, diltiazem, nicardipine, nifedipine, verapamil.
- Cardiac arrhythmia: verapamil.

- Raynaud's disease: nifedipine.
- Prevention of ischaemic neurological damage following subarachnoid haemorrhage: nimodipine.

Adverse effects. Headache, flushing, dizziness, palpitations and hypotension may occur during the first few hours after dosing, as the plasma concentration is increasing, particularly if the initial dose is too high or increased too rapidly. Ankle oedema may also develop. This is probably due to a rise in intracapillary pressure as a result of the selective dilatation by calcium blockers of the precapillary arterioles. Thus the oedema is not a sign of sodium retention. It is not relieved by a diuretic but disappears after lying flat, e.g. overnight. Bradycardia and arrhythmia may occur, especially with the non-dihydropyridines. Gastrointestinal effects include constipation, nausea and vomiting; palpitation and lethargy may be experienced.

There has been some concern that the shorter-acting calcium channel blockers may adversely affect the risk of myocardial infarction and cardiac death. The evidence is based on case–control studies which cannot escape the possibility that sicker patients, i.e. with worse hypertension or angina, received calcium channel blockade. The safety and efficacy of the class has been strengthened by the recent findings of two prospective comparisons with other antihypertensives.

Interactions are numerous. Generally, the drugs in this group are extensively metabolised, and there is risk of decreased effect with enzyme inducers, e.g. rifampicin, and increased effect with enzyme inhibitors, e.g. ketoconazole or cimetidine. Conversely, calcium channel blockers decrease the plasma clearance of several other drugs by mechanisms that include delaying their metabolic breakdown. The consequence, for example, is that diltiazem and verapamil cause increased exposure to carbamazepine, quinidine, statins, ciclosporin, metoprolol, theophylline and (HIV) protease inhibitors. Verapamil increases plasma concentration of digoxin, possibly by interfering with its biliary excretion. β-Adrenoceptor blockers may exacerbate atrioventricular (AV) block and cardiac failure. Grapefruit juice raises the plasma concentration of dihydropyridines (except amlodipine) and verapamil, while St John's wort, as an inducer of CYP3A4, can reduce bio-availability of verapamil and dihydropyridines.

Individual calcium blockers

Nifedipine ($t_{1/2}$ 2 h) is the prototype dihydropyridine. It selectively dilates arteries with little effect on veins; its negative myocardial inotropic and chronotropic effects are much less than those of verapamil. There are sustained-release formulations of nifedipine that permit once-daily dosing, minimising peaks and troughs in plasma concentration so that adverse effects due to rapid fluctuation of concentrations are lessened. Various methods have been used to prolong, and smooth, drug delivery, and bio-equivalence between these formulations cannot be assumed; prescribers should specify the brand to be dispensed. The adverse effects of calcium blockers with a short duration of action may include the hazards of activating the sympathetic system each time a dose is taken. The dose range for nifedipine is 30–90 mg daily. In addition to the adverse effects listed above, gum hypertrophy may occur. Nifedipine can be taken 'sublingually', by biting a capsule and squeezing the contents under the tongue. In point of fact, absorption is still largely from the stomach after this manoeuvre, and it should not be used in a hypertensive emergency because the blood pressure reduction is unpredictable and sometimes large enough to cause cerebral ischaemia.

Amlodipine has a $t_{1/2}$ (40 h) sufficient to permit the same benefits as the longest-acting formulations of nifedipine without requiring a special formulation. Its slow association with L-channels and long duration of action render it unsuitable for emergency reduction of blood pressure where frequent dose adjustment is needed. On the other hand, an occasional missed dose is of little consequence. Amlodipine differs from all other dihydropyridines listed in this chapter in being safe to use in patients with cardiac failure (the PRAISE study).

Verapamil ($t_{1/2}$ 4 h) is an arterial vasodilator with some venodilator effect; it also has marked negative myocardial inotropic and chronotropic actions. It is given thrice daily as a conventional tablet or daily as a sustained-release formulation. Because of its negative effects on myocardial conducting and contracting cells it should not be given to patients with bradycardia, second- or third-degree heart block, or patients with Wolff–Parkinson–White syndrome to relieve atrial flutter or fibrillation. Amiodarone and digoxin increase the AV block. Verapamil increases plasma quinidine concentration and this interaction may cause dangerous hypotension.

Diltiazem ($t_{1/2}$ 5 h) is given thrice daily, or once or twice daily if a slow-release formulation is prescribed. It causes less myocardial depression and prolongation of AV conduction than does verapamil but should not be used where there is bradycardia, second- or third-degree heart block or sick sinus syndrome.

Nimodipine has a moderate cerebral vasodilating action. Cerebral ischaemia after subarachnoid haemorrhage may be partly due to vasospasm; clinical trial evidence indicates that nimodipine given after subarachnoid haemorrhage reduces cerebral infarction (incidence and extent). Although the benefit is small, the absence of any more effective options has led to the routine administration of nimodipine (60 mg every 4 h) to all patients for the first few days after subarachnoid haemorrhage. No benefit has been found in similar trials following other forms of stroke.

Other members include felodipine, isradipine, lacidipine, lercanidipine, nisoldipine.

Angiotensin-converting enzyme (ACE) inhibitors, angiotensin (AT) II receptor blockers (ARBs) and renin inhibitors

Renin is an enzyme produced by the kidney in response to a number of factors, but principally adrenergic (β_1 receptor) activity and sodium depletion. Renin converts a circulating glycoprotein (angiotensinogen) into the biologically inert angiotensin I, which is then changed by angiotensin-converting enzyme (ACE or kininase II) into the highly potent vasoconstrictor angiotensin II. ACE is located on the luminal surface of capillary endothelial cells, particularly in the lungs; and there are also renin–angiotensin systems in many organs, e.g. brain, heart, the relevance of which is uncertain.

Angiotensin II acts on two G-protein-coupled receptors, of which the angiotensin 'AT$_1$' subtype accounts for all the classic actions of angiotensin. As well as vasoconstriction these include stimulation of aldosterone (the sodium-retaining hormone) production by the adrenal cortex. It is evident that angiotensin II can have an important effect on blood pressure. In addition, it stimulates cardiac and vascular smooth muscle cell growth, probably contributing to the progressive amplification in hypertension once the process is initiated. The AT$_2$-receptor subtype is coupled to inhibition of muscle growth or proliferation, but appears of minor importance in the adult cardiovascular system. The recognition that the AT$_1$-receptor subtype is the important target for drugs that antagonise angiotensin II has led, a little confusingly, to alternative nomenclatures for these drugs: angiotensin II blockers, AT$_1$-receptor blockers or the acronym, ARB. The latter abbreviation is used here for consistency.

Bradykinin (an endogenous vasodilator found in blood vessel walls) is also a substrate for ACE. Potentiation of bradykinin contributes to the blood pressure-lowering action of ACE inhibitors in patients with low-renin causes of hypertension. Either bradykinin or one of the neurokinin substrates of ACE (such as substance P) may stimulate cough (below). The ARBs differ from the ACE inhibitors in having no effect on bradykinin and they do not cause cough. ARBs are slightly more effective than ACE inhibitors at preventing angiotensin II vasoconstriction, because angiotensin II can be generated from angiotensin I by non-ACE enzymes such as chymase. ACE inhibitors are more effective at suppressing aldosterone production in patients with normal or low plasma renin levels.

Uses

Hypertension. The antihypertensive effect of ACE inhibitors, ARBs and renin inhibitors results primarily from vasodilatation (reduction of peripheral resistance) with little change in cardiac output or rate; renal blood flow may increase (desirable). A fall in aldosterone production may also contribute to the blood-pressure-lowering action of ACE inhibitors. Both classes slow progression of glomerulopathy. Whether the long-term benefit of these drugs in hypertension exceeds that to be expected from blood pressure reduction alone remains controversial.

ACE inhibitors, ARBs and renin inhibitors are most useful in hypertension when the raised blood pressure results from excess renin production, e.g. renovascular hypertension, or where concurrent use of another drug (diuretic or calcium blocker) renders the blood pressure renin dependent. The fall in blood pressure can be rapid, especially with short-acting ACE inhibitors, and low initial doses of these should be used in patients at risk: those with impaired renal function or suspected cerebrovascular disease. These patients may be advised to omit any concurrent diuretic treatment for a few days before the first dose. The antihypertensive effect increases progressively over weeks with continued administration (as with other antihypertensives) and the dose may be increased at intervals of 2 weeks.

Cardiac failure. ACE inhibitors have a useful vasodilator and diuretic-sparing (but not diuretic-substitute) action that is critical to the treatment of all grades of heart failure. Mortality reduction here may result from their being the only vasodilator that does not reflexly activate the sympathetic system.

The ARBs are at least as effective as ACE inhibitors in patients with heart failure and they can be substituted if patients are intolerant of an ACE inhibitor. Based on the Candesartan in Heart Failure Assessment of Reduction in Mortality and Morbidity (CHARM) trial, they may also benefit patients with heart failure and a low ejection fraction when added to treatment with a β-blocker and ACE inhibitor.

Diabetic nephropathy. In patients with type I (insulin-dependent) diabetes, hypertension often accompanies the diagnosis of frank nephropathy, and aggressive blood pressure control is essential to slow the otherwise inexorable decline in renal function that follows. ACE inhibitors appear to have a specific renoprotective effect, probably because of the role of angiotensin II in driving the underlying glomerular hyperfiltration. These drugs are now first-line treatment for hypertensive type I diabetics, although most patients will need a second or third agent to reach the rigorous blood pressure targets for this condition (see below). Their role in preventing the progression of the earliest manifestation of renal damage, microalbuminuria, is more complicated. Here the evidence suggests that ACE inhibitors do not slow the incidence of microalbuminuria in type I diabetics and an ARB may actually substantially increase it. In contrast, an ACE inhibitor halves the incidence of microalbuminuria in type 2 diabetics with hypertension and normal renal function on follow-up. A parallel group on verapamil did not show any protection confirming that inhibition of the renin–angiotensin–aldosterone (RAAS) axis is required for this effect, not simply lowering the blood pressure. For hypertensive type 2 diabetics with established nephropathy, both ARBs and ACE inhibitors protect against a decline in renal function and reduce macroproteinuria. The evidence suggests they are interchangeable in this respect. Whether combining the two classes of drugs ('dual block') confers further protection of renal function is not yet resolved, although 'dual block' does produce substantially better urine protein sparing than either agent alone.

Myocardial infarction (MI). Following a myocardial infarction, the left ventricle may fail acutely from the loss of functional tissue or in the long term from a process of 'remodelling' due to thinning and enlargement of the scarred ventricular wall. Angiotensin II plays a key role in both of these processes and an ACE inhibitor given after MI markedly reduces the incidence of heart failure. The effect is seen even in patients without overt signs of cardiac failure, but who have low left ventricular ejection fractions (< 40%) during the convalescent phase (3–10 days) following the MI. Such patients receiving captopril in the SAVE trial, had a 37% reduction in progressive heart failure over the 60-month follow-

up period compared with placebo. The benefits of ACE inhibition after MI are additional to those conferred by thrombolysis, aspirin and β-blockers. ARBs also prevent remodelling and heart failure in post-MI patients, but there is no additional benefit from 'dual blockade'.

Cautions

Certain constraints apply to the use of ACE inhibitors:

- Heart failure: severe hypotension may result in patients taking diuretics, or who are hypovolaemic, hyponatraemic, elderly, have renal impairment or with systolic blood pressure of less than 100 mmHg. A test dose of captopril 6.25 mg by mouth may be given because its effect lasts for only 4–6 h. If tolerated, the preferred long-acting ACE inhibitor may then be initiated in low dose.

- Renal artery stenosis (RAS, whether unilateral, bilateral renal or suspected from the presence of generalised atherosclerosis): an ACE inhibitor may cause renal failure and is contraindicated. ARBs are not necessarily any safer in this situation, because angiotensin II- mediated constriction of the efferent arteriole is thought to be crucial to the maintenance of glomerular perfusion in RAS.

- Aortic stenosis/left ventricular outflow tract obstruction: an ACE inhibitor may cause severe, sudden hypotension and, depending on severity, is relatively or absolutely contraindicated.

- Pregnancy represents an absolute contraindication (see below).

- Angioedema may result (see below).

Adverse effects

ACE inhibitors:

- Persistent dry cough occurs in 10%–15% of patients.

- Urticaria and angioedema (less than 1 in 100 patients) are much rarer, occurring usually in the first weeks of treatment. The angioedema varies from mild swelling of the tongue to life-threatening tracheal obstruction, when subcutaneous adrenaline/epinephrine should be given. The basis of the reaction is probably pharmacological rather than allergic, due to reduced breakdown of bradykinin.

- Impaired renal function may result from reduced glomerular filling pressure, systemic hypotension or glomerulonephritis, and plasma creatinine levels should be checked before and during treatment.

- Hyponatraemia may develop, especially where a diuretic is also given; clinically significant hyperkalaemia (see effect on aldosterone above) is confined to patients with impaired renal function.

- ACE inhibitors cause major malformations in the first trimester and are fetotoxic in the second trimester, causing reduced renal perfusion, hypotension, oligohydramnios and fetal death.

- Neutropenia and other blood dyscrasias occur. Other reported reactions include rashes, taste disturbance (dysguesia), musculoskeletal pain, proteinuria, liver injury and pancreatitis.

ARBs are contraindicated in pregnancy as are ACE inhibitors, but avoid the other complications of these drugs – especially the cough and angioedema. They are, in fact, the only antihypertensive drug class for which there is no 'typical' side-effect.

Interactions. Hyperkalaemia can result from use with potassium-sparing diuretics. Renal clearance of lithium is reduced and toxic concentrations of plasma lithium may follow. Severe hypotension can occur with diuretics (above), and with chlorpromazine, and possibly other phenothiazines.

Individual drugs

Captopril (Capoten) has a $t_{1/2}$ of 2 h and is partly metabolised and partly excreted unchanged; adverse effects are more common when renal function is impaired; it is given twice or thrice daily. Captopril is the shortest acting of the ACE inhibitors, one of the few that is itself active by mouth, not requiring de-esterification after absorption.

Enalapril (Innovace) is a prodrug ($t_{1/2}$ 35 h) that is converted to the active enalaprilat ($t_{1/2}$ 10 h). Effective 24-h control of blood pressure probably requires twice-daily administration.

Other members include cilazapril, fosinopril, imidapril, lisinopril, moexipril, perindopril, quinapril, ramipril and trandolapril. Of these, lisinopril has a marginally longer $t_{1/2}$ than enalapril (it is the lysine analogue of enalaprilat), probably justifying its popularity as a once-daily ACE inhibitor. Some of the others are longer acting, with quinapril and ramipril also having a higher degree of binding to ACE in vascular tissue. The clinical significance of these differences is disputed. In the Heart Outcomes Prevention Evaluation (HOPE) study of 9 297 patients, ramipril reduced, by 20%–30%, the rates of death, myocardial infarction and stroke in a broad range of high-risk patients who were not known to have a low ejection fraction or heart failure. The authors considered (probably erroneously) that the results could not be explained entirely by blood pressure reduction.

Losartan was the first ARB to be licensed in the UK. It is a competitive blocker with a non-competitive active metabolite. The drug has a short $t_{1/2}$ (2 h) but the metabolite is much longer lived ($t_{1/2}$ 10 h), permitting once-daily dosing.

Other ARBs in clinical use include candesartan, eprosartan, irbesartan, telmisartan, valsartan and olmesartan. Some of these may be marginally more effective than losartan at lowering blood pressure, but few if any comparisons have been performed at maximal dose of each drug. Losartan is generally used in combination with hydrochlorothiazide. In a landmark study this combination was 25% more effective than atenolol plus hydrochlorothiazide in preventing stroke.

This class of drug is very well tolerated; in clinical trials the side-effect profiles are indistinguishable or even better than those of placebo. Unlike the ACE inhibitors they do not produce cough, and are a valuable alternative for the 10–15% of patients who thereby discontinue their ACE inhibitor. ARBs are used to treat hypertension, left ventricular (LV) failure after MI and established heart failure. With the possible exception of chronic heart failure, they do not appear to be superior to ACE inhibitors.

The cautions listed for the use of ACE inhibitors

(above) apply also to AT1-receptor blockers.

Renin inhibitors share the benefit of ARBs over ACE inhibitors in terms of cough and angioedema. By implication with other agents targeting the RAAS they should not be used in pregnancy.

Aliskiren is the only orally active non-peptide renin inhibitor licensed ($t_{1/2}$ 40 h). The agent is well tolerated apart from dose-dependent diarrhoea; it is not clear if this is class side-effect. It produces additive effects on blood pressure with ACE inhibitors, ARBs, calcium channel blockers and thiazide diuretics. There are currently no outcome data in terms of preventing hypertension-related cardiovascular events, so it should be reserved for inhibiting the RAAS where an ACE inhibitor or ARB is not tolerated.

Interactions. Hyperkalaemia can result from use with potassium-sparing diuretics. Severe hypotension can occur on first dosing if given after agents that increase circulating renin levels such as diuretics (especially loop diuretics) and potent vasodilators.

Other vasodilators

Several older drugs are powerfully vasodilating, but precluded from routine use in hypertension by their adverse effects. Minoxidil and nitroprusside still have special indications.

Minoxidil is a vasodilator selective for arterioles rather than for veins, similar to diazoxide and hydralazine. It acts through its sulphate metabolite as an adenosine triphosphate (ATP)-dependent potassium channel opener. It is highly effective in severe hypertension, but in common with all potent arterial vasodilators its hypotensive action is accompanied by a compensatory baroreceptor-mediated sympathetic discharge, causing tachycardia and increased cardiac output. There is also renin release with secondary salt and water retention, which antagonises the hypotensive effect (so-called 'tolerance' on long-term use). Therefore, it is used in combination with a β-blocker and loop diuretic (as is hydralazine; see below). Hypertrichosis is perhaps the most notorious side-effect of minoxidil. The hair growth is generalised when taken orally and, although a cosmetic problem in women, it has been exploited as a 2%–5% topical solution for the treatment of male-pattern baldness (Regaine).

Sodium nitroprusside is a highly effective antihypertensive agent when given intravenously. Its effect is almost immediate and lasts for 1–5 min. Therefore it must be given by a precisely controllable infusion. It dilates both arterioles and veins, which would cause collapse were the patient to stand up, e.g. for toilet purposes. There is a compensatory sympathetic discharge with tachycardia and tachyphylaxis to the drug.

The action of nitroprusside is terminated by metabolism within erythrocytes. Specifically, electron transfer from haemoglobin iron to nitroprusside yields methaemoglobin and an unstable nitroprusside radical. This breaks down, liberating cyanide radicals capable of inhibiting cytochrome oxidase (and thus cellular respiration). Fortunately, most of the cyanide remains bound within erythrocytes but a small fraction does diffuse out into the plasma and is converted to thiocyanate. Hence, monitoring plasma thiocyanate concentrations during prolonged (days) nitroprusside infusion is a useful marker of impending systemic cyanide toxicity. Poisoning may be obvious as a progressive metabolic acidosis, or may manifest as delirium or psychotic symptoms. Intoxicated subjects are also reputed to have the characteristic bitter almond smell of hydrogen cyanide. Clearly nitroprusside infusion must be used with caution, and outside specialist units it may be safer overall to choose another more familiar drug.

Sodium nitroprusside is used in hypertensive emergencies, refractory heart failure and for controlled hypotension in surgery. An infusion may begin at 0.3–1.0 mg/kg·min, and control of blood pressure is likely to be established at 0.5–6.0 mg/kg·min; close monitoring of blood pressure is mandatory, usually by direct arterial monitoring; rate changes of infusion may be made every 5–10 min.

Diazoxide mimics the actions of other ATP-dependent potassium channel openers or KCOs. The $t_{1/2}$ is 36 h. Diazoxide was used as an intravenous bolus for the emergency treatment of severe hypertension, but this use is now obsolete.

During its use as an antihypertensive it was noted that it caused hyperglycaemia because, unlike other KCOs, it can activate the sulphonylurea-sensitive form of the ATP-potassium channel in the pancreatic islet cells switching off insulin release. Hence it is used in patients with chronic hypoglycaemia from excess endogenous insulin secretion, either from an islet cell tumour or islet cell hyperplasia. Long-term use can cause the same problems of hair growth seen with minoxidil, albeit less consistently.

Hydralazine is now little used for hypertension except for that related to pregnancy (owing to its established lack of teratogenicity), but it may have a role as a vasodilator (plus nitrates) in heart failure. It reduces peripheral resistance by directly relaxing arterioles, with negligible effect on veins; the mechanism of vasorelaxation is unclear. The $t_{1/2}$ is 1 h.

In most hypertensive emergencies (except for dissecting aneurysm) hydralazine 5–20 mg i.v. may be given over 20 min, when the maximum effect will be seen in 10–80 min; it can be repeated according to need and the patient transferred to oral therapy within 1–2 days.

Prolonged use of hydralazine at doses above 50 mg/day may cause a systemic lupus-like syndrome, more commonly in white than in black races, and in those with the slow acetylator phenotype.

Three other vasodilators find a role outside hypertension:

Nicorandil is effective through two actions: it acts as a nitrate by activating cyclic GMP (see above) but also opens the ATP-dependent potassium channel to allow potassium efflux and hyperpolarisation of the membrane, which reduces calcium ion entry and induces muscular relaxation. It is indicated for use in angina, where it has similar efficacy to β-blockade, nitrates or calcium channel blockade. It is administered orally and is an alternative to nitrates when tolerance is a problem, or to the other classes when these are contraindicated by asthma or cardiac failure. Adverse effects to nicorandil are similar to those of nitrates, with headache reported in 35% of patients. It is the only antianginal drug for which at least one trial has demonstrated a beneficial influence on outcome.

Papaverine is an alkaloid present in opium, but is structurally unrelated to morphine. It inhibits phosphodiesterase and its principal action is to relax smooth muscle throughout the body, especially in the vascular system. It is occasionally injected into an area where local vasodilatation is desired, especially into and around arteries and veins to relieve spasm during vascular surgery and when setting up intravenous infusions. It is also used to treat male erectile dysfunction.

Alprostadil is a stable form of prostaglandin E_1. It is effective in psychogenic and neuropathic penile erectile dysfunction by direct intracorporeal injection and is used intravenously to maintain patency of the ductus arteriosus in the newborn with congenital heart disease.

ADRENOCEPTOR-BLOCKING DRUGS

Adrenoceptor-blocking drugs occupy the adrenoceptor in competition with adrenaline/epinephrine and noradrenaline/norepinephrine (and other sympathomimetic amines) whether released from stores in nerve terminals or injected. There are two principal classes of adrenoceptor, α and β.

α-Adrenoceptor-blocking drugs

There are two main subtypes of α adrenoceptor:

- 'Classic' α_1 adrenoceptors, on the effector organ (post-synaptic), mediate vasoconstriction.
- α_2 Adrenoceptors are present both on some effector tissues (post-synaptic) and on the nerve ending (pre-synaptic). The pre-synaptic receptors (or autoreceptors) inhibit release of chemotransmitter (noradrenaline/norepinephrine), i.e. they provide negative feedback control of transmitter release. They are also present in the CNS.

The first generation of α-adrenoceptor blockers were imidazolines (e.g. phentolamine), which blocked both α_1 and α_2 receptors. When subjects taking such a drug stand from the lying position or take exercise, the sympathetic system is physiologically activated (via baroreceptors). The normal vasoconstrictive (α_1) effect (to maintain blood pressure) is blocked by the drug and the failure of this response causes further sympathetic activation and the release of additional transmitter. This would normally be restrained by negative feedback through α_2 autoreceptors, but these are blocked too. The β adrenoceptors, however, are not blocked and the excess transmitter released at adrenergic endings is free to act on them, causing a tachycardia that may be unpleasant. Hence, non-selective α-adrenoceptor blockers are not used on their own in hypertension.

An α_1-adrenoceptor blocker that spares the α receptor, so that negative feedback inhibition of noradrenaline/norepinephrine release is maintained, is more useful in hypertension (less tachycardia and postural and exercise hypotension); prazosin is such a drug (see below).

Uses of α-Adrenoceptor-blocking drugs

- Hypertension
  - essential: doxazosin, labetalol
  - phaeochromocytoma: phenoxybenzamine; phentolamine (for crisis)
- Peripheral vascular disease.
- Benign prostatic hypertrophy (to relax capsular smooth muscle that may contribute tourirary obstruction)

Adverse effects. The converse of the benefit in the treatment of prostatism is the adverse effect of urinary incontinence in women. Other adverse effects of α-adrenoceptor blockade are postural hypotension, nasal stuffiness, red sclerae and, in the male, failure of ejaculation. They may also exacerbate symptoms of angina. Effects peculiar to each drug are mentioned below.

Notes on individual drugs

Prazosin blocks postsynaptic α_1-receptors but not presynaptic α_2 autoreceptors. It has a curious adverse 'first-dose effect': within 2 h of the first dose (rarely after another) there may be a brisk fall in blood pressure sufficient to cause loss of consciousness. Hence the first dose should be small (0.5 mg) and given before going to bed. This unwanted effect, together

with a rather short duration of action ($t_\frac{1}{2}$ 3 h) has led to a sharp decline in its use.

Doxazosin ($t_\frac{1}{2}$ 8 h) was the first α-adrenoceptor blocker suitable for once-daily prescribing. The first-dose effect is also much less marked, although it is still advisable to start patients at a lower dose than is intended for maintenance. It is convenient, for instance, to prescribe 1 mg daily, increasing after 1 week to double this dose without repeating the blood pressure measurement at this stage. A slow-release formulation, doxazosin XL, can be started at the maintenance dose of 4 mg daily.

Other α-adrenoceptor blockers used for prostatic symptoms are *alfuzosin* and *terazosin*.

Indoramin is an older α-blocker, which is a less useful. antihypertensive but still used for prostatic symptoms. It is taken twice or thrice daily.

Phentolamine is a non-selective α-adrenoceptor blocker. It is given intravenously for brief effect in adrenergic hypertensive crises, e.g. phaeochromocytoma or the monoamine oxidase inhibitor–sympathomimetic interaction ('cheese reaction'). In addition to α-receptor block it has direct vasodilator and cardiac inotropic. The dose for hypertensive crisis is 2–5 mg i.v. repeated as necessary (in minutes to hours). This is not a reliable diagnostic test for phaeochromocytoma!

Phenoxybenzamine is an irreversible non-selective α-adrenoceptor-blocking drug whose effects may last for 2 days or longer. The daily dose must therefore be increased slowly. It is impossible to reverse the circulatory effects by secreting noradrenaline/norepinephrine or other sympathomimetic drugs because its effects are insurmountable. This makes it the preferred α-blocker for treating phaeochromocytoma.

It is wise to observe the effects of a single test dose closely before starting regular administration.

Indigestion and nausea can occur with oral therapy, which is best given with food.

Moxisylyte (thymoxamine) is a non-selective α-blocker for which Raynaud's phenomenon is the only extant indication. Labetalol has both α- and β-receptor-blocking actions that are due to different isomers (see β-adrenoceptor block, below). Its parenteral preparation is valuable in the treatment of hypertension emergencies.

Chlorpromazine and amitriptyline, among their other actions, can both produce clinically significant α-blockade, which may be sufficient to cause postural hypotension and falls in the elderly.

β-Adrenoceptor-blocking drugs

Actions

These drugs selectively block the β-adrenoceptor effects of noradrenaline/norepinephrine and adrenaline/epinephrine. They may be pure antagonists or may have some agonist activity in addition (when they are described as partial agonists).

Intrinsic heart rate. Sympathetic activity (through β_1 adrenoceptors) accelerates, and parasympathetic activity (through muscarinic M_2 receptors) slows, the heart. If the sympathetic and the parasympathetic drives to the heart are simultaneously and adequately blocked by β-adrenoceptor blocker plus atropine, the heart will beat at its 'intrinsic' rate. The intrinsic rate at rest is usually about 100 beats/min, as opposed to the usual rate of 80 beats/min, i.e. normally there is parasympathetic vagal 'tone', which decreases with age.

The cardiovascular effects of β-adrenoceptor block depend on the amount of sympathetic tone present. The chief effects result from reduction of sympathetic drive:

- Reduced automaticity (heart rate).
- Reduced myocardial contractility (rate of rise of pressure in the ventricle).
- Reduced renin secretion from the juxtaglomerular apparatus in the renal cortex.

With reduced rate the cardiac output per minute is reduced and the overall cardiac oxygen consumption falls. The results are more evident on the response to exercise than at rest. With acute administration of a pure β-adrenoceptor blocker, i.e. one with no intrinsic sympathomimetic activity (ISA), peripheral vascular resistance tends to rise. This is probably a reflex response to the reduced cardiac

output, but also occurs because the β_1-adrenoceptor (vasoconstrictor) effects are no longer partially opposed by β_2-adrenoceptor (dilator) effects; peripheral flow is reduced. With chronic use peripheral resistance returns to about pre-treatment levels or a little below, varying according to presence or absence of ISA. But peripheral blood flow remains reduced. The cold extremities that accompany chronic therapy are probably due chiefly to reduced cardiac output with reduced peripheral blood flow, rather than to the blocking of peripheral (β_2) dilator receptors.

Hepatic blood flow may be reduced by as much as 30%, prolonging the $t_{1/2}$ of the lipid-soluble drugs whose metabolism is limited by hepatic blood flow, i.e. whose first-pass metabolism is so extensive that it is actually limited by the rate of blood delivery to the liver; these include propranolol, verapamil and lidocaine, which may be used concomitantly for cardiac arrhythmias.

Effects

Within hours of starting treatment with a β-blocker, blood pressure starts to fall. This reflects the acute effect on cardiac output (heart rate and contractility) but this is not sustained and on chronic administration the blockade of renin secretion appears to be the main cause of blood pressure reduction. An additional contributor may be the two- to three-fold increase in natriuretic peptide secretion caused by β-blockade.

A substantial advantage of β-blockade in hypertension is that physiological stresses such as exercise, *upright posture* and *high environmental temperature* are not accompanied by hypotension, as they are with agents that interfere with α-adrenoceptor-mediated homeostatic mechanisms. With β-blockade these necessary adaptive α-receptor constrictor mechanisms remain intact.

At first sight the cardiac effects might seem likely to be disadvantageous rather than advantageous, and indeed maximum exercise capacity is reduced. But the heart has substantial functional reserves so that use may be made of the desired properties in the diseases listed below, e.g. angina, without inducing heart failure. Indeed, β-blockade is now routine practice in patients with established mild to moderate heart failure and usually safe provided uptitration is slow. But heart failure can occur in patients with seriously diminished cardiac reserve.

β-Adrenoceptor selectivity

Some β-adrenoceptor blockers have higher affinity for cardiac β_1 receptors than for cardiac and peripheral β_2 receptors. The ratio of the amount of drug required to block the two receptor subtypes is a measure of the *selectivity* of the drug. (regarding the use of the terms 'β selective' and *'cardioselective'.*) The question is whether the differences between selective and non-selective β-blockers confer clinical advantages. In theory β-blockers are less likely to cause bronchoconstriction, but in practice few available β_1-blockers are sufficiently selective to be safely recommended in asthma. Bisoprolol and nebivolol may be exceptions that can be tried at low doses in patients with mild asthma and a strong indication for β-blockade. There are unlikely ever to be satisfactory safety data to support such use. The main practical use of β-selective blockade is in diabetics, where β_2 receptors mediate both the symptoms of hypoglycaemia and the counter-regulatory metabolic responses that reverse the hypoglycaemia.

Some β-blockers (antagonists) also have agonist action or ISA, i.e. they are partial agonists. These agents cause less fall in resting heart rate than do the pure antagonists and may thus be less effective in severe angina pectoris where reduction of heart rate is particularly important. The fall in cardiac output may be less, and fewer patients may experience unpleasantly cold extremities. Intermittent claudication may be worsened by β-blockade whether or not there is partial agonist effect. Both classes of drug can precipitate heart failure, and indeed no important difference is to be expected because patients with heart failure already have high sympathetic drive (but note that β-blockade can be used to treat cardiac failure).

Abrupt withdrawal may be less likely to lead to a rebound effect if there is some partial agonist action,

as there may be less up-regulation of receptors, such as occurs with prolonged receptor block.

Some β-blockers have a membrane-stabilising (quinidine-like or local anaesthetic) effect, a property that is unimportant at clinical doses but relevant in overdose (see below). Additionally, agents having this effect will anaesthetise the eye (undesirable) if applied topically for glaucoma (timolol is used in the eye and does not have this action).

The ankle jerk relaxation time is prolonged by β_2-adrenoceptor block, which may be misleading if the reflex is being relied on in diagnosis and management of hypothyroidism.

Pharmacokinetics

The plasma concentration of a β-adrenoceptor blocker may have a complex relationship with its effect, for several reasons. First-order kinetics usually apply to elimination of drug from plasma, but the decline in receptor block is zero order. The practical application is important: within 4 h of giving propranolol 20 mg i.v. the plasma concentration falls by 50%, but the receptor block (as measured by exercise-induced tachycardia) falls by only 35%. The relationship between the concentration of the parent drug in plasma and its effect is further obscured if pharmacologically active metabolites are also present. Additionally, for some of the lipid-soluble β-blockers, especially timolol, plasma $t_{1/2}$ may not reflect the duration of β-blockade, because the drug remains bound to the tissues near the receptor when the plasma concentration is negligible.

Most β-adrenoceptor blockers can be given orally once daily in either ordinary or sustained-release formulations because the $t_{1/2}$ of the pharmacodynamic effect exceeds the elimination $t_{1/2}$ of the parent substance in the blood.

Uses of β-adrenoceptor-blocking drugs

Cardiovascular uses: Angina pectoris: β-blockade reduces cardiac work and oxygen consumption.

Hypertension: β-blockade reduces renin secretion and cardiac output; there is little interference with homeostatic reflexes.

Cardiac tachyarrhythmias: β-blockade reduces drive to cardiac pacemakers: subsidiary properties may also be relevant.

Myocardial infarction and β-adrenoceptor blockers: there are two modes of use that reduce acute mortality and prevent recurrence: the so-called 'cardioprotective' effect.

- *Early use* within 6 h (at most 12 h) of onset (intravenously for 24 h then orally for 3–4 weeks). Benefit has been demonstrated only for atenolol. Cardiac work is reduced, resulting in a reduction in infarct size by up to 25% and protection against cardiac rupture. Surprisingly, tachyarrhythmias are not less frequent, perhaps because the cardiac β2 receptor is not blocked by atenolol. Maximum benefit is in the first 24–36 h, but mortality remains lower for up to 1 year. Contraindications to early use include bradycardia<55 beats/min), hypotension (systolic <90 mmHg) and left ventricular failure. A patient already taking a β-blocker may be given additional doses.
- *Late use* for secondary prevention of another myocardial infarction. The drug is started between 4 days and 4 weeks after the onset of the infarct and is continued for at least 2 years.
- *Choice of drug.* The agent should be a pure antagonist, i.e. without ISA.

Aortic dissection and after subarachnoid haemorrhage: by reducing force and speed of systolic ejection (contractility) and blood pressure.

Obstruction of ventricular outflow where sympathetic activity occurs in the presence of anatomical abnormalities, e.g. Fallot's tetralogy (cyanotic attacks): hypertrophic subaortic stenosis (angina); some cases of mitral valve disease.

Hepatic portal hypertension and oesophageal variceal bleeding: reduction of portal pressure.

Cardiac failure: there is now clear evidence from prospective trials that β-blockade is beneficial in terms of mortality for patients with all grades of moderate heart failure. Data support the use of both non-selective (carvedilol, α-blocker as well) and β1-selective (metoprolol and bisoprolol) agents. Survival benefit exceeds that provided by ACE inhibitors

over placebo. The negative inotropic effects can still be significant, so the starting dose is low (e.g. bisoprolol 1.25 mg orally daily in the morning or carvedilol 3.125 mg twice daily, with food) and may be tolerated only with additional antifailure therapy, e.g. diuretic.

Endocrine uses. Hyperthyroidism: β-blockade reduces unpleasant symptoms of sympathetic overactivity; there may also be an effect on metabolism of thyroxine (peripheral de-iodination from T4 to T3). A non-selective agent (propranolol) is preferred to counteract both the cardiac (β1 and β2) effects, and tremor (β2).

Phaeochromocytoma: blockade of β-agonist effects of circulating catecholamines always in combination with adequate α-adrenoceptor block. Only small doses of a β-blocker are required.

Other uses:

- Central nervous system:
  - *anxiety* with somatic symptoms (non-selective β-blockade may be more effective than β1-selective)
  - *migraine prophylaxis*
  - essential tremor, some cases
  - *alcohol and opioid acute withdrawal symptoms*
- Eyes:
  - glaucoma: carteolol, betaxolol, levobunolol and, timolol eye drops act by altering production and outflow of aqueous humour.

Adverse reactions due to β-adrenoceptor blockade

Bronchoconstriction (β receptor) occurs as expected, especially in patients with asthma (in whom even eye drops are dangerous). In elderly chronic bronchitics there may be gradually increasing bronchoconstriction over weeks (even with eye drops). Plainly, risk is greater with non-selective agents, but β1-receptor-selective members can still have significant β2-receptor occupancy and may precipitate asthma.

Cardiac failure may arise if cardiac output is dependent on high sympathetic drive (but β-blockade can be introduced at very low dose to treat cardiac failure; see above). The degree of heart block may be made dangerously worse.

Incapacity for vigorous exercise due to failure of the cardiovascular system to respond to sympathetic drive.

Hypotension when the drug is given after myocardial infarction.

Hypertension may occur whenever blockade of β receptors allows pre-existing α effects to be unopposed, e.g. phaeochromocytoma.

Reduced peripheral blood flow, especially with non-selective members, leading to cold extremities which, rarely, can be severe enough to cause necrosis; intermittent claudication may be worsened.

Reduced blood flow to liver and kidneys, reducing metabolism and biliary and renal elimination of drugs, is liable to be important if there is hepatic or renal disease.

Hypoglycaemia: β_2 receptors mediate both the symptoms of hypoglycaemia and the counter-regulatory metabolic responses that restore blood glucose. Non-selective β-blockers, by blocking β_2 receptors, impair the normal sympathetic-mediated homeostatic mechanism for maintaining blood glucose levels, and recovery from hypoglycaemia is delayed; this is important in diabetes and after substantial exercise. Further, as α adrenoceptors are not blocked, hypertension (which may be severe) can occur as the sympathetic system discharges in an 'attempt' to reverse the hypoglycaemia. The symptoms of hypoglycaemia, in so far as they are mediated by the sympathetic nervous system (anxiety, palpitations), will not occur, except (cholinergic) sweating, and the patient may miss the warning symptoms of hypoglycaemia and slip into coma. β_1-Selective drugs are preferred in diabetes.

Plasma lipoproteins: high-density lipoprotein (HDL) cholesterol falls and triglycerides rise during chronic β-blockade with non-selective agents. β-Selective agents have much less impact overall. Patients with hyperlipidaemia needing a β-blocker should generally receive a β_1-selective one.

Sexual function: interference is unusual and generally not supported in placebo-controlled trials.

Abrupt withdrawal of therapy can be dangerous in angina pectoris and after myocardial infarction, and withdrawal should be gradual, e.g. reduce to a low dose and continue this for a few days. The existence and cause of a β-blocker withdrawal phenomenon is debated, but probably occurs due to up-regulation of β receptors. It is particularly inadvisable to initiate an α-blocker at the same time as withdrawing a β-blocker in patients with ischaemic heart disease, because the β-blocker causes reflex activation of the sympathetic system. The β-blocker withdrawal phenomenon appears to be least common with partial agonists and most common with β-selective antagonists. Rebound hypertension is insignificant.

Adverse reactions not certainly due to β-adrenoceptor blockade

These include loss of general well-being, tired legs, fatigue, depression, sleep disturbances including insomnia, dreaming, feelings of weakness, gut upsets, rashes.

Oculomucocutaneous syndrome occurred with chronic use of practolol (now obsolete) and even occasionally after cessation of use. Other members either do not cause it, or so rarely do so that they are under suspicion only and, properly prescribed, the benefits of their use far outweigh such a very low risk. The mechanism of the syndrome is uncertain but appears immunological.

Pharmacodynamic. The effect on the blood pressure of sympathomimetics having both α- and β-receptor agonist actions is increased by block of β receptors, leaving the α-receptor vasoconstriction unopposed (even adrenaline/epinephrine added to local anaesthetics may cause hypertension); the pressor effect of abrupt clonidine withdrawal is enhanced, probably by this action. Other cardiac antiarrhythmic drugs are potentiated, e.g. hypotension, bradycardia, heart block. Combination with verapamil (i.v.) is hazardous in the presence of atrioventricular nodal or left ventricular dysfunction because the latter has stronger negative inotropic and chronotropic effects than do other calcium channel blockers.

Most non-steroidal anti-inflammatory drugs (NSAIDs) attenuate the antihypertensive effect of β-blockers (but not perhaps of atenolol), presumably due to inhibition formation of renal vasodilator prostaglandins, leading to sodium retention.

β-Adrenoceptor blockers potentiate the effect of other antihypertensives, particularly when an increase in heart rate is part of the homeostatic response (calcium channel blockers and α-adrenoceptor blockers).

Non-selective β-receptor blockers potentiate hypoglycaemia of insulin and sulphonylureas.

Pregnancy

β-Adrenoceptor-blocking agents are used in pregnancy-related hypertension, including pre-eclampsia. Both lipid-and water-soluble members enter the fetus and may cause neonatal bradycardia and hypoglycaemia. They are not teratogenic in pregnancy, but some studies have suggested they cause intrauterine growth retardation.

PERIPHERAL SYMPATHETIC NERVE TERMINAL

Adrenergic neurone-blocking drugs

Adrenergic neurone-blocking drugs are taken up into adrenergic nerve endings by the active noradrenaline/norepinephrine reuptake mechanism (uptake 1). They are relatively ineffective in reducing blood pressure except in the erect position, and their use to control hypertension is now obsolete. Guanethidine is still licensed in the UK as an option for the rapid control of blood pressure, and may also be used for regional intravenous sympathetic blockade in patients with intractable Raynaud's disease.

Metaiodobenzylguanidine (MIBG) is used diagnostically as a radio-iodinated tracer, to locate or confirm chromaffin tumours (phaeochromocytoma and neuroblastoma), which accumulate with drugs in this class.

Depletion of stored transmitter (noradrenaline/norepinephrine)

Reserpine is an alkaloid from plants of the genus Rauwolfia, used in medicine since ancient times for insanity. Reserpine depletes adrenergic nerves of noradrenaline/norepinephrine, primarily by blocking the transport of noradrenaline/norepinephrine into storage vesicles. Its antihypertensive action is chiefly a peripheral action, but it enters the CNS and depletes central catecholamine stores; this explains the sedation, depression and parkinsonian side-effects that can accompany its use. Reserpine is rarely used now that its low cost is matched by many superior classes.

Inhibition of synthesis of transmitter

Metirosine (α-methyl-p-tyrosine) is a competitive inhibitor of the enzyme tyrosine hydroxylase, which converts tyrosine to DOPA. It is occasionally used as an adjuvant (with phenoxybenzamine) to treat phaeochromocytomas that cannot be removed surgically. Catecholamine synthesis is reduced by up to 80% over 3 days. It also enters the CNS and depletes brain noradrenaline/norepinephrine and dopamine, causing reserpine-like adverse effects (see above). Hence, if life expectancy is threatened more by tumour invasion than hypertension, the need for the drug should be weighed carefully.

AUTONOMIC GANGLION-BLOCKING DRUGS

Hexamethonium was the first orally active drug to treat hypertension, but the blockade of both sympathetic and parasympathetic systems caused severe side-effects. Its use in hyperten sion is long obsolete.

Trimetaphan, a short-acting agent, is given intravenously for the emergency control of hypertension; pressure may be adjusted by tilting the body to provide 'minute to minute' control, when the lack of selectivity is useful.

CENTRAL NERVOUS SYSTEM

α₂-Adrenoceptor agonists

Clonidine is an imidazoline that is an agonist to α₂-adrenoceptors (postsynaptic) in the brain, stimulation of which suppresses sympathetic outflow and reduces blood pressure. Drugs of this type are said to be selective for an imidazoline receptor (I_1), rather than the α_2 receptor. In fact, no such receptor has been identified at the molecular level, and genetic knockout experiments have shown that it is the α_2 receptor that is required for the blood pressure-lowering action of imidazoline drugs. At high doses clonidine activates peripheral α_2-adrenoceptors (presynaptic auto receptors) on the adrenergic nerve ending; these mediate negative feedback suppression of noradrenaline/norepinephrine release.

Clonidine was discovered to be hypotensive, not by the pharmacologists who tested it in the laboratory but by a physician who used it on himself as nose drops for a common cold. The $t_{1/2}$ is 6 h. Clonidine reduces blood pressure with little postural or exercise-related drop.

Its most serious handicap is that abrupt or even gradual withdrawal causes rebound hypertension. This is characterised by plasma catecholamine concentrations as high as those seen in hypertensive attacks of phaeochromocytoma. The onset may be rapid (a few hours) or delayed for as long as 2 days; it subsides over 2–3 days. The treatment is either to reinstitute clonidine, intramuscularly if necessary, or to treat as for a phaeochromocytoma (see below). Clonidine should never be used with a β-adrenoceptor blocker that exacerbates withdrawal hypertension. Other common adverse effects include sedation and dry mouth.

Tricyclic antidepressants antagonise the antihypertensive action and increase the rebound hypertension of abrupt withdrawal. Low-dose clonidine (Dixarit 50–75 mg twice daily) also has a minor role in migraine prophylaxis, menopausal flushing and choreas.

Rebound hypertension is a less important problem with longer-acting imidazolines, e.g. moxonidine, and a single dose can be omitted without rebound.

False transmitter

Chemotransmitters and receptors in the CNS are similar to those in the periphery, and the drug in this section also has peripheral actions, as is to be expected.

Methyldopa acts in the brainstem vasomotor centres. It is a substrate (in the same manner as L-dopa) for the enzymes that synthesise noradrenaline/norepinephrine. The synthesis of α-methylnoradrenaline results in tonic stimulation of CNS α_2 receptors because α-methylnoradrenaline cannot be metabolised by monoamine oxidase, and selectively stimulates the α_2-adrenoceptor, i.e. methyldopa acts in the same way as clonidine. Methyldopa is reliably absorbed from the gastrointestinal tract and readily enters the CNS. The $t_{1/2}$ is 1.5 h.

Adverse effects include: sedation (frequent), nightmares and depression. Less common is a positive Coombs' test with haemolytic anaemia, and a rare but life-threatening adverse event is hepatitis.

For these reasons, methyldopa has long been dropped from routine management of hypertension, but remains popular with obstetricians for the hypertension of pregnancy because of its apparent safety for the fetus.

DRUG TREATMENT OF ANGINA, MYOCARDIAL INFARCTION AND HYPERTENSION

ANGINA PECTORIS

An attack of angina pectoris occurs when myocardial demand for oxygen exceeds supply from the coronary circulation. The principal forms relevant to choice of drug therapy are angina of exercise (commonest) and its worsening form, unstable (preinfarction or crescendo) angina (see below), which occurs at rest. Variant (Prinzmetal) angina (very uncommon) results from spasm of a large coronary artery.

Antiangina drugs act as follows:

- *Organic nitrates* reduce preload and afterload and dilate the main coronary arteries (rather than the arterioles).
- *β-Adrenoceptor-blocking drugs* reduce myocardial contractility and slow the heart rate. They may

increase coronary artery spasm in variant angina.

- *Calcium channel-blocking drugs* reduce cardiac contractility, dilate the coronary arteries (where there is evidence of spasm) and reduce afterload (dilate peripheral arterioles).

These classes of drug complement one another and can be used together. The combined nitrate and potassium channel activator *nicorandil* is an alternative when any of the other drugs is contraindicated.

Summary of treatment

- Any contributory cause is treated when possible, e.g.anaemia, arrhythmia.
- Lifestyle is changed so as to reduce the number of attacks. Weight reduction can be very helpful; stop smoking.
- For immediate pre-exertional prophylaxis: glyceryl trinitrate sublingually or nifedipine (bite the capsule and hold the liquid in the mouth or swallow it).
- For an acute attack: glyceryl trinitrate (sublingual) or nifedipine (bite capsule, as above).

For long-term prophylaxis:

- A β_1-adrenoceptor-blocking drug, e.g. bisoprolol, is given regularly (not merely when an attack is expected). Dosage is adjusted by response. Some put an arbitrary upper limit to dose, but others recommend that, if complete relief is not obtained, the dose should be raised to the maximum tolerated, provided the resting heart rate is not reduced below 55 beats/min; or raise the dose to a level at which an increase causes no further inhibition of exercise tachycardia. In severe angina a pure antagonist, i.e. an agent lacking partial agonist activity, is preferred, as the latter may not slow the heart sufficiently. Warn the patient of the risk of abrupt withdrawal.
- A calcium channel-blocking drug, e.g. nifedipine or diltiazem, is an alternative to a β-adrenoceptor blocker; use especially if coronary spasm is suspected or if the patient has myocardial insufficiency or any reversible airflow obstruction. It can also be used with a β-blocker, or
- A long-acting nitrate, isosorbide dinitrate or mono-

nitrate: use so as to avoid tolerance.

- Nicorandil, a long-acting potassium channel activator, does not cause tolerance like the nitrates.
- Drug therapy may be adapted to the time of attacks, e.g. nocturnal (transdermal glyceryl trinitrate, or isosorbide mononitrate orally at night).
- Antiplatelet therapy (aspirin or clopidogrel) reduces the incidence of fatal and non-fatal myocardial infarction in patients with unstable angina, used alone or with low-dose heparin.
- Revascularisation in selected cases (largely by percutaneous coronary intervention (PCI) and stenting).

Newer therapies

Ivabradine causes bradycardia and hence a reduction in myocardial work by slowing the sinus node. It does this by blocking the so-called 'pacemaker' or 'funny' current in sinoatrial (SA) nodal cells. It offers an advantage over β-blockers in being safe to use in asthmatics, but its use is limited by the curious visual disturbance it causes by blocking the same funny current in the retina. Ranolazine blocks the late sodium current and prevents calcium overload in ischaemic cardiac tissue. It also has antiarrhythmic properties and by an unknown mechanism reduces fasting blood glucose and HbA1c levels in diabetics. Nevertheless, the exact role of this agent remains to be determined.

In treating angina, it is important to remember not only the objective of reducing symptoms but also that of preventing complications, particularly myocardial infarction and sudden death. This requires vigorous treatment of all risk factors (hypertension, hyperlipidaemia, and diabetes mellitus) and, of course, cessation of smoking. There is little evidence that the symptomatic treatments, medical or surgical, themselves affect outcome except in patients with stenosis of the main stem of the left coronary artery, who require surgical intervention. Although aspirin has not been studied specifically in patients with stable angina, it is now reasonable therapy, by extrapolation from the studies of aspirin in other patient groups.

ARTERIAL HYPERTENSION

Clinical evaluation of antihypertensive drugs seeks to answer two types of question:

1. Whether long-term reduction of blood pressure benefits the patient by preventing complications and prolonging life; these studies take years, require enormous numbers of patients and are extremely costly.

2. Whether a drug is capable of effective, safe and comfortable control of blood pressure for about 1 year. There is now sufficient evidence of the benefit of reducing raised blood pressure that regulatory authorities do not demand trials of the first kind for all new drugs. Shorter studies are therefore deemed sufficient to allow the introduction of a new drug.

Aims of treatment

The long-term aim is the prevention of stroke, MI and (especially in older patients) heart failure; prevention also requires attention to other risk factors such as smoking and plasma cholesterol. The more immediate aim of treatment is to reduce the blood pressure as near to normal as possible without causing symptomatic hypotension or otherwise impairing well-being (quality of life).

When this aim is achieved in severe cases there is great symptomatic improvement: retinopathy clears and vision improves; headaches are abolished. A variable amount of irreversible damage has often been done by the high blood pressure before treatment is started; so renal failure may progress despite treatment, left ventricular hypertrophy may not fully reverse, and arterial damage leads to ischaemic events (stroke and MI).

It is desirable to start treatment before irreversible changes occur, and in mild and moderately severe cases this usually means advising treatment for symptom-free people whose hypertension was revealed by screening.

Threshold and targets for treatment

The joint NICE/British Hypertension Society guidelines require that antihypertensive drug therapy be initiated:

- when sustained blood pressure exceeds 160/100 mmHg, or
- when blood pressure is in the range 140–159/90–99 mmHg and there is evidence of target organ damage, cardiovascular disease or a 10-year cardiovascular risk greater than 20%
- for diabetics when blood pressure exceeds 140/90 mmHg.
- The optimal *target* is to lower blood pressure to 140/85 mmHg or less in all patients except those with renal impairment, in diabetics or in established cardiovascular disease where there is a lower target of less than 130/80 mmHg.

Drug therapy

Blood pressure may be reduced by any one or more of the actions listed at the beginning of this chapter. The large number of different drug classes for hypertension reduces, paradoxically, the likelihood of a randomly selected drug being the best for an individual patient. Patients and drugs can be divided broadly into two groups depending on their renin status and drug effect on this (Fig. 14.1).

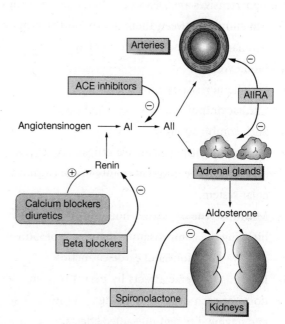

Fig. 14.1 Effects of drugs on the renin–angiotensin system. ARB, angiotensin II receptor blocker; AI/II, angiotensin I/II.

- Type 1, or high-renin patients, who respond better to an ACE inhibitor, ARB, or β-blocker.
- Type 2, or low-renin patients, in whom diuretics or calcium blockers are more likely to be effective as single agents.

As each drug acts on only one or two of the blood pressure control mechanisms, the factors that are uninfluenced by monotherapy are liable to adapt (homeostatic mechanism), to oppose the useful effect and to restore the previous state.

There are two principal mechanisms of such adaptation or tolerance:

1. Increase in blood volume: this occurs with any drug that reduces peripheral resistance (increases intravascular volume) or cardiac output (reduces glomerular flow) due to activation of the renin–angiotensin system. The result is that cardiac output and blood pressure rise. Adding a diuretic in combination with the other drug can prevent this compensatory effect.
2. Baroreceptor reflexes: a fall in blood pressure evokes reflex activity of the sympathetic system, causing increased peripheral resistance and cardiac activity (rate and contractility).

Therefore, whenever high blood pressure is proving difficult to control and whenever a number of antihypertensives are used in combination, the drugs chosen should between them act on all three main determinants of blood pressure, namely:

- Blood volume.
- Peripheral resistance.
- Cardiac output.
- Such combinations will:
- Maximise antihypertensive efficacy by exerting actions at three different points in the cardiovascular system.
- Minimise the opposing homeostatic effects by blocking the compensatory changes in blood volume, vascular tone and cardiac function.
- Minimise adverse effects by permitting smaller doses of each drug each acting at a different site and having different unwanted effects.

First-dose hypotension is now uncommon and occurs mainly with drugs having an action on veins (a adrenoceptor blockers, ACE inhibitors) when baroreflex activation is impaired, e.g. old age or with a contracted intravascular volume following diuretics.

Treating hypertension

A simple stepped regimen in keeping with the 2006 revision of the National Institute for Health and Clinical Excellence (NICE)/British Hypertension Society guidelines is the 'A/CD' schema illustrated in Figure 14.2.

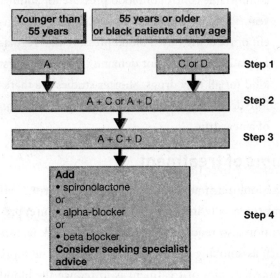

Fig. 14.2 ACD scheme for escalation of antihypertensive therapy. A, ACE inhibitor; C, calcium channel blocker; D, diuretic (see text).

1. If the patient is young (age <55 years) or non-black, use either an **A**CE inhibitor (ARB) (A). For older patients start with either a **C**alcium channel blocker or thiazide **D**iuretic as first-line therapy (C or D). If a drug is effective but not tolerated, switch to the other member of the pair.
2. If the blood pressure is not controlled at 4 weeks, a second agent should be added, using the opposite pair to the first drug, e.g. if the patient is on an ACE inhibitor add a calcium channel blocker or thiazide diuretic (A+C or A+D), as both vasodilatation or diuresis will stimulate the renin–angiotensin system and turn nonrenin-dependent hypertension into renin-dependent hypertension.
3. If blood pressure control is still inadequate on dual therapy, A + C + D is the ideal triple regimen.
4. Patients whose blood pressure remains substan-

tially above target on triple therapy should have either escalated diuretic therapy, e.g. by addition of spironolactone; or addition of α- or β-blockade. There is some evidence that a trial-and-error approach at this point can be avoided by measurement of plasma renin, with low plasma renin indicating the need for further diuretic.

Diuretics and potassium. The potassium-losing (kaliuretic) diuretics used in hypertension can deplete body potassium by up to 10%–15%. However, at low doses, e.g. bendroflumethiazide 2.5 mg/day, significant hypokalaemia is unusual, and should raise suspicion of Conn's syndrome. Vulnerable patients, e.g. the elderly, should be monitored for potassium loss at 3 months and thereafter every 6–12 months. If required, for correction of hypokalaemia, a potassium-sparing Diuretic (amiloride) in a fixed-dose combination with a thiazide (co-amilozide) is preferred over the use of fixed dose diuretic/potassium chloride formulations (most supplements, typically 8 mmol KCl, are in any case inadequate).

A potassium-sparing diuretic should be used with caution in patients who have reduced renal function or diabetes, especially if they are also receiving an ACE inhibitor or ARB.

Compliance. Multi-drug therapy poses a substantial problem of compliance. As treatment will be lifelong, it is worthwhile finding the most convenient regimen for each individual and transferring to a fixed-dose combination where possible. A single daily dose is available for most antihypertensive drugs, where necessary by using sustained-release formulations

Treatment of hypertensive emergencies

It is important to distinguish three circumstances that may exist separately or together; see the Venn diagram (Fig. 14.3) which emphasises the following:

- Severe hypertension is not on its own an indication for urgent (or large) reductions in blood pressure.
- Blood pressure can occasionally require urgent (emergency) reduction even when the hyperten-

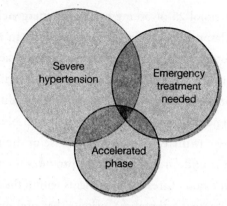

Fig. 14.3 Venn diagram illustrating intersections of three overlapping clinical states defined in the text.

sion is not severe, especially where the blood pressure has risen rapidly.

- Accelerated phase (malignant) hypertension rarely requires urgent reduction, and should instead be regarded as an indication for slow reduction in blood pressure during the first few days. The indications for emergency reduction of blood pressure are rare. They are:
- Hypertensive encephalopathy (including eclampsia).
- Acute left ventricular failure (due to hypertension).
- Dissecting aortic aneurysm.

In these conditions, blood pressure should be reduced over the course of an hour. In patients with a dissecting aneurysm, where the blood pressure may have been completely normal prior to dissection, the target is a blood pressure of about 110/70 mmHg. Otherwise even small reductions will usually remove the emergency.

Accelerated phase hypertension was previously called 'malignant' hypertension because the lack of treatment heralded death within a year of diagnosis. It is characterised pathologically by fibrinoid necrosis of the small arteries. An important consequence is the loss of autoregulation of the cerebral and renal circulation, so that any reduction in blood pressure causes a proportional fall in perfusion of these organs. It is therefore vital not to reduce diastolic blood pressure by more than 20 mmHg on the first day of treatment. To ignore this is to risk cerebral infarction.

Treatment. Unless contraindicated, the best treatment for all circles in the Venn diagram is β-blockade, e.g. Atenolol 25 or 50 mg orally. In emergencies, a vasodilator should be given intravenously in addition. A theoretically preferable, but often impractical, alternative is intravenous infusion of the vasodilator, nitroprusside. In dissecting aneurysm, vasodilators should not be used unless patients are first β-blocked, because any increase in the rate of rise of the pulse stroke is undesirable. Labetalol provides a convenient method of treating all patients within the three circles (except asthmatics), using either oral or parenteral therapy as appropriate. That said, it is not the most effective therapy and should be combined with a long-acting formulation of nifedipine, orally, where further blood pressure reduction is required.

Low doses of all drugs should be used if other antihypertensive drugs have recently been taken or renal function is impaired.

Oral maintenance treatment for severe hypertension should be started at once if possible; parenteral therapy is seldom necessary for more than 48 h.

Pregnancy hypertension

Effective treatment of pregnancy-induced hypertension improves fetal and perinatal survival. There is a lack of good clinical trial evidence on which to base recommendations. Instead, drug selection reflects longevity of use without obvious harm to the fetus and methyldopa is still the drug of choice for many obstetricians. Calcium channel blockers (especially nifedipine) are common second-line drugs; parenteral hydralazine is reserved for emergency reduction of blood pressure in late pregnancy, preferably in combination with a β-blocker to avoid unpleasant tachycardia.

β-blockers (labetalol and atenolol) are often effective and are probably the drugs of choice in the third trimester; there is anecdotal evidence to suggest growth retardation with β-blockade used in the first and second trimesters. Diuretics reduce the chance of developing preeclampsia, but are avoided in preeclampsia itself because these patients already have a contracted circulatory volume.

ACE inhibitors and angiotensin II receptor blockers (ARBs) are absolutely contraindicated during pregnancy They cause major malformations after first-trimester exposure and fetal death, typically mid-trimester. For this reason they are probably best avoided in women of childbearing age, especially where there is no effective contraception, since it is not uncommon for women to discover their pregnancy late into its first trimester. If they are used, women should be counselled to stop an ACE or ARB as soon as they suspect they are pregnant.

Raised blood pressure and proteinuria (pre-eclampsia) complicates 2–8% of pregnancies and may proceed to fitting (eclampsia), a major cause of mortality in mother and child. Magnesium sulphate halves the risk of progress to eclampsia (typically 4 g i.v. over 5–10 min followed by 1 g/h by i.v. infusion for 24 h after the last seizure). Additionally, if a woman has one fit (treat with diazepam), then the magnesium regimen is superior to diazepam or phenytoin in preventing further fits.

Aspirin, in low dose, was reported in early studies to reduce the incidence of Pre-eclampsia in at-risk patients, but a more recent meta-analysis has not supported this. Consequently, it is not routinely recommended.

PULMONARY HYPERTENSION

Idiopathic (primary) pulmonary arterial hypertension (PAH). Verapamil may give symptomatic benefit. Prostanoid formulations used to treat PAH include intravenous epoprostenol (prostacyclin) and inhaled iloprost. The prostanoid formulations have the limitations of a short half-life and a heterogeneous response to therapy. Evidence suggests that endothelin, a powerful endogenous vasoconstrictor, may play a pathogenic role; antagonists, bosentan, ambrisentan and sitoxsentan, improve symptoms and haemodyamic measurements, but dose is limited by hepatic toxicity. The PDE5 inhibitors, sildenafil, tadalafil, and vardenafil, are an alternative. Only tadalafil has been shown to improve survival, although in a comparison of the three drugs only sildenafil increased exercise tolerance. Heart and lung transplantation is recommended for younger patients.

HEART FAILURE AND ITS TREATMENT

Some physiology and pathophysiology

Cardiac output (CO) depends on the rate of contraction of the heart (HR) and the volume of blood that is ejected with each beat, the stroke volume (SV); it is expressed by the relationship:

$$CO = HR \times SV$$

The three factors that regulate the stroke volume are preload, afterload and contractility:

- Preload is the load on the heart created by the volume of blood received into the left ventricle from the left atrium (at the end of ventricular diastole) and that it must eject with each contraction. It can also be viewed as the amount of stretch to which the left ventricle is subject. As the preload rises so also do the degree of stretch and the length of cardiac muscle fibres. Preload is thus a volume load and can be excessive, e.g. when there is valvular incompetence.

- Afterload refers to the load on the contracting ventricle created by the resistance to the blood projected by the ventricle into the arterial system, i.e. the total peripheral resistance. Afterload is thus a pressure load and is excessive, e.g. in arterial hypertension.

- Contractility refers to the capacity of the myocardium to generate the force necessary to respond to preload and to overcome afterload.

Definition of chronic heart failure

As the population ages and the treatment of acute myocardial infarction improves, this condition is becoming increasingly common and there is talk of an 'epidemic' of heart failure. Chronic heart failure is present when the heart cannot provide all organs with the blood supply appropriate to demand. This definition incorporates two elements: firstly, cardiac output may be normal at rest, but secondly, when demand is increased, perfusion of the vital organs (brain and kidneys) continues at the expense of other tissues, especially skeletal muscle. Overall, systemic arterial pressure is sustained until the late stages.

These responses follow neuroendocrine activation when the heart begins to fail.

The therapeutic importance of recognising this pathophysiology is that many of the neuroendocrine abnormalities of heart failure – particularly the increased renin output and sympathetic activity – can be a consequence of drug treatment, as well as the disease. Renal perfusion is normal in early heart failure, whereas diuretics and vasodilators stimulate renin and noradrenaline/norepinephrine production through actions at the juxtaglomerular apparatus in the kidney and on the arterial baroreflex, respectively. The earliest endocrine abnormality in almost all types of cardiac disease is increased release of the heart's own hormones, the natriuretic peptides ANP and BNP (A for atrial, B for brain, where it was first discovered). The concentration in plasma of BNP provides a strong prognostic indicator for patients with all stages of heart failure. These peptides normally sup-press renin and aldosterone production, but heart failure overrides this control, and measurement of BNP now aids the diagnosis of heart failure, with a raised plasma concentration being a sensitive indicator of the disease.

The Starling curve and heart failure

The Starling curve originally described increased contractility of cardiac muscle fibres in response to increased stretch but, applied to the whole ventricle, it can explain the normal relationship between filling pressure and cardiac output (Fig. 14.4). Most patients with heart failure present in phase 'A' of the relationship, and before the 'decompensated' phase (B), in which there is gross dilatation of the ventricle. Diuretic therapy improves the congestive symptoms of heart failure, which are due to the increased filling pressure (preload), but actually reduces cardiac output in most patients. Depending on whether their predominant symptom is dyspnoea (due to pulmonary venous congestion) or fatigue (due to reduced cardiac output), patients feel better or worse. It is likely that a principal benefit of using angiotensin-converting enzyme (ACE) inhibitors in heart failure is their diuretic sparing effect.

Natural history of chronic heart failure

Injury to the heart, e.g. myocardial infarction, hypertension, leads to adaptive ('compensatory') molecular, cellular and interstitial changes that alter its size, shape and function. Myocardial hypertophy and 'remodelling' takes place over weeks or months in response to haemodynamic load, neurohormonal activation and other factors, and the resulting pattern differs according to whether the stimulus is a pressure or volume overload. With the passage of time, and with maladaption, the heart 'decompensates' and heart failure worsens. The process is outlined in Figure 14.5.

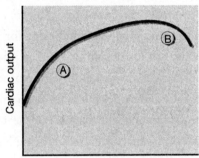

Fig. 14.4 The Starling curve of the relationship between cardiac filling pressure and cardiac output. In phase A, the curve shows that lowering the blood volume (by diuretics) will reduce the filling pressure but the cardiac output will fall. In phase B, lowering the blood volume will reduce the filling pressure but the cardiac output will increase (see text).

Fig. 14.5 Progression of ventricular disease from hypertrophy through to failure following the initial insult. The process is generically referred to as 'cardiac remodelling' and the aim of much drug therapy in heart failure treatment is to try to place a brake on this process.

The degree of activity that the patient can undertake without becoming dyspnoeic provides one useful classification of the severity of heart failure. The New York Heart Association (NYHA) classification offers also an approximate prognosis, with that of the worst grade (Class IV) being as bad as most cancers. Many patients with heart failure die from an arrhythmia, rather than from terminal decompensation, and drugs that avoid increasing the heart's exposure to increased catecholamine concentrations, as do some vasodilators (but see below), appear best for improving prognosis.

Objectives of treatment

As for cardiac arrhythmias, these are to reduce morbidity (relief of symptoms, avoid hospital admission) and mortality.

There is some tension between these two objectives in that the condition is both disabling and deadly, and the action of diuretic and some vasodilator drugs, which temporarily improve symptoms, can jeopardise survival. There is a further tension between the needs of treating the features of forwards failure, or low output, and backwards failure, or the congestive features. The principal symptom of a low cardiac output, fatigue, is difficult to quantify, and patients have tended to have their treatment tailored more to the consequences of venous congestion.

Haemodynamic aims of drug therapy

Acute or chronic failure of the heart usually results from disease of the myocardium itself, mainly ischaemic, or an excessive load imposed on it by arterial hypertension, valvular disease or an arteriovenous shunt. The management of chronic heart failure requires both the relief of any treatable underlying or aggravating cause, and therapy directed at the failure itself.

Distinguishing between the capacity of the myocardium to pump blood and the load against which the heart must work is useful in therapy. The failing myocardium is so strongly stimulated to contract by increased sympathetic drive that therapeutic efforts to induce it to function yet more vigorously are in themselves alone unlikely to be of benefit. Despite numerous candidate drugs introduced over recent years, digoxin remains the only inotropic drug suitable for chronic oral use.

By contrast, agents that reduce preload or afterload can be very effective, especially where the left ventricular volume is increased (less predictably so for failure of the right ventricle). The main hazard of their use is a drastic fall in cardiac output in those occasional patients whose output is dependent on a high left ventricular filling pressure, e.g. who are volume depleted by diuretic use or have severe mitral stenosis.

Classification of drugs

Reduction of preload

Diuretics increase salt and water loss, reduce blood volume and lower excessive venous filling pressure. They are almost invariably required to relieve the congestive features of oedema, in the lungs and the periphery; when the heart is grossly enlarged, cardiac output will also increase (see discussion of Starling curve, above). They are used flexibly, starting with a low dose; the usual sequence would be to begin with a thiazide, then move to furosemide, and in the most extreme cases then judiciously add metolazone.

Nitrates dilate the smooth muscle in venous capacitance vessels, increase the volume of the venous vascular bed (which normally may comprise 80% of the whole vascular system), reduce ventricular filling pressure, thus decreasing heart wall stretch, and reduce myocardial oxygen requirements. Their arteriolar dilating action is relatively slight. Glyceryl trinitrate provides benefit in acute left ventricular failure sublingually or by intravenous infusion. For chronic left ventricular failure nitrates have fallen out of favour, because the ACE inhibitors are more effective.

Reduction of afterload

Hydralazine relaxes arterial smooth muscle and reduces peripheral vascular resistance. Reflex tachycardia limits its usefulness and lupus erythematosus is a risk usually only if the dose exceeds 100 mg per day.

Reduction of preload and afterload

ACE inhibitors and angiotensin receptor II blockers (ARBs) act by:

- reduction of afterload, by preventing the conversion of angiotensin I to the active form, angiotensin II, or byblocking the effects of angiotensin II, which is a powerful arterioconstrictor and is present in the plasma in high concentration in heart failure

- reduction of preload, because the formation of aldosterone, and thus retention of salt and water (increased blood volume), is prevented by reducing the effects of angiotensin II.

ACE inhibitors are the only drugs that reduce peripheral resistance (afterload) without causing a reflex activation of the sympathetic system. The landmark CONSENSUS study compared enalapril with placebo in patients with NYHA class IV heart failure; after 6 months 26% of the enalapril group had died, compared with 44% in the control group. The reduction in mortality occurred among patients with progressive heart failure. There is now strong evidence from long-term studies that ACE inhibitors and ARBs improve survival in and reduce hospital admissions for heart failure.

A common practice has been to give a test dose of a short-acting ACE inhibitor (e.g. ramipril 1.25 mg by mouth) to patients who are in heart failure or on diuretic therapy for another reason, e.g. hypertension. Maintenance of blood pressure in such individuals may depend greatly on an activated renin–angiotensin–aldosterone system, and a standard dose of an ACE inhibitor or ARB can cause a sudden fall in blood pressure. That said, some of the many ACE inhibitors now available have a sufficiently prolonged action that the initial doses have a cumulative effect on blood pressure over several days. Long-acting ACE inhibitors such as lisinopril ($t_\frac{1}{2}$ 12 h) and perindopril ($t_\frac{1}{2}$ 31 h) avoid the risk of sudden falls in blood pressure or renal function (glomerular filtration) after the first dose. Such drugs can be initiated outside hospital in patients who are unlikely to have a high plasma renin (absence of gross oedema or widespread atherosclerotic disease), although it is prudent to arrange for the first dose to be taken just before going to bed. Therapy begins with an ACE inhibitor, and an ARB is substituted if there is intolerance, or added if symptoms continue.

β-Adrenoceptor blockers. The realisation that activation of the renin–angiotensin–aldosterone and sympathetic nervous systems can adversely affect the course of chronic heart failure led to exploration of the possible benefits in heart failure from blockade of β-adrenoceptors. Clinical trials have, indeed, shown that bisoprolol, carvedilol or metoprolol lower mortality and decrease hospitalisation when added to conventional treatment that is likely to include diuretics, digoxin and an ACE inhibitor.

Spironolactone. Plasma aldosterone levels are raised in heart failure. Spironolactone acts as a diuretic by competitively blocking the aldosterone receptor, but in addition it has a powerful effect on outcome in heart failure. Eplerenone, an alternative mineralocorticoid antagonist, also has beneficial effects including in mild to moderate heart failure.

Stimulation of the myocardium

Digoxin improves myocardial contractility (positive inotropic effect) most effectively in the dilated, failing heart and, in the longer term, after an episode of heart failure has been brought under control. This effect occurs in patients in sinus rhythm and is distinct from its (negative chronotropic) action of reducing ventricular rate and thus improving ventricular filling in atrial fibrillation. Over 200 years after the first use of digitalis for dropsy, the DIG trial provided relief for doctors seeking evidence of longterm benefit. Unlike all other positive inotropes, digoxin does not increase overall mortality or arrhythmias.

The phosphodiesterase inhibitors enoximone and milrinone have positive inotropic effects due to selective myocardial enzyme inhibition and may be used for short-term treatment of severe congestive heart failure. Evidence from longer-term use indicates that these drugs reduce survival.

A scheme for the stepwise drug management of chronic heart failure appears in Figure 14.6. Points to emphasise in this scheme are that all patients, even those with mild heart failure, should receive an ACE inhibitor as first-line therapy. Several long-term studies have demonstrated improved survival even when cardiac failure is mild.

Diuretic therapy is very useful for symptom management but has no impact on survival. For most patients the choice will be a loop diuretic, e.g. furosemide starting at 20–40 mg/day. Because of the potassium-sparing effect of ACE inhibition, amiloride (also potassium sparing) is often not required, at least with low doses of a loop diuretic.

There is now overwhelming evidence for the benefit of β-blockers in chronic heart failure, despite the long-held belief that their negative inotropic effect was a contraindication. Early trials were underpowered but a meta-analysis did suggest a 31% reduction in the mortality rate. Subsequently, the CIBIS-2 and MERIT-HF trials, have independently confirmed that chronic β-blockade has a survival effect of this size in moderate to severe (NHYA III/IV) heart failure. Both studies confirmed the one-third reduction in mortality. In MERIT-HF a life was saved for just 27 patient years of treatment, i.e. it was unusually cost effective – more so than ACE inhibitor therapy. The action is probably a class effect of β-blockade, given the divergent pharmacology of the drugs used to date.

The reduction in mortality is additive to ACE inhibition and the survival benefit is largely through a decrease in sudden deaths as opposed to a reduction in progressive pump failure seen with ACE inhibitors. The only cautionary note is that patients must be β-blocked very gradually from low starting doses (e.g. bisoprolol 1.25 mg/day or carvedilol 3.125 mg twice daily) with regular optimisation of the dose of other drugs, especially the loop diuretic, to prevent decompensation of heart failure control.

The use of spironolactone has received considerable support from the RALES trial, which implies that ACE inhibition even at high dose does not effectively suppress hyperaldosteronism in heart failure. The benefit occurs at a surprisingly low dose of spironolactone (25 mg/day); it probably reflects both improved potassium and magnesium conservation

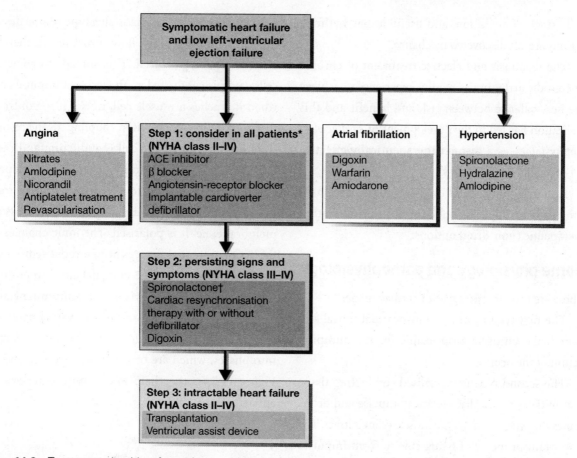

Fig. 14.6 Treatment algorithm for patients with heart failure and reduced left ventricular systolic function. *These treatments generally supplement existing diuretic drugs, with flexible dosing to maintain dry weight; consider hydralazine plus isosorbide dinitrate for patients, as clinical trials indicate a favourable response in this subgroup. † The safety and efficacy of the combination of an ACE inhibitor, an ARB, and an aldosterone antagonist are unknown.

(both are antiarrhythmic) and reversal of fibrosis in the myocardium by aldosterone.

None of the available oral phosphodiesterase inhibitors is established in routine therapy, because the short-term benefit of the increased contractility is offset by an increased mortality rate (presumably due to arrhythmias) on chronic dosing. Their use is restricted to short-term symptom control prior to, for example, transplantation.

Part 2. Cardiac arrhythmia

INTRODUCTION

Objectives of treatment

In almost no other set of conditions is it so clearly obvious to remember the dual objectives, which are to reduce morbidity and mortality.

Arrhythmias are frequently asymptomatic but may be fatal even at first presentation. Antiarrhythmic drugs themselves are also capable of generating arrhythmias (see below) and find use only in the presence of clear indications. In addition, antiarrhythmic agents are to a variable degree negatively inotropic (except for digoxin and possibly amiodarone). These observations provide important primary reasons for caution in the use of these drugs.

A background reason for a careful approach to antiarrhythmic treatment is the gulf between knowledge of their mechanism of action and their clinical uses. On the side of normal physiology, we can see the spontaneous generation and propagation of the cardiac impulse requiring a combination of specialised conducting tissue and inter-myocyte conduction. The heart also has backstops in case of problems with a sequential hierarchy of intrinsic pacemakers. By contrast, the available drugs are at an early stage of evolution, and useful antiarrhythmic actions are yet discovered by chance.

The diagnosis and elective treatment of chronic or episodic arrhythmias require experience to achieve the best balance between risk and benefit and this realization has led to the development of *cardiac electrophysiology* as a distinct therapeutically effective subspeciality of cardiology.

Antiarrhythmic drugs in general have had a hard time proving superior safety or efficacy over other therapeutic (non-drug) options.

Some physiology and pathophysiology

There are broadly two types of cardiac tissue.

The first type is ordinary myocardial (atrial and ventricular) muscle, responsible for the pumping action of the heart.

The second type is specialised conducting tissue that initiates the cardiac electrical impulse and determines the order in which the muscle cells contract. The important property of being able to form impulses spontaneously (automaticity) is a feature of certain parts of the conducting tissue e.g. the sinoatrial (SA) and atrioventricular (AV) nodes. The SA node has the highest frequency of spontaneous discharge, usually around 70 times per minute, and thus controls the contraction rate of the whole heart, making the cells more distal in the system fire more rapidly than they would do spontaneously, i.e. it is the pacemaker. If the SA node fails to function, the next fastest component takes over. This is often the AV node (approx. 45 discharges per min) or sites in the His–Purkinje system (discharge rate about 25 per min).

Altered rates of automatic discharge or an abnormality in the mechanism by which an impulse is generated from a centre in the nodes or conducting tissue, is one cause of cardiac arrhythmia, e.g. atrial fibrillation, atrial flutter or atrial tachycardia.

Ionic movements into and out of cardiac cells

Nearly all cells in the body exhibit a difference in electrical voltage between their interior and exterior, the membrane potential. Some cells, including the conducting and contracting cells of the heart, are excit-

able; an appropriate stimulus alters the properties of the cell membrane, ions flow across it and thereby elicit an action potential. This spreads to adjacent cells, i.e. it is conducted as an electrical impulse and, when it reaches a muscle cell, causes it to contract; this is excitation–contraction coupling. In the resting state the interior of the cell (conducting and contracting types) is electrically negative with respect to the exterior, owing to the disposition of ions (mainly sodium, potassium and calcium) across its membrane, i.e. it is polarised. The ionic changes of the action potential first result in a rapid redistribution of ions such that the potential alters to positive within the cell (depolarisation); subsequent and slower flows of ions then restore the resting potential (repolarisation). These ionic movements separate into phases, which are briefly described here and in Figure 14.7, as they help to explain the actions of antiarrhythmic drugs.

Fig. 14.7 The action potential of a cardiac cell that is capable of spontaneous depolarisation (SA or AV nodal, or His–Purkinje) indicating phases 0–4. The gradual increase in transmembrane potential (mV) during phase 4 is shown; cells that are not capable of spontaneous depolarisation do not exhibit increased voltage during this phase (see text). The modes of action of antiarrhythmic drugs of classes I, II, III and IV are indicated in relation to these phases.

CLASSIFICATION OF ANTIAR-RHYTHMIC DRUGS

The classification still used partially relates to the phases of the cardiac cycle depicted in Figure 14.8.

Phase 0 is the rapid depolarisation of the cell

membrane that is associated with a fast inflow of sodium ions through channels that are selectively permeable to these ions.

Phase 1 is a short initial period of rapid repolarization brought about mainly by an outflow of potassium ions.

Phase 2 is a period when there is a delay in repolarization caused mainly by a slow movement of calcium ions from the exterior into the cell through channels that are selectively permeable to these ions ('long-opening' or L-type calcium channels).

Phase 3 is a second period of rapid repolarisation during which potassium ions move out of the cell.

Phase 4 begins with the fully repolarised state. For cells that discharge automatically, potassium ions then progressively move back into, and sodium and calcium ions move out of, the cell. The result is that the interior becomes gradually less negative until a certain (threshold) potential is reached, which allows rapid depolarisation (phase 0) to occur, and the cycle is repeated; the prevailing sympathetic tone also influences automaticity. Cells that do not discharge spontaneously rely on the arrival of an action potential from another cell to initiate depolarisation.

In phases 1 and 2 the cell is in an absolutely refractory state and is incapable of responding further to any stimulus, but during phase 3, the relative refractory period, the cell will depolarise again if a stimulus is sufficiently strong. The orderly transmission of an electrical impulse (the action potential) throughout the conducting system may be retarded in an area of disease, e.g. localised ischaemia or scar tissue due to previous myocardial infarction. An impulse travelling down a normal Purkinje fibre may spread to an adjacent fibre that has transiently failed to transmit, and pass up it in the reverse direction. Should such a retrograde impulse in turn re-excite the cells that provided the original impulse, re-entrant excitation becomes established and may cause an arrhythmia, e.g. ventricular tachycardia, paroxysmal supraventricular tachycardia, atrial flutter, etc.

Most cardiac arrhythmias are due to either:

- slowed conduction in part of the system leading to the formation of re-entry circuits (more than 90% of tachycardias), or
- altered rate of spontaneous discharge in conducting tissue. Some ectopic pacemakers appear to depend on adrenergic drive.

Classification of drugs

The Vaughan–Williams classification of antiarrhythmic drugs is still commonly used despite its many peculiarities, and on occasion provides a useful shorthand for referring to particular groups or actions of drugs.

Class I: sodium channel blockade. These drugs restrict the rapid inflow of sodium during phase 0 and thus slow the maximum rate of depolarisation. Another term for this property is membrane stabilising activity; the action may contribute to stopping arrhythmias by limiting the responsiveness to excitation of cardiac cells. The class subdivides into drugs that:

I A. lengthen action potential duration and refractoriness (adjunctive class III action), e.g. quinidine, disopyramide, procainamide

I B. shorten action potential duration and refractoriness, e.g. lidocaine and mexiletine

I C. have negligible effect on action potential duration and refractoriness, e.g. flecainide, propafenone.

One value of using the classification is the knowledge that drugs in class 1B are ineffective for supraventricular arrhythmias, whereas they all have some action in ventricular arrhythmias. One feature is that it is not useful in explaining why the classes differ anatomically in their efficacy.

Class II: catecholamine blockade. Propranolol and other b-adrenoceptor antagonists reduce background sympathetic tone in the heart, reduce automatic discharge (phase 4) and protect against adrenergically stimulated ectopic pacemakers.

Class III: lengthening of refractoriness (without effect on sodium inflow in phase 0). Prolongation of the cardiac action potential and increased cellular refractoriness beyond a critical point may stop a re-entrant circuit being completed and thereby prevent or halt a re-entrant arrhythmia (see above), e.g. amiodarone, sotalol. These drugs act by inhibiting I_{Kr}, the rapidly activating component of the delayed rectifier potassium current (phase 3). The gene hERG (*the human ether-à-go-go related gene*) encodes a major subunit of the protein responsible for I_{Kr}. These are the most commonly used antiarrhythmic drugs and while some newer agents in this class, e.g. dofetilide and azimilide, have not achieved wide use, dronedarone is being increasingly prescribed.

Class IV : calcium channel blockade. These drugs depress the slow inward calcium current (phase 2) and prolong conduction and refractoriness particularly in the SA and AV nodes, which helps to explain their effectiveness in terminating paroxysmal supraventricular tachycardia, e.g. verapamil.

Antiarrhythmic drugs are classified here according to a characteristic major action but most have other effects as well. For example, quinidine (class I) has major class III effects, propranolol (class II) has minor class I effects, and sotalol (class III) has major class III effects. Amiodarone and dronedarone both have class I, II, III and IV effects but are usually placed under class III.

PRINCIPAL DRUGS BY CLASS

Class I A (sodium channel blockade with lengthened refractoriness)

Quinidine

Quinidine is considered the prototype antiarrhythmic drug, although it is now used quite rarely and indeed is not available in some jurisdictions. It has a newly identified use that is unique in that it appears to be effective in reducing the risks of sudden cardiac death in those with Brugada syndrome. In addition to its class IA activity, quinidine slightly enhances contractility of the myocardium (positive inotropic effect) and reduces vagus nerve activity on the heart (antimuscarinic effect).

Pharmacokinetics. Absorption of quinidine from the gut is rapid; 75% of the drug is metabolised and the remainder is eliminated unchanged in the urine ($t_{\frac{1}{2}}$ 7 h). Active metabolites may accumulate when renal function is impaired.

Adverse reactions. Quinidine must not be used alone to treat atrial fibrillation or flutter as its antimuscarinic action enhances AV conduction and the heart rate may accelerate. Other cardiac effects include serious ventricular tachyarrhythmias associated with electrocardiographic QT prolongation, i.e. torsade de pointes (Fig. 14.8), the cause of 'quinidine syncope'. Non-cardiac effects, called 'cinchonism', include diarrhoea and other gastrointestinal symptoms, rashes, thromobocytopenia and fever, and these have substantially limited its use.

Disopyramide

Disopyramide was the most commonly used drug in this class but is much less so now. It has significant antimuscarinic activity.

Pharmacokinetics. Disopyramide is used orally and is well absorbed. It is in part excreted unchanged and in part metabolised. The $t_{\frac{1}{2}}$ is 6 h.

Adverse reactions. The antimuscarinic activity is often a significant clinical problem causing dry mouth, blurred vision, glaucoma, micturition hesitancy and retention. Gastrointestinal symptoms, rash and agranulocytosis can also occur. Effects on the cardiovascular system include hypotension and heart failure (negative inotropic effect).

Fig. 14.8 Torsade de pointes ventricular arrhythmia. This patient had received the potassium channel blocking drug, amiodarone, which prolonged the QTc interval and produced this characteristic 'twisting about the points' pattern.

Class I B (sodium channel blockade with shortened refractoriness)

Lidocaine

Lidocaine finds use principally for ventricular arrhythmias, especially those complicating myocardial infarction or occurring, e.g., after cardiothoracic surgery. Its kinetics render it unsuitable for oral administration and its application is restricted to the treatment of acute ventricular arrhythmias.

Pharmacokinetics. Lidocaine is used intravenously and has occasionally been used intramuscularly; dosing by mouth is unsatisfactory because its $t_{1/2}$ is short (1.5 h) and the drug undergoes extensive pre-systemic (first-pass) elimination in the liver.

Adverse reactions are uncommon unless infusion is rapid or there is significant heart failure; they include hypotension, dizziness, blurred sight, sleepiness, slurred speech, numbness, sweating, confusion and convulsions.

Mexiletine. is similar to lidocaine but is effective orally ($t_{1/2}$ 10 h). It has been used for ventricular arrhythmias, especially those complicating myocardial infarction, but is usually poorly tolerated and has been withdrawn in many jurisdictions.

Adverse reactions, almost universal and dose related, include nausea, vomiting, hiccough, tremor, drowsiness, confusion, dysarthria, diplopia, ataxia, cardiac arrhythmia and hypotension.

Class I C (sodium channel blockade with minimal effect on refractoriness)

Flecainide

Flecainide slows conduction in all cardiac cells including the accessory pathways responsible for the Wolff–Parkinson–White (WPW) syndrome.

One common indication – indeed where it is the drug of choice – is atrioventricular (AV) re-entrant tachycardia, such as AV nodal tachycardia or in the tachycardias associated with the WPW syndrome or similar conditions with anomalous pathways. This should be as a prelude to definitive treatment with radiofrequency ablation, which is the overall treatment approach of choice. Flecainide is also very useful in patients with paroxysmal atrial fibrillation, used in conjunction with an agent that blocks the AV node to protect against rapid conduction to the ventricle. Following the salutary findings of the CAST study, flecainide is now restricted to patients without evidence of coronary or structural heart disease. Indeed before it is used an echocardiogram is essential, and in patients at potential risk of coronary artery disease an exercise test or an alternative test of ischaemia is often conducted.

Pharmacokinetics. Metabolism in the liver and renal elimination of unchanged metabolites terminates its action. The $t_{1/2}$ is 14 h in healthy adults but may be over 20 h in patients with heart disease, in the elderly and in those with poor renal function.

Adverse reactions. Flecainide is contraindicated in patients with sinus node disease, heart failure, and in those with a history of myocardial infarction, especially if they have a history of ventricular arrhythmias. Minor adverse effects include blurred vision, abdominal discomfort, nausea, dizziness, tremor, abnormal taste sensations and paraesthesiae.

Propafenone

In addition to the defining properties of this class, propafenone has β-adrenoceptor blocking activity equivalent to a low dose of propranolol. It is occasionally used to suppress non-sustained ventricular arrhythmias in patients whose left ventricular function is normal.

Pharmacokinetics. Propafenone is metabolised by the liver and is a substrate for CYP 2D6. Some 7% of Caucasian patients are poor metabolisers who, for equivalent doses, thus have higher plasma concentrations than the remainder of the population.

Adverse reactions are similar to those of flecainide and are commoner in poor metabolisers. In addition, conduction block may occur, heart failure may worsen and ventricular arrhythmias may be exacerbated, and propafenone should not be used in patients with sustained ventricular tachycardia and poor left ventricular function.

Class II (catecholamine blockade)

β-Adrenoceptor blockers are effective in the prophylaxis of cardiac arrhythmia probably because they counteract the arrhythmogenic effect of catecholamines. The following actions appear to be relevant:

- The rate of automatic firing of the SA node is accelerated by β-adrenoceptor activation and this effect is abolished by β-blockers. Some ectopic pacemakers appear to be dependent on adrenergic drive.
- β-blockers prolong the refractoriness of the AV node, which may prevent re-entrant tachycardias that are dependent on the AV node for their perpetuation.
- Many β-blocking drugs (propranolol, oxprenolol, acebutolol, labetalol) also possess membrane stabilising (class I) properties. Sotalol also prolongs cardiac refractoriness (class III effect) but has no class I effects; it is often preferred when a β-blocker is indicated for arrhythmias, but should be used with care. Esmolol (below) is a short-acting β_1 –selective agent, whose sole use is in the treatment of arrhythmias. Its short duration and β_1 selectivity make it an option for some patients with contraindications to other β-blocking drugs.
- β-Adrenoceptor antagonists are effective for a range of supraventricular arrhythmias, in particular those associated with exercise, emotion or hyperthyroidism. Sotalol finds use to suppress ventricular ectopic beats and ventricular tachycardia although care should be taken with careful monitoring of the QT interval whenever it is used.

Pharmacokinetics. For long-term use, any of the oral preparations of β-blocker are suitable. In emergencies, esmolol is used, its short $t_{1/2}$ (9 min) rendering it suitable for administration by intravenous infusion with rapid alterations in dose, according to response.

Adverse reactions. Cardiac effects from overdosage include heart block or even cardiac arrest. Heart failure may be precipitated in a patient dependent on sympathetic drive to maintain cardiac output.

Interactions. Concomitant intravenous administration of a calcium channel blocker that affects conduction (verapamil, diltiazem) increases the risk of bradycardia and AV block. In patients with depressed myocardial contractility, the combination of oral or intravenous β-blockade and calcium channel blockade (nifedipine, verapamil) may cause hypotension or heart failure.

Class III (lengthening of refractoriness due to potassium channel blockade)

Amiodarone

Amiodarone is the most powerful antiarrhythmic drug available for the treatment and prevention of both atrial and ventricular arrhythmias. Even short-term use can result in serious toxicity, and its use should always follow a consideration or a trial of alternatives. Amiodarone prolongs the effective refractory period of myocardial cells, the AV node and of anomalous pathways. It also blocks β-adrenoceptors non-competitively.

Amiodarone is used in chronic ventricular arrhythmias and in atrial fibrillation, in which condition it both slows the ventricular response and may restore sinus rhythm (chemical cardioversion). It may also be used to maintain sinus rhythm after cardioversion for atrial fibrillation or flutter. Amiodarone has been used for the management of re-entrant supraventricular tachycardias associated with the WPW syndrome, but radiofrequency ablation is now the treatment of choice and amiodarone should not in general be used.

Pharmacokinetics. Amiodarone is effective given orally; its enormous apparent distribution volume (70 L/kg) indicates that little remains in the blood. It is stored in fat and many other tissues and the $t_{1/2}$ of 54 days after multiple dosing signifies slow release from these sites (and slow accumulation to steady state means that a loading dose is necessary). The drug is metabolised in the liver and eliminated through the biliary and intestinal tracts.

Adverse reactions. Cardiovascular effects include bradycardia, heart block and induction of ventricular arrhythmia associated with QT prolongation. Other effects include nausea, vomiting, taste disturbances and the development of corneal microdeposits, which may rarely cause visual halos, night glare and photophobia; the latter are dose related, resolve on discontinuation and do not threaten vision. Sleep disturbance and vivid dreams may be prominent and problematic. Plasma transaminase levels may rise (requiring dose reduction or withdrawal if accompanied by acute liver disorders). Amiodarone contains iodine, and both hyperthyroidism and hypothyroidism are quite common; monitoring thyroid function before and during therapy is essential.

Photosensitivity reactions are common, may be severe and patients should be warned explicitly when starting the drug. Amiodarone may also cause a bluish discoloration on exposed areas of the skin (occasionally reversible on discontinuing the drug). Less commonly, pneumonitis and pulmonary fibrosis occur and hepatitis, sometimes rapidly during short-term use of the drug; these may be fatal, so vigilance should be high. Cirrhosis is reported. Peripheral neuropathy and myopathy occur (usually reversible on withdrawal).

Interaction with digoxin (by displacement from tissue binding sites and interference with its elimination) and with warfarin (by inhibiting its metabolism) increases the effect of both these drugs. β-blockers and calcium channel antagonists augment the depressant effect of amiodarone on SA and AV node function.

Dronedarone

While amiodarone is less pro-arrhythmic than other conventional antiarrhythmic drugs, e.g. flecainide (possibly because it is a 'multi-channel blocker'), it has substantial non-cardiac toxic effects. Dronedarone is structurally similar to amiodarone but has no iodine component and reduced lipophilicity. Dronedarone thus has a shorter half-life and appears better tolerated, with low pro-arrhythmic risk. Dronedarone has been shown to reduce the time to first recurrence of atrial fibrillation. In the EURIDIS and ADONIS clinical trials patients taking dronedarone had a 25% reduction in the risk of AF

recurrence over one year, compared with placebo. In the ATHENA study, dronedarone also reduced the combined risk of cardiovascular hospitalisation or all-cause death by 24% in patients with current or recent AF and an additional risk factor for death, compared with placebo. A post hoc analysis found that dronedarone, compared with placebo, was associated with a significant reduction in the risk of stroke in paroxysmal and persistent AF patients. Data from the DIONYSOS trial suggest that dronedarone may have an improved safety profile when compared to amiodarone, mainly driven by fewer thyroid and neurologic events and less premature discontinuation due to adverse events.

Pharmacokinetics. The absolute bioavailability of dronedarone (given with food) is 15%. It undergoes extensive first-pass metabolism through the CYP 450 3A4 system; hence strong inhibitors of this enzyme should not be coadministered with dronedarone. After oral administration in fed conditions, peak plasma concentrations of dronedarone are reached within 3–6 hours. Steady state is reached within 4–8 days. Dronedarone is mostly excreted in the faeces with only 6% excreted renally, and it has an elimination half-life of 28 h.

Contraindications. Dronedarone is contraindicated in patients with unstable haemodynamic conditions, including patients with symptoms of heart failure at rest or with minimal exertion (corresponding with NYHA class IV and unstable class III patients). Dronedarone is not recommended in stable patients with recent (1–3 months) NYHA class III heart failure, or left ventricular ejection fraction <35%. Patients should consult their doctor if they experience worsening heart failure symptoms.

Due to pharmacokinetic and possible pharmacodynamic interactions, both β-blockers and calcium channel blockers with depressant effects on the sinus and atrioventricular nodes (such as verapamil and diltiazem) should be used with caution when prescribed with dronedarone. They should be initiated at low dose, which should only be increased after ECG assessment. In patients already taking β-blockers or calcium channel blockers, an ECG should be performed and the β-blocker/calcium channel blocker dose should be adjusted if needed.

Unwanted effects. Common side-effects include diarrhoea, abdominal discomfort, nausea, vomiting, and prolonged QT interval. Supportive symptomatic treatment should be provided, and attention should be paid to hydration in those most severely affected. In a proportion of patients, dronedarone may need to be discontinued because of intolerance. There is an increased incidence of skin rash and bradycardia.

Plasma creatinine should be measured 7 days after starting dronedarone, as an increase of approximately 10 micromol/L has been observed with dronedarone 400 mg twice daily in both healthy controls and in patients. This occurs early after treatment initiation and reaches a plateau after 7 days.

Recently released European Society of Cardiology guidelines have included dronedarone as a treatment option for non-permanent AF for rhythm and rate control (Fig. 14.9).

Class IV (calcium channel blockade)

Calcium is involved in the contraction of cardiac and vascular smooth muscle cells, and in the automaticity of cardiac pacemaker cells.. Although the three classes of calcium channel blocker have similar effects on vascular smooth muscle in the arterial tree, their cardiac actions differ. The phenylalkylamine, verapamil, depresses myocardial contraction more than the others, and both verapamil and diltiazem slow conduction in the AV node.

Calcium and cardiac cells

Cardiac muscle cells are normally depolarised by the fast inward flow of sodium ions, following which there is a slow inward flow of calcium ions through the L-type calcium channels (phase 2 in Figure 14.8); the consequent rise in free intracellular calcium ions activates the contractile mechanism.

Pacemaker cells in the SA and AV nodes rely heavily on the slow inward flow of calcium ions (phase 4) for their capacity to discharge spontaneously, i.e. for their automaticity.

Calcium channel blockers inhibit the passage of

calcium through the membrane channels; the result in myocardial cells is to depress contractility, and in pacemaker cells to suppress their automatic activity. Members of the group therefore may have negative cardiac inotropic and chronotropic actions, which can be separated: nifedipine, at therapeutic concentrations, acts almost exclusively on non-cardiac ion channels and has no clinically useful antiarrhythmic activity, whereas verapamil is an effective rate control agent.

Verapamil

Verapamil prolongs conduction and refractoriness in the AV node and depresses the rate of discharge of the SA node. If adenosine is not available, verapamil is a very attractive and, with due care, safe alternative for terminating narrow complex paroxysmal supraventricular tachycardia. Verapamil should not be given intravenously to patients with broad complex tachyarrhythmias whatever the presumptive mechanism, for it may prove lethal.

Adverse effects. include nausea, constipation, headache, fatigue, hypotension, bradycardia and heart block.

Other antiarrhythmics

Digoxin and other cardiac glycosides

Digitalis contains a number of active glycosides (digoxin, lanatosides) whose actions are qualitatively similar, differing principally in rapidity of onset and duration of action; the pure individual glycosides are used. The following account refers to all the cardiac glycosides, but digoxin is the principal one.

Mode of action. Cardiac glycosides affect the heart both directly and indirectly in a series of complex actions, some of which oppose one another. The direct effect is to inhibit the membrane-bound sodium–potassium adenosine triphosphatase (Na^+, K^+-ATPase) enzyme that supplies energy for the system that pumps sodium out of and transports potassium into contracting and conducting cells. By reducing the exchange of extracellular sodium with intracellular calcium, digoxin raises the store of

Fig. 14.9 Algorithm for the management of acute bradycardia. mcg, micrograms. Reproduced with the kind permission of the Resuscitation Council (UK).

intracellular calcium, which facilitates muscular contraction. The indirect effect is to enhance vagal activity by complex peripheral and central mechanisms. The clinically important consequences are on:

- the contracting cells: increased contractility and excitability
- SA and AV nodes and conducting tissue: decreased impulse generation and propagation.

Uses. Digoxin is not strictly an antiarrhythmic agent but rather it modulates the response to arrhythmias. Its most useful property, in this respect, is to slow conduction through the AV node. The main uses are in the following:

- Atrial fibrillation, benefiting chiefly by the vagal effect on the AV node, reducing conduction through it and thus slowing the ventricular rate. Its use in this setting is limited and treatment with β-blockers and calcium channel blockers is generally preferred as they are more effective and less likely to cause adverse effects.
- *Atrial flutter*, benefiting by the vagus nerve action of shortening the refractory period of the atrial muscle so that flutter may occasionally be converted to fibrillation (in which state the ventricular rate is more readily controlled). Electrical cardioversion followed by referral for radiofrequency

ablation is the preferred option when ablation is available.

- *Heart failure*, benefiting chiefly by the direct action to increase myocardial contractility. Digoxin is still used occasionally in chronic heart failure due to ischaemic, hypertensive or valvular heart disease, especially in the short term. This is no longer a major indication following the introduction of other groups of drugs.

Pharmacokinetics. Digoxin is eliminated 85% unchanged by the kidney and the remainder is metabolised by the liver. The $t_{\frac{1}{2}}$ is 36 h. Digoxin is usually administered by mouth.

Adverse effects. Abnormal cardiac rhythms due to digoxin usually take the form of ectopic arrhythmias (ventricular ectopic beats, ventricular tachyarrhythmias, paroxysmal supraventricular tachycardia) and heart block. Gastrointestinal effects include anorexia, which usually precedes vomiting and is a warning that dosage is excessive. Diarrhoea may also occur. Visual effects include disturbances of colour vision, e.g. yellow discolouration (xanthopsia) but also red or green vision, photophobia and blurring. Gynaecomastia in men and breast enlargement in women is seen with long-term use (cardiac glycosides have structural resemblance to oestrogen). Mental effects include confusion, restlessness, agitation, nightmares and acute psychoses.

Acute digoxin poisoning causes initial nausea and vomiting and hyperkalaemia because inhibition of the Na^+, K^+-ATPase pump prevents intracellular accumulation of potassium. The ECG changes of prolonged use of digoxin may be absent. There may be exaggerated sinus arrhythmia, bradycardia and ectopic rhythms with or without heart block.

Treatment of overdose. For severe digoxin poisoning, infusion of the digoxin-specific binding (Fab) fragment of an antibody to digoxin (Digibind) neutralises digoxin in the plasma and is an effective treatment. Because it lacks the Fc segment, this fragment is relatively non-immunogenic and is sufficiently small to be eliminated as the digoxin–antibody complex in the urine. Intravenous phenytoin has been used for ventricular arrhythmias although formal efficacy has not been established, with atropine used for bradycardia. Temporary electrical pacing may be needed.

Interactions. Verapamil, nifedipine and amiodarone raise steady-state plasma digoxin concentrations (see above) and the digoxin dose should be lowered when any of these is added. The likelihood of AV block due to digoxin is increased by verapamil and by β-adrenoceptor blockers.

Adenosine

Adenosine is an endogenous purine nucleotide that slows atrioventricular conduction and dilates coronary and peripheral arteries. It is rapidly metabolised by circulating adenosine deaminase and is also taken up by cells; hence its residence in plasma is brief ($t_{\frac{1}{2}}$ <2 s) and it must be given rapidly intravenously.

Administered as a bolus injection, adenosine is effective for terminating paroxysmal supraventricular (re-entrant) tachycardias, including episodes in patients with Wolff–Parkinson–White syndrome. The initial dose in adults is 6 mg over 2 s with continuous ECG monitoring, with doubling increments every 1–2 min. The average total dose is 125 micrograms/kg.

Adenosine is an alternative to verapamil for supraventricular tachycardia and possibly safer because adenosine is short acting and not negatively inotropic; verapamil is dangerous if used mistakenly in a ventricular tachycardia.

Adverse effects from adenosine are usually not serious because of the brevity of its action, but it may cause distressing dyspnoea, facial flushing, chest pain and transient arrhythmias, e.g. bradycardia. Adenosine should not be given to asthmatics or to patients with second- or third-degree AV block or sick sinus syndrome (unless a pacemaker is in place).

Proarrhythmic drug effects

All antiarrhythmic drugs can also cause arrhythmia; they should be used with care and almost invariably following advice from a specialist (heart rhythm specialist/electrophysiologist). Such proarrhythmic effects most commonly occur with drugs that prolong the QTc interval or QRS complex of the ECG; hypokalaemia aggravates the danger. Quinidine may cause tachyarrhythmias, torsade de pointes (Fig. 14.9) in an estimated 4–6% of patients. The Cardiac Arrhythmia Suppression Trial (CAST) revealed a probable pro-arrhythmic effect of flecainide resulting in fatalities. Digoxin can induce a variety of bradyarrhythmias and tachyarrhythmias (see above).

Choice between drugs and electro-conversion

Direct current (DC) electric shock applied externally is often the best way to convert cardiac arrhythmias to sinus rhythm. Many atrial or ventricular arrhythmias start from transiently operating factors but, once they have begun, the abnormal mechanisms are self-sustaining. With a successful electric shock, the heart is depolarised, the ectopic focus is extinguished and the SA node, the part of the heart with the highest automaticity, resumes as the dominant pacemaker.

Electrical conversion has the advantage that it is immediate, unlike drugs, which may take days or longer to act; also, the effective doses and adverse effects of drugs are largely unpredictable, and can be serious.

Uses of electrical conversion: in supraventricular and ventricular tachycardia, ventricular fibrillation and atrial fibrillation and flutter. Drugs can be useful to prevent a relapse, e.g. sotalol, amiodarone. See also the UK Resuscitation Council's guidelines (Figs 14.10–14.12).

Fig. 14.10 Algorithm for the management of acute tachycardia. Reproduced with the kind permission of the Resuscitation Council (UK).

Adult
Advanced Life
Support

Fig. 14.11 Adult advanced life support. Reproduced with the kind permission of the Resuscitation Council (UK).

Part 3. Hyperlipidaemias

SOME PATHOPHYSIOLOGY

The normal function of lipoproteins is to distribute and recycle cholesterol. The pathways of lipid metabolism and transport and their primary (inherited) disorders are shown in Figure 14.14, and can be summarised thus:

- Cholesterol is absorbed from the intestine within chylomicrons. These are catabolised by lipoprotein lipase (LPL) to remnants, which are taken up by the hepatic low-density lipoprotein (LDL) receptor-related protein (LRP). A specific active transport mechanism also carries cholesterol across the gut mucosa (see below, ezetimibe).
- Cholesterol is synthesised de novo within the liver and peripheral tissues where, for example, it is

converted to steroid hormones or incorporated into cell membranes. Much of the hepatic cholesterol enters the circulation as very-low-density lipoprotein (VLDL) and is metabolised to remnant lipoproteins after LPL removes triglyceride. The remnant lipoproteins are removed by the liver through apolipoprotein E receptors or LDL receptors (LDL-R), or further metabolised to LDL and then removed by peripheral tissues or the liver by LDL receptors.

- The quantity of cholesterol transported from the liver to peripheral tissues exceeds its catabolism there, and mechanisms exist to return about half of the cholesterol to the liver. Through this 'reverse transport', cholesterol is carried by high-density lipoprotein (HDL) from peripheral cells to the liver, where it is taken up by a process involving hepatic lipase. Cholesterol in the plasma is also recycled to LDL and VLDL by cholesterol-ester transport protein (CETP).
- Cholesterol in the liver is reassembled into lipoproteins, or secreted in bile and bile acids (essential for fat digestion and absorption), and then recycled by absorption or excreted in the faeces.

LIPID DISORDERS

Disorders of lipid metabolism are manifest by increased plasma concentrations of the various lipid and lipoprotein fractions (total and LDL cholesterol, VLDL, triglycerides, chylomicrons). They result, predominantly, in cardiovascular disease. This chapter addresses approaches (non-drug as well as drug) to correct abnormal lipid profiles and diminish vascular disease and its consequences. Deposition of cholesterol in the arterial wall is central to the atherosclerotic process. Carriage of VLDL, remnant lipoprotein and LDL to arteries can thus be viewed as potentially atherogenic. In the reverse process, HDL carries cholesterol away from the arterial wall and can be regarded as protective against atherogenesis. Overproduction of VLDL in the liver raises plasma VLDL, remnant lipoprotein and LDL levels if the capacity to metabolise these lipoproteinsis compromised by

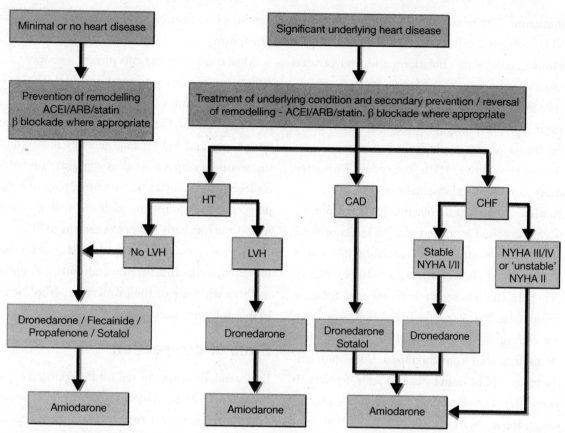

Fig. 14.12 Choice of antiarrhythmic drug for atrial fibrillation according to underlying pathology. ACEI = angiotensin-converting enzyme inhibitor; ARB = angiotensin receptor blocker; CAD = coronary artery disease; CHF = congestive heart failure; HT = hypertension; LVH = left ventricular hypertrophy; NYHA = New York Heart Association; unstable = cardiac decompensation within the prior 4 weeks. Antiarrhythmic agents are listed in alphabetical order within each treatment box. ? = evidence for 'upstream' therapy for prevention of atrial remodelling still remains controversial. Taken from the Task Force for the Management of Atrial Fibrillation of the Eurpean Society of Cardiology (ESC) guidance.

either a primary (inherited) and/or secondary (environmental) abnormality.

Raised levels of LDL cholesterol are associated particularly with risk of coronary heart disease, but it is increasingly clear that moderately raised concentrations of triglycerides, VLDL or remnants in the presence of low HDL cholesterol may also be atherogenic.

There are five primary inherited lipoprotein disorders that disturb lipid metabolism at the points indicated in Figure 14.13. These are:

- Familial hypertriglyceridaemia (FHTG) (rare), including lipoprotein lipase (LPL) deficiency, in which low LPL activity results in decreased removal, and thus increased levels of plasma triglyceride; there is increased hepatic secretion and thus a raised plasma. concentration of tri-

glyceride-rich VLDL. Patients are at risk of recurrent acute pancreatitis when plasma triglyceride exceeds 10 mmol/L, and especially when greater than 20 mmol/L.

- Familial combined hyperlipidaemia (FCHL) (common and most important) in which there is increased hepatic secretion of apolipoprotein B containing VLDL, and conversion to LDL; in consequence plasma LDL and VLDL levels are raised. Patients exhibit macrovascular disease (coronary heart, peripheral and cerebral).

- Remnant removal disease (RRD, also called remnant lipaemia, familial dysbetalipoproteinaemia) (uncommon) in which there is a defect of apolipoprotein E. This is the major ligand that allows internalisation and subsequent metabolism of remnant particles derived from VLDL and chylomicrons. The consequence is accumulation of VLDL remnants called intermediate-density lipo-protein (IDL), with cholesterol and triglycerides usually in the range 6–9 mmol/L. Patients experience severe macrovascular disease (as above).

- Familial hypoalphalipoproteinaemia (FHA, Tangier disease) (rare) in which the serum concentration of (protective) HDL is very low. Coronary heart and peripheral vascular disease result.
- Familial hypercholesterolaemia (FH) (common) is characterised by raised plasma levels of total and LDL cholesterol. It is caused by mutations in either the LDL receptor, Apo B-100 or PCSK9 genes. In the less severe heterozygous form, it affects about 1 in 500 of the population (who carry one copy of the mutant gene). LDL cholesterol levels are increased from childhood. Untreated, half the males will be dead by age 60 years, females 10 years later. The principal consequence is premature coronary heart disease, but occasionally also peripheral and cerebrovascular disease.

Secondary hyperlipidaemias result from liver and biliary disease, obesity, untreated hypothyroidism, diabetes, diet, alcohol excess, renal disease (nephrotic syndrome) and drugs (including etretinate, HIV protease inhibitors, thiazide diuretics, oral contraceptive steroids, glucocorticoids, β-adrenoceptor antagonists, ciclosporin).

Most commonly, patients present with more modestly increased levels of total and LDL cholesterol which result from overproduction of VLDL in the liver due to a combination of high dietary saturated fat, obesity and individual (genetic) susceptibility; the secondary lipaemias thus aggravate underlying dislipaemic tendencies. The resulting picture is called polygenic, manifesting in adult life, with atherosclerosis occurring early but not as early as in FH.

The most severe hyperlipidaemias usually occur in patients with concurrent conditions, e.g. diabetes mellitus with one of the primary hyperlipidaemias, in this polygenic background.

Sites of drug action

In general, drugs act to reduce the concentration of cholesterol within hepatocytes, producing a compensatory increase in LDL receptors on their surface, and increased uptake of cholesterol-rich LDL particles from the blood-stream. Statins decrease the synthesis of cholesterol and hence secretion of VLDL, and increase the surface expression of hepatic LDL receptors. Bile acidbinding (anion exchange) resins deplete the bile acid and thus the cholesterol pool.

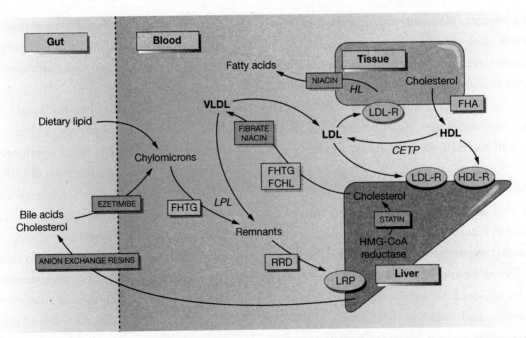

Fig. 14.13 Pathway of lipid transport and sites of drug action. CETP, cholesterol ester transfer protein; HL, hormone-sensitive lipase; LPL, lipoprotein lipase. See text for other abbreviations.

Fibrates decrease the secretion of VLDL and increase the activity of LPL, thereby increasing the removal of triglycerides. Nicotinic acid decreases fatty acid production in the tissues and the secretion of VLDL and clearance of HDL. It also enhances LPL. Ezetimibe blocks the uptake of cholesterol from the gut by targeting a specific cholesterol transporter.

DRUGS USED IN TREATMENT

Statins

These drugs block the rate-limiting enzyme for endogenous hepatic cholesterol synthesis, hydroxy-methylglutaryl coenzyme A (HMG CoA) reductase. This results in increased synthesis of LDL receptors (up-regulation) in the liver and increased clearance of LDL from the circulation; plasma total cholesterol and LDL cholesterol fall, with a maximum effect 1 month after commencing therapy. All statins cause a dose-dependent reduction in total and LDL cholesterol, although there are differences in their therapeutic efficacy; for example, at their starting doses LDL cholesterol falls after 1 month by an average of 17% with fluvastatin (20 mg/day), 28% with simvastatin (10 mg/day) and 38% with atorvastatin (10 mg/day). At higher doses, e.g. 80 mg/day atorvastatin or simvastatin, a 50% or greater reduction in LDL cholesterol is possible. The effects of pravastatin are similar and so-called superstatins (e.g. rosuvastatin) may achieve this level of reduction at lower doses.

There is no tolerance to continued administration of a statin, and because of a circadian rhythm to LDL-receptor synthesis, statins with short $t_{1/2}$ are slightly more effective if given in the evening rather than in the morning. Some effects of statins may be 'lipid independent' and reflect actions on the inflammatory component of atheroma progression (so-called 'pleiotropic' effects). Nevertheless, their efficacy in both primary and secondary prophylaxis of hypercholesterolaemia is probably a class effect; long-term outcome studies have failed so far to differentiate between the various statins. On current information, with no clear advantages or disadvantages between the different statins, the choice of agent to achieve the suggested total or LDL cholesterol levels (see above) is heavily influenced by their relative cost, and the dose likely to achieve the target cholesterol concentration.

Statins are well absorbed by mouth, and are metabolised in the liver. Simvastatin is a prodrug, simvastatin lactone, which is itself inactive. Other statins are prescribed in their active form. Except for rosuvastatin, they are metabolised through CYP pathways (usually 3A4), which is an important source of drug interactions particularly involving simvastatin and atorvastatin. They are well tolerated, the commonest adverse effect being a transient, and usually minor, increase in serum transaminases in some 1% of patients. Asymptomatic increases in muscle enzymes (creatine phosphokinase, CPK) and myositis (with a generalised muscle discomfort) occur more rarely, but are more frequent when statins are combined with other antihyperlidaemic drugs such as fibrates and nicotinic acid; patients should be counselled about myositis when these drugs are co-administered. There is also a genetic predisposition, as carriers of a common variant of the SLCO1B1 gene encoding the OATP1B1 anionic transporter on hepatocytes have a four-fold increased risk of myopathy on simvastatin; this increases to 16-fold if they are carrying two copies of the rs4149056 SNP. Myositis is also more likely with co-administered anti-HIV protease inhibitors, e.g. ritonavir, and with drugs that interfere with metabolism of some statins, e.g. ciclosporin.

Fibric acid derivatives (fibrates)

The class includes bezafibrate, ciprofibrate, fenofibrate and gemfibrozil; the original fibrate, clofibrate, is obsolete. The drugs partly resemble short-chain fatty acids and increase the oxidation of these acids in both liver and muscle. In the liver, secretion of triglyceride-rich lipoproteins falls, and in muscle the activity of lipoprotein lipase and fatty acid uptake from plasma are both increased. Fibrates act through a nuclear transcription factor (peroxisome proliferator-activated receptor (PPAR-α), which up-regulates expression of LPL and apolipoprotein A-I genes, and down-regulates expression of the apolipoprotein C-III gene. The result is that plasma levels of triglyceride decline by 20%–30% and those of cholesterol by 10%–15%; associated with this is a rise in the 'protective' HDL cholesterol. The latter effect may have contributed to the reduction in non-fatal myocardial infarction with gemfibrozil in both the Helsinki Heart Study and more recent Veterans Affairs HDL Intervention Trials (VA-HIT).

Fibrates are the drugs of choice for mixed hyper-lipidaemia raised cholesterol plus triglycerides) but may be used in hypercholesterolaemia, alone or with anion exchange resins or (with care, see above) with statins. There is evidence of varying efficacy among the drugs both in cholesterol-lowering and in additional beneficial effects, such as reduction in blood fibrinogen and urate concentrations; the clinical significance of these differences is not yet known.

Fibric acid derivatives are well absorbed from the gastrointestinal tract, extensively bound to plasma proteins and excreted mainly by the kidney as unchanged drug or metabolites. They are contraindicated where hepatic or renal function is severely impaired (but gemfibrozil has been used in uraemic and nephrotic patients without aggravating deterioration in kidney function). Rarely, fibric acid derivatives may induce a myositis-like syndrome; the risk is greater in patients with poor renal function, and in those who are also receiving a statin; gemfibrizil in particular should never be used with a statin. Fibrates enhance the effect of co-administered oral anticoagulants.

Anion-exchange resins (bile acid sequestrants)

Colestyramine is an oral anion-exchange resin; it binds bile acids in the intestine and depletion of the bile acid pool stimulates conversion of cholesterol to bile acid. The result is a fall in intracellular cholesterol in hepatocytes, and an increase (up-regulation) in both LDL receptors and cholesterol synthesis. Plasma LDL cholesterol concentration falls by 20%–25%. In many patients there is some compen-satory increase in hepatic triglyceride output. Anion exchange resins may be used for hypercholesterolaemia but not when there is significant hypertriglyceridaemia.

Colestyramine is rather unpalatable and poorly tolerated, with up to 50% of patients experiencing constipation and some complaining of anorexia, abdominal fullness and occasionally of diarrhoea, effects that may limit or prevent its use. Because the colestyramine binds anions, drugs such as warfarin, digoxin, thiazide diuretics, phenobarbital and thyroid hormones should be taken 1 h before or 4 h after colestyramine to avoid impairment of their absorption. Binding of fat-soluble vitamins in the gut may be sufficient to cause clinical deficiency, e.g. vitamin K-responsive prolongation of the prothrombin time.

Colestipol is similar to colestyramine but is available in capsule form to increase palatability.

Colesevalam is a bile acid sequestrant (not an anion exchange resin) which binds bile acids and forms an insoluble complex that passes out in the faeces, taking with it bile acid-bound LDL cholesterol.

Ezetimibe

Some 30%–70% of plasma cholesterol is attributable to cholesterol absorbed from the gut. Ezetimibe selectively blocks intestinal cholesterol absorption by inhibition of the Niemann–Pick C1-like 1 (NCPC1L1) transporter, which interrupts the enterohepatic cycling of cholesterol (see above). It is effective when used as monotherapy in a 10-mg dose, producing a 17% fall in LDL cholesterol. Tolerability is similar to that with placebo. Ezetimibe is actually a pro-drug and metabolism in the liver produces the more effective blocker of cholesterol transport, ezetimibe glucuronide ($t_{1/2}$ 22 h).

The real potential of this drug is increased efficacy in combination with statins. Ezetimibe with a low dose of a statin, e.g. simvastatin 10 mg/day, produces a fall in plasma cholesterol similar to that with simvastatin 80 mg/day, providing a possible alternative treatment for patients unable to tolerate high-dose statin monotherapy. Ezetimibe may challenge resins as the agent of choice for patients with hypercholesterolaemia that is not controlled by a statin alone. It remains unclear after a decade of clinical use whether an ezetimibe–statin combination offers any benefit over high-dose statin monotherapy alone in the quest for aggressive reduction in LDL cholesterol levels.

Nicotinic acid and derivatives

Nicotinic acid (also known as niacin or vitamin B$_3$) acts as an antilipolytic agent in adipose tissue, reducing the supply of free fatty acids and hence the availability of substrate for hepatic triglyceride synthesis and the secretion of VLDL. Nicotinic acid lowers plasma triglyceride and cholesterol concentrations, and raises HDL cholesterol levels. It produces a modest reduction in plasma lipoprotein Lp (a), which may contribute to its overall protection against the complications of atheroma. The doses required to do this are well in excess of those required for its vitamin effect and are not shared by nicotinamide. Skin flushing (partially preventable by low-dose aspirin to block prostaglandin production especially of the potent flushing prostaglandin, PGD2) and gastrointestinal upset are common side-effects of nicotinic acid and cause >20% of patients to stop taking it; these are ameliorated by using a slow-release formulation and gradually building up the oral dose over 6 weeks, when tolerance emerges. A further development has been to combine nicotinic acid with a PGD2 antagonist, laropiprant, to reduce the flushing without the gastrointestinal effects of aspirin. Even with this combined formulation 10% of patients cannot tolerate nicotinic acid. Rarely, nicotinic acid can also cause major disturbance of liver function.

Acipimox is better tolerated than nicotinic acid and has a longer duration of action, but is less effective. Unlike nicotinic acid, it does not lower plasma Lp(a) levels.

Other drugs

Omega-3 marine triglycerides (Maxepa) contain the triglyceride precursors of two polyunsaturated fatty acids (eicosapentaenoic acid and docosahexaenoic acid) derived from oily fish. A related product, Oma-

cor, contains omega 3-acid ethyl esters instead of triglycerides. They have no role in treating hypercholesterolaemia, but are taken for CHD prevention (when benefit may be due to an antithrombotic effect). Patients with moderate to severe hypertriglyceridaemia may respond to either agent, although LDL cholesterol levels may rise.

Orlistat, a weight-reducing agent, lowers the glycaemia of diabetes mellitus to a degree that accords with the weight loss, and improves hyperlipidaemia to an extent greater than would be expected.

α-Tocopherol acetate (vitamin E) has no effect on lipid concentrations but is a powerful antioxidant, and oxidation of LDL is an essential step in the development of atheroma. Interest thus focused on a possible role of both endogenous and therapeutic vitamin E in prevention of atheroma, but a recent overview of published outcome trials using vitamin E supplements found no compelling evidence for a-tocopherol in the treatment or prevention of atherosclerosis.

SUMMARY

- The treatment of both hypertension and angina requires drugs that reduce the work of the heart either directly or by lowering peripheral vascular resistance.
- β-Blockade, which acts mainly through reduced cardiac output, and calcium channel blockade, acting by selective arterial dilatation, may be used in either condition.
- Other vasodilators are suited preferentially to hypertension (ACE inhibitors, angiotensin (AT1) receptor blockers (ARBs) and α-adrenoceptor blockers) or to angina (nitrates).
- The treatment of myocardial infarction requires thrombolysis, aspirin and β-adrenoceptor blockade acutely, with the latter two continued for at least 2 years as secondary prevention of a further infarction.
- In chronic heart failure, diuretics and nitrates reduce preload and provide symptomatic relief without affecting outcome.

- ACE inhibitors reduce both preload and after-load, and reduce morbidity and mortality by about one-third in all patients.
- β-Adrenoceptor blockers, gradually introduced, have an effect equivalent to that of ACE inhibitors in patients with moderate or severe heart failure (NYHA Ⅲ or Ⅳ).
- Spironolactone, in low dose, adds further benefit.
- Digoxin improves myocardial contractility most effectively in the dilated, failing heart but also in the longer term, including in patients in sinus rhythm.
- The principal agents for treating acute left ventricular failure are furosemide, diamorphine and oxygen.
- Radiofrequency ablation and devices such as permanent pacemakers and ICDs increasingly provide the preferred approaches in treatment of cardiac arrhythmias. The use of drugs alone is declining but they often constitute adjunctive treatments.
- Adenosine is the treatment of choice for diagnosis and reversal of supraventricular arrhythmias. Verapamil is an alternative for the management of narrow complex tachycardias.
- Amiodarone is the most effective drug for reversing and preventing atrial fibrillation, and for preventing ventricular arrhythmias, but it has notable adverse effects. Dronedarone has been designed to provide the actions of amiodarone without the side-effects but is not so effective.
- All antiarrhythmics can be potentially dangerous, and should be used only in patients who have been properly and fully assessed.
- The most effective cholesterol-reducing drugs are the statins, which inhibit the rate-limiting step in cholesterol synthesis.
- Additional agents may be required for mixed or severe hyperlipidaemia.
- In outcome trials with these drugs, reductions in blood cholesterol by 25%–35% are associated with a 35%–45% reduction in the risk of coronary heart disease.
- The main indications for their use are patients with even slightly increased levels of cholesterol (>5 mmol/L) after a myocardial infarction or any other macrovascular event, in patients with familial hypercholesterolaemia or diabetes, and in patients with a significant absolute CVD risk, especially where there is a family history of premature CVD.

IMPORTANT TERMINOLOGY

adenosine triphosphate (ATP)-dependent potassium channel opener　ATP 敏感钾通道开放药

α₂-Adrenoceptor agonists　α₂ 肾上腺素能受体激动药

angiotensin-converting enzyme (ACE) inhibitors　血管紧张素转化酶抑制药

angiotensin (AT)Ⅱ receptor blockers (ARBs)　血管紧张素Ⅱ受体阻断药

calcium channel blockers　钙通道拮抗药

cardiac glycosides　强心苷类药

digitalis　洋地黄

false transmitter　伪递质

fibric acid derivatives　苯氧酸类药物

hyperthyroidism　甲状腺功能亢进

imidazoline receptor (I₁)　咪唑啉受体

intermittent claudication　间歇性跛行

nitrodilator　硝基扩血管药

renin inhibitors　肾素抑制药

phosphodiesterase inhibitors　磷酸二酯酶抑制药

pleiotropic effects　多效性作用

prophylaxis　预防

statins　他汀类药物

transdermal patch　透皮贴剂

venepuncture　静脉穿刺

CHALLENGE YOURSELF

1. Describe the advantages of the combination of organic nitrates with β-receptor blockers in treatment of angina.
2. Describe the principle of drug selection for hypertension.
3. A 70-year-old male with a history of congestive heart failure, hypertension and coronary artery disease. Maximal ACE inhibitor, β-receptor blocker and diuretics treatment did not significantly ameliorate the depressed ejection fraction, dyspnea and edema. The doctor decided to add digoxin to relieve these symptoms.

1) Do you think the doctor's decision is right?

2) If it is right, describe the evidence to support the prescription.

3) What is the side effects of digoxin?

4. A 72-year-old man has been suffered a myocardiac infarction and has been appropriately managed with oxygen, nitrates, β-receptor blocker and Clopidogrel but has developed ventricular tachycardia.

   1) Which types of drugs are most effective to control the ventricular tachycardia?

   2) Describe the mechanisms of the action of the drug you selected on ventricular tachycardia.

5. The blood pressure of a 55-year-old man with hypertension was under acceptable controlled with ACE inhibitor-thiazide diuretic combination. He was recently diagnosed to have elevated total cholesterol and low-density lipoprotein levels, but triglyceride level is normal.

   1) To reduce the risk of developing coronary artery disease, which type of drugs you will prescribe for this patient? Describe the principle of drug selection.

   2) Describe the mechanism how the drugs you selected reduce the levels of total cholesterol and low-density lipoprotein.

Jiaguo Zhou

Chapter 15

Hematological system

Part 1. Drugs and haemostasis

INTRODUCTION

It is essential that blood remains fluid within the circulation but clots at sites of vascular injury. Injury to blood vessels results in a series of events aimed at preventing blood loss (hemostasis), which include vasoconstriction, platelet aggregation, and the deposition of fibrin. The haemostatic system maintains the integrity of the vascular tree through a complex network of cellular, ligand–receptor and enzymatic interactions. In normal circumstances there is an equilibrium between the natural coagulant–anticoagulant and fibrinolytic–antifibrinolytic systems.

Pathological disruption of the network results in thrombosis or bleeding, or both; the extreme example of haemostatic pathology is a complete breakdown as occurs in disseminated intravascular coagulation (DIC). Drugs that modulate the haemostatic system are valuable in the management of bleeding and thrombotic disorders. Drugs are classified according to the component of the system they affect and their perceived primary mode of action.

THE COAGULATION SYSTEM

The classical view of blood coagulation with separate 'extrinsic' and 'intrinsic' pathways initiated by either *tissue factor* (TF) or contact with an anionic surface does not reflect physiological coagulation. Most non-vascular cells express TF, a cell membrane protein, in a constitutive fashion, whereas de novo TF synthesis can be induced in monocytes and damaged endothelial cells. Injury to the arterial or venous wall exposes extravascular TF-expressing cells to blood. Lipid-laden macrophages in the core of atherosclerotic plaques are particularly rich in TF, thereby explaining the propensity for thrombus formation at sites of plaque disruption. Once bound to TF, factor VIIa activates factor IX and factor X (to IXa and Xa, respectively), leading to thrombin generation and clot formation (Fig. 15.1). It is now evident that coagulation does not occur as linear sequential enzyme activation pathways but rather by a network of simultaneous interactions, which undergo regulation and modulation during the thrombin generation process itself.

In the current model, blood coagulation starts with a transient release of TF by damaged endothelium, resulting in the formation of sub-nanomolar

Fig. 15.1 The blood coagulation network (see text).

amounts of *thrombin* via TF/XIIa-driven Xa formation (extrinsic-tenase). The initial thrombin activity is necessary to prime the system for a full thrombin explosion. Tissue factor pathway inhibitor (TFPI) rapidly shuts down this priming pathway and the full thrombin explosion is then dependent on factor IXa-driven Xa formation. Factor IXa-driven Xa formation (intrinsic-tenase) is amplified by the thrombin explosion itself, as thrombin forms a positive feedback loop by activating factor XIa (not shown in Fig. 15.1), which converts more IX to IXa.

Thrombin converts soluble fibrinogen into insoluble fibrin monomers, which spontaneously polymerise to form the fibrin mesh that is then stabilised and cross-linked by activated factor XIII (factor XIIIa), a thrombin-activated transglutaminase. Thrombin amplifies its own generation by:

- feedback activation of factor V and factor VIII
- activating platelet-bound factor XI, thereby leading to further factor Xa generation
- activating cells that provide the phospholipid surface required for assembly of the macromolecular enzymatic complexes.

PROCOAGULANT DRUGS

Vitamin K

Vitamin K ('Koagulation' vitamin) is essential for normal coagulation. It occurs naturally in two forms. Vitamin K_1 (phylloquinone) is widely distributed in plants and K_2 includes vitamin synthesised in the alimentary tract by bacteria, e.g. *Escherichia coli* (menaquinones). Leafy green vegetables are a good source of vitamin K_1. Bile is required for the absorption of the natural forms of vitamin K, which are fat soluble. The storage pool of vitamin K is modest and can be exhausted in 1 week, although gut flora will maintain suboptimal production of vitamin K-dependent proteins. A synthetic analogue, *menadione* (K_3), is water soluble.

Vitamin K is necessary for the final stage in the synthesis of coagulation proteins in the liver: the *procoagulant* factors II (prothrombin), VII, IX and X,

and *anticoagulant* regulatory proteins, proteins C and S. The vitamin allows γ-carboxylation of glutamic acid residues in their structure; this permits calcium to bind to the molecule, mediating the conformational change required for enzymatic activity, and binding to negatively charged phospholipid surfaces, e.g. platelets. Membrane binding is required for full enzymatic potential.

During γ-carboxylation of the proteins, the *reduced* and *active* form of vitamin KH_2 converts to an epoxide, an *oxidation* product. Subsequently vitamin K epoxide reductase converts oxidised vitamin K back to the active vitamin K, i.e. there exists an interconversion cycle between vitamin K epoxide and reduced vitamin K (Fig. 15.2).

Fig. 15.2 The vitamin K cycle.

When the vitamin is deficient or where drugs (e.g. warfarin) inhibit its action, the coagulation proteins produced are unable to associate with calcium in order to form the necessary three dimensional configuration and associated membrane-binding properties that are required for full enzymatic activity. Their physiologically critical binding to membrane surfaces fails to occur, and this impairs the coagulation mechanism. These proteins are called 'proteins induced in vitamin K absence (PIVKAs)'.

Vitamin K deficiency may arise from:

- dietary deficiency.
- bile failing to enter the intestine, e.g. obstructive jaundice or biliary fistula.
- malabsorption syndromes, e.g. coeliac disease, or after extensive small intestinal resection.

reduced alimentary tract flora, e.g. in newborn infants and rarely after broad-spectrum antibiotics.

The following preparations of vitamin K are available:

Phytomenadione (Konakion), the naturally occurring fat-soluble vitamin K_1, which can be given intravenously, intramuscularly, subcutaneously or orally. The preferred route depends on the degree of coagulopathy and urgency of correcting the haemorrhagic tendency. The intravenous formulation will begin to reverse a vitamin K-deficient coagulopathy within 6 h in a patient with normal liver function. It should be administered slowly to reduce the risk of an anaphylactoid reaction with facial flushing, sweating, fever, chest tightness, cyanosis and peripheral vascular collapse. Oral administration acts within about 12 h and should reduce the anticoagulant effect of warfarin within 24–48 h. The intramuscular route may induce local intramuscular haemorrhage, and subcutaneous absorption is variable.

Menadiol sodium phosphate (vitamin K_3), being water soluble, is preferred in intestinal malabsorption or in states in which bile flow is deficient. The main disadvantage is that it takes 24 h to act, but its effect lasts for several days. Menadiol sodium phosphate in moderate doses causes haemolytic anaemia and, for this reason, neonates should not receive it, especially those that are deficient in glucose 6-phosphate dehydrogenase; their immature livers are unable to cope with the heavy bilirubin load and there is danger of kernicterus.

Vitamin K is used to treat the following:

- Haemorrhage or threatened bleeding due to the coumarin or indanedione anticoagulants. Phytomenadione is preferred for its more rapid action.
- Haemorrhagic disease of the newborn. Prophylaxis is recommended during the period of vulnerability with vitamin K (phytomenadione) 1 mg by single i.m. injection at birth. Alternatively, give vitamin K by mouth as two doses of a colloidal (mixed micelle) preparation of phytomenadione in the first week. Breast-fed babies should receive a further 2 mg at 1 month of age. Formula-fed babies do not need this last supple-

ment as the formula contains vitamin K. Fears that intramuscular vitamin K might cause childhood cancer have been dispelled.

- Intestinal malabsorption syndromes; menadiol sodium phosphate should be used as it is water soluble.

Coagulation factor concentrates

Bleeding due to deficiency of specific coagulation factors is treated by either elevating the deficient factor or replacement of the missing factor. Recombinant factor VIII and IX are now available for patients with congenital deficiency of these factors. For patients with rare coagulation factor deficiencies or multiple acquired deficiencies (liver disease, massive blood loss with dilutional coagulopathy or DIC), replacement therapy requires human-derived fresh frozen plasma (FFP) or factor concentrates containing factors II, VII, IX and X (Beriplex, Octaplex).

FEIBA is a human donor-derived factor concentrate for patients with inhibitory antibodies to factor VIII or IX. It contains a mixture of coagulation factors and produces thrombin generation even in the presence of inhibitors to factor VIII or IX.

Recombinant factor VIIa (NovoSeven) is effective for patients with inhibitory antibodies to factor VIII or IX or deficiency of factor VII. A pure synthetic activated coagulation factor, it generates thrombin even in the presence of inhibitors to factor VIII or IX.

Desmopressin (DDAVP)

Desmopressin is a vasopressin analogue that increases the plasma concentrations of factor VIII and von Willebrand factor, and directly activates platelets. DDAVP is usually given subcutaneously or intravenously, but unwanted effects (headache, flushing and tachycardia) are less severe after subcutaneous use. A concentrated form is available for intranasal use.

DDAVP is useful for treating patients with mild haemophilia A and von Willebrand's disease. For dental extraction, a single injection of 0.3 micrograms/kg 1–2 h before surgery, combined with the oral antifibrinolytic drug, tranexamic acid, for 5–7 days after the procedure, will produce normal haemostasis and prevent secondary haemorrhage.

DDAVP shortens the bleeding time in patients with renal or liver failure.

Adverse effects. Water retention and hyponatraemia may complicate therapy and very young children (<1 year) should not receive DDAVP. Fluid intake should not exceed 1 L in the 8 h following treatment and with repeated doses the plasma sodium should be monitored. Tachyphylaxis (progressively diminishing response to the same dose) can occur.

Other agents

Adrenaline/epinephrine is effective as a topical agent for epistaxis, applied in ribbon gauze that is packed into the nostril, haemorrhage being arrested by local vasoconstriction.

Fibrin glue consists of fibrinogen and thrombin contained in two syringes, the tips of which form a common port that allows delivery of the two components to a bleeding point where fibrinogen converts to fibrin at a rate determined by the concentration of thrombin. Fibrin glue can be used to secure surgical haemostasis, e.g. on a large raw surface, and to prevent external oozing of blood in patients with haemophilia.

Sclerosing agents produce inflammation and thrombosis in veins to induce permanent obliteration, e.g. ethanolamine oleate injection, sodium tetradecyl sulphate (given intravenously for varicose veins) and oily phenol injection (given submucosally for haemorrhoids). Local reactions and tissue necrosis may occur.

ANTICOAGULANT DRUGS

Anticoagulant drugs act principally to reduce the activity of *thrombin*, which do so by:

- *limiting thrombin generation*, either as a result of inhibiting other proteases (clotting factors) involved in its generation or by reducing the activity of zymogens (the precursor inactive forms of the enzymes); or
- *inhibiting (neutralising) thrombin activity*, either directly or indirectly, depending on whether or not they activate the natural serpin-dependent anticoagulant pathway.

Oral vitamin K antagonists (VKA)

Warfarin and other oral vitamin K antagonists (VKA) reduce the activity of zymogens. The anticoagulant effect of oral VKA is expressed as the International Normalised Ratio (INR), which is calculated as follows:

$$INR = (PT_{observed} / PT_{control})^{ISI}$$

where the $PT_{observed}$ and $PT_{control}$ are the prothrombin times of the patient and control, respectively, and the ISI is the international sensitivity index of the thromboplastin reagent be used. For most indications, an INR of 2 to 3 is recommended.

Pharmacokinetics. Warfarin is readily absorbed from the gastrointestinal tract and, like all the current oral anticoagulants, is more than 90% bound to plasma proteins. Metabolism in the liver terminates its action. Warfarin ($t_{1/2}$ 36 h) is a racemic mixture of approximately equal amounts of two isomers, S ($t_{1/2}$ 27 h) and R ($t_{1/2}$ 40 h) warfarin, i.e. it is in effect two drugs. S warfarin is four times more potent than R warfarin. The isomers respond differently to drugs that interact with warfarin.

Pharmacodynamics. Coumarins are structurally similar to vitamin K and competitively inhibit vitamin K epoxide reductase and vitamin K reductase. The overall result is a shift in haemostatic balance in favour of anticoagulation because of the accumulation of clotting proteins with absent or decreased γ-carboxylation sites (PIVKAs).

This shift does not take place until functioning vitamin K-dependent proteins, made before the drug was administered, have been cleared from the circulation. The process occurs at different rates for individual coagulation factors (VII $t_{1/2}$ 6 h, IX and X $t_{1/2}$ 18–24 h, prothrombin $t_{1/2}$ 72 h). The anticoagulant proteins C and S have a shorter $t_{1/2}$ than the procoagulant proteins and their more rapid decline in concentration may create a transient hypercoagulable state. This can be dangerous in individuals with inherited protein C or S deficiency who may develop thrombotic skin necrosis during initiation of oral anticoagulant therapy with vitamin K antagonists. Anticoagulation with heparin until the effect of warfarin is well established reduces the risk of skin necrosis when rapid induction of anticoagulation is required.

The therapeutic anticoagulant effect of warfarin develops only after 4–5 days. Furthermore, the INR does not reliably reflect anticoagulant protection during this initial phase, as the vitamin K-dependent factors diminish at different rates and the INR is particularly sensitive to the level of factor VII, which is not a principal determinant of thrombotic or bleeding risk.

Warfarin is the oral anticoagulant of choice, for it is reliably effective and has the lowest incidence of adverse effects. Because of the delay in onset of anticoagulant effect with oral vitamin K antagonists (VKAs) there is a need for an immediate-acting anticoagulant, such as a heparin, in the first few days of therapy if rapid anticoagulation is required.

The response to warfarin, and other coumarins, varies within and between individuals and therefore regular monitoring of dose is essential.

Dose. There is much inter-individual variation in dose requirements. It is usual to initiate therapy with 10-mg doses, depending on the daily INR, with the maintenance dose then adjusted according to the INR using an established protocol. The target INR for deep vein thrombosis (DVT) is 2.5 (typical range 2.0–3.0).

Adverse effects. The major complication of treatment with warfarin is *bleeding*. As well as a risk of haemorrhage after trauma or surgery, spontaneous bleeding may occur. The risk of bleeding relates to the INR, not the dose of warfarin: the higher the INR, the greater the chance of bleeding. The risk of over-anticoagulation increases with intercurrent illness and interaction with other drugs, and is more likely in patients whose anticoagulant control is unstable. Therefore, it is essential to:

- maintain as stable a level of anticoagulation as possible
- adopt the lowest effective target INR
- educate patients about risk, particularly that associated with additional drug use

Warfarin is a small molecule that crosses the placenta and can produce harmful effects in the developing fetus.

Warfarin embryopathy develops only after exposure to oral anticoagulant during the first trimester of pregnancy. The most common feature is chondrodysplasia punctata, characterised by abnormal cartilage and bone formation (with stippling of epiphyses visible on radiography) in vertebrae and femur, and the bones of the hands and feet during infancy and early childhood; these disappear with age (warfarin is not the only cause of this abnormality). Other less common skeletal abnormalities include nasal hypoplasia and hypertelorism (wide-set eyes).

Bleeding into the central nervous system is a danger throughout pregnancy but particularly at the time of delivery.

As a consequence of the above, warfarin is contraindicated in the first 6–12 weeks of pregnancy and should be replaced by heparin before the anticipated date of delivery, as the action of the latter drug can be terminated rapidly prior to the birth.

Reversal of anticoagulation can be gradual or rapid depending on the circumstances. Vitamin K 5–10 mg is usually adequate for complete reversal, oral administration being less rapid than intravenous. Immediate reversal is more readily achieved with a factor concentrate than fresh frozen plasma.

Drug interactions. Oral anticoagulant control must be precise for safety and efficacy. If a drug that alters the action of warfarin is essential, monitor the INR frequently and adjust the dose of warfarin during the period of institution of the new drug until a new stable therapeutic dose of warfarin results; careful monitoring is also needed on withdrawal of the interacting drug.

Analgesics. Avoid, if possible, non-steroidal anti-inflammatory drugs (NSAIDs) including aspirin because of their irritant effect on gastric mucosa and action on platelets. Paracetamol is acceptable but doses above 1.5 g/day may raise the INR. Dextropropoxyphene inhibits warfarin metabolism, and compounds that contain it, e.g. co-proxamol, should be avoided. Codeine, dihydrocodeine and combinations with paracetamol, e.g. co-dydramol, are preferred. Concomitant use of misoprostol with a NSAID may reduce the risk of gastric bleeding and a selective cyclo-oxygenase (COX)-2 inhibitor may be associated with a lower bleeding risk in patients taking oral anticoagulants.

Antimicrobials. Aztreonam, cefamandole, chloramphenicol, ciprofloxacin, co-trimoxazole, erythromycin, fluconazole, itraconazole, ketoconazole, metronidazole, miconazole, ofloxacin and sulphonamides (including co-trimoxazole) increase anticoagulant effect by mechanisms that include interference with warfarin or vitamin K metabolism. Rifampicin and griseofulvin induce relevant hepatic enzymes and accelerate warfarin metabolism, reducing its effect. Intensive broad-spectrum antibiotics, e.g. eradication regimens for *Helicobacter pylori*, may increase sensitivity to warfarin by reducing the intestinal flora that provide vitamin K.

Anticonvulsants. Carbamazepine, phenobarbital and primidone accelerate warfarin metabolism (by enzyme induction); the effect of phenytoin is variable. Clonazepam and sodium valproate are safe.

Antiarrhythmics. Amiodarone, propafenone and possibly quinidine potentiate the effect of warfarin and dose adjustment is required, but atropine, disopyramide and lidocaine do not interfere.

Antidepressants. Serotonin-reuptake inhibitors may enhance the effect of warfarin, but tricyclics may be useed.

Gastrointestinal drugs. Avoid cimetidine and omeprazole, which inhibit the clearance of R warfarin, and sucralfate, which may impair its absorption. Ranitidine may be used. Most antacids are safe.

Lipid-lowering drugs. Fibrates, and some statins, enhance anticoagulant effect. Avoid colestyramine as it may impair the absorption of both warfarin and vitamin K.

Sex hormones and hormone antagonists. The hormone antagonists danazol, flutamide and tamoxifen enhance the effect of warfarin.

Sedatives and anxiolytics. Benzodiazepines may be used.

Uses of oral VKA

Oral vitamin K antagonist drugs are used to prevent and treat venous thrombosis and pulmonary embolus, and to prevent arterial thromboemboli in patients with atrial fibrillation or cardiac disease, including mechanical heart valves. The following are general indications:

- *Target INR 2.5* is appropriate for treatment of DVT; pulmonary embolism (PE); systemic embolism; prevention of venous thromboembolism in myocardial infarction; mitral stenosis with embolism; transient ischaemic attacks; atrial fibrillation; mechanical prosthetic aortic valves.
- *Target INR 3.5* is preferred for recurrent DVT and PE when already on warfarin with target of 2.5, arterial disease and some mechanical prosthetic mitral valves.
- At least 6 weeks' anticoagulation is recommended after calf vein thrombosis and at least 3 months after proximal DVT or PE. For patients with temporary risk factors and a low risk of recurrence, 3 months of treatment may be sufficient. For patients with idiopathic venous thromboembolism or permanent risk factors, at least 6 months' anticoagulation is usual.

Surgery in patients receiving oral VKA

Elective surgery. Warfarin is withdrawn 5 days before the operation and recommenced when the patient resumes oral intake; heparin (low molecular weight heparin (LMWH) or unfractionated heparin (UFH)) provides cover in the intervening period. In patients with mechanical mitral prosthetic valves, LMWH or UFH is added when the INR is subtherapeutic.

Emergency surgery. Proceed as for bleeding (above).

Dental extractions. Anticoagulation may continue for patients whose INR is less than 4.0. The INR is measured no more than 72 h before the procedure to ensure that the INR will be less than 4.0 on the day of the extraction.

Other vitamin K antagonists

Acenocoumarol (nicoumalone) is similar to warfarin but seldom used; the kidney eliminates it mainly in unchanged form.

Indanedione anticoagulants are rarely used because of allergic reactions unrelated to coagulation; phenindione is still available.

Oral direct thrombin and factor Xa inhibitors

Dabigatran

Dabigatran is a small molecule direct thrombin inhibitor (DTI). Dabigatran etexilate is an oral prodrug of the active compound dabigatran. Dabigatran is a direct specific competitive inhibitor of free and fibrin-bound thrombin. Absorption of the prodrug is rapid (C_{max} <4 h) and the half life of dabigatran is 12–14 h in healthy volunteers and 14–17 h in patients undergoing major orthopaedic surgery. The active compound is not metabolised and is eliminated by renal excretion with 85% of an administered dose detectable in urine. Clearance is significantly prolonged when the glomerular filtration rate is less than 50 mL/min. There is no antidote. There is a significant potentiating drug interaction with amiodarone and other drugs. The drug is approved in many countries for prevention of venous thrombosis in patients undergoing hip or knee replacement.

Rivaroxaban

Rivaroxaban is a small molecule direct competitive inhibitor of factor Xa and limits thrombin generation in a dose dependent manner. Absorption of drug is rapid (C max <4 hours) with a half-life of 7–11 h. Rivaroxaban is metabolised in the liver but can be used in patients with liver disease if there is no coagulopathy. Renal excretion is minimal and there is no accumulation of drug when the glomerular filtration rate is above 15 mL/min. There is no antidote. There are significant potentiating drug interactions with protease inhibitors used to treat HIV infection and with antifungals. The drug is used for prevention

of venous thrombosis in patients undergoing hip or knee replacement.

Parenteral anticoagulants

Heparin

Heparin is a sulphated mucopolysaccharide that is found in the secretory granules of mast cells and is prepared commercially from porcine intestinal mucosa to give preparations that vary in molecular weight from 3 000 to 30 000 Da (average 15 000 Da). It is the strongest organic acid in the body and in solution carries an electronegative charge. The low molecular weight heparins (LMWH, mean mol. wt. 4 000–6 500 Da) are prepared from standard unfractionated (UF) heparin by a variety of chemical techniques. Commercial preparations contain different fractions and display different pharmacokinetics. Some currently available include bemiparin, dalteparin, enoxaparin, reviparin and tinzaparin.

Pharmacokinetics. Heparin is poorly absorbed from the gastrointestinal tract and is given intravenously or subcutaneously; once in the blood its effect is immediate. Heparin binds to several plasma proteins, to endothelial cells, and is taken up by reticuloendothelial cells; the kidney excretes a proportion. Because of these different mechanisms, elimination of heparin from the plasma involves a combination of zero- and first-order processes. The result is that the plasma biological effect $t_{1/2}$ alters disproportionately with dose, being 60 min after 75 units/kg and increasing to 150 min after 400 units/kg.

LMW heparins are less protein bound and have a predictable dose–response profile when administered subcutaneously or intravenously. They also have a longer $t_{1/2}$ than standard heparin preparations.

Pharmacodynamics. Heparin binds to antithrombin (formerly antithrombin III), inducing a conformational change that leads to rapid inhibition of the proteases of the coagulation pathway. Antithrombin is a naturally occurring inhibitor of activated coagulation proteases (factors) that include thrombin, factor Xa and factor IXa in plasma. In the presence of heparin, antithrombin becomes approximately 1000-fold more active and inhibition is essentially instantaneous. Following destruction of the proteases, the affinity of antithrombin for heparin falls; heparin then dissociates from the antithrombin–protease complex and catalyses further antithrombin–protease interactions.

Factor Xa is critical to thrombin generation (Fig. 15.1) and heparin has the capacity to inhibit factor Xa in small quantities by virtue of a specific pentasaccharide sequence. This provides the rationale for using low-dose subcutaneous heparin to prevent thrombus formation.

LMWHs inhibit factor Xa at a dose similar to that for UFH, but have much less antithrombin activity, the principal action of conventional heparin. Fibrin formed in the circulation binds to thrombin and protects it from inactivation by the heparin–antithrombin complex; this may provide a further explanation for the higher doses of heparin needed to stop extension of a thrombus than to prevent it.

Fondaparinux is a synthetic pentasaccharide that inhibits factor Xa by an antithrombin-dependent mechanism. Its specific anti-Xa activity is higher than that of LMWH and its half-life after subcutaneous injection is longer than that of LMWH. Fondaparinux can be administered subcutaneously once daily in fixed doses without coagulation monitoring. Fondaparinux is contraindicated in patients with renal insufficiency (CrCl < 30 mL/min). It is used for prevention and treatment of venous thromboembolism in the same way as traditional LMWHs. The risk of HIT(T) is lower, but the risk of bleeding may be greater than that associated with LMWHs.

Monitoring heparin therapy. Control of standard heparin therapy is by the activated partial thromboplastin time (APTT), the target therapeutic range being 1.5–2.5 times the control. An alternative method is to measure the plasma concentration of heparin by anti-Xa assay. Therapeutic amounts of LMWH do not prolong the APTT and, because the pharmacokinetics are predictable, a safe and effective dose can be calculated without laboratory monitoring, using an algorithm that is adjusted for body-weight.

Adverse effects. Bleeding is the main acute complication of heparin therapy. Patients with impaired hepatic or renal function, with carcinoma, and those aged over 60 years are most at risk. An APTT ratio greater than 3 is associated with an increased risk of bleeding.

Heparin-induced thrombocytopenia (HIT), some times accompanied by *thrombosis* (HIT/T), is due to an autoantibody against heparin in association with platelet factor 4, which activates platelets. It occurs most commonly with heparin derived from bovine lung and is more common with UFHs than with LMWHs. Suspect HIT in any patient in whom the platelet count falls by 50% or more after starting heparin. It usually occurs after 5 days or more of heparin exposure (or sooner if the patient has previously been exposed to heparin). Thrombosis occurs in less than 1% of patients treated with LMWHs but is associated with a mortality and limb amputation rate in excess of 30%. Patients with HIT/T should discontinue all heparin (UF and LMW) and receive an alternative thrombin inhibitor, such as danaparoid or lepirudin. Warfarin should not be commenced until there is adequate anticoagulation with one of these agents and the platelet count has returned to normal.

Osteoporosis may complicate long-term heparin exposure. It is dose related and most frequently observed during pregnancy. The relative risk between LMWHs is not yet established but it appears to be less than with UFHs.

Hypersensitivity reactions and skin necrosis (similar to that seen with warfarin) occur but are rare. Transient alopecia may occur.

Heparin reversal. Protamine, a protein obtained from fish sperm, immediately reverses the anticoagulant action of heparin. It is as strongly basic as heparin is acidic. Protamine sulphate, 1 mg by slow intravenous injection, neutralises 80–100 units UFH. Protamine itself has some anticoagulant effect and overdosage is to be avoided (the maximum must not exceed 50 mg). Its effectiveness in patients treated with LMWH is unknown.

Use of heparin

Treatment of established venous thromboembolism. Patients with acute venous thromboembolism are treated safely and effectively with LMWH as outpatients. Large-scale studies demonstrate that outpatient treatment of acute DVT with unmonitored, body-weight-adjusted LMWH is as safe and effective as inpatient treatment with adjusted-dose i.v. UFH. Further trials confirm the safety and efficacy of LMWH therapy in acute PE.

The traditional regimen for standard UFH is a bolus i.v. injection of 5 000 units (or 10 000 units in major PE) followed by a constant rate i.v. infusion of 1 000–2 000 units/h. The APTT should be measured 6 h after starting therapy and the administration rate adjusted to keep it in the optimal therapeutic range of 1.5–2.5; this usually requires daily measurement of APTT.

Coincident with commencing heparin, patients usually start taking an oral vitamin K antagonist, typically warfarin in the UK. The INR is monitored and loading doses of VKA are given according to a validated loading protocol in order to minimise the risk of over-anticoagulation and bleeding. Ideally the INR should be measured daily during the first 4 days of loading with a VKA.

Prevention of venous thromboembolism. LMWHs are preferred for perioperative prophylaxis because of their convenience. They are as effective and safe as UFH at preventing venous thrombosis. Once-daily subcutaneous administration suffices, as their duration of action is longer than that of UFH and no laboratory monitoring is required.

If UFH is used, 5 000 units should be given subcutaneously every 8 or 12 h without monitoring (this dose does not prolong the APTT), or in pregnancy 5 000–10 000 units subcutaneously every 12 h with monitoring (except for pregnant women with prosthetic heart valves, for whom specialist monitoring is needed).

Cardiac disease. LMWHs are at least as effective as standard heparin for unstable angina. Patients undergoing angioplasty may also receive LMWHs.

Heparin is used to reduce the risk of venous thromboembolism, and the size of emboli from mural thrombi following acute myocardial infarction.

Peripheral arterial occlusion. In the acute phase following thrombosis or arterial embolism, heparin may prevent extension of a thrombus and hasten its recanalisation. Long-term antithrombotic therapy for patients with ischaemic peripheral vascular disease generally requires specific antiplatelet therapy.

Other anticoagulant drugs

Danaparinoid sodium is a mixture of several types of non-heparin glycosaminoglycans extracted from pig intestinal mucosa (84% heparan sulphate). It is an indirect thrombin inhibitor and effective for the treatment of DVT, prophylaxis in high-risk patients and treatment of patients with heparin-associated thrombocytopenia (HIT/T).

Hirudin, a polypeptide originally isolated from the salivary glands of the medicinal leech Hirudo medicalis, is now produced by recombinant technology. It forms an almost irreversible complex with thrombin, causing a potent and specific inhibition of its action. The kidneys are principally responsible for clearing hirudin and the $t_{1/2}$ is 60 min after intravenous administration. No antidote is available for a bleeding patient. It has been used in patients with HIT, thromboprophylaxis in elective hip arthroplasty, unstable angina and myocardial infarction.

Bivalirudin is a bivalent direct thrombin inhibitor produced as a 20-amino-acid recombinant polypeptide. It is a relatively low-affinity inhibitor of thrombin and may thus present a lower bleeding risk, but clinical advantage remains to be shown.

Argatroban, a carboxylic acid derivative, binds non-covalently to the active site of thrombin and is an effective alternative to heparin in patients with HIT.

FIBRINOLYTIC (THROMBOLYTIC) SYSTEM

The system acts to remove intravascular fibrin, thereby restoring blood flow.

Plasminogen activators that convert plasminogen to plasmin initiate the process. A trypsin-like protease, plasmin, then degrades fibrin into soluble fibrin degradation products (Fig. 15.3).

Fig. 15.3 The blood fibrinolytic system. tPA, tissue-type plasminogen activator; uPA, urokinase-type plasminogen activator.

Two immunologically distinct plasminogen activators are found in blood, namely *tissue-type* (tPA) and *urokinase-type* (uPA), both of which are synthesised and released from endothelial cells. Intravascular plasminogen activation is initiated by tPA. In this process, plasminogen and tPA bind to fibrin and the enzymatic activity of tPA is enhanced by fibrin. The result is that plasmin formation takes place only on the fibrin surface and not generally in the circulation, where widespread defibrination would occur and compromise the whole coagulation mechanism. tPA is the plasminogen activator used for the treatment of coronary occlusion.

Plasminogen activator inhibitors. The most important is *endothelial cell-derived type 1 plasminogen activator inhibitor* (PAI-1), which blocks the action of tPA. Another inhibitor, α_2-antiplasmin, rapidly complexes with and inactivates free plasmin. Fibrin-bound plasmin is relatively protected from inactivation so that fibrinolysis can occur despite physiological plasma concentrations of this inhibitor.

An enzyme, known as *thrombin-activatable fibrinolysis inhibitor* (TAFI), attenuates fibrinolysis by cleaving carboxyl terminal lysine residues from fibrin, the removal of which decreases plasminogen and plasmin binding to fibrin, retarding the lytic process. TAFI thus serves as a link between coagulation and fibrinolysis.

DRUGS THAT PROMOTE FIBRINOLYSIS

Recombinant thrombolytic proteins can be reengineered to prolong $t_{1/2}$ and possibly reduce the induced systemic fibrinolytic state. Current drugs possess a broadly equivalent risk of inducing bleeding. Recombinant drugs of human origin are non-antigenic. The $t_{1/2}$ determines whether a drug is suitable for bolus i.v. injection or continuous i.v. infusion. Reteplase and tenecteplase are most appropriate for bolus injection.

Alteplase ($t_{1/2}$ 2–6 min) is a single-chain recombinant tissue-type plasminogen activator (rtPA) that is usually given by continuous i.v. infusion over 30–180 min, according to the indication, i.e. for acute myocardial infarction and acute ischaemic stroke. A bolus dose is recommended for pulmonary embolus.

Reteplase is a deletion mutant of tPA lacking a growth factor and the kringle-binding domain; it possesses a longer $t_{1/2}$ (1.6 h) than alteplase. This permits a double bolus regimen, with completion of treatment in 30 min, rather than the need for administration by infusion. It is licensed for acute myocardial infarction.

Tenecteplase is a tPA variant with amino acid substitutions that confer a longer $t_{1/2}$ (2 h), greater enzymatic efficiency and a more fibrin-specific profile. It is administered as a single i.v. injection over 5–10 s and is licensed for treatment of acute myocardial infarction.

Streptokinase, derived from culture filtrates of *Streptococcus haemolyticus*, is not an enzyme. It binds human plasminogen to produce a plasminogen activator that undergoes a time-dependent change of conformation to create an active site that autocatalytically converts plasminogen to plasmin. The plasmin-complexed streptokinase then decays by proteolytic degradation.

Streptokinase ($t_{1/2}$ 20 min) is given by i.v. infusion, e.g. for up to 72 h when treating patients with venous thromboembolism. It finds use for acute myocardial infarction, deep vein thrombosis and pulmonary embolism, acute arterial thromboembolism, and central retinal venous or arterial thrombosis. The rate of infusion may be limited by tachycardia, fever and muscle aches. Nausea and vomiting may also occur.

Uses of thrombolytic drugs

Coronary artery thrombolysis

The earlier thrombolysis starts, the better the outcome. Benefit is most striking in patients with anterior myocardial infarction treated within 4 h of onset. Contraindications to thrombolytic drug use are those that predispose to intracranial haemorrhage (haemorrhagic stroke, intracranial tumour, recent neurosurgery or brain trauma within the previous 10 days and uncontrolled hypertension) or massive haemorrhage (major surgery of thorax or abdomen within the previous 10 days, current major bleeding such as from the gastrointestinal tract or prolonged cardiopulmonary resuscitation).

Adverse effects. If bleeding occurs, thrombolytic therapy must cease. Depending on the timing of bleeding in relation to therapy, consider antifibrinolytic therapy with aprotonin (for longer-acting drugs) and raising the fibrinogen concentration with fresh frozen plasma or cryoprecipitate (more likely required after streptokinase therapy). Platelet transfusion may be given to correct the platelet function defect induced by plasmin proteolysis of platelet membrane receptors.

Following thrombolytic therapy intramuscular injections are contraindicated, any venepuncture requires at least 10 min of local compression, and arterial puncture must be avoided.

Hypotension can follow treatment with any thrombolytic drug but febrile allergic reactions are about six times more likely with use of a thrombolytic of bacterial origin. Some milder reactions can be managed with paracetamol, an H_1-receptor antihistamine and corticosteroid.

Non-coronary thrombolysis

Pulmonary embolism. Thrombolysis is used in patients with massive pulmonary emboli with cardiovascular compromise; its value in patients with submassive pulmonary embolus is uncertain.

Deep vein thrombosis. Thrombolysis is often not effective in patients with DVT but may be justified when the affected vessels are proximal and risk of pulmonary embolism is high.

Arterial occlusion. Systemic or local thrombolysis may be an option for arterial occlusions distal to the popliteal artery (thrombectomy is the usual therapeutic approach for occlusion of less than 24 h duration proximal to this site). Intravenous streptokinase will lyse 80% of occlusions if infusion begins within 12 h, and 60% if it is delayed for up to 3 days.

Ischaemic stroke. There is little evidence of benefit and most trials have shown increased short-term mortality in patients treated with thrombolysis.

Thrombolysis may also be effective for occluded arteriovenous shunts and for blocked, e.g. central venous, catheters.

DRUGS THAT PREVENT FIBRINOLYSIS

Antifibrinolytics are useful in a number of bleeding disorders.

Tranexamic acid competitively inhibits the binding of plasminogen and tPA to fibrin and effectively blocks conversion of plasminogen to plasmin; fibrinolysis is thus retarded. An intravenous bolus passes largely unchanged in the urine with a $t_{1/2}$ of 1.5 h. Oral and topical formulations are available.

Tranexamic acid is used principally to prevent the *hyperplasminaemic bleeding state* that results from damage to tissues rich in plasminogen activator, e.g. after prostatic surgery, tonsillectomy, uterine cervical cone biopsy and menorrhagia, whether primary or induced by an intrauterine contraceptive device. Tranexamic acid may also reduce bleeding after ocular trauma, and in von Willebrand's disease and haemophilia after dental extraction (normally combined with DDAVP or factor VIII, respectively).

Some patients with *hereditary angioedema* may benefit, presumably by prevention of plasmininduced activation of the complement system.

Tranexamic acid may be of value in *thrombocytopenia* (idiopathic or following cytotoxic chemotherapy). The natural fibrinolytic destabilisation of small platelet plugs is inhibited, reducing the risk of haemorrhage and requirement for platelet transfusion.

Adverse effects are rare but include nausea, diarrhoea and sometimes orthostatic hypotension. Tranexamic acid is contraindicated for patients with haematuria because clot lysis in the urinary tract is prevented and clot colic results.

Aprotinin is a naturally occurring inhibitor of plasmin and other proteolytic enzymes that has been used in the past to limit perioperative bleeding during cardiac bypass and liver transplantation surgery. However, a recently recognised association between aprotonin use and serious end-organ damage has resulted in its withdrawal.

PLATELET FUNCTION

Platelets have a key role in maintaining vascular integrity. They aggregate at and adhere to exposed collagen to form a physical barrier at the site of vessel injury; they accelerate the activation of coagulation proteins; they release stored granules that promote vasoconstriction and wound healing.

Platelets have rightly been termed 'pharmacological packages'. To deliver the above functions, they must first undergo a process of *activation* that involves multiple agonists through numerous intracellular second-messenger pathways and complex networks. These pathways converge on and activate the fibrinogen receptor, *glycoprotein IIbIIIa* (integrin αIIbβ3), inducing a conformational change that results in fibrinogen/fibrin binding. When fibrinogen occupies the receptor, outside-in signalling consolidates platelet activation by up-regulating second-messenger pathways, so providing a positive feedback loop.

In the *coagulation process*, platelets provide an anionic phospholipid surface for assembly of the macromolecular enzymatic complexes required for thrombin generation. Phospholipids in the bilayer membrane of resting platelets are distributed asymmetrically, with anionic phospholipid held in the internal leaflet. Full platelet activation results in scrambling of the membrane with exposure of negatively charged phospholipid on the external leaflet.

This lipid cooperates in the assembly of the thrombin-generating enzymatic complexes.

Receptors on the *platelet membrane* that are known to result in platelet activation through intracellular second messengers include those for thrombin, adenosine diphosphate (ADP), collagen, thromboxane and adrenaline/epinephrine.

Activation is enhanced by occupancy of glycoprotein IIbIIIa (the fibrinogen receptor) and glycoprotein Ib (a component of the Ib/IX/V receptor for von Willebrand protein). The process is mediated primarily through G-coupled second messengers in response to occupancy of the thrombin, ADP and collagen receptors (at high collagen concentration), and through phospholipases and consequent thromboxane generation in response to occupancy of the thromboxane, adrenaline/epinephrine and collagen receptors (at low collagen concentration).

Both thromboxane and ADP are produced in response to platelet activation, and recruit further platelets to activation sites, so providing a positive feedback loop to their respective receptors. There are several ADP receptors on the platelet membrane. Multiple second-messenger pathways are probably involved in their mechanism of activation, not just G-protein-coupled systems. Collagen-induced platelet activation involves at least three receptors with both thromboxane-dependent and thromboxane-independent second-messenger pathways.

High 'shear forces' also activate platelets but the mechanisms are unclear: fibrinogen and its receptor, GPIIbIIIa, are required at low shear rates, and von Willebrand factor and its receptor, GPIb, at high shear rates. ADP and adrenaline/epinephrine are synergistic at high shear and result in larger thrombi for a given rate of shear.

DRUGS THAT INHIBIT PLATELET ACTIVITY (ANTIPLATELET DRUGS)

Aspirin (acetylsalicylic acid) acetylates and thus inactivates cyclo-oxygenase (COX), the enzyme responsible for the first step in the formation of prostaglandins, the conversion of arachidonic acid to prostaglandin H_2. As acetylation of COX is irreversible and the platelet is unable to synthesise new enzyme, COX activity is lost for the platelet lifetime (8–10 days).

Aspirin prevents formation of both thromboxane A_2 (TXA_2) and prostacyclin (PGI_2). Therapeutic interest in the antithrombotic effect of aspirin has centred on separating these actions by using a low dose. In general, 75–100 mg/day by mouth will abolish synthesis of TXA_2 without significant impairment of prostacyclin formation, i.e. amounts substantially below the 2.4 g/day used to control pain and inflammation. Laboratory testing of TXA_2 production or TXA_2-dependent platelet function can provide an assessment of the adequacy of aspirin dose. Among several causes of resistance to aspirin are genetic polymorphisms of COX-1 and other genes involved in thromboxane biosynthesis.

Low-dose aspirin is not without risk: a proportion of peptic ulcer bleeds in people aged over 60 years occur from prophylactic low-dose aspirin.

Dipyridamole reversibly inhibits platelet phosphodiesterase, and consequently cyclic AMP concentration is increased and platelet activity reduced; evidence also suggests that its antithrombotic effect may derive from release of prostaglandin precursors by vascular endothelium. Dipyridamole is bound extensively to plasma proteins and has a $t_{1/2}$ of 12 h.

Clopidogrel is a thienopyridine derivative that inhibits ADP-dependent platelet aggregation. The $t_{1/2}$ of the parent drug is 40 h and metabolism by the liver converts it to its active form. Clopidogrel reduces the risk of the combined outcome of stroke, myocardial infarction (MI) or vascular death in patients with thromboembolic stroke. It decreases vascular death and MI in patients with unstable angina, reduces acute occlusion of coronary bypass grafts, and improves walking distance and decreases vascular complications in patients with peripheral vascular disease. Clopidogrel also finds use in the prevention of stroke in patients who are intolerant of aspirin. An initial dose of 300 mg is followed by a daily dose of 75 mg.

Prasugrel is a thienopyridine derivative like clopidogrel. It inhibits ADP-induced platelet aggregation

more rapidly, more consistently, and to a greater extent than standard dose clopidogrel. A 60-mg loading dose results in at least 50% inhibition of platelet aggregation by 1 h in 90% of patients. The subsequent daily dose is 10 mg.

Epoprostenol (prostacyclin) may be given as an anticoagulant during renal dialysis, with or without heparin; it is infused i.v. and s.c ($t_{1/2}$ 3 min). It is a potent vasodilator.

Glycoprotein (GP) IIb–IIIa antagonists

The platelet glycoprotein IIb–IIIa complex is the predominant platelet integrin, a molecule restricted to megakaryocytes and platelets that mediates platelet aggregation by the binding of proteins such as fibrinogen and von Willebrand factor (vWF) (Fig. 15.4). Hereditary absence of the GP IIb–IIIa complex (Glanzmann's thrombasthenia) results in platelets that are incapable of aggregation by physiological agonists.

GP IIb–IIIa antagonists have been developed as antiplatelet agents. As blockers of the final common pathway of platelet aggregation (the binding of fibrinogen or vWF to the GP IIb–IIIa complex) they are more complete inhibitors of platelets than either aspirin or clopidogrel which act only on the cyclooxygenase or ADP pathway respectively. GP IIb–IIIa antagonists also have an anticoagulant effect by reducing availability of platelet membrane anionic phospholipid. Inhibition of platelet aggregation is dose dependent.

Fig. 15.4 Mechanisms for the activation of platelets. ADP, adenosine diphosphate; GP, glycoprotein.

Abciximab is a human–murinechimeric monoclonal antibody Fab fragment that binds to the GPⅡb–Ⅲa complex with a high affinity and slow dissociation rate. Given intravenously, it is cleared rapidly from plasma ($t_{1/2}$ 20 min). Abciximab (0.25 mg/kg bolus then 0.125 micrograms/kg·min infusion for 12 h) produces immediate and profound inhibition of platelet activity that lasts for 12–36 h after termination of the infusion. The dose causes and maintains blockade of more than 80% of receptors, with a greater than 80% reduction in aggregation. Patients may also receive heparin and an antiplatelet drug, e.g. aspirin. Abciximab is effective in acute coronary syndromes.

Eptifibatide is a cyclic heptapeptide based upon the LysGly-Asp sequence. Tirofiban and lamifiban are non-peptide mimetics. All three are competitive inhibitors of the GPⅡb–Ⅲa complex, with lower affinities and higher dissociation rates than abciximab and relatively short plasma $t_{1/2}$ values (2–2.5 h). Platelet aggregation returns to normal from 30 min to 4 h after discontinuation. Eptifibatide and tirofiban are effective in acute coronary syndromes.

Adverse effects Platelet transfusion after cessation of abciximab is necessary for refractory or life-threatening bleeding. After transfusion, the antibody redistributes to the transfused platelets, reducing the mean level of receptor blockade and improving platelet function. Thrombocytopenia may occur from 1 h to days after commencing treatment in up to 1% of patients. This necessitates platelet counts 2–4 h after commencement and then daily; if severe, therapy must be stopped and, if necessary, platelets transfused. EDTA-induced pseudothrombocytopenia has been reported and a low platelet count should prompt examination of a blood film for agglutination before therapy is stopped.

Other drugs

Dextrans, particularly of mol. wt. 70 000 Da (dextran 70), alter platelet function and prolong the bleeding time. Dextrans differ from the other antiplatelet drugs, which tend to be used for arterial thrombosis; dextran 70 reduces the incidence of postoperative venous thromboembolism if it is given during or just after surgery. The dose should not exceed 10% of the estimated blood volume. Dextrans are rarely used.

USES OF ANTIPLATELET DRUGS

Antiplatelet therapy protects at-risk patients against stroke, myocardial infarction or death. In the first month after an acute myocardial infarction (a vulnerable period) aspirin prevents death, stroke or a further heart attack in about 4 of every 100 patients treated. Continuing treatment from the end of year 1 to year 3 conferred further benefit.

Aspirin is by far the most commonly used antiplatelet agent. The optimal dose is not certain, but one not exceeding aspirin 325 mg/day is acceptable, and 75–100 mg/day may be as effective and preferred where there is gastric intolerance. Aspirin alone (mainly) or aspirin plus dipyridamole greatly reduced the risk of occlusion where vascular grafts or arterial patency were studied systematically.

Many patients who take aspirin for vascular disease may also require a NSAID, e.g. for joint disease. Given their common mode of action by inhibiting prostaglandin synthesis, this raises the issue that NSAIDs may block access of aspirin to active sites on platelets, with loss of cardioprotection. Retrospective cohort and case-control studies suggest no adverse interaction with ibuprofen, but the issue remains unresolved and in the meantime it seems prudent to take aspirin 2 h before a NSAID, e.g. at bedtime.

Part 2. Agents used in anaemias & hematopoietic growth factors

INTRODUCTION

Anaemia due to a haematinic deficiency can be treated with specific replacement therapy (e.g. iron, vitamin B_{12} or folic acid) along with management of the underlying cause. Other secondary anaemias may benefit from haemopoietic growth factor therapy such as erythropoiesis-stimulating agents (e.g. for chronic renal disease), immunosuppression (e.g. for autoimmune haemolytic) or avoidance of specific drugs (e.g. sulfonamides or antibiotics).

IRON

Iron is a trace element that is required for oxygen transport by erythrocytes and for oxidative metabolism in all cells. Up to 75% of body iron is present in haemoglobin (Hb), and the majority of the remainder in myoglobin and enzymes. A normal daily diet contains approximately 10–20 mg iron which is present in meat (heme iron), grains and vegetables. Only 5%–10% of dietary iron is absorbed which is sufficient to compensate for the normal daily loss of iron (1 mg/day) in faeces and desquamation of skin. Iron requirements are greater during periods of growth (i.e. childhood), as a result of blood loss in men-

struation (average menstrual cycle loses 10–15 mg iron) and increased requirements (e.g. pregnancy up to 3 mg iron/day). Gastrointestinal iron absorption can increase up to five-fold with increased demand. Ascorbate increases iron absorption.

Dietary iron is reduced to the ferrous (Fe^{2+}) state at the brush border of the duodenum. *Divalent metal transport 1* (DMT1), located on the membrane of duodenal enterocytes, then transports iron across the intestinal lumen; this is aided by an acidic environment. *Ferroportin*, facilitated by hephaestin, then releases iron into the bloodstream. *Hepcidin* is a key regulator of iron homeostasis and directly inhibits ferroportin release of iron (Fig. 15.5). In the plasma, iron binds to *transferrin* and delivers it to transferrin receptors on developing erythroblasts in the bone marrow. Alternatively, iron may be stored intracel-

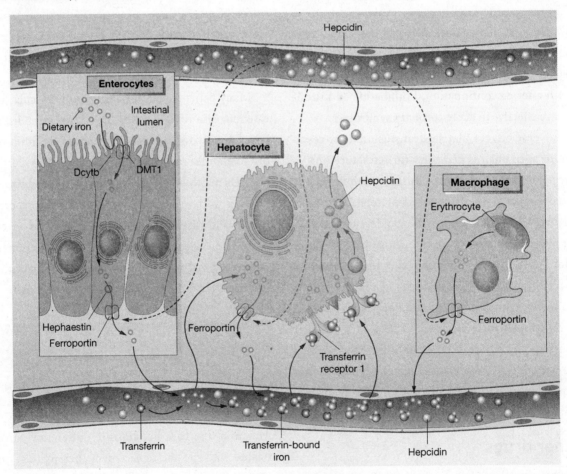

Fig. 15.5 Iron homeostasis. At the brush border, dietary iron is reduced to the ferrous state by duodenal ferric reductase (Dcytb), transported into the mucosal cell by divalent metal transporter 1 (DMT1) and released via ferroportin into the circulation facilitated by hephaestin. Most absorbed iron is delivered to erythroid precursors. Hepatocytes take up iron from the circulation either as free iron or transferrin-bound iron via transferrin receptors 1 and 2. Hepcidin secretion by hepatocytes down-regulates ferroportin-mediated release of iron from enterocytes, macrophages and hepatocytes.

lularly, or excreted in faeces from shed mucosal cells. After 120 days red cells die and the haemoglobin from senescent erythrocytes is released, phagocytosed by macrophages and exported by ferroportin back to plasma transferrin. Excess iron is stored in the bone marrow, hepatocytes and spleen as ferritin (20–300 μg/L).

Iron deficiency

Iron deficiency is the commonest cause of anaemia worldwide. The major causes are:

- Inadequate dietary intake: young infants with inadequate intake of solids (18 months to 3 years), poverty and poor nutrition.
- Increased physiological iron requirements: increased iron demands for growth, i.e. prematurity, rapid growth in adolescence and pregnancy (especially third trimester).
- Reduced iron absorption: coeliac disease, postgastrectomy and gluten-induced enteropathy.
- Blood loss: menstruation, menorrhagia, gastrointestinal malignancy, other causes of chronic haemorrhage (e.g. NSAIDs), hookworm infection and chronic intravascular haemolysis.

The serum ferritin concentration correlates with body iron stores; serum ferritin of < 15 μg/L is virtually specific for iron deficiency. As ferritin is an acute-phase reactant, a normal result does not exclude iron deficiency in the presence of infective and inflammatory conditions. Measurement of serum soluble transferrin receptor (increased in iron deficiency but not by inflammation) may help in differentiating iron deficiency from the anaemia of chronic disease.

Management of iron deficiency and prophylactic iron administration

Management of iron deficiency requires:

1. identification and treatment of the underlying cause, and
2. iron replacement therapy.

Oral iron preparations are the treatment of choice due to their effectiveness, safety and low cost. Iron can be administered as simple iron salts (e.g. ferrous sulphate, fumarate or gluconate) or in saccharated form. Administration of 200 mg ferrous sulphate three times daily provides 180 mg elemental iron per day; up to 30% of the orally administered iron will be absorbed. The haemoglobin will increase by 1 g in the first week; a rise of 2 g/dL after 3 weeks' therapy is evidence of adequate response. Daily administration for 1–3 months will correct anaemia due to iron deficiency. Therapy should be continued for a further 3 months and until the haemoglobin has normalised and iron stores replenished (i.e. serum ferritin > 50 μg/L).

Liquid iron formulations can be used for small children but they stain the teeth. Formulations include ferrous sulphate solution (5 mL contains 12 mg elemental iron), iron polymaltose solutions and polysaccharide–iron complex (5 mL contains 100 mg elemental iron). *Prophylactic oral iron* is appropriate in pregnancy, menorrhagia, following partial or complete gastrectomy, for patients with chronic renal disease receiving erythropoietin, in the early treatment of severe pernicious anaemia (rapid erythropoiesis may exhaust iron stores) and for low-birth-weight or premature infants. Lower doses of oral iron (e.g. 200 mg ferrous sulphate daily) are generally prescribed.

Adverse effects of oral iron (e.g. nausea, epigastric pain, diarrhoea and constipation) are related to the amount of available iron. These effects can generally be ameliorated by reducing the dose, using divided doses, switching to an alternative iron salt (e.g. ferrous gluconate), and/or taking the iron with food. Oral iron may not be well absorbed in patients who have had a partial or complete gastrectomy or coeliac disease. Folate deficiency may be unmasked by effective iron therapy. Where there is a deficiency of both iron and folate, the latter may not be obvious until iron is administered.

Parenteral iron is rarely indicated and should only be administered if there is:

- Proven iron deficiency and oral iron cannot be tolerated.
- Ongoing blood loss so severe that oral therapy is insufficient to maintain iron stores.
- Inadequate gastrointestinal iron absorption.

Parenteral iron formulations include:

- *Iron dextran* (ferric hydroxide complexed with dextrans, 50 mg/mL) which can be administered by deep intramuscular injection, slow intravenous injection or infusion.
- *Iron sucrose* (ferric hydroxide complexed with sucrose, 20 mg/mL) which is delivered by slow intravenous injection or infusion (not recommended for children).

The dose of parenteral iron is based on body weight and the haemoglobin (Hb) deficit, as follows:

Dose of iron (mg) = {Target Hb (g/dL) – Actual Hb × weight (kg) × 2.4} + 500 mg

Adverse effects of intravenous iron include immediate, severe and potentially life-threatening anaphylactoid reactions, fever and arthropathy. Patients should therefore be closely monitored during administration and facilities for cardiopulmonary resuscitation should be available. A history of allergic disorders including asthma, eczema and anaphylaxis is a contraindication to parenteral iron. Intramuscular iron can be painful and may permanently stain the skin. Less severe manifestations include urticaria, rashes and nausea; delayed reactions such as arthralgia, myalgia and fever can also occur. Intramuscular iron has also been associated with soft tissue sarcomas. Oral iron preparations should not be given for 24 h prior to parenteral therapy or for 5 days after the last intravenous injection. This is to prevent adverse reactions as a result of saturation of transferrin binding capacity leading to a high, unbound plasma iron concentration.

Iron poisoning and acute overdose

Iron poisoning is commonest in children, is usually accidental and particularly dangerous. The phases in acute oral iron poisoning are shown in Box 15.1. Ferrous sulphate is the most toxic, while sustained-release iron preparations and multivitamins cause less severe poisoning. Poisoning is severe if the plasma iron concentration exceeds the total iron binding capacity (upper limit 75 mmol/L) or plasma becomes pink due to the formation of ferrioxamine. Treatment is urgent and involves chelating iron in plasma. As an immediate measure, raw egg and milk help bind iron in the stomach. Iron chelation therapy is required for severe toxicity. Desferrioxamine is administered by intravenous infusion (not exceeding 15 mg/kg·h and maximum 80 mg/kg in 24 h) to chelate serum free iron.

Box 15.1 Acute Iron Poisoning

Phase 1

0.5–1 h after ingestion: Abdominal pain, grey-black vomit, diarrhoea, leucocytosis and hyperglycaemia. Severe cases have acidosis and cardiovascular collapse which may proceed to coma and death.

Phase 2

Improvement occurs, lasting 6–12 h; may be sustained or may deteriorate to next phase.

Phase 3

Jaundice, hypoglycaemia, bleeding, encephalopathy, metabolic acidosis and convulsions are followed by cardiovascular collapse, coma and sometimes death 48–60 h after ingestion. Severe brain and liver damage is seen at autopsy.

Phase 4

1–2 months later: scarring and stricture may cause upper gastrointestinal obstruction.

VITAMIN B$_{12}$

The cobalamins are a family of compounds (cyano-, hydroxyo-, methyl- and adenosylcobalamin) that have vitamin B$_{12}$ activity. They have the same basic structure with cobalt within a central corrin ring. Vitamin B$_{12}$ is produced only by microorganisms and humans obtain it by ingesting foods of animal origin. Vitamin B$_{12}$ is required by all cells for DNA synthesis; it is also required for red cell production, methylation and myelin synthesis. A normal diet contains 5–30 µg vitamin B$_{12}$ per day and 1–3 µg is absorbed. Ingested vitamin B$_{12}$ binds to intrinsic factor (IF) synthesised by gastric parietal cells. The cobalamin–IF complex passes to the terminal ileum where it is absorbed. Newly absorbed vitamin B$_{12}$ binds to transcobalamin to form holotranscobalamin (20%–30% of plasma vitamin B$_{12}$); this is the biologically active form which is available for delivery to cells. Most vitamin B$_{12}$ (70%) in the blood is bound to haptocorrin (holohaptocorrin, formerly transcobalamin I) which is taken up by and stored in the liver. The liver stores up to 2–5 mg of vitamin B$_{12}$, which is sufficient for 2–4 years after absorption ceases. Cobalamin is not metabolised significantly and passes into bile and urine.

Vitamin B$_{12}$ deficiency

The most common causes of vitamin B$_{12}$ deficiency are:

- Inadequate dietary intake: the elderly and vegans.
- Pernicious anaemia. Autoimmune destruction of gastric parietal cells produces atrophic gastric mucosa and reduced secretion of intrinsic factor. Vitamin B$_{12}$ deficiency results from failure to absorb cobalamin in the terminal ileum.
- Malabsorption syndromes. Intestinal disease affecting the terminal ileum can interrupt the normal enterohepatic circulation of vitamin B$_{12}$ and result in vitamin B$_{12}$ deficiency. Malabsorption can also result from poor release of vitamin B$_{12}$ from food as a consequence of impaired secretion of acid and pepsin by the stomach.
- Drugs. A number of drugs can reduce vitamin B$_{12}$ absorption, including metformin, aminosalicylic acid, nicotine, phenytoin and large doses of vitamin C.

Vitamin B$_{12}$ deficiency can result in:

- Subclinical disease: mild anaemia without clinical symptoms or signs.
- Megaloblastic anaemia (macrocytic anaemia with oval macrocytes and hypersegmented neutrophils).
- Subacute combined degeneration of the brain, spinal cord and peripheral nerves.
- Abnormalities of epithelial tissue, particularly the alimentary tract, e.g. sore tongue and malabsorption.

Cobalamin deficiency is diagnosed by measuring total plasma vitamin B$_{12}$ (normal 150–450 pmol/L); this includes holotranscobalamin and holohaptocorrin. Holotranscobalamin (normal level 33–91 ng/L), the active portion of vitamin B$_{12}$, is more sensitive and specific for vitamin B$_{12}$ deficiency. In vitamin B$_{12}$ deficiency the serum folate may be elevated and

red cell folate reduced due to disturbance of normal absorption and metabolism (Fig. 15.6). Methylmalonic acid levels may be elevated and are relatively specific for vitamin B$_{12}$ deficiency whereas elevated homocysteine levels are not.

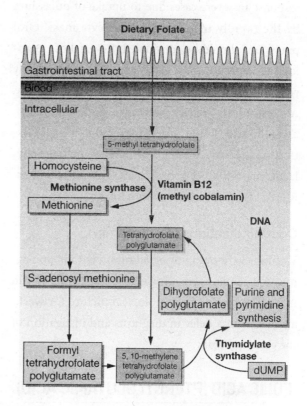

Fig. 15.6 Schematic diagram showing the link between vitamin B$_{12}$ and folate metabolism.

Management of vitamin B$_{12}$ deficiency and prophylactic administration

Vitamin B$_{12}$ administration is indicated for the prevention and treatment of deficiency. *Hydroxocobalamin* is the preferred form of vitamin B$_{12}$ for clinical use. In vitamin B$_{12}$ deficiency, hydroxocobalamin should be given at a dose of 1 mg intramuscularly three times per week for 2 weeks (6 doses) to replenish body vitamin B$_{12}$ stores. Maintenance therapy (1 mg every 3 months) is required if the underlying cause cannot be corrected, such as in pernicious anaemia which requires lifelong vitamin B$_{12}$ therapy. After commencing therapy, there is a blood reticulocyte peak at 5–7 days, and the haemoglobin, red cell count and haematocrit rise after 1 week. The blood indices normalise within 2 months. Failure to respond implies an incorrect or incomplete diagnosis (e.g. additional haematinic deficiency). Stimulation of erythropoiesis may deplete iron and folate stores and these may require supplementation. Hypokalaemia may occur at the height of the erythrocyte response in severe cases due to uptake of potassium by the rapidly increasing erythrocyte mass. Oral potassium should be considered. Reversal of neurological damage is slow, rarely marked, and inversely related to the extent and duration of neuropathy. Adverse effects are extremely rare. Both vitamin B_{12} and folic acid should be administered in megaloblastic anaemia while plasma levels are awaited. Prophylactic vitamin B_{12} (e.g. for vegans) should be administered at a dose of 1 mg every 3 months.

Contraindications to cobalamin

Vitamin B_{12} should not be administered for undiagnosed anaemia. Even a single dose of vitamin B_{12} can interfere with the haematological picture for weeks and result in a delay in diagnosis and instigation of the correct therapy.

FOLIC ACID (PTEROYLGLUYAMIC ACID)

Folic acid is one of the B group vitamins and is widely distributed, particularly in green vegetables, fruits, yeast and liver. A normal adult diet contains approximately 400 µg of folic acid (one-third in monoglutamate and two-thirds polyglutamate form) and 100–200 µg is absorbed. Daily requirements are 50–100 µg. Folate polyglutamate is deconjugated to the monoglutamate form prior to absorption in the proximal jejunum. Within the plasma folate is present mainly as 5-methyl tetrahydrofolate. This enters the cell and is demethylated to tetrahydrofolate, a process that requires vitamin B_{12} (Fig. 15.6). Total folate content of the body is 6–10 mg, stores which will last for only 3–4 months on a folate-deficient diet. Folate is required for amino acid and DNA synthesis and cell division.

Folic acid deficiency

Deficiency of folic acid causes megaloblastic anaemia as a result of impaired production of purines and pyrimidines, essential for DNA synthesis. The haematological features are indistinguishable from vitamin B_{12} deficiency. It is critical to determine which of these haematinics is deficient, as incorrect therapy can have severe ramifications; specifically, folic acid supplements may accelerate progression of subacute combined degeneration of the spinal cord due to vitamin B_{12} deficiency.

In *pregnancy* daily folate requirements increase to 400 µg/day in the third trimester to meet the demands of the developing fetus and placenta. *Premature neonates* require folate supplementation because they lack the build-up of folate stores that normally occurs in the last weeks of pregnancy and hence are commonly deficient. In *chronic haemolytic anaemia* (e.g. autoimmune haemolytic anaemia; sickle cell anaemia; hereditary spherocytosis) the compensatory increased bone marrow erythroid activity results in increased folate demand. Renal dialysis removes folate and therefore chronic haemodialysis or peritoneal dialysis can result in folate depletion. A number of *drugs* interfere with folate absorption, inhibit the activity of folate dependent enzymes or displace folate from transport proteins. Dihydrofolate reductase is inhibited by methotrexate, trimethoprim and pyrimethamine. The antidote to these drugs is folinic acid (5-methyl tetrahydrofolate).

Management of folic acid deficiency and prophylactic administration

Large doses of synthetic folic acid (5 mg orally daily for 4 months) are used to treat folate deficiency irrespective of the cause; up to 15 mg may be required if there is malabsorption. Long-term use may be required if the underlying condition cannot be controlled and/or folate deficiency is likely to recur (e.g. sickle cell disease). It is critical that vitamin B_{12} deficiency be excluded and treated prior to commencement of folic acid therapy. If not, cobalamin neuropathy may develop. Adverse reactions are rare; allergy occurs, and status epilepticus may be precipitated. There is no advantage in giving folinic acid instead of folic acid, except in the treatment of the toxic effects of folic acid antagonists such as methotrexate.

Assessment of folate status before conception should be considered and folate supplementation (400 µg/day orally) given if required. In women hoping to conceive who have had a previous neural tube defect fetus, 5 mg folate daily is recommended. Prophylactic folic acid (200–500 µg daily) should be taken throughout pregnancy; this is generally administered together with prophylactic iron.

HAEMOPOIETIC GROWTH FACTORS

Haemopoietic growth factors, such as ESA and granulocyte colony-stimulating factor (G-CSF), are produced by recombinant DNA technology. These can be administered to stimulate erythroid and myeloid lineages in the bone marrow and are potentially useful for secondary anaemias (e.g. chronic renal failure) and neutropenia due to disease or chemotherapy.

Erythropoiesis-stimulating agents (ESA)

Erythropoietin (EPO), a glycoprotein hormone encoded by a gene on chromosome 7 (7q), controls and regulates erythropoiesis. The kidneys produce 90% and the liver the majority of the remainder. EPO binds to receptors on erythrocyte progenitors in the bone marrow and stimulates their proliferation, differentiation and survival. Normal EPO production increases with hypoxia and decreases with polycythaemia. The anaemia of chronic renal failure is largely due to failure of erythropoietin production.

Therapeutic EPO agents are classified as ESA. Recombinant human erythropoietin (*epoetin*) can be given subcutaneously or intravenously and has a $t_{1/2}$ of 4 h. The dose and frequency of administration is dependent on the indication and response. For optimal erythropoietic response there must be adequate iron and folate stores (as above). The maximum reticulocyte response is seen at 4 days. Epoetin-α and -β are two recombinant forms of EPO available for the treatment of EPO-responsive anaemia and these have equal clinical efficacy. *Darbepoetin* is a hyperglycosyl-ated EPO-derivative with a longer t½ than epoetin. This allows less frequent administration.

Clinical uses of ESA

Anaemia of chronic renal failure. EPO is effective (50–150 units/kg) in chronic renal failure patients with symptoms attributable to anaemia and a Hb <11 g/dL. The aim of EPO therapy is to restore the haemoglobin to 11–12 g/dL. Higher target Hb levels ≥13 g/L are reported to result in risk of stroke, serious cardiovascular events and death. It is critical that plentiful iron is available and the serum ferritin should be maintained > 200 µg/L. Intravenous iron may be required to optimise iron stores prior to EPO administration. In patients with renal failure, a dose-dependent increase in arterial blood pressure follows the rise in red cell mass, and encephalopathy may occur in some hypertensive patients. Arteriovenous shunts of dialysis patients, especially those that are compromised, may thrombose because of increased blood viscosity.

Anaemia due to cancer chemotherapy. ESA have been used in the management of chemotherapy-induced anaemia (Hb <10 g/dL). There is clinical trial evidence that ESA administration increases tumour progression, tumour recurrence, serious cardiac and thrombotic events and death. These serious safety concerns have restricted the use of ESA in oncology.

Other clinical uses of EPO. In symptomatic chronic heart failure with mild anaemia (Hb <10 g/dL) ESA treatment can reduce symptoms, and improve the anaemia and exercise tolerance. Epoetin has also been effective for anaemia of prematurity, rheumatoid arthritis myelodysplasia and HIV patients treated with zidovudine. In all of these settings higher doses of epoetin are required than in renal failure. EPO may be administered to reduce the need for blood transfusion in elective non-cardiac, non-vascular surgery, and can be considered before surgery for patients who decline blood transfusion.

Adverse effects of ESA. Venous thromboembolism is a well-recognised risk. Transient influenza-like symptoms may accompany initial intravenous injections of ESA. Pure red cell aplasia due to development of antibodies may occur after epoetin-α. As increased erythropoiesis outstrips iron and folate stores, iron and folate deficiency may develop, especially in dialysis patients.

Granulocyte colony-stimulating factor

Granulocyte colony-stimulating factor (G-CSF) is a glycoprotein cytokine that stimulates the growth, differentiation and activity of myeloid cells. Recombinant G-CSF, administered intravenously or subcutaneously (5–10 µg/kg per dose), has the following applications:

- Haemopoietic stem cell mobilisation into the peripheral blood for autologous or allogeneic transplantation. Blood mobilised progenitor cells are associated with earlier neutrophil and platelet recovery, fewer transfusions and shorter hospitalisation than those from bone marrow.

- To hasten neutrophil recovery following myelosuppressive chemotherapy, after autologous and allogeneic bone marrow transplantation, in aplastic anaemia and AIDS. G-CSF increases the neutrophil count four- to five-fold within hours of administration, shortens the duration of neutropenia and reduces infections in patients who have received cytotoxic myelosuppressive chemotherapy.

- To improve the neutrophil count in myelodysplastic syndromes, and congenital, cyclical and idiopathic neutropenia. G-CSF can reduce the risk of life- threatening infections and prolong survival.

G-CSF is rapidly cleared after intravenous injection ($t_{1/2}$ 2 h). *Pegfilgrastim*, which has polyethylene glycol covalently bound to G-CSF, has a longer $t_{1/2}$ (40 h) allowing for less frequent dosing, e.g. once per chemotherapy cycle. High concentrations of G-CSF are found in plasma, bone marrow and kidneys; it is degraded to amino acids and excreted in urine.

Adverse effects of G-CSF are medullary bone pain which occurs with high intravenous doses, musculoskeletal pain, dysuria, splenomegaly, allergic reactions and raised liver enzymes. If administered to patients with sickle cell anaemia it may precipitate painful crises. There is an increased risk of acute myeloid leukaemia with chronic G-CSF administration in children with congenital neutropenia.

SUMMARY

- Procoagulant drugs is used to treat haemorrhagic disease. Vitamin K is necessary for the final stage in the synthesis of coagulant factors II (prothrombin), VII, IX and X, and anticoagulant regulatory proteins, proteins C and S. Desmopressin increases the plasma concentration of factor VIII and von Willebrand factor, directly activates platelets, and is useful in patients with mild haemophilia A and von Willebrand's disease.

- The predominant effect of anticoagulant drugs is to limit thrombin generation, or to neutralise thrombin. Warfarin and other oral vitamin K antagonists act by reducing the activity of vitamin K-dependent clotting factors; they take 4–5 days to produce a therapeutic effect. Oral direct thrombin and anti-Xa inhibitors have a fast pharmacodynamic effect in parallel with their pharmacokinetic profile; their anticoagulant effect cannot be reversed. Heparin depends for its anticoagulant action on the presence in plasma of antithrombin, a naturally occurring inhibitor of activated coagulation proteases that include thrombin, factor Xa and factor IX a.

- Fibrinolytic drugs dissolve thrombi in acutely occluded coronary arteries, thereby restoring blood flow to ischaemic myocardium and improving prognosis. Thrombolysis is also effective for massive pulmonary emboli with cardiovascular compromise.

- Antiplatelet therapy protects at-risk patients against stroke, myocardial infarction or death. Aspirin acetylates and thus inactivates cyclo-oxygenase (COX) to inhibit the formation of prostaglandins, and in low dose reduces platelet activity by preventing the formation of thromboxane. Clopidogrel inhibits ADP-dependent platelet aggregation. GP IIb–IIIa antagonists block the final common pathway of platelet aggregation (the binding of fibrinogen or vWF to the GPⅡb–Ⅲa complex) and are more complete inhibitors of platelets than either aspirin or clopidogrel.

- Iron-deficiency anemia is characterized by decreased levels of ferritin (most sensitive marker) and serum iron, as well as decreased transferrin saturation. Most patients are adequately treated with oral iron therapy, although parenteral iron therapy is necessary in selected patient populations.

- Macrocytic anemia can be due to the deficiency of vitamin B_{12} or folic acid, which results from inadequate intake, decreased absorption, and increased requirements. Neurologic symptoms can be present and can become irreversible if the vitamin B_{12} deficiency is not treated promptly. Adequate folic acid intake is essential in women of childbearing age to decrease the risk of neural tube defects in their children.

- Haemopoietic growth factors, such as ESA and G-CSF, can be administered to stimulate erythroid and myeloid lineages in the bone marrow and are potentially useful for secondary anaemias (e.g. chronic renal failure) and neutropenia due to disease or chemotherapy.

IMPORTANT TERMINOLOGY

adverse effects　不良反应

allergic reaction　过敏反应；变态反应

anaemia　贫血

anaphylactoid reaction　类过敏反应，过敏样反应

aplastic anaemia　再生障碍性贫血

atherosclerotic Plaques　动脉粥样硬化斑块

autoimmune haemolytic anaemia (AIHA)　自身免疫性溶血性贫血

biliary fistula　胆瘘

broad-spectrum antibiotic　广谱抗生素

coagulation system　凝血系统

coeliac disease　乳糜泻

disseminated intravascular coagulation (DIC)　弥散性血管内凝血

divalent metal transport 1 (DMT1)　二价金属离子转运蛋白 1

erythropoiesis　红细胞生成

erythropoietin (EPO)　促红细胞生成素

extrinsic-tenase　外源性活化因子 X 酶复合物

ferroportin　铁转运蛋白，铁蛋白

fibrinolytic system　纤维蛋白溶解系统

glucose 6-phosphate dehydrogenase　葡萄糖 6-磷酸脱氢酶

granulocyte colony-stimulating factor (G-CSF)　粒细胞集落刺激因子

haematocrit　红细胞压积；血细胞比容；血细胞容积

haemolytic anaemia　溶血性贫血

haemophilia B (Christmas disease)　B 型血友病（克雷司马斯病）

haemophilic arthropathy　血友病性关节炎

haemopoietic growth factor　造血生长因子

haemorrhoids　痔疮

haemostatic system　凝血系统

helicobacter pylori　幽门螺杆菌

hematologic system　血液系统

hemostasis　止血；止血法

heparin-induced thrombocytopenia (HIT)　肝素诱导性血小板减少症

hepcidin　铁调素

intrinsic-tenase　内源性活化因子 X 酶复合物

kernicterus　核黄疸

malabsorption syndromes　吸收不良综合征

obstructive jaundice　梗阻性黄疸；阻塞性黄疸

plasminogen activator inhibitors　纤溶酶原激活物抑制物

reduced vitamin K　还原型维生素 K

serotonin-reuptake inhibitors　5- 羟色胺再摄取抑制剂

serpin　丝氨酸蛋白酶抑制剂

tachyphylaxis　（因连续服用同一种药物而产生的）快速抗药反应；快速耐受

thrombotic thrombocytopenic purpura　血栓性血小板减少性紫癜

tissue factor (TF)　组织因子

transferrin　转铁蛋白

von Willebrand factor (vWF)　血管假性血友病因子

von Willebrand's disease (vWD)　维勒布兰德氏病（血管性血友病）

Warfarin embryopathy　华法林胚胎病

CHALLENGE YOURSELF

1. Please list 3 classes of anticoagulants and describe their mechanisms of action.
2. Compare the mechanisms of action, pharmacokinetics, clinical uses, and toxicities of the major antiplatelet drugs.
3. List the acute toxicities of iron and urgent treatment for iron poisoning.
4. Explain the major hazard involved in the use of folic acid as sole therapy for megaloblastic anemia.
5. Describe the clinical uses and toxicity of hematopoietic growth factors, EPO and G-CSF.

Fenfei Gao

Chapter | 16 |

Endocrine system, metabolic conditions

Part 1. Adrenal corticosteroids, antagonists, corticotropin

ADRENAL STEROIDS AND THEIR SYNTHETIC ANALOGUES

The adrenal is a composite endocrine gland, and each zone of the cortex synthesises a different predominant steroid; a mnemonic is offered in Figure 16.1 in which the first letter of each word is the first letter of each zone and its corresponding steroid product. The principal synthetic pathways are illustrated in Figure 16.2.

The principal hormone is the glucocorticoid cortisol secreted from the largest zone, the fasciculata; the mineralocorticoid aldosterone is secreted by the glomerulosa, and a number of androgens and oestrogens are secreted by the zona reticularis. The hypothalamic–pituitarys system, through corticotropin releasing factor (CRF) and ACTH, controls cortisol and, to a lesser extent, aldosterone secretion; synthesis and secretion of aldosterone is regulated mainly by the renin–angiotensin system, and by variation in plasma K^+ levels.

Adrenal corticosteroids are available for physiological replacement therapy, in primary (Addison's disease), secondary adrenal insufficiency and congenital adrenal hyperplasia, but their chief use in medicine is for their anti-inflammatory and immunosuppressive effects (pharmacotherapy). Supraphysiological doses are generally required to achieve these pharmacological effects. Chronic use of supraphysiological doses has many adverse effects. Much successful effort has gone into separating glucocorticoid from mineralocorticoid effects.

In the account that follows, the effects of hydrocortisone will be described and then other steroids in so far as they differ. In the context of this chapter, 'adrenal steroid' means a substance with hydrocortisone-like activity.

- **Cortex**

- 'Go Find Rex, Make Good Sex'
  Glomerulosa
  Fasciculata
  Reticularis
  Mineralocorticoids
  Glucocorticoids
  Androgens

- **Medulla**
  Epinephrine
  Norepinephrine

Fig.16.1 The zones of the adrenal gland and the hormones they secrete.

Mechanism of action

Glucocorticoids stimulate the cell through both a classical cytosolic receptor that, on binding with agonist, translocates to the nucleus, and an unidentified membrane-bound receptor. The classical receptor is responsible for so-called genomic effects through either activation or repression of DNA transcription. Up-regulation of gene transcription occurs when the receptor dimerises on specific DNA glucocorticoid response elements (GREs) with consequent recruitment of coactivator proteins. Many of the undesired effects of glucocorticoid occur through this pathway.

Repression of DNA transcription occurs at slightly lower cortisol concentrations than required for transactivation. Through protein–protein interaction, the glucocorticoid– receptor complex inactivates pro-inflammatory transcription factors such as nuclear factor (NF)-κB and activator protein 1 (AP-1), preventing their stimulation of inflammatory mediators: prostaglandins, leukotrienes, cytokines and platelet-activating factor. These mediators would normally contribute to increased vascular permeability and subsequent changes including oedema, leucocyte migration and fibrin deposition.

There is a distinction between replacement therapy (physiological effects) and the higher doses of pharmacotherapy. However, the distinction is not absolute because cortisol is a stress hormone, and some of its physiological actions are triggered by the increased secretion of cortisol during acute or chronic stress. In the list that follows, the main physiological effects are those concerned with elimination of a water load, and mobilisation of glucose. The suppression of inflammatory mediators may also be seen as part of physiological homeostasis.

On inorganic metabolism. Cortisolis required for excretion of a water load. This action is due to maintenance of glomerular filtration, activation of atrial natriuretic factor, and inhibition of vasopressin secretion. These physiological effects are unrelated to the mineralocorticoid (Na⁺-retaining) action of cortisol that occurs at supraphysiological concentrations.

On organic metabolism

- Carbohydrate metabolism, Glycogenolysis and gluconeogenesis are increased and peripheral glucose utilisation is decreased (due to insulin antagonism).
- Protein metabolism, Anabolism (conversion of amino acids to protein) decreases but catabolism continues, so that there is a negative nitrogen balance with muscle wasting. The skin atrophies and this, with increased capillary fragility, causes bruising and striae. Healing of peptic ulcers or of wounds is delayed, as is fibrosis.
- Bone metabolism, Cortisol inhibits the number and function of osteoblasts, and the synthesis of collagen. Osteoporosis (reduction of bone protein matrix) is the main consequence of chronic glucocorticoid administration. Growth slows in children.
- Fat metabolism, Lipolysis is increased, and the secretion of leptin (the appetite suppressant) is inhibited. These actions lead to increased appetite and deposition of adipose tissue, particularly on shoulders, face and abdomen.
- Inflammatory response is depressed, Neutrophil and macrophage function are depressed, including the release of chemical mediators and the effects of these on capillaries.
- Allergic responses are suppressed. The antigen-antibody interaction is unaffected, but its injurious inflammatory consequences do not follow.
- Antibody production is lessened by heavy doses.
- Lymphoid tissue is reduced (including leukaemic lymphocytes).
- Renal excretion of urate is increased.
- Blood eosinophils reduce in number and neutrophils increase.
- Euphoria or psychotic states may occur, perhaps due to central nervous system (CNS) electrolyte changes.
- Anti-vitamin D action.
- Reduction of hypercalcaemia, chiefly where this is due to excessive absorption of calcium from the gut (sarcoidosis, vitamin D intoxication).
- Urinary calcium excretion is increased and renal stones may form.
- Growth reduces where new cells are being added (growth in children), but not where they are replacing cells as in adult tissues.
- Suppression of hypothalamic–pituitary–adreno-cortical feedback system, (with delayed recovery) occurs with chronic use, so that abrupt withdrawal leaves the patient in a state of adrenocortical insufficiency.

The average daily secretion of cortisol is normally 10 mg (5.7 mg/m²). The exogenous daily dose that completely suppresses the cortex is hydrocortisone 40–80 mg, or prednisolone 10–20 mg, or its equivalent of other agents. Recovery of function is quick after a few days' use, but when used over months, recovery takes months. A steroid-suppressed adrenal gland continues to secrete aldosterone.

Individual adrenal steroids

The selectivity of hydrocortisone for the glucocorticoid receptor is due not to a different binding affinity of hydrocortisone to the two receptors but to the protection of the mineralocorticoid receptor by locally high concentrations of the enzyme 11 β-hydroxysteroid dehydrogenase, which converts cortisol to the inactive cortisone. This enzyme satu-

Fig. 16.2 Adrenal. corticosteroid biosynthesis

rates at concentrations of cortisol (and some synthetic glucocorticoids) just above the physiological range, which explains the onset of mineralocorticoid action with pathological secretion of cortisol, and pharmacological use of glucocorticoids.

Hydrocortisone (cortisol) is the principal naturally occurring steroid; it is taken orally; a soluble salt can be given intravenously for rapid effect in emergency whether due to Deficiency, allergy or inflammatory disease. A suspension (Hydrocortisone Acetate Inj.) is available for intra-articular injection.

Parenteral preparation for systemic effect: the soluble Hydrocortisone Sodium Succinate Inj. gives quick (1–2 h) effect; for continuous effect, about 6-hourly administration is appropriate. Prednisolone Acetate Inj. i.m. is an alternative, once or twice a week.

Prednisolone is predominantly anti-inflammatory (glucorticoid), biologically active, and has little sodium-retaining activity; it is the standard choice for anti-inflammatory pharmacotherapy, orally or intramuscularly.

Methylprednisolone is similar to prednisolone; it is used intravenously for pulse therapy.

Fluorinated corticosteroids (triamcinolone, fludrocortisone)

Triamcinolone has virtually no sodium-retaining (mineralocorticoid) effect. Muscle wasting may occasionally be severe, and chronic administration is therefore contraindicated. Anorexia and mental depression can occur at high dose.

Fludrocortisone is a synthetic mineralocorticoid, which stimulates sodium retention. It can replace aldosterone when the adrenal cortex is destroyed (Addison's disease). Fludrocortisone is also the drug of choice in most patients with autonomic neuropathy, in whom volume expansion is easier to achieve than a sustained increase in vasoconstrictor tone. Much higher doses of fludrocortisone (0.5– 1.0 mg) are required when the cause of hypotension is a salt-losing syndrome of renal origin, e.g. after an episode of interstitial nephritis.

Dexamethasone and betamethasone are similar, powerful, predominantly anti-inflammatory steroids.

They are longer acting than prednisolone and are used for therapeutic adrenocortical suppression.

Aldosterone ($t_{1/2}$ 20 min), is the principal natural salt-retaining hormone. After oral administration, it is rapidly inactivated in the first pass through the liver and is not available for therapeutic use.

Spironolactone is a competitive mineralocorticoid (aldosterone) antagonist. It is used in the treatment of primary hyperaldosteronism, as a diureticin resistant hypertension, and when severe oedema is due to secondary hyperaldosteronism, e.g. cirrhosis, congestive cardiac failure. Long-term treatment increases survival in cardiac failure, possibly through blocking the fibrotic effect of aldosterone upon the heart. The dose of spironolactone is limited by its anti-androgen activity. Eplerenone has greater selectivity than spironolactone for the mineralocorticoid than androgen receptor, but has lower efficacy in blocking aldosterone and may need to be used together with amiloride.

Beclometasone, budesonide, fluticasone, mometasone and ciclesonide are potent soluble steroids suitable for use by inhalation for asthma and intranasally for hay fever. Patients swallow about 90% of an inhalation dose, which is then largely inactivated by hepatic first-pass. The drugs are listed in order of development; some newer agents possess properties (first-pass metabolism, high protein binding and lipophilicity) that may increase pulmonary residence time and reduce systemic effects. The main protection against these effects is simply that absorption through mouth, lungs and gut is low relative to the amounts used in systemic administration. The risk of suppression of the hypothalamic–pituitary–adrenal (HPA) axis is infrequent and dose dependent. The greatest risk of suppression appears to occur with high-dose fluticasone usage in children, who may present with hypoglycaemia and acute adrenal insufficiency.

Pharmacokinetics of corticosteroids

Absorption of the synthetic steroids given orally is rapid. The plasma $t_{1/2}$ of most is 1–3h but the maximum biological effect occurs after 2– h. Administration is usually two or three times a day. They are metabolised principally in the liver (some undergoing hepatic first-pass metabolism, see above) and some pass unchanged into the urine. Hepatic and renal disease prolongs, and enzyme induction shortens, to an extent that can be clinically important.

Topical application (skin, lung, joints) allows absorption, which can be enough to cause systemic effects.

In the blood, adrenal steroids circulate in both free and bound forms. Only the free form is biologically active. In the case of hydrocortisone, 95% is bound to cortisol-binding globulin (CBG). This has high affinity, but low capacity; when CBG is saturated, hydrocortisone is 80% bound to albumin.

Because CBG is saturated at peak diurnal levels of cortisol, the free cortisol concentration ranges from approximately 1 nanomol/L at the diurnal trough to approximately 100 nanomol/L at the diurnalpeak. CBG concentrations increase in the presence of oestrogens, e.g. pregnancy, oral contraceptives.

In patients with very low serum albumin, the steroid dose should be lowered to allow for reduced binding capacity. In liver disease, low albumin concentration may be accompanied by slow metabolism ($t_{1/2}$ of prednisolone may be doubled).

Dosage schedules

Various dosing schedules have attempted to limit HPA suppression by allowing the plasma steroid concentration to fall between doses in order to provide time for pituitary recovery. These have not been successful. Daily administration, preferably as a single morning dose, is required for the shortest time necessary. For some indications, e.g. use of methylprednisolone in collagen diseases, pulsed administration of high doses is employed at intervals of weeks or months.

Choice of adrenal steroid: summary
- For oral replacement therapy in adrenocortical insufficiency, use hydrocortisone as the glucocorticoid. In primary adrenal failure (Addison's disease and congenital adrenal hyperplasia), use fludrocortisone as the mineralocorticoid to replace aldosterone.

- For anti-inflammatory and antiallergic (immunosuppressive) effect, use prednisolone or dexamethasone. For inhalation, more potent adrenal steroids are required, e.g. beclometasone or budesonide.
- In diagnostic testing use dexamethasone. In adults with congenital adrenal hyperplasia use hydrocortisone, prednisolone or dexamethasone and hydrocortisone in children.

Adverse effects of systemic adrenal steroid pharmacotherapy

These arise from an excess of the physiological or pharmacological actions of hydrocortisone. Adverse effects are dependent on the corticosteroid used, and on dose and duration. Some occur only with systemic use and for this reason local therapy, e.g. inhalation, intra-articular injection, is preferred where practicable.

The principal adverse effects of chronic corticosteroid administration are:

Endocrine. Chronic dosing leads to features of Cushing's syndrome: moon face, central obesity, oedema, hypertension, striae, bruising, acne, hirsutism. Diabetes mellitus may occur.

Musculoskeletal. Proximal myopathy and tendon rupture may occur. Osteoporosis develops insidiously leading to fractures of vertebrae, ribs, femora and feet. Pain and restriction of movement may occur months in advance of radiographic changes. A bisphosphonate, with vitamin D and calcium supplements, is useful for prevention and treatment. Daily subcutaneous injections of teriparatide (human parathyroid hormone 1-34) increase bone formation and bone density and prevent fractures in glucocorticoid treated patients with osteoporosis. Growth in children is impaired. Avascular necrosis of bone (femoral heads) is a serious complication (at higher doses); it appears to be due to restriction of blood flow through bone capillaries.

Immune. Suppression of the inflammatory response to infection and immunosuppression can mask typical symptoms and signs, and cause more rapid deterioration than usual. The incidence of infection increases with high-dose therapy, and any infection can be more severe when it occurs. The main infections of which patients are at increased risk are fungal, especially candidiasis, and activation of previously dormant tuberculosis. Pneumocystis carinii can occur in the absence of other forms of immunosuppression. Intra-articular injections demand strict asepsis. Live vaccines become dangerous. Developing chickenpox may result in a severe form of the disease, and patients who have not had chickenpox should receive varicella zoster immune globulin within 3 days of exposure. Similarly, avoid exposure to measles.

Gastrointestinal. Patients taking steroid regularly, especially in combination with a non-steroidal anti-inflammatory drug (NSAID), have an excess incidence of peptic ulcer and haemorrhage of about 1%–2%. Prophylactic treatment with a proton pump inhibitor is appropriate when ulcer is particularly likely, e.g. in rheumatoid arthritis, or patients with a history of peptic ulcer disease. There is increased incidence of pancreatitis.

Central nervous system. Depression and psychosis can occur during the first few days of high-dose administration, especially in those with a history of mental disorder. Other effects include euphoria, insomnia, and aggravation of schizophrenia and epilepsy. Long-term treatment may result in raised intracranial pressure with papilloedema, especially in children.

Ophthalmic effects may include posterior subcapsular lens cataract (risk when dose exceeds prednisolone 10 mg/day or equivalent for more than a year), glaucoma (with prolonged use of eye drops), and corneal or scleral thinning.

Other effects include menstrual disorders, delayed tissue healing (including myocardial rupture after myocardial infarction), thromboembolism and, paradoxically, hypersensitivity reactions including anaphylaxis.

Adrenal steroids and pregnancy

Adrenal steroids are teratogenic in animals. A three- to fourfold relative risk of cleft palate is observed in the offspring of mothers receiving steroid pharmacotherapy during early pregnancy. Adrenal insufficiency due to hypothalamic– pituitary suppression in the newborn occurs only with high doses to the mother. Dosage during pregnancy should be kept as low as practicable and fluorinated steroids are best avoided as they are more teratogenic in animals. Hypoadrenal women who become pregnant may require an increase in hydrocortisone replacement therapy by about 10 mg/day to compensate for the increased binding by plasma proteins that occurs in pregnancy. Manage labour as for major surgery (below).

Precautions during chronic adrenal steroid therapy

The most important precaution during replacement and pharmacotherapy is regular review for adverse effects including fluid retention (weight gain), hypertension, glycosuria, hypokalaemia (potassium supplements may be necessary) and back pain (osteoporosis). The main hazard is patient non-compliance.

Patients must always:

- carry a steroid card giving details of therapy
- be impressed with the importance of compliance
- know what to do if they develop an intercurrent illness or other severe stress, i.e. double their next dose and consult their doctor. If a patient omits a dose, a replacement dose should be taken as soon as possible to maintain the same total daily intake, because every patient should be taking the minimum dose necessary to control the disease
- have access to parenteral hydrocortisone (their own supply for i.m. injection, if urgent medical referral is not always possible).

Membership of one of the self-help patient groups can be helpful.

Treatment of intercurrent illness

The normal adrenal cortex responds to severe stress by secreting more than 300 mg hydrocortisone daily. During intercurrent illness, or any other form of severe stress, escalation of steroid dose, and treatment of the underlying problem, is urgent. Effective chemotherapy of bacterial infections is especially important.

Viral infections contracted during steroid therapy (prednisolone20mg/day, or the equivalent) can be overwhelming. Immunosuppressed patients exposed to varicella/herpes zoster virus may need passive protection with varicella zoster immunoglobulin (VZIG) as soon as practicable. However, corticosteroid may sometimes be useful therapy for some viral diseases (e.g. thyroiditis, encephalitis) once there has been time for the immune response to occur. Corticosteroid then acts by suppressing unwanted effects of immune responses and excessive inflammatory reaction.

Vomiting warrants parenteral steroid.

Surgery requires that patients receive hydrocortisone 100mg i.m. or i.v. (hydrocortisone 20 mg orally) with premedication. If there are any signs of cardiovascular collapse during the operation, infuse hydrocortisone (100 mg) i.v. at once. If surgery is uncomplicated, hydrocortisone 50–100 mg i.v.or i.m.every 6h for 24–72h is adequate for most patients on replacement therapy. Then reduce the dose by half every 24 h until the normal dose is reached.

Minor operations, e.g. dental extraction, may be covered by hydrocortisone 20 mg orally 2–4 h before operation, and the same dose afterwards.

In all of these situations, an intravenous infusion should be available for immediate use in case the recommendations above are insufficient. These precautions are particularly relevant for patients who have received substantial corticosteroid treatment within the previous year, because their HPA system may fail to respond adequately to severe stress. If steroid therapy has been very prolonged, and in patients undergoing adrenalectomy for Cushing's syndrome for adrenal adenoma (because the remaining adrenal gland is atrophic), the precautions apply for as long as 2 years afterwards, or until there is evidence of recovery of normal adrenal function.

Dosage and routes of administration

No single schedule suits every case, but examples appear below.

Systemic commencing doses:

- For a serious disease such as systemic lupus, der-matomyositis: prednisolone up to 0.5–1.5 mg/kg daily, orally in divided doses. There is no evidence of increased benefit above 60–80 mg/day.
- If the condition is life-threatening, give prednisolone up to 60 mg, or its equivalent of another steroid.
- Cyclophosphamide or azathioprine are valuable adjuncts which may enhance the initial control of the disease and have a sparing effect on the maintenance dose of prednisolone.
- Alternatively, high dose pulses (methylprednisolone 1.0g i.v. daily for 3 days) maybe used, followed by oral maintenance with prednisolone and/or a steroid-sparing agent (above).
- For less dangerous disease, e.g. rheumatoid arthritis, give prednisolone 7.5–10.0 mg daily, adjusted later according to the response.
- In particular cases, including replacement of adrenal insufficiency, the dosage appears in the account of the disease.
- For continuous therapy, give the minimum amount to produce the desired effect. Imperfect control may have to be accepted by the patient if full control, e.g. of rheumatoid arthritis, though obtainable, involves doses that will lead to toxicity, e.g. osteoporosis, if continued for years.

Topical applications (creams, intranasal, inhalations, enemas) are used in order to obtain local effect, while avoiding systemic effects; suspensions of solutions are also injected into joints, soft tissues and subconjunctivally. All can, in heavy dose, be absorbed sufficiently to suppress the hypothalamus and cause other unwanted effects. Individual preparations appear in the text where appropriate.

Contraindications to adrenal steroids for suppressing inflammation are all relative. Where the patient has diabetes, a history of mental disorder or peptic ulcer, epilepsy, tuberculosis, hypertension or heart failure, the reasons for use must be compelling. The presence of any infection demands that effective chemotherapy be begun before the corticosteroid, but there are exceptions. Topical corticosteroid applied to an inflamed eye can be disastrous if the inflammation is due to herpes virus.

Adrenal steroids containing fluorine intensify diabetes more than do others and are to be avoided in that disease.

Long-term use of adrenal steroids in children presents essentially the same problems as in adults with the addition of growth retardation. This is unlikely to be important unless therapy exceeds 6 months; there is a growth spurt after withdrawal. The dose should be reduced to the minimum required to maintain immunosuppression and be given daily or alternate days.

Common childhood viral infections may be more severe, and if a non-immune child taking steroids is exposed to virus infection it is wise to try to prevent the disease with the appropriate specific immuno-globulin.

Live virus vaccination is unsafe in immunosup-pressed subjects, e.g. systemic prednisolone, more than 2 mg/kg·day for more than1 week in the preced-ing 3 months, as it may cause the disease, but active immunisation with killed vaccines or toxoids will give normal response unless the dose of steroid is high, when the response maybe suppressed.

Raised intracranial pressure may occur more readily in children than in adults.

> **Indications for use of adrenal steroids**
> - Replacement of hormone deficiency.
> - Inflammation suppression.
> - Immunosuppression.
> - Suppression of excess hormone secretion.

USES OF ADRENOCORTICAL STEROIDS

Replacement therapy

Acute adrenocortical insufficiency (Addisonian crisis)

This is an emergency; hydrocortisone sodium succi-nate 100 mg is given i.v. immediately it is suspected.

- An intravenous infusion of sodium chloride solu-tion (0.9%) is set up immediately and a second 100 mg hydrocortisone is added to the first litre, which should be given as quickly as the cardio-vascular status permits (2–3L of sodium chloride may be infused in the first 1–2h and 5–6L may be needed in the first 24 h).
- The patient should then receive hydrocortisone 50 mg i.v. or i.m. 6-hourly for 24–72 h; thereafter a total of 30–40 mg/day orally in two or three divided doses usually suffices.

Treatment to restore electrolyte balance will depend on the circumstances. Seek and treat the cause of the crisis; it is often an infection. When the dose of hydrocortisone falls below 40 mg/day, supplementary mineralocorticoid (fludrocortisone) may be needed.

The hyperkalaemia of Addison's disease will respond to the above regimen and must not be treated with insulin.

Chronic primary adrenocortical insufficiency (Addison's disease)

Hydrocortisone is given orally (15–25 mg total daily) in two to three divided doses, according to the algo-rithm in Figure 16.3 Some patients working under increased physical activity or mental stress may require higher doses up to 40 mg daily. The aim is to mimic the natural diurnal rhythm of secretion. All patients also require mineralocorticoid replacement, and fludrocortisone; 50200 micrograms orally once a day is the usual dose.

The dose of the hormones is determined in the individual by following general clinical progress and particularly by observing: weight, blood pressure, appearance of oedema, serum sodium and potassium concentrations, and haematocrit. In addition, mea-surement of cortisol levels at critical points in the day as a day curve can be done and the information used to adjust the hydrocortisone dose. Where available, plasma renin assay is useful for titration of fludro-cortisone dose. If any complicating disease arises, e.g. infection, a need for surgery or other stress, the hydrocortisone dose is immediately doubled.

If there is vomiting, the parenteral replacement hormone must be given without delay.

Chronic secondary adrenocortical insufficiency

This occurs in hypopituitarism. The need for hydrocortisone may be less than in primary insufficiency, especially when ACTH deficiency is partial. Some patients with borderline adrenocortical insufficiency may require steroid supplementation only during periods of stress, such as infection or surgery. Mineralocorticoid replacement is seldom required, for the pituitary has little control over aldosterone production. Other pituitary replacement is given as appropriate.

Iatrogenic adrenocortical insufficiency: abrupt withdrawal

This occurs in patients who have recently received prolonged pharmacotherapy with a corticosteroid that inhibits hypothalamic production of the corticotropin releasing hormone and so results in secondary adrenal failure. Treat by reinstituting the original therapy or manage as for acute adrenal insufficiency, as appropriate. To avoid an acute crisis on discontinuing therapy, the corticosteroid must be withdrawn gradually to allow the hypothalamus, the pituitary and the adrenal to regain normal function. Treat patients taking corticosteroids who have an infection or surgical operation (major stress) as for primary insufficiency.

Sudden withdrawal of large doses of steroid hormone. used to suppress inflammation or allergy may

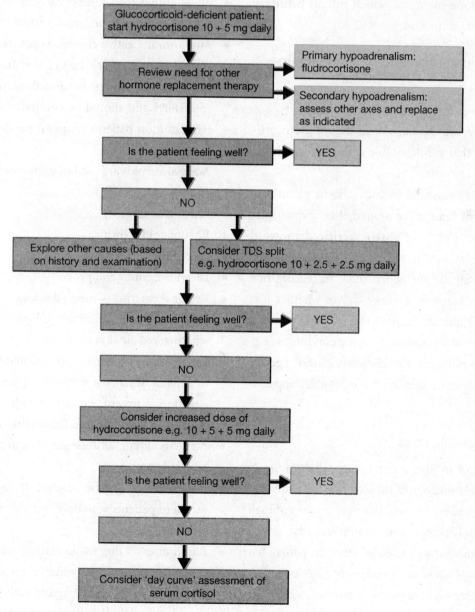

Fig. 16.3 Algorithm for treatment of the glucocorticoid-deficient patient. Patients should be reassessed at 6–8-week intervals while their treatment is optimised.

lead not only to an adrenal insufficiency crisis but also to relapse of the disease that is suppressed, not cured. Such relapse can be extremely severe, and sometimes life-threatening. Secondary adrenal insufficiency can occur after high-dose inhaled potent glucocorticoids in the treatment of asthma.

Pharmacotherapy

Suppression of adrenocortical function

In congenital adrenal hyperplasia, excess adrenal androgen secretion is suppressed by hydrocortisone in children, and hydrocortisone or prednisolone or dexamethasone in adults, which inhibit pituitary corticotropin production.

Use in inflammation and for immunosuppression

Drugs with primarily glucocorticoid effects, e.g. prednisolone, are chosen, so that the mineralocorticoid effects that are inevitable with hydrocortisone do not limit the dose.

It remains essential to use only the minimum dose that will achieve the desired effect. Sometimes therapeutic effects are partly sacrificed to avoid adverse effects, as it has not so far proved possible to separate all the glucocorticoid effects from one another; for example, it is not known whether it is possible to eliminate catabolic effects and yet retain anti-inflammatory action. In some conditions, e.g. nephrotic syndrome, the clinician cannot specify exactly what action they want the drug developer to provide.

Further specific uses

The decision to give a corticosteroid commonly depends on knowledge of the likelihood and amount of benefit (bearing in mind that very prolonged high dose inevitably brings serious complications), on the severity of the disease and on whether the patient has failed to respond usefully to other treatment.

Adrenal steroids are used in nearly all cases of the following:

- Exfoliative dermatitis and pemphigus, if severe.
- Connective tissue diseases, if severe, e.g. lupus erythematosus (systemic), polyarteritis nodosa, polymyalgia rheumatica and cranial giant cell arteritis (urgent therapy to save sight), dermatomyositis.
- Severe asthma.
- Acute lymphatic leukaemia.
- Acquired haemolytic anaemia.
- Severe allergic reactions of all kinds, e.g. serum sickness, angioedema, trichiniasis. Alone, they will not control acute manifestations of anaphylactic shock as they do not act quickly enough.
- Organ transplant rejection.
- Acute spinal cord injury: early, brief, and high dose (to reduce the oedema/inflammation).
- Autoimmune active chronic hepatitis: a corticosteroid improves well-being, liver function and histological findings; prednisolone will benefit some 80% and should be continued in the long term, as most patients relapse if the drug is withdrawn.

Adrenal steroids are used in some cases of the following:

- Rheumatic fever.
- Rheumatoid arthritis.
- Ankylosing spondylitis.
- Ulcerative colitis and proctitis.
- Regional enteritis (Crohn's disease).
- Hay fever (allergic rhinitis); also some bronchitics with marked airways obstruction.
- Sarcoidosis. If there is hypercalcaemia or threat to a major organ, e.g. eye, adrenal steroid administration is urgent. Pulmonary fibrosis may be delayed and CNS manifestations may improve.
- Acute mountain/altitude sickness, to reduce cerebral oedema.
- Prevention of adverse reaction to radiocontrast media in patients who have had a previous severe reaction.
- Blood diseases due to circulating antibodies, e.g. thrombocytopenic purpura (there may also be a decrease in capillary fragility with lessening of purpura even though thrombocytes remain few); agranulocytosis.

- Eye diseases. Allergic diseases and non-granulomatous inflammation of the uveal tract. Bacterial and viral infections may be made worse and use of corticosteroids to suppress inflammation of infection is generally undesirable, is best left to ophthalmologists and must be accompanied by effective chemotherapy; this is of the greatest importance in herpes virus infection. Corneal integrity should be checked before use (by instilling a drop of fluorescein). Prolonged use of corticosteroid eye drops causes glaucoma in 1 in 20 of the population (a genetic trait). Application is generally as hydrocortisone, prednisolone or fluorometholone drops, or subconjunctival injection.

- Nephrotic syndrome. Patients with minimal change disease respond well to daily prednisolone, 2 mg/kg, for 6weeks followed by 1.5 mg/kg on alternate days. Relapses are treated with the higher dose until proteinuria is trace level only, and then the lower dose for a month. Multiple relapses then require a tapering dose over several months rather than complete withdrawal. In such patients, steroid sparing agents, ciclosporin, tacrolimus, and mycophenolate, may be used to reduce long-term dosing.

- A variety of skin diseases, such as eczema. Severe cases may involve occlusive dressings if a systemic effect is undesirable, though absorption can be substantial.

- Aphthous ulcers. Hydrocortisone 2.5 mg oromucosal tablets are allowed to dissolve next to the ulcer; beclometasone dipropionate inhaler 50-100 micrograms may be sprayed on the oral mucosal, or betamethasone soluble talet 500 miligrams dissolved in water may be used, without swallowing, as a mouth wash. Triamcinolone acetonide in Orabase, or fluocinonide gel covered by Orabase may be used where available. Early initiation of treatment may accelerate healing.

- Acute gout resistant to other drugs.

- Hypercalcaemia of sarcoidosis and of vitamin D intoxication responds to prednisolone 30 mg daily (or its equivalent of other adrenal steroid) for 10 days. Hypercalcaemia of myeloma and some other malignancies responds more variably. Hyperparathyroid hypercalcaemia does not respond.

- Raised intracranial pressure due to cerebral oedema, e.g. in cerebral tumour or encephalitis. This is probably an anti-inflammatory effect, which reduces vascular permeability and acts in 12–24 h. Give dexamethasone 10 mg i.m. or i.v. (or equivalent) initially and then 4 mg 6-hourly by the appropriate route, reducing the dose after 2–4 days and withdrawing over 5– days. Much higher doses may be used in palliation of inoperable cerebral tumour.

- Preterm labour: (to mother) to enhance fetal lung maturation.

- Aspiration of gastric acid (Mendelsohn's syndrome).

- Myasthenia gravis.

- Cancer.

Use in diagnosis. Dexamethasone suppression test. Dexamethasone acts on the hypothalamus to reduce output of corticotropin releasing hormone (CRH), but it does not interfere with measurement of cortisol in blood or urine. Normal suppression of cortisol production after administering low dexamethasone (0.5 mg 6-hourly) indicates that the HPA axis is intact. Failure of suppression implies pathological hypersecretion of ACTH by the pituitary, ectopic ACTH or autonomous secretion of cortisol by the adrenal. Dexamethasone is used because its action is prolonged (24 h). There are several ways of carrying out the test.

Withdrawal of pharmacotherapy

The longer the duration of therapy, the slower must be the withdrawal.

If use is less than 1 week, e.g. for acute asthma, although some hypothalamic suppression will have occurred, withdrawal can be safely accomplished in a few steps.

After use for 2 weeks, for rapid withdrawal, a 50% reduction in dose each day is reasonable.

If the duration of treatment is longer, dose reduction is accompanied by the dual risk of resurgence of the disease and iatrogenic hypoadrenalism; withdrawal should then proceed very slowly, e.g. 2.5–5 mg prednisolone or equivalent at intervals of 3–7 days.

An alternative scheme is to halve the dose weekly until it is 25 mg/day of prednisolone or equivalent, then to make reductions of about 1 mg/day every third to seventh day. Paediatric tablets (1 mg) can be useful during withdrawal.

These schemes may yet be too rapid (with the occurrence of fatigue, 'dish-rag' syndrome or relapse of disease). The rate of reduction may then need to be as slow as prednisolone 1mg/day (or equivalent) per month, particularly as the dose approaches the level of physiological requirement (equivalent of prednisolone 5–7.5 mg daily).

The long tetracosactide test or plasma corticotropin concentration is useful to assess recovery of adrenal responsiveness. A positive result does not necessarily indicate full recovery of the patient's ability to respond to stressful situations; the latter is best shown by an adequate response to insulin-induced hypoglycaemia (which additionally tests hypothalamic–pituitary capacity to respond).

Corticotropin should not be used to hasten recovery of the atrophied cortex because its effects further suppress the hypothalamic–pituitary axis, on recovery of which the patient's future depends. Complete recovery of normal HPA function sufficient to cope with severe intercurrent illnesses or surgery is generally complete in 2 months but may take as long as 2 years.

There are many reports of collapse, even coma, occurring within a few hours of omission of adrenal steroid therapy, e.g. due to patients' ignorance of the risk to which their physicians are exposing them, or failure to carry their tablets with them. Patients must be instructed on the hazards of omitting therapy and, during intercurrent disease, intramuscular preparations should be freely used. For anaesthesia and surgery in adrenocortical insufficiency.

INHIBITION OF SYNTHESIS OF ADRENAL AND OTHER STEROID HORMONES

These agents have use in diagnosis of adrenal disease and in controlling excessive production of cortico-

steroids, e.g. by corticotropin-producing tumours of the pituitary (Cushing's syndrome) or by adrenocortical adenoma or carcinoma where the cause cannot be removed. Use of these drugs calls for special care as they can precipitate acute adrenal insufficiency. Hydrocortisone replacement in a block and replace regimen may be given. Some members inhibit other steroid synthesis.

Metyrapone inhibits the enzyme, steroid11b-hydroxylase, which converts 11-deoxy precursors into hydrocortisone, corticosterone and aldosterone. It affects synthesis of aldosterone less than that of glucocorticoids.

Trilostane blocks the synthetic path earlier (3β-hydroxysteroid dehydrogenase) and thus inhibits aldosterone synthesis as well.

Formestane is a specific inhibitor of the aromatase that converts androgens to oestrogens. A depot injection of 250 mg i.m. is given twice a month to treat some patients with carcinoma of the breast who have relapsed on tamoxifen.

Aminoglutethimide blocks at an even earlier stage, preventing the conversion of cholesterol to pregnenolone. It therefore stops synthesis of all steroids, hydrocortisone, aldosterone and sex hormones (including the conversion of androgens to oestrogens); it has a use in breast cancer.

Ketoconazole inhibits several cytochrome P450 enzymes, including those involved in steroid synthesis. It is an effective antifungal agent by virtue of its capacity to block ergosterol synthesis. In humans it inhibits steroid synthesis in gonads and adrenal cortex. Its principal P450 target in the adrenal is the enzyme CYP 11B1 (11β-hydroxylase), which catalyses the final step in cortisol synthesis. CYP 11B1 inhibition by ketoconazole renders it a useful treatment for Cushing's syndrome, while testosterone synthesis inhibitors may be useful in advanced prostatic cancer.

Anastrozole is an adrenal aromatase inhibitor that finds use as adjuvant treatment of oestrogen receptor-positive early breast cancer in postmenopausal women. It is used as sole therapy, following 2–3 years of tamoxifen, in advanced breast cancer in postmenopausal women that is oestrogen receptor positive or responsive to tamoxifen. Letrozole and exemestane are similar.

COMPETITIVE ANTAGONISM OF ADRENAL STEROIDS

Spironolactone antagonises the sodium-retaining effect of aldosterone and other mineralocorticoids. It is used to treat primary and secondary hyperaldosteronism.

ADRENOCORTICOTROPHIC HORMONE (ACTH) (CORTICOTROPIN)

Natural corticotropin is a 39-amino-acid polypeptide secreted by the anterior pituitary gland; it is obtained from animal pituitaries.

The physiological activity resides in the first 24 amino acids (which are common to many species) and most immunological activity lies in the remaining 15 amino acids.

The pituitary output of corticotropin responds rapidly to physiological requirements by the familiar negative-feedback homeostatic mechanism. As the $t_{1/2}$ of corticotropin is 10 min and the adrenal cortex responds within 2 min, corticosteroid output can adjust rapidly.

Synthetic corticotropins have the advantage of shorter amino acid chains (they lack amino acids 25–39) which are less likely to cause serious allergy, although this does occur. Additionally, they are devoid of animal proteins, which are potent allergens.

Tetracosactide (tetracosactrin) consists of the biologically active first 24 amino acids of natural corticotropin (from humans or animals) and so it has similar properties, e.g. $t_{1/2}$ 10 min.

Actions

Corticotropin stimulates the synthesis of corticosteroids (of which the most important is cortisol) and to a lesser extent of androgens, by the cells of the adrenal cortex. It has only a minor (transient) effect on aldosterone production, which proceeds independently; in the absence of corticotropin the cells of the inner cortex atrophy.

The release of natural corticotropin by the pituitary gland is controlled by the hypothalamus through corticotropin releasing hormone (CRH, or corticoliberin), production of which is influenced by environmental stresses as well as by the level of circulating cortisol. High plasma concentration of any adrenal steroid with glucocorticoid effect prevents release of CRH and so of corticotropin, lack of which in turn results in adrenocortical hypofunction. This is why catastrophe may accompany abrupt withdrawal of long-term adrenal steroid therapy with adrenal atrophy.

The effects of corticotropin are those of the steroids (hydrocortisone, androgens) liberated by its action on the adrenal cortex. Prolonged heavy dosage causes the clinical picture of Cushing's syndrome.

Uses. Corticotropin is used principally in diagnosis and rarely in treatment. It is inactive if taken orally and has to be injected like other peptide hormones.

Diagnostic use is to test the capacity of the adrenal cortex to produce cortisol. With the short synacthen test, the plasma cortisol concentration is measured before and 30 min and 60 min after an intramuscular injection of 250 micrograms of tetracosactide (Synacthen); a normal response is a rise in plasma cortisol concentration of more than 200 nmol/L or a peak of greater than 500 nmol/L at 30 or 60 min.

Therapeutic use is seldom appropriate, as the peptide hormone must be injected. Selective glucocorticoid (without mineralocorticoid) action is not possible, and clinical results are irregular. Corticotropin cannot be relied on to restore adrenal cortisol output when a steroid is being withdrawn after prolonged therapy, as it does not restore function in the suppressed hypothalamic–pituitary part of the HPA axis.

Preparations

- Tetracosactide Injection is supplied as an ampoule for injection i.v., i.m. or s.c.
- Tetracosactide Zinc Injection (Synacthen Depot)

i.m. in which the hormone is adsorbed on to zinc phosphate from which it is slowly released. This is the form used in the long tetracosactide test.

SUMMARY

- Physiological concentrations of cortisol are essential for supporting the circulation and glucose production. Physiological concentrations of aldosterone are essential to prevent excessive sodium loss.
- For systemic pharmacological uses, prednisolone or other synthetic adrenocorticosteroids are used because they are more selective glucocorticoids, i.e. have less sodiumretaining activity.
- For local administration (skin, lung), more potent, fluorinated steroids may be required.
- Glucocorticoids inhibit the transcriptional activation of many of the inflammatory cytokines, giving them a versatile role in the treatment of many types of inflammation.
- Fludrocortisone is a valuable treatment for many sodiumlosing states, and for most causes of autonomic neuropathy.
- Corticotropin is used to test the capacity of the adrenal gland to produce cortisol.

Part 2. Diabetes mellitus, insulin, oral antidiabetes agents, obesity

DIABETES OVERVIEW

Diabetes mellitus affects at least 2% of many national populations. Its successful management requires close collaboration between the patient and healthcare professionals.

Diabetes is best regarded as a group of related conditions in which blood glucose levels tend to rise. Diabetes is common and increasing. In large part, this global increase in diabetes may be related to increased levels of obesity. Diabetes can lead to serious medical complications – blindness from retinopathy, renal failure, gangrene and limb amputation, cardiovascular disease and premature death. Aggres-

sive therapy with a combination of pharmacological therapies aimed at lowering blood glucose and blood pressure and optimising lipids can reduce risk of these complications.

HISTORY OF INSULIN THERAPY IN DIABETES

Diabetes was known to ancient Greek medicine with the description of 'a melting of the flesh and limbs into urine... the patients never stop making water but the flow is incessant... their mouth becomes parched and their body dry'.

Insulin (as pancreatic islet cell extract) was first administered to a 14-year-old insulin-deficient patient on 11 January 1922 in Toronto, Canada. R.D. Lawrence, an adult sufferer from diabetes who developed the disease in 1920 and who, because of insulin, lived until 1968, has told how:

Many doctors, after they have developed a disease, take up the speciality in it... But that was not so with me. I was studying for surgery when diabetes took me up. The great book of Joslin said that by starving you might live four years with luck. [He went to Italy and, whilst his health was declining there, he received a letter from a biochemist friend which said] there was something called 'insulin' appearing with a good name in Canada, what about going there and getting it. I said 'No thank you; I've tried too many quackeries for diabetes; I'll wait and see'. Then I got peripheral neuritis... So when [the friend] cabled me and said, 'I've got insulin – it works – come back quick', I responded, arrived at King's College Hospital, London, and went to the laboratory as soon as it opened... It was all experimental for [neither of us] knew a thing about it... So we decided to have 20 units a nice round figure. I had a nice breakfast. I had bacon and eggs and toast made on the Bunsen. I hadn't eaten bread for months and months...by 3 o'clock in the afternoon my urine was quite sugar free. That hadn't happened for many months. So we gave a cheer for Banting and Best.

But at 4 pm I had a terrible shaky feeling and a terrible sweat and hunger pain. That was my first experience of hypoglycaemia. We remembered that Banting and Best had described an overdose of insulin in dogs. So I had some sugar and a biscuit and soon got quite well, thank you.

Diabetes mellitus is classified broadly as:

- **Type 1** (formerly, insulin dependent diabetes mellitus, IDDM) which typically occurs in younger people who cannot secrete insulin.
- **Type 2** (formerly, non-insulin dependent diabetes mellitus, NIDDM), which usually occurs in older people who are typically (although not always) obese. Type 2 diabetes is best thought of as a group of conditions characterised by a variable combination of reduced insulin secretion and resistance to insulin's blood glucose lowering action.
- **Other causes:** including gestational diabetes, disease processes affecting the liver or pancreas such as cystic fibrosis causing a 'secondary' diabetes, monogenic forms (maturity onset diabetes of the young, MODY). These terms and abbreviations are used in this chapter.

Sources of insulin

Insulin is synthesised and stored (bound to zinc) in granules in the β-islet cells of the pancreas. Daily secretion typically amounts to 30–40 units, which is about 25% of total pancreatic insulin content. The principal factor that evokes insulin secretion is a high blood glucose concentration. In addition, insulin release following oral intake of carbohydrate is facilitated by the action of 'incretin factors' such as GLP-1 released from specialised neuroendocrine cells in the small bowel.

Insulin is a polypeptide with two peptide chains (A chain, 21 amino acids; B chain, 30) linked by two disulphide bridges. The basic structure having metabolic activity is common to all mammalian species but there are minor species differences:

- Bovine insulin differs from human insulin by three amino acids.
- Porcine insulin differs from human by only one amino acid.
- Human insulin is made either by enzyme modification of porcine insulin, or by using recombinant DNA to synthesise the pro-insulin precursor molecule for insulin. This is done by artificially introducing the DNA into either Escherichia coli or yeast.
- Insulin analogues are now widely used and have modifications introduced to the A and/or B chains, which result in more rapid onset and offset of action (rapidly acting analogues), or slower offset (long acting analogues) than naturally occurring insulin.

Insulin receptors

Insulin receptors (comprising 2 αand 2 β subunits) are present on the surface of target cells such as liver, muscle and fat. Insulin binding results in tyrosine autophosphorylation of the β subunit. This then phosphorylates other substrates so that a signalling cascade is initiated and biological responses ensue. Downstream effects of stimulation of the insulin receptor include both immediate/short-term actions (for example translocation of the glucose transporter GLUT4 to the surface of target cell) and longer-term actions (for example increased expression of glucokinase and reduced expression of gluconeogenic and ketogenic enzymes in the liver).

Actions of insulin

- Reduction in blood glucose is due to increased glucose uptake in peripheral tissues (which oxidise glucose or convert into glycogen or fat), and a reduction in hepatic output of glucose (diminished breakdown/increased synthesis of glycogen and diminished gluconeogenesis).
- Other metabolic effects. Although, therapeutically, insulin is thought of as a blood glucose lowering hormone, it has a number of other cellular actions. Insulin is an anabolic hormone, enhancing protein synthesis (which has resulted in cases of misuse by bodybuilders). It also inhibits both breakdown of fats (lipolysis) and ketogenesis. Insulin also has actions on electrolytes, stimulating potassium uptake into cells and renal sodium retention (anti-natriuretic effect). Within brain,

insulin may have actions to stimulate memory and act as a nutritional signal to help control appetite/food intake.

USES

- Diabetes mellitus is the main indication.
- Insulin promotes the passage of potassium into cells by stimulating cell surface Na/K ATPase action, and this effect is utilised to correct hyperkalaemia.
- Insulin-induced hypoglycaemia can also be used as a stress test of anterior pituitary function (growth hormone and corticotropin and thus cortisol are released).

Pharmacokinetics

In health, insulin is secreted by the pancreas, enters the portal vein and passes straight to the liver, where half of it is taken up. The rest enters and is distributed in the systemic circulation so that its concentration (in fasting subjects) is only about 15% of that entering the liver. Insulin is released continuously and rhythmically from the healthy pancreas with additional increases following carbohydrate ingestion. As described below, modern insulin regimens in diabetes aim to match this pattern as far as possible.

In contrast to the natural pancreatic release, when insulin is injected subcutaneously during the treatment of diabetes, it enters the systemic circulation so that both liver and other peripheral organs receive the same concentration. It is inactivated in the liver and kidney; about 10% appears in the urine. The plasma $t_{1/2}$ is only 5 min although clearance of 'tissue' insulin levels lags behind this; this is noteworthy when stopping intravenous insulin infusions as it may take 60 min for effects to wear off.

Most commonly, insulin is self-delivered by patients using either a syringe with a fixed needle (after drawing up insulin from a vial) or an insulin pen device (supplied as a preloaded disposable pen or with replaceable cartridges). Within hospital, soluble insulin may be delivered by intravenous infusion. Typically, 50 units soluble insulin is dissolved in 50 mL isotonic saline (i.e. insulin concentration 1 unit/mL).

An alternative and increasingly popular method for delivering insulin, especially in type 1 diabetes, is for patients to use continuous subcutaneous insulin infusion devices ('insulin pumps'). These small cellphone-size personal devices provide a continuous basal delivery of soluble insulin with an additional insulin bolus when needed to cover meals or to correct high blood glucose values. Insulin pumps have become more sophisticated over the last decade, with patients able to set multiple pre-programmed basal insulin rates, and/or temporary infusion rates for such things as exercise or illness. Most pumps now have inbuilt software to calculate bolus doses from blood glucose/carbohydrate data. Some of the currently available insulin pumps link to subcutaneous continuous glucose monitors and, excitingly, the expectation is that this hardware will allow the development of an 'artifical pancreas' with insulin delivery controlled partially or totally by real-time glucose sensing.

Preparations of insulin

Dosage is measured in international units standardised by chemical assay. There are three major factors:
- Strength (concentration).
- Source (human, porcine, bovine).
- Formulation (short acting vs delayed action).

Broadly speaking, four different types of insulin with differing time-courses of action are available for treating diabetes.

1. Short duration of action (and rapid onset). Soluble insulin (also called neutral or regular insulin). The most recent additions to this class of insulin, lispro, aspart and glulisine, are modified human insulins with changes in the B chain resulting in more rapid absorption after subcutaneous injection and thus a faster onset and shorter duration of action.

2. Intermediate duration of action (and slower onset). Preparations in which the insulin has been modified physically by combination with protamine or zinc to give an amorphous or crystalline suspension; this is given subcutaneously and

slowly dissociates to release insulin in its soluble form. Isophane (NPH) insulin, a suspension with protamine, is still widely used. Insulin Zinc Suspensions (amorphous or a mixture of amorphous and crystalline) are now rarely used.

3. Longer duration of action. Newer analogues glargine and detemir (Fig. 16.4) have become widely used, especially in type 1 diabetes. Small changes in the amino acid structure of glargine result in a significant slowing of absorption from subcutaneous depots. In contrast, detemir owes its protracted action to fatty acylation. After absorption, detemir is thus bound to circulating albumin which delays its action.

4. A biphasic mixture of soluble or short acting analogue insulin with isophane insulin.

Notes for prescribing insulin

Allergy to purified or analogue insulins is very rare.

Antibodies to insulin do occur, but are largely of no clinical significance.

Compatibility. Soluble insulin may be mixed in the syringe with insulin zinc suspensions (amorphous, crystalline) and with isophane and mixed (biphasic) insulin, and used at once. Long acting analogue insulins, and protamine insulin suspensions, should not be mixed in a syringe with short acting insulins.

Intravenous insulin. Only soluble (neutral) insulin should be used. Analogue and regular insulin have identical action profiles when given i.v. although the latter tends to be more widely used.

The standard strength of insulin preparations is 100 units/mL (U100). Solutions of 40 and 80 units/mL remain available in some countries, and healthcare providers should be aware of this. Biological standardisation of insulin has been replaced by physicochemical methods (high-performance liquid chromatography, HPLC).

Adverse effects of insulin

Hypoglycaemia

Hypoglycaemia is the main adverse effect of the therapeutic use of insulin. It occurs with excess insulin dosing. Common causes are misjudging or missing meals, activity/exercise and alcohol. Hypoglycaemia is problematic because the brain relies largely, if not exclusively, on circulating glucose as its source of fuel. A significant fall in blood glucose can result in impaired cognition, lethargy, coma, convulsions and perhaps even death (hypoglycaemia was implicated

Fig. 16.4 Amino acid alterations in insulin analogues. The diagram shows the structure of native insulin, and the modifications of this structure in a number of commercially available alternatives.

in one series in 4% of deaths aged less than 50 years in patients with type 1 diabetes). Hypoglycaemia is a major factor for insulin-treated patients, with fear of hypoglycaemia being rated as highly as fear of other complications of diabetes such as blindness or limb amputation. Hypoglycaemia is a particular problem for some patients who lose symptomatic awareness of (and associated counter regulatory neurohumoral defences against) hypoglycaemia.

Prevention of hypoglycaemia depends largely upon patient education, but regular mild episodes of hypoglycaemia are an almost unavoidable aspect of intensive glycaemic control, at least with currently available insulin replacement regimens. Patients should be vigilant, particularly if they have reduced symptomatic awareness of hypoglycaemia, carry rapid acting carbohydrates with them and monitor blood glucose regularly, especially with exercise and before driving a motor vehicle. Where the conscious level is impaired, rescue needs to be non-oral therapy with either i.v. glucose (dextrose) or glucagon.

Lipohypertrophy may occur if an injection site is repeatedly used, because of the local anabolic effects of insulin. Aesthetics aside, lipohypertrophy is a practical issue as insulin absorption from injection into areas of fatty hypertrophy becomes more variable and unpredictable, resulting in both hyperglycaemia and hypoglycaemia. Lipoatrophy at injection sites is rare (but still occurs) with modern, purified insulins and is thought to be related to a local immune reaction to insulin. More generalised allergic reactions to insulin are fortunately rare. If either lipodystrophy or lipoatrophy are present, the site should be avoided.

ORAL ANTIDIABETES DRUGS

Oral antidiabetes drugs are either ① secretagogue therapy to increase endogenous insulin release, or ② insulin sensitisers to reduce insulin resistance, or ③ drugs aimed at modifying absorption of glucose.

(i) Insulin secretagogues

Sulfonamide derivatives (sulfonylureas) act to increase endogenous insulin secretion by blocking ATP-sen-

sitive potassium channels on the β-islet cell plasma membrane. This results in the release of stored insulin in response to glucose. The discovery of sulfonylureas was serendipitous. In 1930 it was noted that sulfonamides could cause hypoglycaemia, and in 1942 severe hypoglycaemia was found in patients with typhoid fever during a therapeutic trial of sulfonamide. Sulfonylureas were introduced into clinical practice in 1954 and continue to be widely used in type 2 diabetes. Sulfonylureas are ineffective in totally insulin-deficient patients; successful therapy probably requires at least 30% of normal β-cell function to be present. Secondary failure (after months or years) occurs due to declining β-cell function.

Their main adverse effects are hypoglycaemia and weight gain. Hypoglycaemia can be severe and prolonged (for days), and may be fatal in 10% of cases, especially in the elderly and patients with heart failure in whom long-acting agents should be avoided. Erroneous alternative diagnoses such as stroke may be made. Sulfonamides, as expected, potentiate sulfonylureas both by direct action and by displacement from plasma proteins.

Choice is determined by the duration of action as well as the patient's age and renal function, and unwanted effects. The long acting sulfonylureas, e.g. glibenclamide, are associated with a greater risk of hypoglycaemia; for this reason they should be avoided in the elderly, for whom shorter acting alternatives, such as gliclazide, are preferred. In patients with impaired renal function, gliclazide, glipizide and tolbutamide are preferred as they are not excreted by the kidney. Gliclazide is a commonly used second-generation agent. If the dose exceeds 80 mg, the drug should be taken twice daily before meals, or once daily if prescribed as a modified-release preparation. Glimepiride is designed to be used once daily and provokes less hypoglycaemia than glibenclamide.

Meglitinides such as repaglinide ($t_{1/2}$ 1 h) are short-acting oral hypoglycaemic agents that have not been widely used in clinical practice. Like sulfonylureas, they act by blockade of ATP-dependent potassium channels. The shorter action profile of meglitinides compared with sulfonylureas should in theory reduce risk of hypoglycaemia.

Incretin analogues and mimetics. Exenatide and liraglutide are functional analogues of incretin, a glucagon-like peptide-1 (GLP-1), and naturally occurring peptide that enhances insulin secretion in response to rise in blood glucose. Aside from boosting insulin secretion, they have other actions which offer potential advantages over other insulin secretagogues in diabetes: reducing glucagon secretion, slowing gastric emptying and acting on brain GLP-1 receptors to reduce appetite. Animal studies suggest that there may be a stimulatory effect of GLP-1 analogues on beta cell mass although this has not yet been demonstrated reliably in humans. GLP-1 therapy is currently aimed at overweight patients with type 2 diabetes where sulfonylureas or insulin therapy may promote weight gain. Exenatide and liraglutide are administered subcutaneously twice or once daily although longer-acting analogues are likely to be available soon, allowing a regimen with injections no more often than once weekly. The main adverse effect is nausea, which may be sufficient to prevent use. Rarely, pancreatitis has been reported in patients using GLP-1 agonists.

Dipeptidyl peptidase-4 (DPP-4) inhibitors (vildagliptin and sitagliptin) offer an alternative strategy for targeting the GLP-1 pathway, in this case by inhibiting breakdown of native GLP-1. The main advantage these agents offer over injectable GLP-1 agonists is that they are orally active but are generally less potent.

(ii) Insulin sensitisers

Biguanides Metformin is now the only biguanide in use, and is a major agent in the management of type 2 diabetes. The most important physiological effect appears to be an increase in hepatic insulin sensitivity/reduction of hepatic glucose production. Recent studies have suggested that the intracellular target of metformin in the liver is the enzyme adenosine monophosphate-activated protein kinase (AMPK) system. AMPK is a conserved regulator of the cellular response to low energy, being activated when intracellular ATP levels decrease and AMP concentrations increase.

Metformin ($t_{1/2}$ 5h) is taken with or after meals. Metformin can be used in combination with either insulin or other oral hypoglycaemic agents. Its chief use is in the obese patient with type 2 diabetes, either alone or in combination with a sulfonylurea or insulin. The drug is ineffective in the absence of insulin.

Minor adverse reactions are common, including nausea, diarrhoea and a metallic taste in the mouth. These symptoms are usually transient or subside after reduction of dose and can be minimised by building doses up slowly and ensuring that metformin is taken with or after food. A modified release preparation, Metformin MR, is reported to be better tolerated in some patients who suffer gastrointestinal side-effects with regular metformin.

More serious, but rare, is lactic acidosis. When this condition does occur, it is usually against the background of significant medical illnesses which tend to increase circulating lactic acid levels, particularly renal impairment, liver failure, or cardiogenic or septic shock. Metformin is therefore contraindicated in these conditions, including relatively mild renal impairment and use should be reviewed when plasma creatinine is >130 mmol/L (or eGFR <45 mL/min·1.73 m^2) and stopped when plasma creatinine is >150 mmol/L (or eGFR <30 mL/min·1.73 m^2).

Metformin should also be withdrawn temporarily before general anaesthesia and administration of iodine-containing contrast media, which might precipitate renal impairment. During pregnancy, metformin use is unlicensed and current advice is that it should be substituted by insulin. Lactic acidosis may require treatment with i.v. isotonic sodium bicarbonate.

Apart from diabetes, the insulin-sensitising effects of metformin may also be useful in polycystic ovary syndrome, a condition in which insulin resistance occurs and may contribute to the hyperandrogenism and consequent hirsutism and disordered menstrual cycles which characterise this condition.

Thiazolidinediones. Pioglitazone reduces peripheral insulin resistance, leading to a reduction of blood glucose concentration. This class of drugs stimulate the nuclear hormone receptor, peroxisome proliferator-activated receptor (PPARγ), which causes differentiation of adipocytes. The major action is to stimulate peripheral insulin sensitivity and thus glucose uptake in skeletal muscle, although the mechanism by which this 'cross-talk' from adipocytes to muscle occurs is unclear. They are slower to act than either metformin or sulfonylureas.

The main adverse effects of thiazolidinediones are weight gain (typically 3–4 kg of weight gain in the first year of use), fluid retention (with peripheral oedema in 3%–4% of patients) and decreased bone density.

(iii) Agents which reduce glucose absorption

Acarbose is an a-glucosidase inhibitor that reduces the digestion of complex carbohydrates and slows their absorption from the gut and thus reduces post-prandial glycaemia. The usual dose is 50–300 mg/day. Adverse effects are common, mainly flatulence and diarrhoea, which lead to a high discontinuation rate. In high doses it may cause frank malabsorption. Acarbose may be combined with a sulfonylurea.

Dietary fibre and diabetes. The addition of gel-forming (soluble) but unabsorbable fibre (guar gum, a hydrocolloidal polysaccharide of galactose and mannose from seeds of the 'cluster bean') to the diet of diabetics reduces carbohydrate absorption and flattens the postprandial blood glucose curve. Reduced need for insulin and oral agents has been reported, but adequate amounts (taken with lots of water) are unpleasant (flatulence) and patient compliance is therefore poor.

Choice of oral antidiabetic drugs in type 2 diabetes

In general terms, a hierarchy of therapies exists for type 2 diabetes, progressing from diet and lifestyle alone (described later), through monotherapy with oral agents, combinations of oral therapies and then onto insulin/injection therapy either alone or in combination with oral treatment. The nature of 'typical' type 2 diabetes is that glucose intolerance tends to progress so that many patients will need to escalate therapy with time to avoid worsening glycaemia (and warning patients of this early after diagnosis

helps avoid subsequent disappointment and demotivation). It is also worth emphasising that this 'typical' time-course is not universal. Analogous to type 1 diabetes, some patients may present with marked symptomatic hyperglycaemia requiring immediate insulin therapy (and indeed some of these may have an unrecognised late onset of type 1 diabetes).

The evidence base for the most effective strategies for using antidiabetic therapy continues to evolve and the following is UK NICE guidance set out as a guide for readers. Current advice is that metformin (where not contraindicated and if tolerated) is useful primary monotherapy for overweight patients and many who are not overweight. Sulfonylurea therapy is now less often used as first-line therapy but is an alternative to metformin or can be added in to dual therapy as needed. Thiazolidinediones can also be used in combination with the above. GLP-1 agonists may be considered where overweight is a consideration. The therapeutic target is to maintain the HbA1c (glycosylated haemoglobin) below 7.0% and insulin may eventually be required, either alone or in combination with metformin (and/or sulfonylurea or pioglitazone).

Diet and diabetes

Specialised diet and lifestyle advice is of paramount importance in managing diabetes. Patients should be allowed to follow their own preferences as far as is practicable. They should receive dietary advice on a high complex carbohydrate diet (approx. 65% of total calories) with low fat (<30% of calories) and an emphasis on reduction in saturated fat in favour of mono-and polyunsaturates. Caloric intake may need to be restricted and patients encouraged to achieve an ideal body-weight. Although certain foods are marketed as 'diabetic', there are concerns about whether these may be low in glucose but high in calories. Diet should be high in fibre with plenty of fresh fruit and vegetables. Advice about alcohol intake and smoking should be given (and where appropriate, information about what to do when/after drinking alcohol because of the effects causing delayed hypoglycaemia). This should be combined with advice about activity/exercise levels.

As earlier indicated, increasing numbers of patients with type 1 diabetes are now taught how to count dietary carbohydrates, allowing them to adjust their insulin doses around dietary intake/activity/alcohol.

The advice above may need further modifying in those with ischaemic heart disease and/or established nephropathy.

Interactions with non-diabetes drugs

Some examples are listed below to show that the possibility of interactions of practical clinical importance is a real one. In general, whenever a patient with diabetes takes other drugs it is prudent to be on the watch for disturbance of glycaemic control.

β-adrenoceptor-blocking drugs may impair the sympathetically mediated (β_2 receptor) release of glucose from the liver in response to hypoglycaemia and also reduce the adrenergically mediated symptoms of hypoglycaemia (except sweating). Insulin hypoglycaemia may thus be more prolonged and/or less noticeable. Ideally, a patient with diabetes needing a β-adrenoceptor blocker should be given a β_1-selective member, e.g. bisoprolol.

Thiazide diuretics at a higher dose than those now generally used in hypertension can precipitate/worsen diabetes, probably by reducing insulin secretion.

Hepatic enzyme inducers may enhance the metabolism of sulfonylureas that are metabolised in the liver (tolbutamide). Cimetidine, an inhibitor of drug-metabolising enzymes, increases metformin plasma concentration and effect.

Monoamine oxidase inhibitors potentiate oral agents and perhaps also insulin. They can also reduce appetite and so upset control.

Interaction may occur with alcohol (hypoglycaemia with any antidiabetes drug).

Salicylates and fibrates can increase insulin sensitivity, resulting in lower blood glucose.

The action of sulfonylureas is intensified by heavy sulfonamide dosage, and some sulfonamides increase free tolbutamide concentrations, probably by competing for plasma protein-binding sites.

The use of glucagon as rescue therapy for hypoglycaemia is described above. Adrenaline/epinephrine raises the blood sugar concentration by mobilising liver and muscle glycogen (a β_2-adrenoceptor effect), and suppressing secretion of insulin (an a-adrenoceptor effect). Hyperglycaemia may occur in patients with phaeochromocytoma, and is usually reversed by a-adrenoceptor blockade.

Adrenal steroids, either endogenous or exogenous, antagonise the actions of insulin. Although this effect is only slight with mineralocorticoids, glucocorticoid hormones increase gluconeogenesis and reduce glucose uptake and utilisation by the tissues. The therapeutic use of high dose glucocorticoids may precipitate frank diabetes in some patients or worsen blood glucose control in those with established diabetes. Steroid-induced diabetes often requires insulin rather than oral hypoglycaemic therapy, particularly for flexibility if steroid doses are being tapered down. Similarly, patients with Cushing's syndrome may also develop 'secondary diabetes' with a marked resistance to insulin. In contrast, patients with hypoadrenalism from Addison's disease, hypopituitarism, or following steroid withdrawal after prolonged glucocorticoid therapy may be abnormally sensitive to insulin action and prone to recurrent hypoglycaemia.

Growth hormone antagonises the actions of insulin in the tissues. Like Addison's disease, growth hormone deficiency may cause increased insulin sensitivity and/or a tendency for hypoglycaemia. Acromegalic patients may develop insulin-resistant diabetes.

Oral contraceptives can impair carbohydrate tolerance although the effects are usually relatively mild.

Thyroid hormone excess may increase the requirements for insulin.

Drug-induced diabetes

Diazoxide is chemically similar to thiazide diuretics, but stimulates the ATP-dependent K^+ channel that is blocked by the sulfonylureas. Although formerly used as an antihypertensive agent, its current use in therapeutics is confined to the rare indication of treating hypoglycaemia due to islet cell tumour (insulinoma). Adrenocortical steroids are also diabetogenic.

Pregnancy and diabetes

During (and indeed before) pregnancy, close control of diabetes is critical. Ideally, pregnancy should be planned and women should be seen in a preconception clinic to optimise care. Glycaemic targets are tight, aiming for HbA1c values as close to the non-diabetic range (4.0%–5.9%) as possible. Current practice is for women on oral hypoglycaemic agents who are planning, or starting, a pregnancy to change to insulin and continue on it throughout pregnancy. There is no definitive evidence that oral drugs are associated with fetal malformations. Other drugs (blood pressure and lipid lowering) should be reviewed and stopped or altered to agents judged safe in pregnancy as appropriate. Oral folic acid should be started.

Diabetes can present de novo during pregnancy. Although this is usually gestational diabetes which resolves after delivery, it is worth remembering that rarely type 2 or type 1 diabetes can present in pregnancy.

Risks of pregnancy in diabetes include an increased rate of fetal loss and malformations. Maternal hyperglycaemia can lead to fetal hyperglycaemia with consequent fetal islet cell hyperplasia, high birth-weight babies (leading to mechanical obstetric challenges) and postnatal hypoglycaemia.

Note that glycosuria is not a reliable guide of blood glucose values in pregnancy. The renal threshold for glucose (also of lactose) falls, so that glycosuria and lactosuria may occur in the presence of a normal blood glucose.

Insulin requirements increase steadily after the third month. Some women develop a marked intolerance of oral carbohydrates with a tendency for large postprandial rises in blood glucose. During labour, i.v. insulin infusion may be needed. Use of β_2-adrenoceptor agonists and of dexamethasone (to prevent respiratory distress syndrome in the prematurely newborn) causes hyperglycaemia and increased insulin (and potassium) needs.

Of note, insulin requirements reduce immediately after delivery and may remain low during the following weeks, particularly with lactation/breast feeding.

SUMMARY

- Diabetes mellitus is important in global terms because of its chronicity, and high incidence and frequency of major complications. It is generally divided into two kinds: type 1 (previously, insulin dependent diabetes mellitus) and type 2 (previously, non-insulin dependent diabetes, essentially an umbrella term for a group of conditions which are non-type 1).

- Type 1 diabetes is commoner in those with onset before age 30 whereas type 2 diabetes prevails in older patients. Increasingly, insulin therapy is required in type 2 diabetes when glycaemic control is not optimised by oral drugs.

- Insulin is usually self-administered subcutaneously to stable patients, with a variety of regimens which can be tailored to the needs of a particular patient. Modern practice in type 1 diabetes is to educate patients in flexible insulin dosing which is adjusted for differing meals, activity levels, etc.

- If a drug is required in type 2 diabetes, metformin (a biguanide) is now widely used as first-line therapy, especially for the obese. Other monotherapy options include a sulfonylurea in the non-obese or a thiazolidinedione in patients intolerant of, or uncontrolled by, metformin or sulfonylurea. Many patients with type 2 diabetes will need treatment escalation with time to multiple combination therapy and/or insulin.

Part 3. Thyroid hormones, antithyroid drugs

THYROID HORMONES

L-thyroxine (T_4 or tetra-iodo-L-thyronine) and lio-L-thyronine (T_3 or tri-iodo-L-thyronine) are the natural hormones of the thyroid gland. T_4 is a less active precursor of T_3, which is the major mediator of physiological effect. In this part, T_4 for therapeutic use is referred to as levothyroxine.

For convenience, the term 'thyroid hormone' is used to comprise T_4 plus T_3. Both forms are available for oral use as therapy.

Physiology and pharmacokinetics

Thyroid hormone synthesis requires oxidation of dietary iodine, followed by iodination of tyrosine to mono-and di-iodotyrosine; coupling of iodotyrosines leads to formation of the active molecules, tetra-iodothyronine (T_4 or L-thyroxine) and tri-iodothyronine (T_3 or L-thyronine).

These active thyroid hormones are stored in the gland within the molecule of thyroglobulin, a major component of the intrafollicular colloid. They are released into the circulation following reuptake of the colloid by the apical cells and proteolysis. The main circulating thyroid hormone is T_4. About 80% of the released T_4 is deiodinated in the peripheral tissues to the biologically active T_3 (30%–35%) and biologically inactive 'reverse' T_3 (45%–50%); thus most circulating T_3 is derived from T_4. Further de-iodination, largely in the liver, leads to loss of activity.

In the blood both T_4 and T_3 are extensively (99.9%) bound to plasma proteins (thyroxine binding globulin (TBG) and transthyretin (TTR), albumin and lipoproteins). The concentration of TBG is raised by oestrogens (physiological or pharmacological) and prolonged use of neuroleptics. The concentration of TBG is lowered by adrenocortical and androgen (including anabolic steroid) therapy and by urinary protein loss in the nephrotic syndrome. Phenytoin and salicylates compete with thyroid hormone for TBG binding sites. Effects such as these would interfere with the assessment of the clinical significance of measurements of total thyroid hormone concentration but the availability of free thyroid hormone assay largely avoids such complicating factors. Normal values are: free T_4 9–25 picomol/L, free T_3 3–9 picomol/L.

T_4 and T_3 are well absorbed from the gut, except in myxoedema coma when parenteral therapy is required.

T_4 **(levothyroxine).** A single dose reaches its maximum effect in about 10 days (its binding to plasma proteins is strong as well as extensive) and passes off in 2–3 weeks ($t_{1/2}$ 7 days in euthyroid, 14 days in hypothyroid and 3 days in hyperthyroid subjects).

T_3 **(liothyronine)** is about five times as biologically potent as T_4; a single dose reaches its maximum effect in about 24 h (its binding to plasma proteins is weak) and passes off in 1 week ($t_{1/2}$ 2 days in euthyroid subjects).

Pharmacodynamics

Thyroid hormone passes into the cells of target organs. T_4 is de-iodinated to T_3, which combines with specific nuclear receptors and induces characteristic metabolic changes:

- Protein synthesis during growth.
- Increased metabolic rate with raised oxygen consumption.
- Increased sensitivity to catecholamines with proliferation of β-adrenoceptors (particularly important in the cardiovascular system).

LEVOTHYROXINE FOR HYPOTHYROIDISM

The main indication for levothyroxine is treatment of thyroxine deficiency (cretinism, adult hypothyroidism) from any cause. The adult requirement of hormone is remarkably constant, and dosage does not usually have to be altered once the optimum has been found. Patients should be monitored annually. Monitoring needs to be more frequent in children, who may need more as they grow. Similarly, pregnant women should be monitored monthly, and require a 50–100% increase in their normal dose of levothyroxine.

Early treatment of neonatal hypothyroidism (cretinism) (1 in 5 000 births) is important if permanent mental defect is to be avoided. It must be lifelong.

Hypothyroidism due to panhypopituitarism requires replacement with glucocorticoids as well as with thyroid hormone. Use of levothyroxine alone can cause acute adrenal insufficiency.

Small doses of levothyroxine in normal subjects merely depress pituitary thyroid-stimulating hormone (TSH) production and consequently reduce the output of thyroid hormone by an equivalent amount.

Levothyroxine is used in some countries for the treatment of non-toxic nodular goitre, on the assumption that nodular thyroid tissue growth is dependent on TSH. The treatment is not curative. Levothyroxine should not be used to treat obesity.

Treatment of hypothyroidism

Levothyroxine tablets contain pure L-thyroxine sodium and should be used.

The initial oral dose in healthy patients under the age of 60, without cardiac disease, is 50–100 micrograms/day. In the old and patients with heart disease or multiple coronary risk factors, this level should be achieved gradually (to minimise cardiovascular risk due to a sudden increase in metabolic demand), starting with 12.5–25 micrograms daily for the first 2–4 weeks, and then increasing by 12.5 micrograms monthly until normal TSH levels are achieved.

The usual replacement dose at steady state in patients with complete thyroid failure, is 1.6 micrograms/kg·day, 100–200 micrograms per day given as a single dose. This is usually sufficient to reduce plasma TSH to normal (0.3–3.5 mU/L), which is the best indicator of adequate treatment. Patients who appear to need increasing doses with fluctuating TSH levels, are probably not taking their tablets consistently; the possibility of malabsortion or other drug interaction should be excluded. The maximum effect of a dose is reached after about 10 days and passes off over about 2–3 weeks. Absorption is more complete and less variable if levothyroxine is taken at the same time every day, one hour before breakfast.

Tablets containing physiological mixtures of levothyroxine and liothyronine are not sufficiently evaluated to recommend in preference to levothyroxine alone.

Hypothyroid patients tend to be intolerant of drugs in general owing to slow metabolism.

Liothyronine tabs. Liothyronine is the most rapidly effective thyroid hormone, a single dose giving maximum effect within 24 h and passing off over 24–48 h. It is not routine treatment for hypothyroidism because its rapid onset of effect can induce heart failure. Its main uses are myxoedema coma and psychosis, both rare conditions. A specialised use is during the withdrawal of levothyroxine replacement (to permit diagnostic radioiodine scanning) in patients with thyroid carcinoma.

Myxoedema coma follows prolonged total hormone deficiency and constitutes an emergency. Liothyronine 5–20 micrograms is given intravenously every 12 h. Intravenous therapy is mandatory because drug absorption is impaired. Intravenous hydrocortisone should be given to cover the possibility of coexisting adrenocortical insufficiency.

Subclinical hypothyroidism. Subclinical hypothyroidism is defined as an elevated serum TSH concentration in the presence of normal free T_4 and free T_3. Although termed subclinical, 25% of patients have symptoms of hypothyroidism and cognitive disturbance. Meta-analyses of population based studies show a higher incidence of ischaemic heart disease and mortality in subjects younger than 65 years. Indications for treatment are pregnancy, ovarian dysfunction/infertility, symptoms of hypothyrodism, TSH 210 mU/L, TSH <10 mU/L and positive thyroid antibodies and patients with high risk of cardiovascular disease.

Adverse effects of thyroid hormone parallel the increase in metabolic rate. The symptoms and signs are those of hyperthyroidism. Symptoms of myocardial ischaemia, atrial fibrillation or heart failure are liable to be provoked by too vigorous therapy or in patients having serious ischaemic heart disease who may even be unable to tolerate optimal therapy. Should they occur, discontinue levothyroxine for at least a week, and recommence at lower dose. Only slight overdose may precipitate atrial fibrillation in patients aged over 60 years.

In pregnancy a hypothyroid patient on thyroxine replacement should be assessed with a preconception TSH level measurement and free T_4 and TSH should be checked once pregnancy is confirmed. Monthly measurements of free T_4 and TSH are recommended. Optimal replacement therapy is essential in the first trimester when the athyroid fetus is dependent on maternal supply to ensure normal neurointellectual development. An average 50% increase in dose of levothyroxine is required and ideally patients should anticipate this increase. Some endocrinologists advise patients to increase their daily dose by 30% or 25–50 micrograms per day. Post delivery, patients revert to their preconception dose. Breast feeding is not contraindicated.

ANTITHYROID DRUGS AND HYPER-THYROIDISM

Drugs used for the treatment of hyperthyroidism include:

- Thionamides, which block the synthesis of thyroid hormone.
- Iodine: radioiodine, which destroys the cells that make thyroid hormone; iodide, an excess of which reduces the production of thyroid hormone temporarily (it is also necessary for the formation of hormone, and both excess and deficiency can cause goitre).

Thionamides (thiourea derivatives) carbimazole, methimazole, propylthiouracil

Mode of action (Fig. 16.5)

The major action of thionamides is to reduce the formation of thyroid hormone by inhibiting oxidation and organification (incorporation into organic form) of iodine (iodotyrosines) and coupling of iodotyrosines. Maximum effect is delayed until existing hormone stores are exhausted (weeks, see below). With high dose, reduced hormone synthesis leads to hypothyroidism.

Carbimazole and methimazole (the active metabolite of carbimazole) ($t_{1/2}$ 6 h) and propylthiouracil ($t_{1/2}$ 2 h) are commonly used, but the $t_{1/2}$ matters little because the drugs accumulate in the thyroid and act there for 30–40 h; thus a single daily dose suffices.

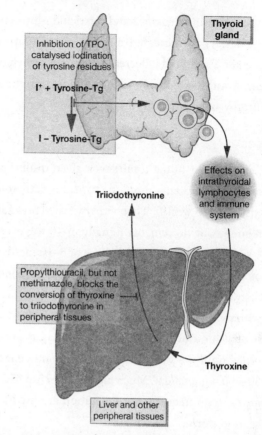

Fig. 16.5 Effects of antithyroid drugs. The multiple effects of antithyroid drugs include inhibition of thyroid hormone synthesis and a reduction in both intrathyroid immune dysregulation and (in the case of propylthiouracil) the peripheral conversion of thyroxine to triiodothyronine. Tyrosine-Tg, tyrosine residues in thyroglobulin; 1$^+$, the iodinating intermediate; TPO, thyroid peroxidase.

Propylthiouracil (PTU) differs from other members of the group in that it also inhibits peripheral conversion of T_4 to T_3, but only at high doses used in treatment of thyroid storm PTU differs from the other thionamides in its apparent radio-protective effect when used prior to radioiodine treatment.

Carbimazole is the drug of choice in the UK. PTU is used when a patient develops side-effects to carbimazole. PTU is not recommended in children because of the increased risk of severe hepatotoxicity and death.

Immunosuppression

In patients taking antithyroid drugs, serum concentrations of antithyrotropin receptor antibodies decrease with time, as do other immunologically important molecules, including intracellular adhesion molecule

1, and soluble interleukin-2 and interleukin-6 receptors. There is an increased number of circulating suppressor T cells and a decreased number of helper T cells. Antithyroid drugs may also induce apoptosis of intrathyroidal lymphocytes.

Doses

- Carbimazole 40 mg total/day is given orally (or methimazole 30 mg) until the patient is euthyroid (usually 4–6 weeks). Then either titrate (titration regimen) by decrements initially of 10 mg every 4–6 weeks to a maintenance dose of 5–10 mg/day, or continue (block–replace regimen) 40 mg once daily, and add levothyroxine 100 micrograms/day, with monitoring of free T_4 and TSH.
- Propylthiouracil 300–450 mg total/day is given orally until the patient is euthyroid: maintenance 50–100 mg total/day. Much higher doses (up to 2.4 g/day) with frequent administration are used for thyroid storm.

Use

It is probable that no patient is wholly refractory to these drugs. Failure to respond is likely to be due to the patient not taking the tablets or to wrong diagnosis. The drugs are used in hyperthyroidism:

- As principal therapy.
- As adjuvant to radioiodine, before and after administration, to control the disease until the radiation achieves its effect.
- To prepare patients for surgery.

Clinical improvement is noticeable in 2–4 weeks, and the patient should be euthyroid in 4–6 weeks.

The best guides to therapy are the patient's symptoms (decreased nervousness and palpitations), increased strength and weight gain, and decreased pulse rate.

Symptoms and signs are, of course, less valuable as guides if the patient is also taking a β-adrenoceptor blocker, and reliance then rests on biochemical tests.

With optimal treatment the gland decreases in size, but over-treatment leading to low hormone concentrations in the blood activates the pituitary feedback system, inducing TSH secretion and goitre.

Adverse reactions

The thionamide drugs are all liable to cause adverse effects. Minor reactions include maculopapular or urticarial rash, pruritus, arthralgia, fever, anorexia, nausea, abnormalities of taste and smell. Major effects include agranulocytosis, aplastic anaemia, thrombocytopenia, acute hepatic necrosis, cholestatic hepatitis, lupus-like syndrome, vasculitis.

Blood disorders (<3 per 10 000 patient-years) are most common in the first 2 months of treatment. Routine leucocyte counts to detect blood dyscrasia before symptoms develop are unlikely to protect, as agranulocytosis may be so acute that blood counts give no warning. Patients must be given written warning to stop the drug and have a leucocyte count performed if symptoms of a sore throat, fever, bruising or mouth ulcers develop. Any suggestion of anaemia should be investigated.

Cross-allergy between the drugs sometimes occurs, but is not to be assumed for agranulocytosis. Treatment of agranulocytosis consists of drug withdrawal, admission to hospital, and administration of broad-spectrum antibimicrobials plus granulocyte colony-stimulating factor.

Pregnancy. If a pregnant woman has hyperthyroidism (2 per 1 000 pregnancies), she should be treated with the smallest possible amount of these drugs because they cross the placenta; over-treatment causes fetal goitre. Meticulous control is essential and thyroid test should be monitored monthly. Surgery in the second trimester may be preferred to continued drug therapy. Ideally, patients should be rendered euthyroid prior to pregnancy.

Both PTU and carbimazole are considered safe in nursing mothers but because of the risk of hepatotoxicity carbimazole is preferred.

Control of antithyroid drug therapy

The aim of drug therapy is to control the hyperthyroidism until a natural remission takes place. The recommended duration of therapy is 12–18 months. Longer treatment is usual for young patients with large, vascular goitres, because of the higher risk of recurrence (2–3 years). A shorter course (6–9 months) is recommended for the block–replace regimen. Most patients enter remission, but some will relapse – usually during the first 3 months after withdrawal from treatment. Approximately 30–40% of patients remain euthyroid 10 years later. If hyperthyroidism recurs, there is little chance of a second course of thionamide achieving long-term remission. In such patients, indefinite low-dose antithyroid treatment is an alternative option to radioiodine or surgery.

The use of levothyroxine concurrently with an antithyroid drug ('block and replace regimen') facilitates maintenance of a euthyroid state and reduces the frequency of clinic visits. There is a higher risk of the dose-related adverse effects of carbimazole, and no compensatory reduction in the incidence of relapse. Therefore, the 'titration' regimen is regarded as first-line treatment.

β-Adrenergic blockade. There is increased tissue sensitivity to catecholamines in hyperthyroidism with a rise in either the number of β-adrenoceptors or the second-messenger response (i.e. intracellular cyclic AMP synthesis) to their stimulation. Therefore, some of the unpleasant symptoms are adrenergic.

Quick relief can be obtained with a b-adrenoceptor blocking drug (judge the dose by heart rate), although these do not block all the metabolic effects of the hormone, e.g. on the myocardium, and the basal metabolic rate is unchanged. For this reason, b-blockade is not used as sole therapy except in mild thyrotoxicosis in preparation for radioiodine treatment, and in these patients it should be continued until the radioiodine has taken effect. β-blockers do not alter the course of the disease, or affect biochemical tests of thyroid function. Any effect on thyroid hormonal action on peripheral tissues is clinically unimportant. Although atenolol is widely used, it is preferable to choose a drug that is non-selective for b1 and $β_2$ receptors and lacks partial agonist effect (e.g. propranolol 20–80 mg 6–8-hourly, or timolol 5 mg once daily). The usual contraindications to b-blockade apply, especially asthma.

Iodine (iodide and radioactive iodine)

Iodide is well absorbed from the intestine, distributed like chloride in the body, and rapidly excreted by the kidney. It is selectively taken up and concentrated (about × 25) by the thyroid gland, more in hyperthyroidism and less in hypothyroidism. A deficiency of iodide reduces the amount of thyroid hormone produced; this stimulates the pituitary to secrete TSH. The result is hyperplasia and increased vascularity of the gland, with eventual goitre formation.

Effects

The effects of iodide are complex and related to the dose and thyroid status of the subject.

In hyperthyroid subjects, a moderate excess of iodide may enhance hormone production by providing 'fuel' for hormone synthesis. But a substantial excess inhibits hormone release and promotes storage of hormone and involution of the gland, making it firmer and less vascular so that surgery is easier. The effect is transient and its mechanism uncertain.

In euthyroid subjects with normal glands an excess of iodide from any source can cause goitre (with or without hyperthyroidism), e.g. use of iodide-containing cough medicines, iodine-containing radiocontrast media, amiodarone, seaweed eaters.

A euthyroid subject with an autonomous adenoma (hot nodule) becomes hyperthyroid if given iodide.

Uses

Iodide (large dose) is used for thyroid storm (crisis) and in preparation for thyroidectomy because it rapidly benefits the patient by reducing hormone release and renders surgery easier and safer (above).

Potassium iodate in doses of 85 mg orally 8-hourly (longer intervals allow some escape from the iodide effect) produces some effect in 1–2 days, maximal after 10–14 days, after which the benefit declines as the thyroid adapts. A similar dose used for 3 days covers administration of some ^{131}I- or ^{123}I-containing preparations, for instance meta- iodobenzylguanidine (^{123}I-MIBG).

Iodine therapy maximises iodide stores in the thyroid, which delays response to thionamides. Prophylactic iodide (1 part in 100 000) may be added to the salt, water or bread where goitre is endemic.

In economically deprived communities, a method of prophylaxis is to inject iodised oil intramuscularly every 3–5 years; given early to women, this prevents endemic cretinism but occasional hyperthyroidism occurs.

As an antiseptic for use on the skin, povidone–iodine (a complex of iodine with a sustained-release carrier, povidone or polyvinyl–pyrrolidone) can be applied repeatedly and used as a surgical scrub.

Bronchial secretions. Iodide is concentrated in bronchial and salivary secretions. It acts as an expectorant.

Organic compounds containing iodine are used as contrast media in radio-imaging. It is essential to ask patients specifically whether they are allergic to iodine before such contrast media are used. Severe anaphylaxis, even deaths, occur every year in busy imaging departments; iodine-containing contrast media are being superseded by so-called non-ionic preparations.

Adverse reactions

Patients vary enormously in their tolerance of iodine; some are intolerant or allergic to it both orally and when it is applied to the skin.

Symptoms of iodism include: a metallic taste, excessive salivation with painful salivary glands, running eyes and nose, sore mouth and throat, a productive cough, diarrhoea, and various rashes that may mimic chickenpox. A saline diuresis enhances elimination.

Goitre can occur with prolonged use of iodide-containing expectorant by bronchitics and asthmatics. Such therapy should therefore be intermittent, if it is used at all.

Topical application of iodine-containing antiseptics to neonates has caused hypothyroidism. Iodide intake above that in a normal diet will depress thyroid uptake of administered radioiodine, because the two forms will compete.

In the case of diet, medication, and water-soluble radio-diagnostic agents, interference with thyroid function will cease 2–4 weeks after stopping the source, but with agents used for cholecystography it may last for 6 months or more (because of tissue binding).

Radioiodine (^{131}I)

^{131}I is treated by the body just like the ordinary non-radioactive isotope, so that when swallowed it is concentrated in the thyroid gland. It emits mainly β radiation (90%), which penetrates only 0.5 mm of tissue and thus allows therapeutic effects on the thyroid without damage to the surrounding structures, particularly the parathyroids. It also emits some g-rays, which are more penetrating and are detectable with a radiation counter. ^{131}I has a physical (radioactive) $t\frac{1}{2}$ of 8 days.

^{131}I is the preferred initial treatment for hyperthyroidism caused by Graves' disease in North America. It is contraindicated in children and pregnant or breast-feeding women, and can induce or worsen ophthalmopathy. It is used in combination with surgery in thyroid carcinoma.

In hyperthyroidism, the beneficial effects of a single dose may be felt in 1 month, and patients should be reviewed at 6 weeks to monitor for onset of hypothyroidism. The maximal effect of radioiodine may take 3 months to achieve. β-Adrenoceptor blockade and, in severe cases, an antithyroid drug will be needed to render the patient comfortable while waiting; this is more likely when radioiodine is used for patients with relapsing thyrotoxicosis. Very rarely radiation thyroiditis causes excessive release of hormone and thyroid storm. Repeated doses may be needed.

Adverse effects of radioiodine are as for iodism, above. In the event of inadvertent overdose, large doses of sodium or potassium iodate should be given to compete with the radioiodine for thyroid uptake and to hasten excretion by increasing iodide turnover (increased fluid intake and a diuretic are adjuvants).

Radioiodine offers the advantages that treatment is simple and carries no immediate mortality, but it is slow in acting and the dose that will render the patient euthyroid is difficult to judge. In the first year after treatment, 20% of patients will become hypothyroid. Thereafter, 5% of patients become hypothyroid annually, perhaps because the capacity of thyroid cells to divide is permanently abolished so that cell renewal ceases. There is therefore an obligation to monitor patients indefinitely after radioiodine treatment, for most are likely to need treatment for hypothyroidism eventually.

Risks

Experience had eliminated the fear that radioiodine causes carcinoma of the thyroid, and led to its use in patients of all ages. The Chernobyl disaster subsequently revived concern about exposure of children and it would be wise again to restrict radioiodine treatment to adults. Pregnant women should not be treated with radioiodine (^{131}I) because it crosses the placenta.

There is a theoretical risk of teratogenic effect and women are advised to avoid pregnancy for an arbitrary 12 months after treatment.

Treatment of thyroid carcinoma requires larger doses of radioiodine than are used for hyperthyroidism, and there is an increased incidence of late leukaemia in these patients. The management of thyroid carcinoma is highly specialised, and extends beyond the scope of this textbook.

Radioisotope tests

Radioiodine uptake can be used to test thyroid function, although it has now been superseded by technetium-99m. Scanning the gland may be useful to identify solitary nodules and in the differential diagnosis of Graves' disease from the less common thyroiditides, e.g. de Quervain's thyroiditis. In thyroiditis, excessive thyroid hormone release caused by follicular cell damage can cause clinical and biochemical features of hyperthyroidism, but radionuclide uptake is reduced.

Choice of treatment of hyperthyroidism
- Antithyroid drugs.
- Radioiodine.
- Surgery.

Antithyroid drugs are generally preferred provided the goitre is small and diffuse. They may be used in pregnancy.

Radioiodine is an alternative first-line treatment for adult patients, but not in pregnancy. It may be preferred to antithyroid drugs in patients with large or multinodular goitres, and in patients with a single hyperfunctioning adenoma ('hot nodule'). Preparation with antithyroid drugs is recommended in severe thyrotoxicosis.

Surgery is generally a second choice for thyrotoxicosis. It may be indicated if the thyroid contains a nodule of uncertain nature, or in patients with large, multinodular goitre causing tracheal compression.

Preparation for surgery

Routine preparation of hyperthyroid patients for surgery can be achieved satisfactorily by making them euthyroid with one of the above drugs plus a β-adrenoceptor blocker for comfort and safety, and adding iodate for 7–10 days before operation (not sooner) to reduce the surgically inconvenient vascularity of the gland.

In an emergency, the patient is prepared with a β-adrenoceptor blocker (e.g. propranolol 6-hourly, with dose titration to eliminate tachycardia) for 4 days, continued through the operation and for 7–10 days afterwards. Iodide is also given. The important differences with this second technique are that the gland is smaller and less friable but the patient's tissues are still hyperthyroid and, to avoid a hyperthyroid crisis or storm, it is essential that the adrenoceptor blocker continue as above without the omission of even a single 6-hourly dose of propranolol.

Thyroid storm

Thyroid crisis, or storm, is a life-threatening emergency owing to the liberation of large amounts of hormone into the circulation. Surgical storm is rare with modern methods of preparing hyperthyroid patients for surgery. Medical thyroid storm may occur in patients who are untreated or incompletely treated. It may be precipitated by infection, trauma, surgical emergencies or operations, radiation thyroiditis, toxaemia of pregnancy or parturition.

Treatment is urgently required to save life. Propranolol should be given immediately, 60–80 mg orally every 6 h or i.v. slowly, initially 0.5–1 mg over 10 min with continuous cardiac rhythm monitoring; the i.v. dose may be repeated every few hours until the oral dose takes effect. Large doses of an antithyroid agent, preferably propylthiouracil 300–400 mg 4-hourly are required, down a nasogastric tube or per rectum. Thereafter, iodide is used to inhibit further hormone release from the gland (potassium iodide/iodate 600 mg to 1.0 g orally in the first 24 h). Lithium carbonate may be used particularly in cases of iodide allergy. Large doses of adrenocorticoids, e.g. dexamethasone 4 mg 6-hourly, are given to inhibit both release of thyroid hormone from the gland and peripheral conversion of T_4 to T_3. Hyperthermia may be treated by cooling and aspirin; heart failure in the ordinary way; fluid deficit by a combination of normal saline and 5% dextrose.

Graves' ophthalmopathy

Graves' ophthalmopathy is characterized by inflammation of periorbital and retroorbital connective tissue, fat and muscle. It is associated with Graves' thyrotoxicosis; it may also occur in patients with euthyroid or hypothyroid chronic autoimmune thyroiditis.

It is an autoimmune disease which appears now to be due in part to the expression of the TSH receptor on orbital cells such as preadipocytes and fibrobalsts and probably myocytes.

Antithyroid drugs do not help directly. Nevertheless, it is important that any thyroid dysfunction is treated meticulously, and the TSH concentration held within the low normal range. Mild to moderate cases regress spontaneously. Artificial tears (hypromellose) are useful when natural tears and blinking are inadequate to maintain corneal lubrication. In severe cases, high doses of systemic prednisolone, alone or in combination with another immunosuppressive (azathioprine), may help. A course of low-dose orbital radiation achieves rapid regression of oph-

thalmopathy, and may avoid the need for prolonged immunosuppressive therapy. In severe cases with optic neuropathy decompressive surgery is indicated to relieve pressure of the optic nerve.

Treatment of subclinical hyperthyroidism

Subclinical hyperthyroidism is defined biochemically by normal serum free T_4 and free T_3 but suppressed TSH concentrations. Some 5% of patients per annum progress to frank hyperthyroidism, and there is an increased risk of atrial fibrillation, stroke and osteoporosis. The treatment of endogenous subclinical hyperthyroidism should be considered when the TSH level is less than 0.1 mU/L, especially in patients aged over 60 years, those with an increased risk for heart disease, osteopenia or osteoporosis, or with clinical symptoms suggestive of hyperthyroidism. Other patients should be monitored 6-monthly; eventually 50% become euthyroid.

SUMMARY

- Autoimmune disease of the thyroid can cause over- or under-production of thyroid hormone.
- Hypothyroidism is readily treated with levothyroxine 50–200 micrograms daily orally, continued indefinitely.
- The treatment of hyperthyroidism due to Graves' disease is either 12–18 months' treatment with carbimazole or propylthiouracil, or a (usually) single dose of [131]I.
- The natural history of Graves' disease is of alternating remission and relapse. Progression to hypothyroidism can occur, especially after ^{131}I treatment. All patients require long-term follow-up.

Part 4. Sex hormones

SEX (GONADAL) HORMONES AND ANTAGONISTS: STEROID HORMONES

Steroid hormone receptors (for gonadal steroids and adrenocortical steroids) are complex proteins inside the target cell. The steroid penetrates, binds to the receptor and translocates into the cell nucleus, which is the principal site of action and where RNA synthesis occurs. Compounds that occupy the receptor without causing translocation into the nucleus or the replenishment of receptors act as antagonists, e.g. spironolactone to aldosterone, cyproterone to androgens, clomifene to oestrogens.

Selectivity. Many synthetic analogues, although classed as, e.g. androgen, anabolic steroid, progestogen, are nonselective and bind to several types of receptor as agonist, partial agonist, antagonist. The result is that their effects are complex. The selective oestrogen receptor modulators (SERMS) may be antagonists to the oestrogen receptors in the breast, while being agonists in bone. Tamoxifen and raloxifene are such SERMS, which therefore increase bone density (as normal oestrogen does) but reduce the risk of breast cancer (by blocking the breast receptor to estradiol).

Pharmacokinetics. Steroid sex hormones are well absorbed through the skin (factory workers need protective clothing) and the gut. Most are subject to extensive hepatic metabolic inactivation (some so much that oral administration is ineffective or requires very large doses, if a useful amount is to pass through the liver and reach the systemic circulation).

There is some enterohepatic recirculation, especially of oestrogen, and this may be interrupted by severe diarrhoea, with loss of efficacy. Some nonsteroidal analogues are metabolised more slowly. Sustained-release (depot) preparations are used. The hormones are carried in the blood extensively bound to sex hormone binding globulin.

In general the plasma t½ relates to the duration of cellular action, which is implied in the recommended dosage schedules.

ANDROGENS

Testosterone is the predominant natural androgen secreted by the Leydig cells of the testis; in a normal adult male testosterone production amounts to 4 –9 mg/24 h. It circulates highly bound to a hepatic gly-

coprotein called sex hormone binding globulin (65%) and loosely bound to albumin (33%). Only 1%–2% of circulating testosterone is unbound and freely available to tissues. It is converted by hydroxylation to the active dihydrotestosterone (DHT). Testosterone is necessary for normal spermatogenesis, for the development of the male secondary sex characteristics, sexual potency and for the growth, at puberty, of the genital tract.

Protein anabolism is increased by androgens, i.e. androgens increase the proportion of protein laid down as tissue, especially muscle and (combined with training, increase strength). Growth of bone is promoted, but the rate of closure of the epiphyses is also hastened, causing short stature in cases of precocious puberty or of androgen overdose in the course of treating hypogonadal children.

Indications for androgen therapy

Indications for testosterone treatment are primary testicular failure such as a result of bilateral anorchia, Klinefelter's (XXY) karyotype, surgery, chemotherapy and radiotherapy, or secondary testicular failure as a result of hypothalamic– pituitary disease.

Other conditions that require testosterone treatment are delayed puberty in boys aged 16 years or older, angioneurotic oedema and adrenal insufficiency in females.

Testosterone replacement improves libido and overall sexual performance in hypogonadal men. Its effect on erectile response to sexual arousal is less clear and sildenafil and its analogues are more appropriate for patients complaining of erectile dysfuntion.

Preparations and choice of androgens

Testosterone given orally is subject to extensive hepatic first-pass metabolism and it is therefore usually given by other routes. Androgens are available for oral, buccal, transdermal or depot administration.

Oral preparations

Testosterone undecanoate is highly lipophilic. When given orally it is absorbed through the intestinal lymphatics, thereby bypassing otherwise extensive hepatic first-pass metabolism. Yet bioavailability is poor and variable. The $t_{\frac{1}{2}}$ is short and the dose is 40–120 mg three times daily. It is converted to DHT before being absorbed, so monitoring should be by measuring DHT, not testosterone levels.

Mesterolone is a DHT derivative.

Parenteral preparations

Sustanon is a mixed testosterone ester preparation normally given 2–4 weekly by deep intramuscular injection; the usual dose is 250 mg (range 100–250 mg). Other preparations, testosterone enanthate and testosterone epionate, are given at 1–2-week intervals. These preparations are widely used and have a good safety profile. Their main disadvantage is fluctuation of plasma testosterone concentrations, causing swings of mood and well-being. But testosterone undecanoate (1 000 mg in 4 mL castor oil given by a depot intramuscular injection) achieves stable physiological concentrations lasting for 3 months.

Transdermal preparations

Patches are available for scrotal and non-scrotal sites; they provide stable pharmacokinetics and are an alternative to painful injections. Absorption is superior at the scrotum because of its high skin vascularity. High concentrations of DHT are achieved because 5α-reductase is present in scrotal skin.

Non-scrotal patches are applied to the skin of the upper arms, back, abdomen and thighs.

Local skin reactions occur in 10% of cases and they are secondary to absorption enhancers. Application of corticosteroid ointment improves tolerability. Patches must be changed every 24 h.

Transdermal gels are hydroalcoholic gels for delivering testosterone transdermally. They are applied daily on the skin of the arms and torso. Showering must be avoided for 6 h, as well as intimate skin contact with others, as transfer of testosterone may occur.

Buccal preparations

These are available in a sustained-release form. A tablet is placed in the small depression above the incisor tooth twice daily. Testosterone is absorbed and delivered into the superior vena cava, thereby bypassing hepatic first-pass metabolism. Steady-state testosterone and DHT concentrations are achieved in 24 h.

Testosterone implants

Pellets of crystallised testosterone are implanted subcutaneously under local anaesthesia by a small incision in the anterior abdominal wall, using a trocar and cannula. Three implanted pellets (total 600 mg) give hormone replacement for about 6 months. There is an approximately 10% risk of extrusion of the pellets; infection and haemorrhage are uncommon.

Adverse effects

Increased libido may lead to undesirable sexual activity, and virilisation is undesired by most women. Androgens have a weak salt and water retaining activity, which is not often clinically important. Liver injury (cholestatic) can occur, particularly with 17α-alkyl derivatives (ethylestrenol, danazol, oxymetholone); it is reversible but these agents should be avoided in hepatic disease. As androgens are contraindicated in carcinoma of the prostate, monitoring during treatment includes regular measurement of prostate specific antigen (PSA). Haemoglobin should also be monitored to avoid polycythaemia.

Effects on blood lipids are complex and variable, and the balance may be to disadvantage.

In patients with malignant disease of bone, androgen administration may be followed by hypercalcaemia. The less virilising androgens are used to promote anabolism and are discussed below.

ANTIANDROGENS (ANDROGEN ANTAGONISTS)

Oestrogens and progestogens are physiological antagonists to androgens. But compounds that compete selectively for androgen receptors have been made.

Cyproterone

Cyproterone is a derivative of progesterone; its combination of structural similarities and differences results in the following:

- Competition with testosterone for receptors in target peripheral organs (but not causing feminisation as do oestrogens); it reduces spermatogenesis even to the level of azoospermia (reversing over about 4 months after the drug is discontinued); abnormal sperm occurs during treatment.
- Competition with testosterone in the CNS, reducing sexual drive and thoughts, and causing impotence.
- Some agonist progestogenic activity on hypothalamic receptors, inhibiting gonadotrophin secretion, which also inhibits testicular androgen production.

Uses. Cyproterone is used for reducing male hypersexuality, and in prostatic cancer and severe female hirsutism. A formulation of cyproterone plus ethinylestradiol (Dianette, which contains only 2 mg of cyproterone acetate) is offered for this latter purpose as well as for severe acne in women; this preparation acts as an oral contraceptive but does not have a UK licence, and should not be used primarily for this purpose.

Flutamide and bicalutamide are non-steroidal antiandrogens available for use in conjunction with the gonadorelins (e.g. goserelin) in the treatment of prostatic carcinoma.

Finasteride and dutasteride which inhibit conversion of testosterone to dihydrotestosterone, have localised antiandrogen activity in tissues where dihydrotestosterone is the principal androgen; they are therefore useful drugs in the treatment of benign prostatic hypertrophy.

Spironolactone also has antiandrogen activity and may help hirsutism in women (as an incidental benefit to its diuretic effect). Androgen secretion may be diminished by continued use of a gonadorelin (LHRH) analogue.

Ketoconazole (antifungal) interferes with androgen and corticosteroid synthesis by inhibiting several of the cytochrome P450 enzymes involved in steroid biosynthesis and may be used in prostatic carcinoma and Cushing's syndrome (400 mg twice daily).

Metyrapone inhibits one enzyme on the cortisol and aldosterone synthetic pathway, 11 hydroxylase, and is therefore also used in the treatment of Cushing's syndrome while awaiting definitive surgical (either bilateral adrenalectomy or transphenoidal pituitary hypophysectomy) treatment.

OESTROGENS

Estrone and estradiol are both natural oestrogens. Oestrogens are responsible for the development of normal secondary sex characteristics in women, uterine growth, thickening of vaginal mucosa and the ductal breast system.

Preparations of oestrogens

The dose varies according to whether replacement of physiological deficiencies is being carried out (replacement therapy) or whether pharmacotherapy is being used.

- Ethinylestradiol ($t_{1/2}$ 13 h) is a synthetic agent of first choice for pharmacological uses (mainly contraceptive, female hypogonadism and menstrual disorders); it is effective by mouth, dose 20–50 micrograms/day.
- Estradiol and estriol are orally active mixed natural oestrogens, dose 1–2 mg/day.
- Conjugated oestrogens (Premarin) are orally active mixed natural oestrogens containing 50%–65% estrone obtained from the urine of pregnant mares, dose 0.625–1.25 mg.
- Estropipate (piperazine estrone sulphate) is an orally active synthetic conjugate.
- Diethylstilbestrol (stilboestrol) is the first synthetic oestrogen; it is used (rarely) in prostatic cancer, and occasionally in post-menopausal women with breast cancer.

Indications for oestrogen therapy

Replacement therapy in hypooestrogenaemia

This term refers to decreased oestrogen production due to ovarian disease, or to hypothalamic–pituitary disease (hypogonadotrophic hypogonadism). Treatment is by cyclic oestrogen (estradiol 1–2 mg, conjugated oestrogens 0.625/1.25 mg daily or ethinylestradiol 20–30 micrograms continuously) plus a progestogen, medroxyprogesterone 2.5–10 mg daily for the last 10–14 days of oestrogen treatment. An alternative treatment is the oral contraceptive.

Post-menopausal hormone replacement therapy (HRT)

HRT refers to the use of oestrogen treatment in order to reverse or prevent problems due to the loss of ovarian hormone secretion after the menopause, whether physiological or induced. The tissues sensitive to oestrogen include brain, bone, skin, cardiovascular and genitourinary. The goal of HRT is to reduce the vasomotor symptoms of oestrogen loss (hot flushes, sleeplessness and vaginal dryness) without causing disorders that may be more common with oestrogen treatment such as breast and endometrial cancer.

All types of HRT (oestrogen with or without progestogen) are effective at reducing the hot flushes experienced by more than 50% of post-menopausal women. The benefit is most during the first year of treatment when 75% of women report a reduced likelihood. By year 3 of treatment the reduction in frequency decreases by 65% in comparison to placebo. The other major value of HRT is the relief of vaginal dryness. Vaginal administration is the most effective route for treatment of dyspareunia and related symptoms. Urinary incontinence does not respond to HRT.

The clinical evidence base for prescribing HRT has changed since the publication of trials showing excess risks of breast cancer and stroke that outweigh small benefits in reduction of fractures and risk of colonic cancer. HRT should not be used in the treatment of osteoporosis or for prevention of coronary heart disease.

Preparations used for HRT. There are three types of regimen:

1. Women without a uterus take continuous oestrogen alone.
2. Women with a uterus require oestrogen combined with progestogen to prevent endometrial proliferation and risk of endometrial cancer.

- In the commonest, 'sequential', regimen women take oestrogen without a break and add a progestogen from day 12–14 to day 28 of each cycle (different preparations vary in the exact length of progestogen prescribing). The first course is started on the first day of menstruation (if present), and 28-day cycles of treatment follow thereafter without interval.

- In the 'continuous' regimen (appropriate only for women who have been amenorrhoeic for more than 1 year) fixed-dose combinations of oestrogen and progestogen are taken without a break. Continuous combination HRT regimens will eventually induce amenorrhoea in most women, thereby eliminating one of the major deterrents to HRT use, withdrawal bleeding.

Calendar packs are available. The oral preparations, Prempak-C and Femoston, use, respectively, conjugated oestrogen and estradiol as their oestrogen. Oral progestogens include dihydrogesterone, medroxyprogesterone, norgestrel and norethisterone. Individual progestogens can be given orally in combination with an oestrogen, assubcutaneous depot injection or by transdermal patch. Some patches provide both hormones but obviously lack the facility for doses to be separately titrated to provide the minimum necessary to prevent both flushing and (if undesired) withdrawal bleeding.

An alternative to oestrogen therapy is tibolone 2.5 mg, which is a synthetic oral steroid with weak oestrogenic, progestogenic and androgenic properties. Its main adverse effect is vaginal bleeding, which needs investigation if persistent. Vasomotor menopausal symptoms may occasionally be helped by low doses of clonidine (Dixarit).

Contraception. HRT in routine use does not provide contraception and any potentially fertile woman who requires HRT should take appropriate precautions. A woman is considered potentially fertile for 2 years after her last menstrual period if she is under 50 years of age, and for 1 year if she is aged over 50 years. A woman who is under 50 years and free of all risk factors for venous and arterial disease can use a low-oestrogen combined oral contraceptive pill to provide both relief of menopausal symptoms and contraception; it is recommended that the oral contraceptive be stopped at 50 years of age as there are more suitable alternatives.

Adverse effects of HRT. The commonest reasons for withdrawal are irregular or withdrawal bleeding and breast pain. Concerns about musculoskeletal symptoms and weight gain have not been substantiated in the long-term trials. Transdermal patches were associated with skin reactions but as the alcohol content has been reduced in the newer formulations the incidence has been reduced.

The more serious complications are venous thromboembolism and cancer of the endometrium or breast. These risks are small in absolute terms, particularly so for the risks of cancer during the first 5 years of treatment.

For venous thromboembolism, the excess risk is 4 per 1 000 woman-years, which may be considered clinically insignificant except in women with predisposing factors, e.g. previous personal or family history of thromboembolism, or recent surgery.

The risk of carcinoma of the endometrium is increased two-fold during 5 years, rising to seven-fold with longer treatment. Because endometrial cancer is uncommon, the absolute risk is about one-tenth that of thromboembolic disease; the risk subsides over 5–10 years after stopping treatment.

Carcinoma of the breast can occur with any type of HRT. Some 45 in every 1 000 women aged 50 years will have breast cancer over the next 20 years, rising by only 2, 6 and 12 cases, respectively, for women who take HRT for 5, 10 or 15 years. A family history of breast cancer does not increase the risks from HRT.

The risk of gallstones may be increased up to two-fold. HRT does not increase risk of ovarian cancer.

Blood lipids: the effect of oestrogens is on balance favour-able, but the addition of a progestogen (unless gestodene or desogestrel) reverses the balance.

Contraindications to oestrogen therapy include recent arterial or venous thromboembolic disease, and history of oestrogen-dependent neoplasm, e.g.

breast cancer. Hypertension, liver disease or gallstones, migraine, diabetes, uterine fibroids or endometriosis may all be made worse by oestrogen. These are very variable, and are not absolute contraindications.

ANTI-OESTROGENS

Selective antagonists of the oestrogen receptor are used either to induce gonadotrophin release in anovulatory infertility or to block stimulation of oestrogen receptor-positive carcinomas of the breast.

Clomifene is structurally related to diethylstilbestrol; it is a weak oestrogen agonist having less activity than natural oestrogens, so that its occupation of receptors results in antagonism, i.e. it is a partial agonist. Clomifene blocks hypothalamic oestrogen receptors so that the negative feedback of natural oestrogens is prevented and the pituitary responds by increased secretion of gonadotrophins, which may induce ovulation.

Clomifene is administered during the early follicular phase of the menstrual cycle (50 mg daily on days 2–6) and is successful in inducing ovulation in about 85% of women. Multiple ovulation with multiple pregnancy may occur and this is its principal adverse effect, which can be limited by using ultrasonography. There have been reports of an increased incidence of ovarian carcinoma following multiple exposure, and the number of consecutive cycles for which clomifene may be used to stimulate ovulation should be limited to 12.

Cyclofenil acts similarly to clomifene.

Tamoxifen is a non-steroidal competitive oestrogen antagonist on target organs. Although available for anovulatory infertility (20 mg daily on days 2, 3, 4 and 5 of the cycle), its main use now is in the treatment of oestrogen-dependent breast cancer. Treatment with tamoxifen delays the growth of metastases and increases survival; if tolerated it should be continued for 5 years.

Tamoxifen is also the hormonal treatment of choice in women with oestrogen receptor-positive metastatic breast cancer. Approximately 60% of such patients respond to initial hormonal manipulation, whereas less than 10% of oestrogen receptor-negative tumours respond.

Severe adverse effects are unusual with tamoxifen but patients with bony metastases may experience an exacerbation of pain, sometimes associated with hypercalcaemia; this reaction commonly precedes tumour response. Amenorrhoea commonly develops in pre-menopausal women. Patients should be told of the small risk of endometrial cancer and encouraged to report relevant symptoms early. They can be reassured that the benefits of treatment far outweigh the risks. Tamoxifen is now considered a SERM.

PROGESTERONE AND PROGESTOGENS

Progesterone ($t_{1/2}$ 5 min) is produced by the corpus luteum and converts the uterine epithelium from the proliferative to the secretory phase. It is thus necessary for successful implantation of the ovum and is essential throughout pregnancy, in the last two-thirds of which it is secreted in large amounts by the placenta. It acts particularly on tissues that are sensitised by oestrogens. Some synthetic progestogens are less selective, having varying oestrogenic and androgenic activity, and these may inhibit ovulation, though not very reliably. Progestogens are of two principal kinds:

- Progesterone and its derivatives: dydrogesterone, hydroxyprogesterone, medroxyprogesterone ($t_{1/2}$ 28 h).
- Testosterone derivatives: norethisterone and its prodrug ethynodiol ($t_{1/2}$ 10h), levonorgestrel, desogestrel, gestodene, gestronol, norgestimate.

Drospirenone isa derivativeofthe syntheticaldosteroneantagonist, spironolactone. It therefore has antimineralocorticoid activity, reducing salt retention and blood pressure. Italso exhibits partialantiandrogenicactivity, about 30% of that of cyproterone acetate. It is available as a combination with ethinylestradiol for use as a contraceptive.

Most progestogens can virilise directly or by metabolites (except progesterone and dydrogesterone), and fetal virilisation to the point of sexual ambiguity has occurred with vigorous use during pregnancy.

Uses

The clinical uses of progestational agents are ill defined, apart from contraception, the menopause and post-menopausal hormone replacement therapy.

Other possible uses include: menstrual disorders, e.g. menorrhagia, endometriosis, dysmenorrhoea and premenstrual syndrome (doubtful efficacy), breast and endometrial cancer.

Preparations

Available progestogens (some used only in combined formulations) include:

- Oral: norethisterone, dydrogesterone, gestodene, desogestrel, levonorgestrel, megestrol, medroxyprogesterone.
- Suppositories or pessaries: progesterone.
- Injectable: progesterone, hydroxyprogesterone, medroxyprogesterone.

Adverse effects of prolonged use include virilisation, raised blood pressure and an adverse trend in blood lipids. Gestodene, desogestrel and norgestimate may have less affinity for androgen receptors and therefore fewer unfavourable effects on blood lipids; the first two of these may have a higher risk of thrombosis.

ANTIPROGESTOGENS

Menstruation (in its luteal phase) is dependent on progesterone, and uterine bleeding follows antagonism of progesterone. Pregnancy is dependent on progesterone (for implantation, endometrial stimulation, suppression of uterine contractions and placenta formation), and abortion follows progesterone antagonism in early pregnancy.

Mifepristone is a pure competitive antagonist at progesterone and glucocorticoid receptors. Clinical trials of oral use in hospital outpatients have shown it to be safe and effective in terminating pregnancy. Efficacy is enhanced if its use is followed by vaginal administration of a prostaglandin (gemeprost) to produce uterine contractions (the success rate is raised from 85% to more than 95%).

Adverse effects of the combined treatment include nausea and vomiting, dizziness, asthenia, abdominal pain; uterine bleeding may be heavy. Mifepristone also offers the opportunity for mid-trimester terminations. These are likely to become more frequent with rise in the number of inherited syndromes amenable to antenatal diagnosis at this stage.

Guidelines may vary in detail and the following are general regimens:

- For gestation of up to 1 week where the fetus is deemed viable, mifepristone 600 mg by mouth followed 36–48 h later by gemeprost 1 mg by vagina.
- For mid-trimester medical abortion (13–24 weeks), mifepristone 600 mg by mouth followed 36–48 h later by gemeprost 1 mg every 3 h by vagina to a maximum of 5mg.

Other progesterone derivatives

Danazol (Danol) is a derivative of the progestogen, ethisterone. It has partial agonist androgen activity and is described as an 'impeded' androgen; it has little progestogen activity. It is a relatively selective inhibitor of pituitary gonadotrophin secretion (LH, FSH) affecting the surge in the mid-menstrual cycle more than basal secretion. This reduces ovarian function, which leads to atrophic changes in endometrium, both uterine and elsewhere (ectopic), i.e. endometriosis. In males it reduces spermatogenesis. Unwanted androgenic effects occur in women (acne, hirsutism and, rarely, enlargement of the clitoris).

It is used chiefly for: endometriosis, fibrocystic mastitis, gynaecomastia, precocious puberty, menorrhagia and hereditary angioedema.

Gestrinone is similar.

FERTILITY REGULATION

CONTRACEPTION BY DRUGS AND HORMONES

The requirements of a successful hormonal contraceptive are stringent, for it will be used by millions of healthy people who wish to separate sexual relations from physical reproduction. The following represent the ideal:

- It must be extremely safe as well as highly effective.
- Its action must be quick in onset and quickly and completely reversible, even after years of continuous use.
- It must not affect libido. The fact that alternative methods are less reliable implies that their use will lead to more unwanted pregnancies with their attendant inconvenience, morbidity and mortality, and this must be taken into account in deciding what risks of hormonal contraception are acceptable.

Hormonal contraception in women comprises:

- Oestrogen and progestogen (combined and phased administration).
- Progestogen alone.

Combined contraceptives (the 'pill')

Combined oestrogen–progestogen oral contraceptives (COCP) have been used extensively since 1956. The principal mechanism is inhibition of ovulation through suppression of LH surge by hypothalamus and pituitary. In addition the endometrium is altered, so that implantation is less likely and cervical mucus becomes more viscous and impedes the passage of the spermatozoa.

The combination is conveniently started on the first day of the cycle (first day of menstruation) and continued for 21 days (this is immediately effective, inhibiting the first ovulation). It is followed by a period of 7 days when no pill is taken, and during which bleeding usually occurs. Thereafter, regardless of bleeding, a new 21-day course is begun, and so on, i.e. active tablets are taken daily for 3 weeks out of 4. For easy compliance, some combined pills are packaged so that the woman takes one tablet every day without interruption (21 active then 7 dummy).

In some instances, the course is not started on the first day of menstruation but on the second to the fifth day (to give a full month between the menses at the outset). An alternative method of contraception should then be used until the seventh pill has been taken, as the first ovulation may not have been suppressed in women who have short menstrual cycles.

The pill should be taken at about the same time (to within 12 h) every day to establish a routine. The monthly bleeds that occur 1–2 days after the cessation of active hormone administration are hormone withdrawal bleeds not natural menstruation. They are not an essential feature of oral contraception, but women are accustomed to monthly bleeds and they provide monthly reassurance of the absence of pregnancy.

Numerous field trials have shown that progestogen– oestrogen combinations, if taken precisely as directed, are the most reliable reversible contraceptive known. (The only close competitors are depot progestogens and progestogenreleasing intrauterine devices.)

Important aspects

Subsequent fertility. After stopping the pill, fertility that is normal for the age the woman has now reached is restored, although conception may be delayed for a few months longer in younger, and for as much as a year in older, users than if other methods had been used.

Effect on an existing pregnancy. Although progestogens can masculinise the female fetus, the doses for contraception are so low that risk of harming an undiagnosed pregnancy is extremely small, probably less than 1 in 1000 (the background incidence of birth defects is 1%–2%).

Carcinomas of the breast and cervix are slightly increased in incidence; the incidence of hepatoma (very rare) is increased. The risk to life seems to be less than that of moderate smoking (10 cigarettes/day) and than that of a normal pregnancy, as the risks of pulmonary embolus are higher in a normal pregnancy. The risk of carcinoma of the ovary and endometrium is substantially reduced. The overall incidence of cancer is unaltered.

The effect on menstruation is generally to regularise it, and often to diminish blood loss, but amenorrhoea can occur. In some women 'breakthrough' intermenstrual bleeding occurs, especially at the outset, but this seldom persists for more than a few cycles. Premenstrual tension and dysmenorrhoea are much reduced.

Libido is greatly subject to psychosocial influences, and removal of fear of pregnancy may permit enthusiasm for the first time. It is likely that direct pharmacological effect (reduction) is rare. There is evidence that the normal increase in female-initiated sexual activity at time of ovulation is suppressed.

Cardiovascular complications. The incidence of venous thromboembolism is increased in pill users. It is lowest in the 20–35-microgram pill and rises progressively with the 50-and 100-microgram preparations; it is not known whether there is any difference between doses of 20 and 35 micrograms. The small increase in hypertension, cerebrovascular events and acute myocardial infarction is confined principally to smokers.

Increased arterial disease also appears to be associated with the type of progestogen in the combined pill. The 'third-generation' pills appear to carry a higher risk of venous thrombosis, but may have a lower risk of arterial thrombosis because their lower androgen activity leads to slightly higher high-density lipoprotein (HDL) levels than older pills. The progestogen-only pill does not significantly affect coagulation.

Major surgery (in patients taking oestrogen–progestogen contraceptives and post-menopausal hormone replacement therapy). Because of the added risk of venous thromboembolism (surgery causes a fall in antithrombin levels), oral contraceptives should be withdrawn, if practicable, 4 weeks before all lower limb operations or any major elective surgery (and started again at the first menstruation to occur more than 2 weeks after surgery). But increase in clotting factors may persist for many weeks and there is also the risk of pregnancy to be considered. An alternative for emergencies is to use low molecular weight heparin (although this may not reverse all the oestrogenic effects on coagulation) and other means (mechanical stimulation of venous return) to prevent postoperative thrombosis.

Plasma lipoproteins may be adversely affected; least where the progestogen is desogestrel or low-dose norethisterone.

Plasma proteins. Oestrogens cause an increase in proteins, particularly the globulins that bind hydrocortisone, thyroxine and iron. As a result, the total plasma concentration of the bound substances is increased, although the concentration of free and active substance remains normal. This can be misleading in diagnostic tests, e.g. of thyroid function. This effect on plasma proteins passes off about 6 weeks after cessation of the oestrogen.

Other adverse effects

Often more prominent at the outset and largely due to oestrogen, these include: nausea and, rarely, vomiting; breast discomfort, fluid retention, headache (including increase in migraine), lethargy, abdominal discomfort, vaginal discharge or dryness. Depression may occur but most depression in pill users is not due to the contraceptive.

The above account gives rise to guidelines for use: **Absolute contraindications** include:

- A personal history of thromboembolic venous, arterial or cardiac disease, or severe or multiple risk factors for these.
- Transient cerebral ischaemic attacks without headache.
- Infective hepatitis, until 3 months after liver function test results have become normal, and other liver disease including disturbances of hepatic excretion, e.g. cholestatic jaundice, Dubin–Johnson and Rotor syndromes.
- Migraine, if there is a typical aura, focal features, or if it is severe and lasts for more than 72 h despite treatment, or is treated with an ergot derivative (use with caution is acceptable if there is no aura, focal features, or if it is controlled with a 5-HT$_1$ receptor agonist).
- Carcinoma of the breast or genital tract, past or present.
- Other conditions including: systemic lupus erythematosus, porphyria, following evacuation of a hydatidiform mole (until urine and plasma

gonadotrophin concentrations are normal), undiagnosed vaginal bleeding.

Relative contraindications or uses with caution, include:

- Family history of venous thromboembolism, arterial disease or a known prothrombotic condition, e.g. factor V Leiden (pretreatment coagulation investigation is advised).
- Diabetes mellitus, which may be precipitated or become more difficult to control (avoid if there are diabetic complications).
- Hypertension (avoid if blood pressure exceeds 160/100 mmHg).
- Smoking more than 40 cigarettes per day (15 cigarettes/ day enhances the risks of circulatory disease three-fold, and constitutes an absolute contraindication for women over 35 years).
- Age over 35 years (avoid if older than 50 years).
- Obesity (avoid if body mass exceeds 39 kg/m^2).
- Long-term immobility, e.g. due to leg plaster, confinement to bed.
- Breast feeding (until weaning or for 6 months after birth).

Duration of use does not enhance risks of itself. The increase in risk with increased duration of use is due to increasing age. The approaching menopause presents an obvious problem. Cyclical bleeding will continue to occur under the influence of the drugs even after the natural menopause. Thus the only way of deciding whether contraception can be permanently abandoned is by discontinuing it (and using another technique) for 3 months annually to see whether natural menstruation is resumed, or by stopping the combined pill for 1 month and measuring luteinising hormone (LH)/follicle stimulating hormone (FSH) concentration in the blood, which indicates the state of pituitary function.

Benefits additional to contraception

Menses are accompanied by less premenstrual tension and dysmenorrhoea. When oestrogen is combined with the antiandrogen cyproterone acetate as the progestogenic agent Dianette, the combined pill is useful treatment for acne in young women.

Formulations of oestrogen–progestogen combination

Oestrogen: ethinylestradiol or mestranol.

Progestogen:
- Second generation: norethisterone, levonorgestrel.
- Third generation: desogestrel, gestodene, norgestimate.

Combined oral contraceptives are defined as second or third generation by the progestogen component (firstgeneration progestogens are obsolete). Those containing a fixed amount of oestrogen and progestogen in each active tablet are termed 'monophasic'. Other pills employ variable ratios between oestrogen and progestogen, in two (biphasic) or three (triphasic) periods within the menstrual cycle. The dose of progestogen is low at the beginning and higher at the end, the oestrogen remaining either constant or rising slightly in mid-cycle. The objective is to achieve effective contraception with minimal distortion of natural hormonal rhythms.

The advantages claimed for these techniques are diminished adverse metabolic changes, e.g. blood lipids, and a particularly reliable monthly bleeding pattern without loss of contraceptive efficacy. Preparations include BiNovum, TriNovum, Logynon.

It is now appreciated that the earlier preparations had much more oestrogen than was necessary for efficacy. It seems probable that 20 micrograms is about the limit below which serious loss of efficacy can be expected. Indeed, in patients whose hepatic enzymes are likely to be induced, e.g. those taking antiepileptic or some anti-rheumatic drugs, it is advisable to use a preparation containing 50 micrograms oestrogen or more to avoid loss of efficacy due to increased oestrogen metabolism (elimination of breakthrough bleeding is a guide to adequacy of dose).

Choice of oestrogen–progestogen combination

There is a wide choice of formulations, with the dose of ethinylestradiol varying from 20 to 35 micrograms. In general, users should be prescribed the lowest total hormone dose that suits them (good cycle control and minimal unwanted effects) and should make a start with the first preparation given above, recognising that compliance is particularly important with the 20-microgram dose.

Common problems

Missed pill. The following refers to the combined pill:
- If an omitted dose is remembered within 12 h, it should be taken at once and the next dose at the usual time, and all should be well.
- If more than 12 h have elapsed, the above procedure should be followed but an additional barrier method of contraception should be used for 7 days. Although the protective effect of cervical mucus returns within 48 h, this 7-day period is needed to ensure effective suppression of an ovulation that may have been initiated by the missed pill.

Intercurrent gut upset. If vomiting occurs more than 3 h after a pill, behave as for a missed pill (above). The hormones are rapidly absorbed and only severe diarrhoea would interfere significantly with efficacy. In case of doubt, it would be prudent to use a barrier method during and for 7 days after the episode.

Changing of preparation. If a woman is unhappy on one preparation she may be changed to another containing a different dose of oestrogen and/or progestogen. The new preparation should start the day after she has finished a cycle on the previous preparation. If this is done no extra risk of pregnancy occurs.

Breakthrough bleeding (bleeding on days of active pill taking) can mean that a higher dose of oestrogen or progestogen is required. Note that missed or late pills, drug interaction or sexually transmitted infection, e.g. due to chlamydia, can also cause breakthrough bleeding.

Progestogen-only contraception

Progestogen-only pills (POPs) are indicated where oestrogen is contraindicated and in lactating women. Progestogens render cervical mucus less easily penetrable by sperm and induce a premature secretory change in the endometrium so that implantation does not occur. Older POPs became unreliable if not taken at the same time of day, because their effect on cervical mucus wears off after 3 h and their additional action to inhibit ovulation occurs in only 40% of cycles. There is also liability to breakthrough bleeding.

A newer POP containing 75 micrograms desogestrel inhibits ovulation in 97%–99% of cycles, resulting in an efficacy similar to that of the COCP. A further advantage of the newer POP is that no extra contraceptive cover is required if the exact time of dose is missed, provided the delay is no more than 12 h. Ectopic pregnancy may be more frequent due to a fertilised ovum being held up in a functionally depressed fallopian tube.

Medroxyprogesterone acetate and its metabolites are excreted in breast milk, so women who breastfeed should wait until 6 weeks postpartum before starting Depo-Provera, when the infant's enzyme system should be more mature. Norethisterone enantate 200 mg (Noristerat) is shorter-acting than Depo-Provera, 8 weeks, and is used to provide contraception after administration of the rubella vaccine, and until a partner's vasectomy has taken effect. It can also be used in the longer-term but only on a 'named patient' basis.

Subdermal implantations that release hormone for several years are in use; they can be removed surgically if adverse effects develop or pregnancy is desired. For example, a flexible rod containing etonorgestrel (Implanon) inserted into the lower surface of the upper arm provides contraception for 3 years (2 years for overweight women because they have lower blood concentrations). The rod must be removed when its effective period has elapsed.

Two depot injections of intramuscular progestogen are available, equal in efficacy to the combined pill. Medroxyprogesterone (Depo-Provera) ($t_{1/2}$ 28 h) is a sustained-release (aqueous suspension) deep intramuscular injection given 3-monthly. When injected between day 1 and day 5 of the menstrual cycle, contraception starts immediately. If given after day 5, a barrier contraceptive is needed for7 days.

Postcoital ('morning after pill') and emergency contraception

The overall risk of pregnancy following a single act of unprotected intercourse on any day in the menstrual cycle is 2%–4%. The risk from a single act is highest (20%–30%) in the days before and just after ovulation. Pregnancy may be prevented before implantation by disrupting the normal hormonal arrangements; the mode of action is probably by delaying or preventing ovulation or by preventing implantation of the fertilised ovum.

Progestogen-only treatment is preferred. Levonorgestrel 1500 micrograms is taken within 72 h of unprotected sexual intercourse. It can be taken more than once in a cycle, if required, and there is no upper limit to how many times it can be taken in a year. Contraindications to hormonal emergency contraception include current or suspected pregnancy, unprotected sexual intercourse more than 72 h earlier, and sensitivity to the components of the progestogen-only preparation. Some women complain of nausea and vomiting, which responds best to domperidone.

Drug interaction with steroid contraceptives

Particularly now that the lowest effective doses are in use there is little latitude between success and failure if absorption, distribution and metabolism are disturbed. Any additional drug-taking must be looked at critically lest it reduces efficacy.

Enzyme induction. The rifamycins, rifampicin and rifabutin, are potent inducers of hepatic drug-metabolising enyzmes. The classic example of failure with the combined pill is breakthrough bleeding and pregnancy in young women being treated with rifampicin for tuberculosis, or meningitis including eradication of the carrier state. The enhanced metabolism of the steroids results in contraceptive failure.

Antiepileptics (phenytoin and carbamazepine but not sodium valproate) create a similar risk. Indeed, all drugs that induce metabolising enzymes, whether prescribed or self-administered (alcohol, tobacco smoking), constitute a risk to contraceptive efficacy and prescribing should be specifically reviewed for the effect.

Broad-spectrum antimicrobials, e.g. ampicillin,

doxycycline, can reduce the efficacy of combined oral contraceptives by diminishing the bacterial flora that metabolise ethinylestradiol in the large bowel and make it available for recycling. Additional contraceptive measures should be taken during a short course of antimicrobial, and for 7 days thereafter. When the course is long, i.e. more than 3 weeks, the bacteria have time to recover by developing resistance, and additional precautions are unnecessary after the first 14 days.

Hypothalamic/pituitary hormone approach to contraception

Other methods of contraception

Copper intrauterine devices are widely used and highly effective (>99% at 1 year) for 5 years, and some for 10 years. They are especially useful in the over-40s, in whom oral contraceptives may become progressively contraindicated and for whom one IUD will last into the menopause. The IUD prevents implantation of the fertilised ovum, and has an additional antifertilisation effect enhanced by the toxic effect of copper ions on the gametes.

The intrauterine levonorgestrel system Mirena is used as a contraceptive, as a medical treatment for idiopathic menorrhagia and as the progestogen component of hormone replacement therapy. It is popular because of reduced dysmenorrhoea and lighter menses. Mirena contains 52 mg levonorgestrel surrounded by a Silastic capsule, and releases 20 micrograms/day over 5 years, after which the device should be changed.

Vaginal preparations, used to immobilise or kill (spermicide) spermatozoa, are used to add safety to various mechanical contraceptives. They are very unreliable and should be used alone only in an emergency. Substances used include non-oxinols (surfactants that alter the permeability of the sperm lipoprotein membrane) as pessary, gel or foam.

Oil-based lubricants cause failure of rubber condoms and contraceptive diaphragms; many 'lubricants', e.g. hand or baby creams, wash off readily, but are nevertheless oil-based. Barrier contraceptive devices made of polyurethane, e.g. the female condom (Femidom), are not so affected.

Risks of contraception in relation to benefit

Despite the small risk of thromboembolism, the death rate from taking oral contraceptives is less than that pregnancy.

MENSTRAL DISORDERS

Amenorrhoea, primary or secondary, requires specialist endocrinological diagnosis. Where the cause is failure of hormone production, cyclical replacement therapy is indicated.

Menorrhagia can be associated with both ovulatory and anovulatory ovarian cycles. It is important to distinguish the menstrual consequences of each cycle. Ovulatory ovarian cycles give rise to regular menstrual cycles, whereas anovulatory cycles result in irregular menstruation or, extremely, amenorrhoea. This distinction is critical in management.

Both ovulatory and anovulatory cycles can give rise to excessive menstrual loss in the absence of any other abnormality, so-called dysfunctional uterine bleeding. Endocrine disorders do not cause excessive menstrual loss, with the exception of the endocrine consequences of anovulation. Equally, haemostatic disorders are rare causes of menorrhagia. One consequence of excessive menstrual loss is iron deficiency anaemia. In the Western world, menorrhagia is the commonest cause of iron deficiency anaemia.

Medical treatment of menorrhagia is either non-hormonal or hormonal therapy. As there is no hormonal defect, the use of hormonal therapy does not correct an underlying disorder but merely imposes an external control of the cycle. For many women, cycle control is as important an issue as the degree of menorrhagia.

The two main first-line treatments for menorrhagia associated with ovulatory cycles are non-hormonal, namely tranexamic acid (an antifibrinolytic) and a non-steroidal anti-inflammatory drug (NSAID), e.g. mefenamic acid 500 mg when the blood loss becomes heavy, followed by 250 mg three times daily for 3 days. The effectiveness of these treatments has been shown in randomised trials and reported in systematic reviews of treatment. Tranexamic acid reduces menstrual loss by about a half and NSAIDs reduce it by about a third. Both have the advantage of being taken only during menstruation itself and are particularly useful in women who either do not require contraception or do not wish to use a hormonal therapy. They are also of value in treating excessive menstrual blood loss associated with the use of non-hormonal intrauterine contraceptive devices.

Hormonal therapy should be regarded as a third-choice treatment only in women not requiring contraception as a parallel objective. Progestogens are effective only when given for 21 days in each cycle. Combined oral contraceptives are useful for anovulatory bleeding as they impose a cycle. The levonorgestrel releasing intrauterine system (Mirena) is advocated as an alternative to surgery.

The timing of menstruation. Sometimes there are pressing reasons to prevent menstruation at the normal time but obviously this cannot be done at the last moment.

Menstruation can be postponed by giving oral norethisterone 5 mg three times daily, starting 3 days before the expected onset; bleeding occurs 2–3 days after withdrawal. Users of the combined oral contraceptive pill (having a 7-day break) can simply continue with active pills where they would normally stop for 7 days.

Although there is no evidence that harm follows such manoeuvres, it is obviously imprudent to practise them frequently.

Note. These uses of progestogen should not be undertaken if there is any possibility of pregnancy.

Endometriosis. Medical treatments for endometriosis have focused on the hormonal alteration of the menstrual cycle in an attempt to produce a pseudo-pregnancy, pseudo-menopause or chronic anovulation. Each of these situations is believed to cause a suboptimal milieu for the growth and maintenance of endometrium and, by extension, of implants of endometriosis. Danazol 600– 800 mg/day causes anovulation by attenuating the mid-cycle surge of luteinising hormone secretion, inhibiting multiple enzymes in the steroidogenic pathway, and increasing plasma free testosterone concentrations.

Medroxyprogesterone causes the decidualisation of endometrial tissue, with eventual atrophy.

Adverse effects occur at low (20–30 mg/day) or high (100 mg/day) dose, and include abnormal uterine bleeding, nausea, breast tenderness, fluid retention and depression. These resolve after the discontinuation of the drug.

Gestrinone 5–10 mg/week is an antiprogestational steroid that causes a decline in the concentrations of oestrogen and progesterone receptors, and a 50% decline in plasma estradiol concentrations. Androgenic adverse effects, such as a deepening of the voice, hirsutism and clitoral hypertrophy, are potentially irreversible. A combination of an oestrogen and a progestogen induces a hormonal pseudo-pregnancy. The oral contraceptive is used either continuously or cyclically (21 active pills followed by 7 days of placebo). Both regimens are effective; the amenorrhea of continuous administration is advantageous for women with dysmenorrhoea.

Gonadotrophin releasing hormone (GnRH) agonists diminish the secretion of follicle stimulating hormone and luteinising hormone, resulting in hypogonadotrophic hypogonadism, endometrial atrophy and amenorrhoea. The GnRH agonist can be given intranasally, subcutaneously or intramuscularly, with a frequency of administration ranging from twice daily to every 3 months. The unwanted effects are the menopausal-type symptoms of hypo-oestrogenism (such as transient vaginal bleeding, hot flushes, vaginal dryness) and can be prevented by concurrent administration of HRT in post-menopausal doses.

Although most treatments for endometriosis are directed at the hormones themselves, the symptoms can be also treated directly. NSAIDs such as diclofenac, ibuprofen and mefenamic acid are often given to relieve the pain associated with endometriosis. These drugs are frequently the first-line treatment in women with pelvic pain whose cause has not yet been proved to be endometriosis.

Dysmenorrhoea is due to uterine contractions resulting from excess prostaglandins in the uterus during ovulatory cycles. It can be treated by suppressing ovulation (using the combined pill or norethisterone), or by using inhibitors of prostaglandin synthesis, e.g. aspirin, indometacin, naproxen. The analgesic prostaglandin synthase inhibitor (NSAID) may need to be given for several days before menstruation, or only at the time of the pain.

Premenstrual tension syndrome may be due to an imbalance of natural oestrogen and progesterone secretion, but knowledge of the syndrome remains imprecise. Psychosocial factors can be important. Placebo effects are strong. Drugs are not necessarily the preferred treatment.

Cyclical breast pain or mastalgia, when severe, may respond to continuous use of gamolenic acid (Efamast) by mouth; it is an essential unsaturated fatty acid for cell membranes (patients have low concentrations); it may act by reducing cellular uptake of prolactin and ovarian hormones. Danazol and bromocriptine also help.

MYOMETRIUM

Oxytocics, i.e. drugs that hasten childbirth, and prostaglandins induce uterine contractions. They are used to induce abortion, to induce or augment labour, and to minimise blood loss from the placental site.

Oxytocics

Oxytocin is a peptide hormone of the posterior pituitary gland. It stimulates the contractions of the pregnant uterus, which becomes much more sensitive to it at term. Patients with posterior pituitary disease (diabetes insipidus) can go into labour normally.

Oxytocin is released reflexly from the pituitary following suckling (also by manual stimulation of the nipple) and produces an almost immediate contraction of the myoepithelium of the breast; it can be used to enhance milk ejection (nasal spray). The only other clinically important effect is on the blood pressure, which may fall if an overdose is given.

Synthetic oxytocin (Syntocinon) is pure and is not contaminated with vasopressin as is the natural product, which is obsolete.

Oxytocin is used intravenously in the induction of labour and sometimes for uterine inertia, haemorrhage or during abortion. It produces, almost immediately, rhythmic contractions with relaxation between, i.e. it mimics normal uterine activity.

The decision to use oxytocin requires special skill. It has a $t_{1/2}$ of 6 min and is given by intravenous infusion using a pump; it must be closely supervised; the dose is adjusted by results; overdose can cause uterine tetany and even rupture. The utmost care is required.

Oxytocin is structurally close to vasopressin and it is no surprise that it also has antidiuretic activity. Serious water intoxication can occur with prolonged intravenous infusions, especially where accompanied by large volumes of fluid. The association of oxytocin with neonatal jaundice appears to be due to increased erythrocyte fragility causing haemolysis.

Oxytocin has been supplanted by the ergot alkaloid, ergometrine, as prime treatment of postpartum haemorrhage.

Ergometrine is used to contract the uterus. It is an α-adrenoceptor and dopamine receptor agonist and acts almost immediately when injected intravenously. The uterus is stimulated at all times, but is much more sensitive in late pregnancy.

Ergometrine and oxytocin differ in their actions on the uterus. In moderate doses, oxytocin produces slow generalised contractions with full relaxation in between; ergometrine produces faster contractions superimposed on a tonic contraction. High doses of both substances produce sustained tonic contraction. It will be seen, therefore, that oxytocin is more suited to induction of labour and ergometrine to the prevention and treatment of postpartum haemorrhage, the incidence of which is reduced by its routine prophylactic use (generally intramuscularly).

There are advantages in a mixture of oxytocin and ergometrine (Syntometrine).

Prostaglandins

Prostaglandins that soften the uterine cervix (by an action on collagen) and have a powerful oxytocic effect include:

Dinoprost (prostaglandin $F_2\alpha$; $PGF_2\alpha$) (Prostin F2 alpha) and dinoprostone (prostaglandin E_2; PGE_2) (Prostin E2). They are used to induce labour and to terminate pregnancy, including missed or partial abortion and in the treatment of hydatidiform mole; they are given by intra-or extra-amniotic injection, by vaginal tablet, or intracervical gel, by intravenous infusion or by mouth. Their safe and effective use (including choice of route) requires special skill.

Adverse effects include vomiting, diarrhoea, headache, pyrexia and local tissue reaction.

Gemeprost (prostaglandin E_1 analogue) (Cervagem) is used intravaginally to soften the cervix before operative procedures in the first trimester of pregnancy and for abortion, alone and in combination with an antiprogestogen.

Carboprost (prostaglandin F_2 analogue) is used for postpartum haemorrhage (resistant to ergometrine and oxytocin) for its oxytocin action. It is highly effective. Adverse effects include hypertension, asthma and pulmonary oedema.

Induction of abortion

Gemeprost, administered vaginally as pessaries, is the preferred prostaglandin for the medical induction of late therapeutic abortion. Gemeprost ripens and softens the cervix before surgical abortion, particularly in primigravida. Misoprostol by mouth or by vaginal administration, or gemeprost, may be given to induce medical abortion (an unlicensed indication in the UK). Pretreatment with mifepristone can facilitate the process, by sensitising the uterus to the prostaglandin so that abortion occurs in a shorter time and with a lower dose of prostaglandin.

Induction and augmentation of labour

Oxytocin is administered by slow intravenous infusion as below, usually in conjunction with amniotomy, and dinoprostone by vaginal tablets, pessaries and vaginal gels. Misoprostol may be used orally or vaginally to induce labour (an unlicensed indication in the UK).

The UK National Institute for Health and Clinical Excellence has recommended that:

- Dinoprostone is preferable to oxytocin for induction of labour in women with intact membranes, regardless of parity or cervical favourability.
- Dinoprostone and oxytocin are equally effective for the induction of labour in women with ruptured membranes, regardless of parity or cervical favourability.
- Intravaginal dinoprostone preparations are preferable to intracervical preparations.
- Oxytocin should not be started for 6 h following administration of vaginal prostaglandins.
- When used to induce labour, the recommended dose of oxytocin by intravenous infusion is initially 0.001–0.002 units/min, increased at intervals of at least 30 min until a maximum of three to four contractions occurs every 10 min (0.012 units/min is often adequate); the maximum recommended rate is 0.032 units/min (licensed max. 0.02 units/min).

Prevention and treatment of uterine haemorrhage

Bleeding due to incomplete abortion can be controlled with ergometrine and oxytocin (Syntometrine) given intramuscularly. Their combination is more effective in early pregnancy than either drug alone.

For the routine management of the third stage of labour ergometrine 500 micrograms with oxytocin 5 units (Syntometrine 1 mL) is given by intramuscular injection on delivery of the anterior shoulder or, at the latest, immediately after the baby is delivered. In pre-eclampsia, oxytocin may be given alone by intramuscular injection. These regimens are also used for the treatment of postpartum haemorrhage. The same drugs may be given i.v. for excessive uterine bleeding caused by uterine atony. Carboprost is an alternative for haemorrhage unresponsive to ergometrine and oxytocin.

Uterine relaxants

β$_2$-Adrenoceptor agonists relax the uterus and are given by i.v. infusion by obstetricians to inhibit premature labour, e.g. isoxsuprine, terbutaline, ritodrine, salbutamol. Their use is complicated by the expected cardiovascular effects, including tachycardia, hypotension. Less easy to explain, but more devastating on occasion to the patient, is severe left ventricular failure. The combination of fluid overload (due to the vehicle) and increased oxygen demand by the heart are possible factors; the risk is higher in multiple pregnancy, pre-existing cardiac disease or maternal infection. It is important to administer the β$_2$ agonist with minimum fluid volume using a syringe pump with 5% dextrose (not saline) as diluent, and to monitor the patient closely for signs of fluid overload.

The dose of ritodrine for i.v. administration is: initially 50 micrograms/min, increased gradually according to response by 50 micrograms/min every 10 min until contractions stop or maternal heart rate reaches 140 beats per min; continue for 12–48 h after contractions cease (usual rate 150–350 micrograms/min).

SUMMARY

- The hypothalamus releases a number of locally active hormones such as CRH, TRH and GnRH that stimulate or inhibit pituitary hormone release such as ACTH, TSH, LH and FSH. They regulate adreanal cortex, Thyroid gland and gonadal function.
- Sex hormons, including oestrogen, progesterone and androgen secreted by the gonadal glands. Oestrogen is used for Replacement therapy in hypooestrogenaemia, Chemotherapy and contraception. Progesterone, apart from contraception, the menopause and post-menopausal hormone replacement therapy. Menstrual disorders, endometriosis, breast and endometrial cancer are also it's indications.
- Hormonal contraception in women comprises oestrogen–progestogen combination and Progestogen-only contraceptives.
- Oxytocics, i.e. prostaglandins and oxytocin induce uterine contractions. They are used to induce or augment labour, and to minimise blood loss from the placental site. Ergometrineis only used for Prevention and treatment of uterine haemorrhage and promotion of uterusre naturation.

IMPORTANT TERMINOLOGY

adrenal corticosteroids 肾上腺皮质激素

glucocorticoid 糖皮质激素

mineralocorticoid 盐皮质激素

replacement therapy 替代疗法

insulin 胰岛素

insulin secretagogues 胰岛素促泌剂

sulfonylureas 磺脲类

meglitinides 氯茴苯酸类

incretin analogues and mimetics 肠降血糖素类似物

dipeptidyl peptidase-4 (DPP-4) inhibitors 二肽基肽酶-4 抑制剂

insulin sensitisers 胰岛素增敏剂

biguanides 双胍类

thiazolidinediones 噻唑烷二酮类

thyroid hormones 甲状腺素

antithyroid drugs 抗甲状腺药

thiourea derivatives 硫脲类

iodine 碘

radioiodine 放射性碘

growth hormone (GH) 生长激素

vasopressin (antidiuretic hormone) 加压素, 抗利尿激素

oestrogen 雌二醇

androgen 雄激素

contraceptives 避孕药

adrenocorticotrophic hormone (ACTH) 促肾上腺皮质激素

corticotropin releasing hormone (CRH) 促肾上腺皮质激素释放激素

follicle stimulating hormone (FSH) 卵胞刺激素

growth hormone releasing hormone (GHRH) 生长激素释放激素

gonadotrophin releasing hormone (GnRH) 促性腺激素释放激素

thyrotrophin releasing hormone (TRH) 促甲状腺激素释放激素

thyroid stimulating hormone (TSH) 促甲状腺激素

vasoactive intestinal peptide (VIP) 肠道血管活性肽

oxytocics 催产药

CHALLENGE YOURSELF

1. What are the pharmacology action of glucocorticoid?
2. What are the clinical use of insulin?
3. Please introduce the classification of Oral antidiabetes drugs.
4. What are the pharmacology action of thiourea derivatives?
5. What kinds of hormones can be releases by hypothalamus and pituitary?

Li Chen

Chapter 17

Respiratory system

INTRODUCTION

The vital functions of respiratory system include the conduction of air, the exchange of oxygen and carbon dioxide, and protecting the respiratory surfaces from infection and exposure to noxious elements. The respiratory tract is commonly divided into upper and lower respiratory tract. Disorders of the upper respiratory tract are those associated with infections and seasonal allergies. Disorders of the lower respiratory tract may be broadly classified as parenchymal infections and obstructive airway conditions. Drugs that are used for treatment of respiratory diseases include antitussives, bronchodilators, respiratory stimulants, pulmonary surfactant, oxygen, antihistamine, β-adrenoceptor agonist, corticosteroids, antimicrobials and antivirals. There are multiple drug administration routes which allow flexibility for the clinician and reduce systemic side effects. Successful use of these various agents requires a thorough understanding of their mechanisms of actions, potential side effects and limitations.

COUGH

There are two sorts of cough: the useful and the useless. Cough is useful when it effectively expels secretions or foreign objects from the respiratory tract, i.e. when it is *productive*; it is useless when it is unproductive and persistent. Useful cough should be allowed to serve its purpose and suppressed only when it is exhausting the patient or is dangerous, e.g. after eye surgery. Useless persistent cough should be stopped. Asthma, rhinosinusitis (causing postnasal drip) and oesophageal reflux are the commonest causes of persistent cough. Recently, *eosinophilic bronchitis* has been recognised as a possibly significant cause; it responds well to inhaled or oral corticosteroid. Clearly the overall approach to persistent cough must involve attention to underlying factors. The British Thoracic Society publishes guidelines on cough and its management that are available online.

Sites of action for treatment

Peripheral sites

On the *afferent* side of the cough reflex: by reducing input of stimuli from throat, larynx, trachea, a warm moist atmosphere has a demulcent effect on the pharynx.

On the *efferent* side of the cough reflex: measures to render secretions more easily removable (mucolytics, postural drainage) will reduce the amount of coughing needed, by increasing its efficiency.

The best antitussive of all is removal of the cause of the cough itself, i.e. treatment of underlying conditions (above). In patients with hypertension or cardiac failure, a common cause of a dry cough is treatment with an angiotensin-converting enzyme (ACE) inhibitor. This can be stopped by switching to an angiotensin II receptor blocker (ARB), e.g. losartan.

Central nervous system

Agents may act on the:

- medullary paths of the cough reflex (opioids)
- cerebral cortex
- subcortical paths (opioids and sedatives in general)

Cough is also under substantial voluntary control and can be inducible by psychogenic factors (e.g. the anxiety not to cough during the quiet parts of a musical concert) and reduced by a placebo. Considerations such as these are relevant to practical therapeutics.

Cough suppression

Antitussives that act peripherally

Smokers should stop smoking.

Cough originating above the larynx often benefits from syrups and lozenges that glutinously and soothingly coat the pharynx (demulcents), e.g. simple linctus (mainly sugar-based syrup). Small children are prone to swallow lozenges, so a sweet on a stick may be preferred.

Linctuses are demulcent preparations that can be used alone and as vehicles for other specific antitussive agents.

Cough originating below the larynx is often relieved by water aerosol inhalations and a warm environment – the archetypal 'steam' inhalation. Compound benzoin tincture may be used to give the inhalation a therapeutic smell (aromatic inhalation). This manoeuvre may have more than a placebo effect by promoting secretion of a dilute mucus that gives a protective coating to the inflamed mucous membrane. Menthol and eucalyptus are alternatives. The efficacy of menthol may be explained by the discovery that it can block the ion channel TRPV1, which is activated by capsaicin, the 'hot chilli' component of *Capsicum* species and a potent trigger for cough.

Local anaesthetics can also be used topically in the airways to block the mucosal cough receptors (modified stretch receptors and C-fibre endings) directly. Nebulised lidocaine, for example, reduces coughing during fibreoptic bronchoscopy and is also effective in the intractable cough that may accompany bronchial carcinoma.

Antitussives that act centrally

The most consistent means of suppressing cough irrespective of its cause is blockade of the *medullary cough centre* itself. *Opioids*, such as methadone and codeine, are very effective, although part of this antitussive effect could reflect their sedatory effect on higher nervous centres; nevertheless antitussive potency of an opiate is generally poorly correlated with its potency at causing respiratory depression.

As *dextromethorphan* (the d-isomer of the codeine analogue levorphanol) and *pholcodine* also have an antitussive effect that is not blocked by naloxone, non-μ-type opiate receptors are probably involved (and dubbed σ-type). It is not surprising, then, that these opiates also have no significant analgesic or respiratory-depressant effects at the doses required for their antitussive action.

Opioids are usually formulated as *linctuses* for antitussive use. Deciding on which agent to use depends largely on whether sedation and analgesia may be useful actions of the linctus. Hence methadone or diamorphine linctus may be preferred in patients with advanced bronchial carcinoma. In contrast, dextromethorphan, being non-sedating and non-addictive, is widely incorporated into over-the-counter linctuses.

Sedation generally reduces the sensitivity of the cough reflex. Hence older sedating antihistamines, e.g. diphenhydramine, can suppress cough by non-H_1-receptor actions; often the doses needed cause substantial drowsiness so that combination with other drugs, such as pholcodine and dextromethorphan, is common in over-the-counter cough remedies.

Mucolytics and expectorants

Normally about 100 mL fluid is produced from the respiratory tract each day and most of it is swallowed. Respiratory mucus consists largely of water and its slimy character is due to glycoproteins cross-linked together by disulphide bonds. In pathological states much more mucus may be produced; an exudate of plasma proteins that bond with glycoproteins and form larger polymers results in the mucus becoming more viscous. Patients with chest diseases such as cystic fibrosis (CF) and bronchiectasis have difficulty in clearing their chest of viscous sputum by cough because the bronchial cilia are rendered ineffective. Drugs that liquefy mucus can provide benefit.

Mucolytics

Carbocisteine and *mecysteine* have free sulphydryl groups that open disulphide bonds in mucus and reduce its viscosity. They are given orally or by inhalation (or instillation) and may be useful chiefly where particularly viscous secretion is a problem (cystic fibrosis, care of tracheostomies). Mucolytics may cause gastrointestinal irritation and allergic reaction.

Water inhalation via an aerosol (breathing over a hot basin) is a cheap and effective expectorant therapy in bronchiectasis. Simply hydrating a dehydrated patient can also have a beneficial effect in lowering sputum viscosity.

Dornase α is phosphorylated glycosylated recombinant human deoxyribonuclease. It is given daily by inhalation of a nebulised solution containing 2 500 units (2.5 mg). It is of modest value only in patients with cystic fibrosis, whose genetic defect in chloride transport causes particularly viscous sputum. The blocked airways, as well as the sputum itself, are a trap for pathogens, and the lysis of invading neutrophils leads to substantial levels of free and very viscous DNA within the CF airways.

Expectorants

These are said to encourage productive cough by increasing the volume of bronchial secretion; there is little clinical evidence to support this, and they may be of no more value than placebo. The group includes squill, guaiphenesin, ipecacuanha, creosotes and volatile oils.

Cough mixtures

Every formulary is replete with combinations of antitussives, expectorants, mucolytics, bronchodilators and sedatives. Although choice is not critical, knowledge of the active ingredients is important, as some contain sedative antimuscarinic antihistamines or phenylpropanolamines (which may antagonise antihypertensives). Use of glycerol or syrup as a demulcent cough preparation, or of simple linctus (citric acid), is probably defensible.

Choice of drug therapy for cough

As always, it is necessary to have a clear idea of the underlying problem before starting any therapy. For example, the approach to cough due to invasion of a bronchus by a neoplasm differs from that due to postnasal drip from chronic sinusitis or to that due to chronic bronchitis. The following are general recommendations.

Simple suppression of useless cough

Codeine, pholcodine, dextromethorphan and methadone linctuses can be used in large, infrequent doses. In children, cough is nearly always useful and sedation at night is more effective to give rest. A sedative antihistamine is convenient (e.g. promethazine), although sputum thickening may be a disadvantage. In pertussis infection (whooping cough), codeine and atropine methonitrate may be tried.

To increase bronchial secretion slightly and to liquefy what is there

Water aerosol with or without menthol and benzoin inhalation, or menthol and eucalyptus inhalation may provide comfort harmlessly.

Carbocysteine or another mucolytic orally may occasionally be useful.

Preparations containing any drug with antimuscarinic action are undesirable because this thickens bronchial secretion. Oxygen inhalation dries secretions, so rendering them even more viscous; oxygen must be bubbled through water, and patients having oxygen may need measures to liquefy sputum.

Cough originating in the pharyngeal region

Glutinous sweets or lozenges (demulcents), incorporating a cough suppressant or not, as appropriate, are used.

RESPIRATORY STIMULANTS

The drugs used (analeptics) are central nervous system (CNS) stimulants capable of causing convulsions in doses just above those used therapeutically. Hence, their use must be monitored carefully.

Doxapram increases the rate and depth of respiration by stimulating the medullary respiratory centres both directly and reflexly through the carotid body. A continuous i.v. infusion of 1.5–4.0 mg/min is given according to the patient's response. Coughing and laryngospasm that develop after its use may represent a return of normal protective responses. Doxapram is also an effective inhibitor of shivering following general anaesthesia.

Adverse effects include restlessness, twitching, itching, vomiting, flushing, bronchospasm and cardiac arrhythmias, and in addition doxapram causes patients to experience a feeling of perineal warmth; in high doses it raises blood pressure.

Aminophylline (a complex of theophylline and EDTA) in addition to its other actions is a respiratory stimulant and may be infused slowly i.v. (500 mg in 6 h).

Uses

Respiratory stimulants have a considerably reduced role in the management of acute ventilatory failure, following the increased use of non-invasive nasal positive-pressure ventilation for respiratory failure. Situations where they may still be encountered are:

- Acute exacerbations of chronic lung disease with *hypercapnia*, drowsiness and inability to cough or to tolerate low (24%) concentrations of inspired oxygen (air is 21 % oxygen). A respiratory stimulant can arouse the patient sufficiently to allow effective physiotherapy and, by stimulating respiration, can improve ventilation–perfusion matching. As a short-term measure, this may be used in conjunction with assisted ventilation without tracheal intubation (BIPAP), and thereby 'buy time' for chemotherapy to control infection and avoid full tracheal intubation and mechanical ventilation.
- *Apnoea* in premature infants; aminophylline and caffeine may benefit some cases.
- The manufacturer's data sheet suggests the use of doxapram for buprenorphine overdoses where the respiratory depression is not responsive to naloxone.

Avoid respiratory stimulants in patients with epilepsy (risk of convulsions). Other relative contraindications include ischaemic heart disease, acute severe asthma ('status asthmaticus'), severe hypertension and thyrotoxicosis.

Irritant vapours, to be inhaled, have an analeptic effect in fainting, especially if it is psychogenic, e.g. aromatic solution of ammonia (Sal Volatile). No doubt they sometimes 'recall the exorbitant and deserting spirits to their proper stations'.

PULMONARY SURFACTANT

The endogenous surfactant system produces stable low surface tension in the alveoli, preventing their collapse. Failure of production of natural surfactant occurs in respiratory distress syndrome (RDS), including that in the neonate. Synthetic phospholipids are now available for intratracheal instillation to act as surfactants: *colfosceril palmitate, poractant-α* and *beractant*. These need to be stored chilled, and the manufacturers' instructions followed carefully, because on reaching body temperature their physicochemical properties change rapidly. Their function is to coat the surface of the alveoli and maintain their patency, and their administration to premature neonates with RDS is a key part in reducing mortality and long-term complications in this condition.

OXYGEN THERAPY

Oxygen used in therapy should be prescribed with the same care as any drug, including its specific inclusion on the patient's drug chart; there should be a well-defined purpose and its effects should be monitored objectively.

The absolute indication to supplement inspired air is *inadequate tissue oxygenation*. As clinical signs may be imprecise, arterial blood gases should be measured whenever suspicion arises. An elevated serum lactate is also a useful marker. Nevertheless, tissue hypoxia should be assumed when the PaO_2 falls below 6.7 kPa (50 mmHg) in a previously normal acutely ill patient, e.g. with myocardial infarction, acute pulmonary disorder, drug overdose, musculoskeletal or head trauma. Chronically hypoxic patients may maintain adequate tissue oxygenation with a PaO_2 below 6.7 kPa by compensatory adaptations, including an increased red cell mass and altered haemoglobin–oxygen binding characteristics. Oxygen therapy is used as follows:

- *High-concentration* oxygen therapy is reserved for a state of low PaO_2 in association with *normal* or *low* $PaCO_2$ (*type I respiratory failure*), as in: pulmonary embolism, pneumonia, pulmonary oedema, myocardial infarction and young patients with acute severe asthma. Concentrations of oxygen up to 100% may be used for short periods, as there is little risk of inducing hypoventilation and carbon dioxide retention.

- *Low-concentration* oxygen therapy is reserved for a state of low PaO_2 in association with a *raised* $PaCO_2$ (*type II failure*), typically seen during exacerbations of chronic obstructive pulmonary disease. The normal stimulus to respiration is an increase in $PaCO_2$, but this control is blunted in chronically hypercapnic patients whose respiratory drive comes from *hypoxia*. Increasing the PaO_2 in such patients by giving them high concentrations of oxygen removes their stimulus to ventilate, exaggerates carbon dioxide retention and may cause fatal respiratory acidosis. The objective of therapy in such patients is to provide just enough oxygen to alleviate hypoxia without exaggerating the hypercapnia and respiratory acidosis; normally the inspired oxygen concentration should not exceed 28%, and in some 24% may be sufficient.

- *Continuous long-term domiciliary oxygen therapy* (LTOT) is given to patients with severe persistent hypoxaemia and cor pulmonale due to chronic obstructive pulmonary disease. Patients are provided with an oxygen concentrator. Clinical trial evidence indicates that taking oxygen for more than 15 h per day improves survival.

HISTAMINE, ANTIHISTAMINES AND ALLERGIES

Histamine is a naturally occurring amine that has long fascinated pharmacologists and physicians. It is found in most tissues in an inactive bound form, and pharmacologically active free histamine, released in response to stimuli such as physical trauma or immunoglobulin (Ig) E-mediated activation, is an important component of the acute inflammatory response.

The physiological functions of histamine are suggested by its *distribution in the body*, in:

- *body epithelia* (the gut, the respiratory tract and in the skin), where it is released in response to invasion by foreign substances
- *glands* (gastric, intestinal, lachrymal, salivary), where it mediates part of the normal secretory process
- *mast cells* near blood vessels, where it plays a role in regulating the microcirculation.

Actions. Histamine acts as a local hormone (autacoid) similarly to serotonin or prostaglandins, i.e. it functions within the immediate vicinity of its site of release. With gastric secretion, for example, stimulation of receptors on the histamine-containing cell causes release of histamine, which in turn acts on receptors on parietal cells which then secrete hydrogen ions. The actions of histamine that are clinically important are those on:

Smooth muscle. In general, histamine causes smooth muscle to contract (excepting arterioles, but including the larger arteries). Stimulation of the pregnant human uterus is insignificant. A brisk attack of bronchospasm may be induced in subjects who have any allergy, particularly asthma.

Blood vessels. Arterioles are dilated, with a consequent fall in blood pressure. This action is due partly to nitric oxide release from the vascular endothelium of the arterioles in response to histamine receptor activation. Capillary *permeability* also increases, especially at postcapillary venules, causing oedema. These effects on arterioles and capillaries represent the *flush* and the *wheal* components of the triple response described by Thomas Lewis. The third part, the *flare*, is arteriolar dilatation due to an axon reflex releasing neuropeptides from C-fibre endings.

Skin. Histamine release in the skin can cause itch.

Gastric secretion. Histamine increases the acid and pepsin content of gastric secretion.

As may be anticipated from the above actions, *anaphylactic shock*, which is due in large part to histamine release, is characterised by circulatory collapse and bronchoconstriction. The most rapidly effective antidote is adrenaline/epinephrine, and an antihistamine (H_1 receptor) may be given as well.

Various chemicals can cause release of histamine. The more powerful of these (proteolytic enzymes and snake venoms) have no place in therapeutics, but a number of useful drugs, such as D-tubocurarine and morphine, and even some antihistamines, cause histamine release. This *anaphylactoid* (i.e. IgE independent) effect is usually clinically mild with a transient reduction in blood pressure or a local skin reaction, but significant bronchospasm may occur in asthmatics.

Metabolism. Histamine is formed from the amino acid histidine and is inactivated largely by deamination and methylation. In common with other local hormones, this process is extremely rapid.

Histamine receptors. Histamine binds to H_1, H_2 and H_3 receptors, all of which are G-protein coupled. The H_1 receptor is largely responsible for mediating its pro-inflammatory effects, including the vasomotor changes, increased vascular permeability and up-regulation of adhesion molecules on vascular endothelium, i.e. it mediates the oedema and vascular effects of histamine. H_2 receptors mediate release of gastric acid. Blockade of histamine H_1 and H_2 receptors has substantial therapeutic utility.

H_3 receptors are expressed in a wide range of tissues including brain and nerve endings, and function as feedback inhibitors for histamine and other neurotransmitters. More recently identified is the H_4 receptor, which is involved in leucocyte chemotaxis.

Histamine antagonism and H_1- and H_2-receptor antagonists

The effects of histamine can be opposed in three ways:

- *By using a drug with opposing effects.* Histamine constricts bronchi, causes vasodilatation and

increases capillary permeability; adrenaline/epinephrine, by activating α- and $β_2$-adrenoceptors, produces opposite effects–referred to as *physiological antagonism*.

- *By blocking histamine binding* to its site of action (receptors), i.e. using competitive H_1-and H_2-receptor antagonists.
- *By preventing the release of histamine from storage cells.* Glucocorticoids and sodium cromoglicate can suppress IgE-induced release from mast cells; $β_2$ agonists have a similar effect.

Drugs that competitively block H_1-histamine receptors were the first to be introduced and are conventionally called the 'antihistamines'. They effectively inhibit the components of the triple response and partially prevent the hypotensive effect of histamine, but they have no effect on histamine-induced gastric secretion which is suppressed by blockade of histamine H_2 receptors. Thus, histamine antagonists are classified as:

- histamine H_1-receptor antagonists
- histamine H_2-receptor antagonists: cimetidine, famotidine, nizatidine, ranitidine

The selectivity implied by the term 'antihistamine' is unsatisfactory because the older first-generation antagonists show considerable blocking activity against muscarinic receptors, and often serotonin and α-adrenergic receptors as well. These features are a disadvantage when H_1 antihistamines are used specifically to antagonise the effects of histamine, e.g. for allergies. Hence the appearance of second-generation H_1 antagonists that are more selective for H_1 receptors and largely free of antimuscarinic and sedative effects has been an important advance. They can be discussed together.

Actions. H_1-receptor antihistamines oppose, to varying degrees, the effects of liberated histamine. They are generally competitive, surmountable inhibitors and strongly block all components of the triple response (a pure H_1-receptor effect), but only partially counteract the hypotensive effect of high-dose histamine (a mixed H_1- and H_2-receptor effect). H_1 antihistamines are of negligible use in asthma, in which non-histamine mediators, such as the cysteinyl-leukotrienes, are the predominant constrictors. They are more effective if used before histamine has been liberated, and reversal of effects of free histamine is more readily achieved by physiological antagonism with adrenaline/epinephrine, which is used first in life-threatening allergic reactions.

The older *first-generation* H$_1$ antihistamines cause drowsiness and patients should be warned of this, e.g. about driving or operating machinery, and about additive effects with alcohol. Paradoxically, they can increase seizure activity in epileptics, especially children, and can cause seizures in non-epileptic subjects if taken in overdose. The newer *second-generation* H$_1$ antihistamines penetrate the blood–brain barrier less readily and are largely devoid of such central effects. Antimuscarinic effects of first-generation H$_1$ antihistamines are sometimes put to therapeutic advantage in parkinsonism and motion sickness.

Pharmacokinetics. H$_1$ antihistamines taken orally are readily absorbed. They are metabolised mainly in the liver. Excretion in the breast milk may be sufficient to cause sedation in infants. They are generally administered orally and can also be given intramuscularly or intravenously.

Uses. The H$_1$ antihistamines are used for symptomatic relief of allergies such as hay fever and urticaria. They are of broadly similar therapeutic efficacy.

Individual H$_1$-receptor antihistamines

Non-sedative second-generation drugs

These newer drugs are relatively selective for H$_1$ receptors, enter the brain less readily than do the earlier antihistamines, and lack the unwanted antimuscarinic effects. Differences lie principally in their duration of action.

Cetirizine ($t_{1/2}$ 7 h), *loratadine* ($t_{1/2}$ 15 h) and *terfenadine* ($t_{1/2}$ 20 h) are effective taken once daily and are suitable for general use. *Acrivastine* ($t_{1/2}$ 2 h) is so short acting that it is best reserved for intermittent therapy, e.g. when breakthrough symptoms occur in a patient using topical therapy for hay fever. Other non-sedating antihistamines are desloratadine, fexofenadine, levocetirizine and mizolastine.

Adverse effects. The second-generation antihistamines are well tolerated but an important adverse effect occurs with terfenadine. This drug can prolong the QTc interval on the surface ECG by blocking a potassium channel in the heart (the rapid component of delayed rectifier potassium current, I$_{Kr}$), which triggers a characteristic ventricular tachycardia (torsade de pointes) and probably explains the sudden deaths reported during early use of terfenadine (and prompted its withdrawal from North American markets). It is associated with either high doses of terfenadine or inhibition of its metabolism. Terfenadine depends solely on the 3A4 isoform of cytochrome P450, and inhibiting drugs include erythromycin, ketoconazole and even grapefruit juice. Fexofenadine, the active metabolite, has a much lower affinity for the I$_{Kr}$ channel and does not cause QTc prolongation.

Sedative first-generation agents

Chlorphenamine ($t_{1/2}$ 20 h) is effective when urticaria is prominent, and its sedative effect is then useful.

Diphenhydramine ($t_{1/2}$ 32 h) is strongly sedative and has antimuscarinic effects; it is also used in parkinsonism and motion sickness.

Promethazine ($t_{1/2}$ 12 h) is so strongly sedative that it is used as a hypnotic in adults and children.

Alimemazine, azatadine, brompheniramine, clemastine, cyproheptadine, diphenylpyraline, doxylamine, hydroxyzine and *triprolidine* are similar.

Adverse effects. Apart from sedation, these include: dizziness, fatigue, insomnia, nervousness, tremors and antimuscarinic effects, e.g. dry mouth, blurred vision and gastrointestinal disturbance. Dermatitis and agranulocytosis can occur. Severe poisoning due to overdose results in coma and sometimes in convulsions.

Drug management of some allergic states

Histamine is released in many allergic states, but it is not the sole cause of symptoms, other chemical mediators, e.g. leukotrienes and prostaglandins, also being involved. Hence the usefulness of H$_1$-receptor antihistamines in allergic states is variable, depending on the extent to which histamine, rather than other mediators, is the cause of the clinical manifestations.

Note also that H_2-receptor antagonists (separate from their role in reducing gastric acid secretion) can be used to reduce the effects of a type I hypersensitivity response, e.g. rhinitis, urticaria and conjunctivitis.

Hay fever. If symptoms are limited to rhinitis, a glucocorticoid (beclometasone, betamethasone, budesonide, flunisolide or triamcinolone), ipratropium or sodium cromoglicate applied topically as a spray or insufflation is often all that is required. Ocular symptoms alone respond well to sodium cromoglicate drops. When both nasal and ocular symptoms occur, or there is itching of the palate and ears as well, a systemic non-sedative H_1-receptor antihistamine is indicated. Sympathomimetic vasoconstrictors, e.g. ephedrine, are immediately effective when applied topically, but rebound swelling of the nasal mucous membrane occurs when medication is stopped. Rarely, a systemic glucocorticoid, e.g. prednisolone, is justified for a severely affected patient to provide relief for a short period, e.g. during academic examinations.

Hyposensitisation, by subcutaneous injection of graded and increasing amounts of grass and tree pollen extracts, is an option for seasonal allergic hay fever due to pollens (which has not responded to antiallergy drugs), and of bee and wasp allergen extracts for people who exhibit allergy to these venoms (exposure to which can be life-threatening). If hyposensitisation is undertaken, facilities for immediate cardiopulmonary resuscitation must be available because of the risk of anaphylaxis. A sublingual tablet containing a very low dose grass pollen extract (Grazax) is also now available to effect similar desensitisation. It has to be taken daily before and throughout the grass pollen season but does not cause anaphylaxis. Another strategy for subjects with very severe atopic and extrinsic asthma is to use a monocloncal antibody against IgE (omalizumab), which causes a rapid, dose-related and sustained fall in plasma IgE concentrations. The antibody is designed to bind to the part of the IgE molecule that interacts with the high-affinity IgE receptor (FcRI) on mast cells and basophils, thus preventing the activation of these cells by cross-linking of bound IgE.

BRONCHIAL ASTHMA

Asthma affects 10%–15% of the UK population; this figure is increasing.

Some pathophysiology

The bronchi become hyperreactive as a result of a persistent *inflammatory* process in response to a number of stimuli that include biological agents, e.g. allergens, viruses, and environmental chemicals such as ozone and glutaraldehyde. Inflammatory mediators are liberated from mast cells, eosinophils, neutrophils, monocytes and macrophages. Some mediators such as histamine are preformed and their release causes an immediate bronchial reaction. Others are formed after activation of cells and produce more sustained bronchoconstriction; these include metabolites of arachidonic acid from both the cyclo-oxygenase, e.g. prostaglandin D_2 and lipo-oxygenase, e.g. cysteinyl-leukotrienes C_4 and D_4, pathways. In addition platelet activating factor (PAF) is being recognised increasingly as an important mediator.

The relative importance of many of the mediators is not defined precisely but they interact to produce mucosal oedema, mucus secretion and damage to the ciliated epithelium. Breaching of the protective epithelial barrier allows hyperreactivity to be maintained by bronchoconstrictor substances or by local axon reflexes through exposed nerve fibres. Wheezing and breathlessness result. The bronchial changes also obstruct access of inhaled drug to the periphery, which is why they can fail to give full relief.

Asthma, like many of the common chronic disorders (hypertension, diabetes mellitus), is a polygenic disorder, and already genetic loci linked to either increased production of IgE or bronchial hyperreactivity have been reported in some families with an increased incidence of asthma.

Early in an attack there is hyperventilation so that Pao_2 is maintained and $Paco_2$ is lowered, but with increasing airways obstruction the Pao_2 declines and $Paco_2$ rises, signifying a serious asthmatic episode.

Types of asthma

Asthma associated with specific allergic reactions

This *extrinsic* type is the commonest and occurs in patients who develop allergy to inhaled antigenic substances. They are also frequently atopic, showing positive responses to skin prick testing with the same antigens. The hypersensitivity reaction in the lung (and skin) is of the immediate type (type I) involving IgE-mediated mast cell activation. Allergen avoidance is particularly relevant to managing this type of asthma.

Asthma not associated with known allergy

Some patients exhibit wheeze and breathlessness in the absence of an obvious allergen or atopy. They are considered to have *intrinsic* asthma and, because of a lack of an identifiable allergen, allergen avoidance has no place in their management.

Exercise-induced asthma

Some patients develop wheeze that regularly follows within a few minutes of exercise. A similar response occurs following the inhalation of cold air, as the common mechanism appears to be airway drying. Inhalation of a β_2-adrenoceptor agonist, sodium cromoglicate or one of the newer leukotriene receptor antagonists prior to either challenge prevents bronchoconstriction.

Asthma associated with chronic obstructive pulmonary disease

A number of patients with persistent airflow obstruction exhibit substantial variation in airways resistance and in the extent to which they benefit from bronchodilator drugs. It is important to recognise that asthma may coexist with chronic obstructive pulmonary disease, and to assess their responses to bronchodilators or glucocorticoids over a period of time (as formal tests of respiratory function may not reliably predict clinical response in this setting).

Approaches to treatment

With the foregoing discussion in mind, the following approaches to treatment are logical:

- Prevention of exposure to allergen(s).
- Reduction of the bronchial inflammation and hyperreactivity.
- Dilatation of narrowed bronchi.

These objectives may be achieved as follows:

Prevention of exposure to allergen(s)

This approach is appropriate for extrinsic asthmatics. Identification of an allergen may be aided by the patient's history (wheezing in response to contact with grasses, pollens, animals), by intradermal skin prick injection of selected allergen or by demonstrating specific IgE antibodies in the patient's serum, i.e. the RAST test (RadioAllergoSorbent Test). Avoiding an allergen may be feasible when it is related to some specific situation, e.g. occupation, but is less feasible if it is widespread, as with house-dust mite.

Reduction of the bronchial inflammation and hyperreactivity

As persistent inflammation is central to bronchial hyperreactivity, the use of anti-inflammatory drugs is logical.

Glucocorticoids bring about a gradual reduction in bronchial hyperreactivity. They are the mainstay of asthma treatment. The exact mechanisms are still disputed but probably include: inhibition of the influx of inflammatory cells into the lung after allergen exposure; inhibition of the release of mediators from macrophages and eosinophils; and reduction of the microvascular leakage that these mediators cause. Glucocorticoids used in asthma include prednisolone (orally), and beclometasone, fluticasone and budesonide (by inhalation).

Sodium cromoglicate (cromolyn, Intal) impairs the immediate response to allergen and was formerly thought to act by inhibiting the release of mediators from mast cells. Evidence now suggests that the late allergic response and bronchial hyperreactivity are also inhibited, and points to effects of cromoglicate on other inflammatory cells and also on local axon reflexes. Cromoglicate is poorly absorbed from the gastrointestinal tract but well absorbed from the lung, and it is given by inhalation (as powder, aerosol or nebuliser); it is eliminated unchanged in the urine and bile.

As it does not antagonise the bronchoconstrictor effect of the mediators after they have been released, cromoglicate is not effective at terminating an existing attack, i.e. it *prevents* bronchoconstriction rather than inducing bronchodilation. Special formulations are used for *allergic rhinitis* and *allergic conjunctivitis*.

Sodium cromoglicate is effective in extrinsic (allergic) asthma, including asthma in children and exercise-induced asthma, but its use has declined since the efficacy and safety of low-dose inhaled corticosteroid have become apparent.

It is remarkably non-toxic. Apart from cough and bronchospasm induced by the powder it may rarely cause allergic reactions. Application to the eye may produce a local stinging sensation and the oral form may cause nausea.

Nedocromil sodium (Tilade) is structurally unrelated to cromoglicate but has a similar profile of actions and can be used by metered aerosol in place of cromoglicate.

Other drugs. Ketotifen is a histamine H_1-receptor blocker that may also have some anti-asthma effects but its benefit has not been demonstrated conclusively. In common with other antihistamines it causes drowsiness.

Dilatation of narrowed bronchi

This is achieved most effectively by *physiological antagonism* of bronchial muscle contraction, namely by stimulation of adrenergic bronchodilator mechanisms. Pharmacological antagonism of specific bronchoconstrictors is less effective, either because individual mediators are not on their own responsible for a large part of the bronchoconstriction (acetylcholine, adenosine, leukotrienes) or because the mediator is not even secreted during asthma attacks (histamine).

β_2-Adrenoceptor agonists. The predominant adrenoceptors in bronchi are of the β_2 type and their stimulation causes bronchial muscle to relax. β_2-Adrenoceptor activation also stabilises mast cells. Agonists in widespread use include salbutamol, terbutaline, fenoterol, eformoterol and salmeterol. Salmeterol is longer acting because its lipophilic side-chain anchors the drug in the membrane adjacent to the receptor, slowing tissue washout.

Less selective adrenoceptor agonists such as adrenaline/epinephrine, ephedrine, isoetharine, isoprenaline and orciprenaline are less safe, being more likely to cause cardiac arrhythmias. α-Adrenoceptor activity contributes to bronchoconstriction, but α-adrenoceptor antagonists have not proved effective in practice.

Theophylline, a methylxanthine, relaxes bronchial muscle, although its precise mode of action is still debated. Inhibition of phosphodiesterase (PDE), especially its type 4 isoform, now seems the most likely explanation for its bronchodilating and more recently reported anti-inflammatory effects. Blockade of adenosine receptors is probably unimportant. Other actions of theophylline include chronotropic and inotropic effects on the heart and a direct effect on the rate of urine production (diuresis).

Absorption of theophylline from the gastrointestinal tract is usually rapid and complete. Some 90% is metabolised by the liver and there is evidence that the process is saturable at therapeutic doses. The $t_{\frac{1}{2}}$ is 8 h, with substantial variation. It is prolonged in patients with severe cardiopulmonary disease and cirrhosis; obesity and prematurity are associated with reduced rates of elimination; tobacco smoking enhances theophylline clearance by inducing hepatic P450 enzymes. These pharmacokinetic factors and the low therapeutic index render necessary the therapeutic monitoring of the plasma theophylline to achieve the best outcome; the desired concentration range is 10–20 mg/L (55–110 micromol/L).

Theophylline is relatively insoluble and is formulated either as a salt with choline (choline theophyllinate) or complexed with EDTA (aminophylline). *Aminophylline* is sufficiently soluble to permit intravenous use of theophylline in acute severe asthma (status asthmaticus). Rapid intravenous injection will induce unwanted effects (below) by exposing the heart and brain to high concentrations before distribution is complete. Intravenous injection must be slow (a loading dose of 5 mg/kg over 20 min followed by an infusion of 0.9 mg/kg·h, adjusted according to subsequent plasma theophylline concentrations). The loading dose should be avoided in any patient who is already taking a methylxanthine preparation (always enquire about this before injecting the loading dose!).

There are numerous sustained-release oral forms for use in chronic asthma, but because they are not bio-equivalent patients should not switch between them once they are stabilised on a particular preparation.

Adverse effects. At high therapeutic doses some patients experience nausea and diarrhoea, and plasma concentrations above the recommended range risk cardiac arrhythmia and seizures. Enzyme inhibition by erythromycin, ciprofloxacin, allopurinol or oral contraceptives increases the plasma concentration of theophylline; enzyme inducers such as carbamazepine, phenytoin and rifampicin reduce the concentration.

Overdose with theophylline has assumed greater importance with the advent of sustained-release preparations that prolong toxic effects, with peak plasma concentrations being reached 12–24 h after ingestion. Vomiting may be severe but the chief dangers are cardiac arrhythmia, hypotension, hypokalaemia and seizures. Activated charcoal should be given every 2–4 h until the plasma concentration is below 20 mg/L. Potassium replacement is important to prevent arrhythmias, and a benzodiazepine (e.g. diazepam) is used to control convulsions.

Antimuscarinic bronchodilators. Release of acetylcholine from vagal nerve endings in the airways activates muscarinic (M_3) receptors on bronchial smooth muscle causing bronchoconstriction. Blockade of these receptors with atropine causes

bronchodilatation, although the preferred antimuscarinics in clinical practice are inhaled ipratropium, oxitropium or the long-acting tiotropium (its effects last for up to 24 h). These synthetic compounds, unlike atropine, are permanently charged molecules that resist significant absorption after inhalation and thus minimise antimuscarinic effects outside of the lung. They are used mostly in older patients with chronic obstructive pulmonary disease, but are useful in acute severe asthma when combined with β_2-adrenoceptor agonists. Vagally mediated bronchoconstriction appears to be important in acute asthma, but relatively unimportant for most chronic stable asthmatics.

Leukotriene receptor antagonists, e.g. montelukast and zafirlukast, competitively prevent the bronchoconstrictor effects of cysteinyl-leukotrienes (C_4, D_4 and E_4) by blocking their common cysLT1 receptor. They have similar efficacy to low-dose inhaled glucocorticoid. The scarcity of comparisons with established medications consigns them to a second- or third-line role in treatment. They could be substituted at Step 2 or later stages of the current five-step regimen for asthma (Fig. 17.1). There are no studies to justify their use as steroid-sparing (far less, replacement) therapy. When used occasionally in this way in patients unwilling or unable to use metered-dose inhalers, serial monitoring of spirometry is essential.

Fig. 17.1 A five-step management scheme for chronic asthma. β_2, β_2-Adrenoceptor agonist; GCC, glucocorticoid, e.g. beclometasone, budesonide or fluticasone.

Montelukast is given once per day and zafirlukast twice daily. Leukotriene receptor antagonists are generally well tolerated, although Churg–Strauss syndrome has been reported rarely with their use. This probably represents unmasking of the disease as glucocorticoids are withdrawn following addition of the leukotriene receptor antagonist. Alerting features to this development are vasculitic rash, eosinophilia, worsening respiratory symptoms, cardiac complications and peripheral neuropathy.

Drug therapy by inhalation

The inhaled route has been developed to advantage because the undesirable effects of systemic exposure to drugs, especially glucocorticoids, are substantially reduced. The pharmacokinetic advantages of using the inhaled versus the oral route are apparent from the substantially reduced dose requirement: salbutamol 100 micrograms from an aerosol inhaler will provide bronchodilatation similar to 2 000 micrograms by mouth.

Before a drug can be inhaled, it must first be converted into particulate form; the optimum particle size to reach and be deposited in the small bronchi is around 2 μm. Such particles are delivered to the lung as an aerosol, i.e. dispersed in a gas, which can be produced in a number of different ways:

Pressurised aerosol. Drug is dissolved in a low boiling point liquid in a canister under pressure. Opening the valve releases a metered dose of liquid that is ejected into the atmosphere; the carrier liquid evaporates instantly, leaving an aerosol of the drug that is inhaled. Until recently the vehicle has been a CFC (chlorofluorocarbon), but due to concerns over depletion of atmospheric ozone these are being replaced by hydrofluoroalkanes (HFAs), which are ozone friendly. This switch has introduced a noticeable change in the taste of some inhalers, but more importantly it has changed the bio-equivalence of inhaled glucocorticoids. HFA-based glucocorticoid inhalers are generally more potent than a CFC-based inhaler delivering the same dose at the lips (typically the efficacy is doubled).

To ensure optimal drug delivery, it is necessary to coordinate activation of the inhaler with inspiration and a final hold of breath. Many patients, especially the young and the elderly, find this very difficult and 'spacer' devices are often used between the inhaler and lips; these act as an aerosol reservoir and also reduce impaction of aerosol in the oropharynx. Topical deposition can cause local side-effects in the mouth, particularly candida with inhaled glucocorticoids; a spacer abolishes this problem.

Nebulisers convert a solution or suspension of drug into an aerosol. Jet nebulisers require a driving gas, usually air from a compressor unit for home use, or oxygen in hospital; the solution in the nebulising chamber is broken into droplets by the jet and the larger droplets are filtered off leaving the smaller ones to be inhaled. Ultrasonic nebulisers convert a solution into particles of uniform size by vibrations created by a piezoelectric crystal (which converts electricity into mechanical vibration). With either method the aerosol is delivered to the patient by a mouthpiece or facemask, so no coordination is called for, and the dose can be altered by changing the strength of the solution. Much larger doses can be administered by nebuliser than by pressurised aerosol.

Dry powder inhalers. The drug is formulated as a micronised powder and placed in a device, e.g. a spinhaler or diskhaler, from which it is inhaled. Patients can often use these when they fail with metered-dose aerosols. Inhalation of powder occasionally causes transient bronchoconstriction.

Drug treatment

This varies with the severity and type of asthma. It is a general rule that the effectiveness of changes in drug and dose should be monitored by serial measurements of the simple respiratory function tests such as peak expiratory flow rate (PEFR) or forced expiratory volume in 1 s (FEV_1). Neither the patient's feelings nor physical examination are alone sufficient to determine whether there is still room for improvement. When an asthmatic attack is severe, arterial blood gases must also be measured.

Constant and intermittent asthma

The 2008 British Thoracic Society guidelines recommend a five-step approach (summarised in Fig. 17.1) to the drug management of chronic asthma. The scheme starts with a patient requiring occasional β_2-adrenoceptor agonist and follows an escalating plan of add-on anti-inflammatory treatment. Points to emphasise are:

1. Short-acting β_2-adrenoceptor agonists are used throughout as rescue therapy for acute symptoms.
2. Patients must be reviewed regularly as they can move up or down the scheme.
3. Particular attention should be paid to inhaler technique, as this is an important cause of treatment failure. Patients who cannot manage inhaled therapy, even with the addition of a spacer device or use of a dry-powder device, can be given oral therapy, although this will be accompanied by more systemic side-effects.

An inhaled β_2-adrenoceptor agonist should be used initially. Salbutamol or terbutaline (1–2 puffs up to four times daily) are typical short-acting β_2-adrenoceptor agonists whose bronchodilator effect is prompt in onset (within a few minutes) and lasts 4–6 h. Salmeterol and formoterol have a much longer duration of effect (12–24 h), making them useful for nocturnal symptoms; they should not be used as 'rescue' bronchodilator (salmeterol in particular, because its bronchodilating action takes 15–30 min to emerge) nor as a replacement for inhaled glucocorticoid. β_2-Adrenoceptor agonists all cause dose-dependent tremor, especially if given orally rather than inhaled.

Anti-inflammatory agents can commence either with sodium cromoglicate or low-dose inhaled glucocorticoid (Step 2). The inhaled glucocorticoids in current use (beclometasone, budesonide and fluticasone) are characterised by low oral bio-availability because of high first-pass metabolism in the liver (almost 100% for fluticasone). This property is important, as it minimises the systemic effects of inhaled glucocorticoid, 80%–90% of which is actually swallowed. Precisely for this reason, prednisolone or hydrocortisone would have less advantage (over oral administration) if inhaled, because they are absorbed from the gut and enter the circulation with relatively little pre-systemic metabolism. Inhaled glucocorticoids also exhibit higher lipid solubility and potency than those usually administered orally. Potency (the physical mass of drug in relation to its effect) is generally unimportant in comparisons of oral drugs, but is essential for locally administered drugs.

Inhaled glucocorticoids are generally safe at low doses. Topical effects (oral candida and hoarseness) are eliminated by using a spacer device and rinsing the mouth. High doses (> 2 000 micrograms/day) are reported to carry a slightly increased risk of cataract and glaucoma; this may reflect local aerosol deposition rather than a true systemic effect. Bone turnover is also increased in adults, suggesting a long-term risk of accelerated osteoporosis, and bone growth may be reduced in children (although evidence indicates that normal adult height can be attained). Therefore, it is important that patients are maintained on the minimum dose of inhaled glucocorticoid necessary for symptom control.

Oral prednisolone is very effective for severe exacerbations and short courses (e.g. 30 mg daily for 5–7 days) are frequently given. Provided symptoms and peak flows respond promptly, more prolonged courses or prolonged reduction of dose are unnecessary. When oral glucocorticoids are used long term (Step 5), doses should be adjusted much more slowly. Adverse corticosteroid effects may also be minimised by administering a single morning dose to coincide with the normal peak cortisol concentration (and thus the least suppression of feedback to the hypothalamic–adrenal axis). This is possible because of the long duration of their biological effect (18–36 h) compared with plasma $t_{1/2}$ (3 h for prednisolone). Morning dosing with inhaled glucocorticoid may also have a prednisolone-sparing effect. Some patients may get further prednisolone-sparing by addition of nebulised high-dose budesonide, 1–2 mg twice daily or fluticasone 500 micrograms twice daily.

Chest infections in asthma

Antimicrobials are over-prescribed for exacerbations of asthma. Respiratory tract infections do cause increased airflow obstruction and bronchial hyperresponsiveness, but viral not bacterial pathogens are the commonest culprits. Antimicrobials should be prescribed only if there is high suspicion of a bacterial respiratory tract infection, e.g. purulent sputum. Note that macrolide antibiotics, such as erythromycin and clarithromycin, interfere with theophylline metabolism.

Acute severe asthma ('status asthmaticus')

This is a life-threatening emergency requiring rapid aggressive treatment. The airways may become refractory to β_2-adrenoceptor agonists after 36–48 h, partly for pharmacological reasons (possibly receptor desensitisation) and partly due to the prolonged respiratory acidosis. The mucous plugs, which are the hallmark of the condition, may also prevent inhaled drugs from reaching the distal airways.

The following lists, with some explanation, the recommendations of the British Thoracic Society for managing acute severe asthma:

Immediate treatment

- *Oxygen* by mask (humidified, to help liquefy mucus). Carbon dioxide narcosis is rare in asthma and 60% can be used if the diagnosis is not in doubt. In older patients, or when there is any concern about chronic carbon dioxide retention, start with 28% oxygen and check that the Paco$_2$ has not risen before delivering 35% oxygen.
- *Salbutamol* by nebuliser in a dose of 2.5–5 mg over about 3 min, repeated in 15 min. Terbutaline 5–10 mg is an alternative.
- *Prednisolone* 30–60 mg by mouth or hydrocortisone 100 mg i.v.
- *Avoid sedation* of any kind.
- Chest radiography is required to exclude pneumothorax.

If life-threatening features are present (absent breath sounds, cyanosis, bradycardia, exhausted appearance, PEFR < 33% predicted or best, arterial oxygen saturation of < 92%):

- Ipratropium 0.5 mg should be added to the nebulised β_2 agonist.
- Consider i.v. magnesium sulphate (1.2–2 g over 20 min).

- Alert the intensive care unit.

Subsequent management. If the patient is improving, continue:

- 40%–60% oxygen.
- Prednisolone 30–60 mg daily or hydrocortisone 100–200 mg 6-hourly.
- Nebulised salbutamol or terbutaline 4-hourly.

If the patient is *not improving* after 15–30 min:

- Continue oxygen and glucocorticoid.
- Give *nebulised* β_2-adrenoceptor agonist more frequently, e.g. salbutamol up to 10 mg/h.
- Add ipratropium 0.5 mg to nebuliser and repeat 6-hourly until patient is improving.

If the patient is *still not improving*:

- Consider intravenous infusion of aminophylline (0.9 micrograms/kg·min) or
- Consider as an alternative *intravenous* β_2-adrenoceptor agonist (as above), e.g. salbutamol 250 micrograms over 10 min, then up to 20 micrograms/min as an infusion (as nebulised salbutamol may not be reaching the distal airways).
- Contact the intensive care unit to discuss intubation and mechanical ventilation.

Monitoring response to treatment

- By peak expiratory flow rate (PEFR) every 15–30 min.
- Oxygen saturation: maintain > 92%. Repeat blood gas measurements if initial Pao$_2$ < 8 kPa (60 mmHg) and/or initial Paco$_2$ is normal or raised (the tachypnoea is expected to reduce Paco$_2$ in most patients).

Treatment in intensive care unit. Transfer (accompanied by doctor with facilities for intubation) is required if:

- any of the above deteriorates, despite maximal treatment
- the patient becomes exhausted, drowsy, or confused
- coma or respiratory arrest occurs

Treatment at discharge from hospital. Patients should:

- continue high-dose inhaled glucocorticoid and complete course of oral prednisolone
- be instructed to monitor their own PEFR and not to reduce dose if the PEFR falls, or there is a recurrence of early morning dipping in the reading

(patients should not generally be discharged until there is less than 25% diurnal variation in PEFR readings)

Warnings

Asthma may be precipitated by β-adrenoceptor blockade and the use of β-adrenoceptor antagonists is *contraindicated* in asthmatics; fatal asthma has been precipitated by β-blocker eye drops, even allegedly β_1-selective agents.

Overuse of β2-adrenergic agonists is dangerous. In the mid-1960s, there was an epidemic of sudden deaths in young asthmatics outside hospital. It was associated with the introduction of a high-dose, metered aerosol of isoprenaline (β1 and β2 agonist); it did not occur in countries where the high concentration was not marketed. The epidemic declined in Britain when the profession was warned, and the aerosols were restricted to prescription only. Though the relationship between the use of β2-receptor agonists and death is presumed to be causal, the actual mechanism of death is uncertain; overdose causing cardiac arrhythmia is not the sole factor. The subsequent development of selective β2-receptor agonists was a contribution to safety, but a review in New Zealand during the 1980s found that the use of fenoterol (β2 selective) by metered-dose inhalation was associated with increased risk of death in severe asthma, and later analysis concluded that it was the most likely cause. A further cause for concern comes from a meta-analysis of 19 clinical trials which concluded that long-acting β agonists (LABAs) increased severe and life-threatening asthma exacerbations, as well as asthma-related deaths. The US Food and Drug Administration has recently confirmed their belief that the benefits of LABAs still outweigh these risks but have opted for a more cautious labelling policy.

CHRONIC OBSTRUCTIVE PULMONARY DISEASE (COPD)

Whereas asthma is characterised by *reversible* airways obstruction and bronchial hyperreactivity, COPD is characterised by *incompletely reversible* airways obstruction and *mucus hypersecretion*; it is predominantly a disease of the smaller airways. Nevertheless, distinguishing the two can be difficult in some patients, and one view is that asthma predisposes smokers to COPD (the Dutch hypothesis). In practice, even though – indeed precisely because–most of the airway obstruction is fixed in COPD, it is important to maximise the reversible component. This can be assessed by measuring FEV_1 (forced expiratory volume in 1 s) before and after a course of oral prednisolone, e.g. at least 30 mg/day for 2 weeks; reversibility is arbitrarily defined as a rise in FEV_1 of more than 15% (and greater than 200 mL). An important caveat is that patients' symptoms sometimes improve despite little or no demonstrable reversibility, because FEV_1 measures large airways function, and in COPD mainly the small airways are affected.

Drugs used to treat COPD are exactly as for asthma, except that antimuscarinics, such as ipratropium or the longer-acting tiotropium, are often more effective bronchodilators than β_2 agonists. Patients with reversible airways obstruction should also receive an inhaled glucocorticoid and its combination with a long-acting β_2 agonist may improve control, especially in moderate or severe disease ($FEV_1 < 50\%$ predicted), e.g. fluticasone + salmeterol (Seretide). This strategy is designed to reduce the frequency of disease exacerbations rather than affect the decline in lung function perse.

A theophylline may also be effective in patients with severe disease, but requires special care in the elderly, including monitoring of plasma theophylline. Mucolytic drugs reduce acute episodes of COPD and days of illness; they are best reserved for patients with recurrent, prolonged or severe exacerbations of the disease. Quitting smoking remains the only action of proven benefit in preserving lung function in COPD.

Long-term oxygen therapy improves survival in hypoxic patients. It is indicated when:

- PaO_2 is less than 7.3 kPa (56 mmHg) when stabilised on optimal medical treatment.
- PaO_2 is 7.3–8.0 kPa and there is evidence of right-sided cardiac failure (cor pulmonale).

SUMMARY

- Drugs that block the actions of acetylcholine and histamine are weak or ineffective in the treatment of asthma.
- Most anti-asthma treatment is therefore aimed either at reducing release of inflammatory cytokines (glucocorticoids and sodium cromoglicate) or at direct bronchodilatation by stimulation of the bronchial β_2-adrenoceptors.
- Aggressive use of glucocorticoids, especially by the inhaled route, is the keystone of the modern stepped approach to asthma management.
- Antihistamines conventionally refer to antagonists of the H_1 receptor, and have wide applications in the treatment of allergic disorders, and in anaphylaxis.
- The principal adverse effect of older first-generation antihistamines, sedation, is avoided by use of newer second-generation drugs which do not enter the CNS.
- Smoking cessation and long-term treatment with oxygen are the only interventions that are known to improve survival in chronic obstructive pulmonary disease.

IMPORTANT TERMINOLOGY

allergy   过敏

antihistamine   抗组胺

antitussive   镇咳药

asthma   哮喘

β_2-adrenoceptor agonist β_2- 肾上腺素受体激动剂

bronchial inflammation   气道炎症

bronchoconstriction   支气管狭窄

bronchodilator drugs   支气管扩张剂

bronchospasm   支气管痉挛

chronic obstructive pulmonary disease   慢性阻塞性肺疾病

cough   咳嗽

expectorants   祛痰药

histamine H_1-receptor blocker   组胺 H_1 受体阻滞剂

leukotriene receptor antagonists   白三烯受体拮抗剂

long-acting β agonists (LABAs)   长效 β 激动剂

mucolytics   黏液溶解剂

pulmonary surfactant   肺表面活性物质

respiatory distress syndrome (RDS)   呼吸窘迫综合征

respiratory stimulants   呼吸兴奋药

theophylline   茶碱

CHALLENGE YOURSELF

1. Please compare risks and benefits of common medications used for cough.
2. Please compare the advantages and disadvantage of epinephrine, isoprenaline and salbutamol when they are used to treat asthma.

Rong Xu

Chapter | 18 |

Clinical medication for digestive system disease

Part 1 Clinical medication for Oesophagus, stomach and duodenum diseases

SYNOPSIS

'Dyspepsia' is a non-specific term which encompasses a number of symptoms attributable to the upper gastrointestinal (GI) tract, and may include anything from acid reflux to abdominal bloating. Approximately one third of the population in Western societies experiences regular dyspepsia, although the majority self-medicate with over-the-counter antacid preparations and do not seek medical advice. Up to 50% of those who do will have demonstrable pathology, most commonly gastro-oesophageal reflux or peptic ulceration. The remainder, in whom no abnormality is found, are diagnosed as having non-ulcer dyspepsia. Finally, nausea and vomiting are deeply unpleasant sensations with a number of causes and, fortunately, a number of effective therapies.

GASTRIC ACID SECRETION AND MUCOSAL PROTECTION

In the normal upper GI tract, the destructive effects of gastric hydrochloric acid are balanced by a variety of mucosal protective mechanisms. Duodenal and gastric ulceration results from an imbalance between these two opposing forces. *Helicobacter pylori* (*H. pylori*) infection and use of non-steroidalanti-inflammatory drugs (NSAIDs) play an important role in upsetting this fine balance. Other digestive enzymes such as pepsinogen/pepsin also contribute to the gastric phase of digestion but are qualitatively of less importance.

Gastric acid secretion

Acid secretion by parietal cells in the gastric mucosa is regulated by four main neurohumoral mediators: gastrin, acetylcholine (ACh), histamine, and prostaglandins.

Gastrin

Gastrin is a peptide hormone secreted by neuroendocrine G cells in response to a variety of physical and neurohumoral stimuli such as gastric distension, the presence of amino acids, vagal stimulation and histamine. Gastrin activates gastrin receptors on the basolateral aspect of the parietal cell, stimulating acid secretion.

Acetylcholine (ACh)

ACh, secreted by parasympathetic vagal efferents, activates muscarinic M_3 receptors on parietal cells and also on mast cell-like histamine secreting cells in the gastric mucosa. Both of these actions result in acid secretion.

Histamine

Histamine is secreted by enterochromaffin-like cells (mast cell-like cells in the gastric mucosa) at a basal rate, and secretion is augmented by gastrin and ACh from parasympathetic stimulation. Histamine secreted into the portal circulation stimulates H_2 receptors on parietal cells, promoting acid secretion.

Prostaglandins

Locally produced prostaglandins E_2 and I_2 inhibit parietal cell acid secretion. Prostaglandins are produced by the cyclo-oxygenase enzyme. In the stomach, these prostaglandins are produced by the constitutively expressed COX-1 enzyme isoform.

Mucosal protective mechanisms

Mucus and bicarbonate is secreted by cells in the gastric and duodenal mucosa and provides a protective relatively alkaline physical barrier against the otherwise destructive intragastric environment. Secretion is promoted by prostaglandins, which also inhibit gastric acid secretion. Numerous lifestyle factors adversely affect the mucosal barrier, including smoking and alcohol.

Helicobacter pylori (*H. pylori*): an occasionally silent killer

It is now known that a large majority of benign gastric and duodenal ulceration is due to *H. pylori* infection (following Marshall and Warren's Nobel prize-winning experiments); *H. pylori* appears to stimulate increased acid secretion. All patients colonised with *H. pylori* develop gastritis, but only about 20% have ulcers or other lesions. As yet incompletely understood host factors and differences in strain of the organism are likely to explain this discrepancy. *H.pylori* infection is carcinogenic and is the leading cause of gastric carcinoma. It is also highly associated with gastric MALT lymphoma. Eradication of the organism can lead to regression and even resolution of this latter malignancy.

NSAIDs: enemies of the gut

All NSAIDs are ulcerogenic, but ibuprofen is less prone to cause these problems than other non-selective NSAIDs. NSAIDs are weak organic acids and the acid milieu of the stomach facilitates their non-ionic diffusion into gastricmucosal cells. Here the neutral intracellular pH causes the drugs to become ionised and trapped in the mucosa because they cannot diffuse out in this form. Aspirin and the other NSAIDs inhibit cyclo-oxygenase (COX). In the stomach, the constitutively expressed COX-1 isoform is responsible for the production of the gastroprotective prostaglandins E2 and I2. Inhibition of the inducible COX-2 isoform (which is normally up-regulated in activated inflammatory cells) is responsible for NSAIDs' anti-inflammatory properties. Most NSAIDs inhibit both isoforms unselectively, so the beneficial anti-inflammatory effect is offset by the potential for mucosal injury by depletion of protective prostaglandins. Aspirin is particularly potent in this respect, perhaps because it inhibits COX irreversibly, unlike the other NSAIDs where inhibition is reversible and concentration dependent.

For years, the treatment of peptic ulceration centred around measures to neutralise gastric acid, to inhibit its secretion or to enhance mucosal defences, but recognition of the central role of *H. pylori* revolutionised the approach. Haemorrhage is one of the feared complications of peptic ulceration. The treatment of choice is endoscopic therapy, but Proton pump inhibitors (PPIs), usually given as an intravenous infusion for 72 h to guarantee high and constant plasma levels, have a role as an adjunctive treatment. Reduction of gastric acid and raising of gastric pH results in clot stabilisation, thus promoting haemostasis.

DRUGS TO REDUCE OR NEUTRALISE GASTRIC ACID

Antacids

Antacids directly neutralise secreted acid and raise intragastric pH. They protect the gastric mucosa against acid (by neutralisation) and pepsin (which is inactive above pH 5, and which in addition is inactivated by aluminium and magnesium). Most commonly they are magnesium or aluminium salts. The hydroxide is the most common base, but trisilicate, carbonate and bicarbonate are also used.

Antacids relieve mild dyspeptic symptoms and they are taken intermittently when symptoms occur.

Individual antacids

Sodium bicarbonate can release sufficient carbon dioxide in the stomach to cause discomfort and belching. Magnesium oxide and magnesium trisilicate cause an osmotic diarrhoea.

Aluminium hydroxide tends to constipate, which reacts with hydrochloric acid to form aluminium chloride and in turn reacts with intestinal secretions to produce insoluble salts, especially phosphate.

Some antacid mixtures contain sodium, may be dangerous for patients with cardiac, renal or liver disease. For example, a 10-mL dose of magnesium carbonate mixture or of magnesium trisilicate mixture contains about 6 mmol sodium (normal daily dietary intake is approximately 120 mmol sodium).

Aluminium- and *magnesium*-containing antacids may interfere with the absorption of other drugs by binding with them or by altering gastrointestinal pH or transit time. It is probably advisable not to co-administer antacids with drugs that are intended for systemic effect by the oral route.

However, unwanted effects and inconvenience limit their regular use. Antacid is not of clinical significance if used on an intermittent, short-term basis but if given regularly over a period of time (days to weeks or longer) or in large doses will result in a potentially dangerous metabolic alkalosis.

H$_2$ receptor antagonists (H$_2$RAs)

Pharmacokinetics and dosage. H$_2$RAs are given orally and are well absorbed. Since there is anecdotal evidence that peptic ulcer healing with H$_2$-receptor antagonists correlates best with suppression of nocturnal acid secretion, many prefer to give these drugs as a single evening dose (e.g. ranitidine 150–300 mg).

Pharmacology. H$_2$RAs are less potent than the PPIs, as alternative pathways of parietal cell activation remain uninhibited. They competitively inhibit histamine binding at H$_2$ receptors on the basolateral aspect of parietal cells, resulting in a reduction of gastric acid secretion. The inhibitory effect can be overcome with high gastrin levels, as occurs post-prandially. Tolerance may develop, probably due to down-regulation of receptors.

Adverse effects and interactions are few with short-term use. Cimetidine is a weak anti-androgen, and may cause gynaecomastia and sexual dysfunction in males. Cimetidine inhibits cytochromes P450 and there is potential for increased effect from any drug with a low therapeutic index that is inactivated by these isoenzymes, e.g. warfarin, phenytoin. Ranitidine and famotidine largely avoid these unwanted effects. A potential danger is that patients with serious pathology such as gastric carcinoma will self-medicate, allowing their disease to progress. The inhibitory effect can be overcome with high gastrin levels, as occurs postprandially. Tolerance may develop, probably due to down-regulation of receptors.

Proton pump inhibitors (PPIs)

Pharmacokinetics. PPIs are available in oral and intravenous formulations. Oral PPIs are degraded at low pH and must be given in enteric-coated forms. Systemic availability increases with dose and also with time, owing to decreased inactivation of the prodrug as gastric acidity is reduced. Maximum efficacy occurs after up to 5 days of therapy. Uninhibited Na$^+$/K$^+$-ATPase will regenerate when the PPI is discontinued; this may take 2–3 days.

Pharmacology. As can be deduced from the above, the most effective site of action for antisecretory drugs is the proton pump. PPIs are taken up by parietal cells from the portal circulation and are then excreted into the acid milieu around the secretory canaliculus. The resulting ionised form binds irreversibly to the proton pump, resulting in virtual total inhibition of acid secretion.

Adverse reactions and interactions. PPIs are as a rule well tolerated and serious adverse effects are unusual. Given their mechanism of action, there are theoretical concerns about cancer (due to the stimulatory effect of the hypergastrinaemia resulting from the loss of negative feedback), mineral deficiencies (due to loss of acid-related absorption of iron, calcium and B_{12}, for example) and enteric infections (due to the loss of the antibacterial properties of a strongly acidic environment). Although an increased incidence of osteoporotic fractures and *Clostridium difficile* (*C. diff*) colitis has been noted in some observational studies, there has been no good evidence that these risks are significant, even after almost 20 years of clinical experience.

Examples of PPIs are omeprazole (10–20 mg daily), lansoprazole (15–30 mg daily) and pantoprazole. All are similar in pharmacokinetics, efficacy and adverse effect profile.

Other targets for acid suppression

Gastrin inhibitors exist as experimental tools only as they are not effective acid suppressants. Antimuscarinic treatments for peptic ulceration are obsolete, but underlie the rationale for the surgical vagotomy which is now rarely performed.

DRUGS TO ENHANCE MUCOSAL PROTECTION

Sucralfate (SUCRose sulFATE and ALuminium hydroxide complex)

Pharmacology. Sucralfate provides a physical barrier to gastric acid. It is activated by acid to produce a viscous gel, and will therefore be ineffective if given with therapies that inhibit acid release or raise gastric pH. In the acid environment of the stomach, the aluminium moiety is released so that the compound develops a strong negative charge and binds to positively charged protein molecules that transude from damaged mucosa. The result is a viscous paste that adheres selectively and protectively to the ulcer base. It also binds to and inactivates pepsin and bile acids, which has the added benefit of reducing mucus degradation. Its therapeutic efficacy in healing gastric and duodenal ulcers is approximately equal to that of the histamine H_2-receptor antagonists.

Adverse effects and interactions. Sucralfate may cause constipation but is otherwise well tolerated. The concentration of aluminium in the plasma may be raised but this appears to be a problem only with long-term use by uraemic patients, especially those undergoing chronic intermittent haemodialysis. As the sucralfate is effective only in acid conditions, an antacid should not be taken 30 min before or after a dose. Sucralfate interferes with absorption of several drugs, including ciprofloxacin, theophylline, digoxin, phenytoin and amitriptyline, possibly by binding due to its strong negative charge.

Bismuth chelate (tripotassium dicitratobismuthate, bismuth subcitrate, bismuth potassium citrate)

Pharmacology. This substance was thought to act by chelating with protein in the ulcer base to form a protective coating against adverse influences of acid, pepsin and bile. It may also promote protective prostaglandin, mucus and bicarbonate synthesis. Probably more importantly, bismuth chelate is now known to suppress *H. pylori* growth, especially when combined with an antimicrobial. Bismuth chelate finds use for benign gastric and duodenal ulcer, and has a therapeutic efficacy approximately equivalent to that of histamine H_2-receptor antagonists. Ulcers remain healed for a longer time after bismuth chelate than after H_2-receptor antagonists, probably due to its ability to eradicate *H.pylori*.

Adverse effects. Bismuth chelate, particularly as a liquid formulation, darkens the tongue, teeth and stool; the effect is less likely with the tablet, which is thus more acceptable. Systemic absorption of bismuth from the chelated preparation is small but it does pass into the urine and it is prudent to avoid the drug for patients with impaired renal function. Urinary elimination continues for months after bismuth is discontinued. Bismuth toxicity causes encephalopathy.

Misoprostol

Pharmacology. Misoprostol is a synthetic analogue of the protective prostaglandin E1 and therefore has the same antisecretory and cytoprotective properties. Traditionally it has been coadministered with NSAIDs to counteract the latter's effects on endogenous prostaglandin synthesis.

Adverse effects. Diarrhoea and abdominal pain, transient and dose related, are the commonest. Women may experience gynaecological disturbances such as vaginal spotting and dysmenorrhoea; the drug is contraindicated in pregnancy or for women planning to become pregnant, as the products of conception may be aborted. Indeed, women have resorted to using misoprostol (illicitly) as an abortifacient in parts of the world where provision of contraceptive services is poor.

Alginate

Alginate is a common and harmless component of antacids. It forms a viscous raft which forms a physical barrier between the gastric contents and the oesophageal, gastric and duodenal mucosa.

THE OESOPHAGUS IN HEALTH AND DISEASE

The normal oesophagus effortlessly transfers food and drink from the benign environment of the mouth through the gate of the lower oesophageal sphincter into the harsh acidic environment of the stomach. Transient gastrooesophageal reflux occurs in almost everybody and it is only when episodes become frequent, with prolonged exposure of the oesophageal mucosa to acid and pepsin, that problems develop.

The physiological lower oesophageal sphincter (LOS), normally located at the gastrooesophageal junction at the level of the diaphragm, allows solid and liquid boluses to pass into the stomach while preventing acidic gastric contents refluxing into the oesophagus. Intrinsic tonic contraction of the LOS is interrupted by normal transient lower oesophageal relaxation as well as coordinated relaxation when swallowing is initiated. Numerous neurohumoral intermediaries are involved in these processes, including parasympathetic efferents, Ach, g-aminobutyric acid (GABA) and glutamate. The integrity of the sphincter can be compromised by the presence of a hiatus hernia, which disrupts its anatomical and physiological components.

Excessive or inappropriate relaxation of the LOS results in gastrooesophageal reflux disease, oesophagitis and oesophageal ulceration, stricturing resulting in mechanical obstruction and sometimes a secondary oesophageal dysmotility and spasm. Reduced oesophageal clearance of acid may also contribute. In susceptible individuals, acid reflux triggers columnar metaplasia of the native squamous epithelium (also known as Barrett's oesophagus). This is a pre-malignant condition for oesophageal adenocarcinoma.

Oesophageal dysmotility tends to produce symptoms of dysphagia to both solids and liquids, as opposed to mechanical obstruction which results in dysphagia to solids unless very advanced. A high sphincter tone and uncoordinated oesophageal contractions can cause dysphagia and pain. Achalasia is a motility disorder of unknown aetiology characterised by oesophageal hypomotility, a hypertonic LOS and a failure of relaxation of the LOS.

DRUGS AFFECTING OESOPHAGEAL MOTILITY AND THE LOWER OESOPHAGEAL SPHINCTER

The D_2 agonist drugs *domperidone* and *metoclopramide* can have a beneficial effect on reflux symptoms, firstly by enhancing gastric emptying and thus reducing the volume of acid available to reflux up the oesophagus, and secondly by increasing LOS basal tone. A number of drugs reduce tonic lower oesophageal sphincter tone or increase transient lower oesophageal sphincter relaxation and thus promote reflux, including *nitrates*, *theophyllines*, drugs with *antimuscarinic* activity or unwanted effects, and *calcium channel antagonists*. These agents may occasionally be useful in alleviating the symptoms of oesophageal spasm, although the effect is usually disappointing. They are rarely potent enough to be of significant use in achalasia. Commonly used examples include *nifedipine*, *diltiazem*, and *modified-release nitrates*. Newer therapies being explored in the treatment of GORD include GABA inhibition to reduce transient lower oesophageal sphincter relaxations. *Baclofen* is clinically effective but has limiting CNS unwanted effects, and more tolerable compounds are being investigated. Other pharmacological targets which are showing potential in early clinical research include *cannabinoid agonists*.

Oesophageal dysmotility

This can be notoriously difficult to treat satisfactorily. Prokinetic drugs can be tried in cases of confirmed oesophageal hypomotility; conversely, a calcium channel antagonist or a long-acting nitrate can be tried if the problem is predominantly one of spasm. Treatment of coexistent reflux may improve spasm secondary to reflux. Pharmacological management of achalasia (Characterised by incomplete relaxation of LOS, increased LOS tone, lack of peristalsis in the oesophagus and consequent inability of smooth muscle to move food down the oesophagus) is best viewed as a temporary measure and drugs which reduce LOS tone rarely provide effective symptomatic improvement. Botulinum toxin, which inhibits cholinergic transmission by reducing ACh release from pre-synaptic motor neurones, can be injected endoscopically into the LOS and results in medium-term (3–6 months) relaxation of the LOS and symptomatic improvement. Endoscopic dilatation or surgical correction results in longer-term improvement. Relaxation of the LOS results in potentially free reflux of gastric acid contents and must therefore be accompanied by a PPI.

Drugs to treat Gastro-oesophageal reflux

The mainstay of medical treatment of acid reflux disease is the neutralization or reduction of gastric acid production, and is therefore most easily achieved with PPIs, although H$_2$RAs (e.g. ranitidine 150–300 mg daily) may be sufficient. Endoscopically proven oesophagitis may require 4–6 weeks of PPI therapy to heal (e.g. omeprazole 20 mg once daily; lansoprazole 30 mg once daily). If symptoms recur, the lowest effective antacid dose should be used to maintain remission. Doses may need to be doubled in severe or refractory cases. Prokinetic drugs such as domperidone 10–20 mg four times daily or meto-

clopramide 10 mg three times daily can improve symptoms, best in conjunction with an antisecretory agent.

Reflux-like symptoms unresponsive to PPI therapy are unlikely to be due to acid reflux and alternative causes require exploration. Biliary reflux can produce identical symptoms to acid reflux, and is unresponsive to PPI therapy due to its alkaline nature. It may respond to prokinetic therapy.

Lifestyle modification includes reduction in habits that promote acid reflux. Caffeine, alcohol, smoking and obesity relax the lower oesophageal sphincter and should be substituted or discontinued if possible. Avoid late evening meals to allow time for the stomach to empty before lying supine. Minor occasional symptoms are effectively managed with over-the-counter alginate-containing antacids.

Eosinophilic oesophagitis

This is increasingly recognised as an important cause of oesophageal symptoms. It is a disorder of unknown aetiology characterised by substantial eosinophilic submucosal infiltrates in the absence of significant acid reflux and may be associated with other atopic conditions. Treatment options are limited, but topically applied corticosteroids (e.g. swallowing inhaled steroids) can be helpful in inducing and maintaining remission.

Other disorders of acid secretion

The Zollinger–Ellison syndrome is a rare disorder due to a gastrin-secreting tumour which may arise anywhere in the GI tract, but most commonly in the pancreas, duodenum or stomach. High levels of serum gastrin cause hyperstimulation of parietal cells and hypersecretion of gastric acid, leading to multiple gastric and small bowel ulcers. Very high doses of PPI, up to 120 mg of omeprazole or greater per day, may be required to counteract this.

NAUSEA AND VOMITING

The physiology of nausea and vomiting is complex and incompletely understood. Vomiting can be protective, e.g. when it expels toxins (such as food poisoning and alcohol) from the GI tract. Suppressing nausea and vomiting is important in the management of other conditions including chemotherapy, general anaesthesia, morning sickness of pregnancy and when it accompanies other disease states (e.g. cardiac ischaemia, migraine).

A number of stimuli are integrated in the chemoreceptor trigger zone (CTZ) and vomiting centre located in the floor of the fourth ventricle, including blood-borne molecules (especially toxins, peptides and drugs), sensory and psychological stimulation from higher centres, physical signals such as distension from the stomach and GI tract, other autonomic inputs, and vestibular feedback. Implicated neurotransmitter mediators include ACh (acting on muscarinic receptors), HA (H_1 receptors), DA (D_2 receptors), 5-HT (5-HT_3 receptors) and Substance P (NK_1 receptors).

Drugs used in nausea and vomiting

Antimuscarinics

Hyoscine is still the most common drug of its class used as an antiemetic. It suffers from all the side-effects of antimuscarinic agents.

H₁-receptor antagonists

Examples include *cyclizine*, *promethazine* and *cinnarizine*. They do not have significant action at the CTZ. Drowsiness is a significant side-effect.

D₂-receptor antagonists

These include the *phenothiazines*, also used as antipsychotics, such as chlorpromazine and haloperidol. They are powerful antiemetics but have relatively common and significant CNS side-effects including drowsiness and extrapyramidal movement disorders.

Metoclopramide and *domperidone* are D_2-receptor antagonists without antipsychotic activity which have prokinetic properties, which can augment their antiemetic effect. They act *centrally* by blocking dopamine D_2 receptors in the CTZ, and metoclopramide also acts *peripherally* by enhancing the action of acetylcholine at muscarinic nerve endings in the gut. They raise the tone of the lower oesophageal sphincter, relax the pyloric antrum and duodenal cap, and increase peristalsis and emptying of the upper gut. The peripheral actions are utilised to empty the stomach before emergency anaesthesia and in labour. Metoclopramide can cause the same side-effects as the phenothiazines. Domperidone does not readily cross the blood-brain barrier and consequently has fewer CNS effects.

5-HT₃-receptor antagonists

Drugs such as ondansetron are powerful and well tolerated agents which act at the CTZ.

Corticosteroids

Corticosteroids are particularly useful in chemotherapy-associated nausea and vomiting. Their mechanism of action is unclear. Newer therapies, at present only licensed in the context of chemotherapy-associated symptoms, include the cannabinoid receptor agonist *nabilone* and the neurokinin-1 antagonist *aprepitant*.

Choice of antiemetic

Muscarinic and H_1 antagonists and the D_2 antagonists domperidone and metoclopramide are useful for general use, including motion sickness. Promethazine is used frequently to treat morning sickness. The 5-HT_3 antagonists can be used in cases unresponsive to these first-line therapies, and are particularly useful in postoperative nausea and vomiting. Corticosteroids are used primarily in the context of chemotherapy-associated nausea and vomiting, either alone or in conjunction with one or more of drugs such as a phenothiazine, 5-HT_3 antagonist, nabilone or aprepitant.

NON-ULCER DYSPEPSIA AND FUNCTIONAL DISORDERS

Up to a third of patients presenting to secondary care with dyspeptic symptoms have no pathological cause identified and have 'non-ulcer dyspepsia'. Management of these patients can be challenging and requires a comprehensive approach. Many patients with non-ulcer dyspepsia have abnormalities of gastric emptying and increased pain perception in the gastrointestinal tract, suggesting that the condition is part of the spectrum of irritable bowel syndrome.

Acid-predominant symptoms such as heartburn and epigastric discomfort may respond to anti-acid or antisecretory therapy. Although a minority of patients may respond to *H. pylori* eradication, there is no evidence that there is a causative link and the response rate is not greater than that seen with placebo.

The sensation of bloating is poorly understood but may involve visceral afferent hypersensitivity and hypomotility. Motility-predominant symptoms such as bloating may respond to prokinetic drugs. Antispasmodics such as peppermint oil can help, as can tricyclic antidepressants in low-dose, as for neuropathic pain.

Part 2. Clinical medication for intestinal disease

SYNOPSIS

Problems of constipation, diarrhea and irritable bowel syndrome are extremely common. Worldwide, infective diarrhoeal diseases are the third leading cause of death, a result of fluid, electrolyte and nutrient depletion. Around 1.5 million children under the age of 5 die due to diarrhoea, almost exclusively in the developing world. The management of these conditions is reviewed.

- Diarrhoea (drug treatment, importance of fluid and electrolyte replacement).
- Constipation: mode of action and use of drugs.
- Inflammatory bowel disease.
- Irritable bowel syndrome.

DIARRHOEA

A patient complaining of 'diarrhoea' may in fact describe a wide variety of colorectal symptoms. The World Health Organization defines diarrhoea as the passage of three or more loose or liquid stools per Day (or more frequent liquid passage than is normal for the individual). Diarrhoea ranges from a mild and socially inconvenient symptom to a major cause of death and malnutrition in the developing world. The first priority of therapy is to preserve fluid and electrolyte balance.

Some physiology

Diarrhoea results from an imbalance between secretion and reabsorption of water. The absorption of water is a passive phenomenon, and is reliant on the presence of a solute gradient across the cell allowing water to follow by osmosis. Sodium is the most important solute in this regard. Sodium gradients are established by active transporters and co-transporters linked to a variety of solutes and nutrients, including other electrolytes, amino acids and simple saccharides.

Mechanism of diarrhoea

Osmotic diarrhoea

The presence of indigestible or unabsorbed osmotically active molecules in the intestine results in water retention in the lumen. Many laxatives work on this principle. The diarrhoea of lactose intolerance is an example of an osmotic diarrhoea; lactase deficiency results in osmotically active lactose remaining in the bowel as it cannot be absorbed. Furthermore, any disease which results in damage to the small or large bowel mucosa (such as coeliac disease) will impair the intestine's ability to absorb solutes, thus effectively causing an osmotic diarrhoea.

Secretory diarrhoea

This results from the abnormal secretion of osmotically active solutes. Normally, in response to various stimuli, crypt cells actively transport chloride into the gut lumen, and sodium and water follow. This stimulus–secretion coupling is modulated by cyclic AMP and GMP, calcium, prostaglandins and leukotrienes. Numerous enteric hormones stimulate secretion, including vasoactive intestinal peptide secretin. Rarely neuroendocrine tumours secrete large amounts of these hormones, resulting in a profuse secretory diarrhoea. Numerous intestinal microbes including Vibriocholerae and enterotoxigenic Escherichia coli (ETEC) produce enterotoxins which cause unregulated electrolyte excretion by interfering with this process.

Increased gut transit

This is generally idiopathic but is rarely due to secretory tumours of the alimentary tract, i.e. neuroendocrine tumours which can secrete peptides such as histamine, 5-HT and VIP (vasoactive intestinal peptide) which have prokinetic effects on the bowel. Idiopathic cases are commonly seen in patients with irritable bowel syndrome (IBS), if ever, severe enough to produce clinically significant fluid or electrolyte disturbance or malabsorption.

Treatments Of Diarrhoea

Fluid and electrolyte treatment

Oral rehydration therapy (ORT). Oral rehydration therapy (ORT) with glucose– electrolyte solution is sufficient to treat the vast majority of episodes of watery diarrhoea from acute gastroenteritis. As a simple, effective, cheap and readily administered therapy for a potentially fatal condition, ORT is one of the major advances in therapy and one of the more successful global public health interventional strategies. It is effective because glucose-coupled sodium transport continues during diarrhoea, allowing sodium and water absorption to continue via an alternative pathway.

Oral rehydration salts (ORSs). The World Health Organization/UNICEF -recommended formulation is: Sodium chloride 3.5 g/L. Potassium chloride 1.5 g/L.

Sodium citrate 2.9 g/L. Anhydrous glucose 20.0 g/L. This provides sodium 90 mmol/L, potassium 20 mmol/L, chloride 80 mmol/L, citrate 10 mmol/L, glucose 111 mmol/ L (total osmolarity 311 mmol/L). Several other formulations exist, some with less sodium. Of note, it can be seen that attempted rehydration

therapy with commercial soft drinks alone will fail because their sodium content is too low (usually less than 4 mmol/L). Most cases respond adequately with assiduous attention to oral intake but fluid and electrolyte depletion are especially dangerous in children and the elderly, who may need intravenous fluid replacement. Antimotility drugs are inappropriate for severe diarrhoea; hazardous adverse effects counterbalance any marginal benefit.

Antimotility drugs

Codeine, diphenoxylate and loperamide all activate opiate receptors on the smooth muscle of the bowel to reduce peristalsis and increase segmentation contractions. The actions of all three drugs are antagonised by naloxone. Loperamide and diphenoxylate are relatively enterospecific and do not cross the blood–brain barrier (except diphenoxylate in large doses). These drugs should also be avoided in patients with active inflammatory bowel disease for they may cause paralytic ileus and toxic megacolon.

Infectious diarrhoea

This includes travellers'diarrhoea which is associated with enterotoxigenic strains of Escherichia coli; other bacteria including Shigella and Salmonella spp., viruses including the Norwalk family, and parasites (particularly Giardia lamblia) have also been implicated.

Transmission is almost invariably by ingestion of contaminated food and water, which indicates the most effective way of reducing risk. Infectious diarrhoea as a rule is self-limiting and oral rehydration is generally all that is required.

Antimotility agents are relatively contraindicated due to concerns of reduced pathogen clearance and toxic megacolon but may be permissible in mild cases.

Antibiotics is controversial as even in cases of bacterial dysentery they do not reduce duration of symptoms by more than 48 hours, and there is hard in vitro as well as anecdotal evidence that their use in patients with certain bacterial infections (e.g. E.coli O175) can precipitate haemolytic-uraemic syndrome (HUS), which can be life-threatening. Antibiotics may be indicated if the patient is toxic or immunosuppressed, or if invasive infections (e.g. Shigella) are suspected or confirmed. Many regimens are used (commonly ciprofloxacin) but macrolides are theoretically less prone to precipitating HUS in susceptible patients.

Chemotherapy is available for certain specific organisms if enteric infection is confirmed on stool culture, e.g. amoebiasis, giardiasis.

Diarrhoea due to *Clostridium difficile* ('*C.diff*')

Aetiology. *C. diff* infection may range from an offensive but limited diarrhoeal illness to a life-threatening toxic pseudomembranous colitis, and for this reason occupies such a prominent place in the public consciousness. The major risk factors for infection are older age, recent antibiotic use and a history of recent (within 3 months) hospitalisation. Virtually all antibiotics have been implicated as a risk factor for C. diff infection (including, rarely, metronidazole, one of the mainstays of treatment), but clindamycin, quinolones, cephalosporins and other β-lactams are particularly notorious.

Treatment. First-line treatment has traditionally consisted of 7–14 days of metronidazole by mouth. There is better evidence for a prolonged (4-week) tapering course of oral vancomycin, although this tends to be reserved for severe, refractory or relapsed infections. The tapering course allows the killing of reactivated spores which may have survived initial treatment. Vancomycin not absorbed from the GI tract is excreted renally; it must therefore be given orally (125 mg four times daily initially; occasionally doubled) and monitoring of serum levels is unnecessary. There are also some data supporting the use of more novel treatments, although solid evidence is lacking. Probiotics and faecal enemas (prepared using normal faeces from unaffected donors), for example, are thought to work by recolonising the bowel with non-pathogenic bacterial flora, whereas intravenous immunoglobulin probably works by neutralising pathogenic toxins.

Drug-induced diarrhoea

Innumerable drugs have diarrhoea as a side-effect.

Antimicrobials are the commonest drugs that cause diarrhoea. This is usually due to a benign alteration of bowel flora, but occasionally this will allow latent C. diff colonisation to result in overt colitis.

Bile acid malabsorption (BAM)

BAM is increasingly recognised as an important cause of irritable bowel syndrome (IBS) and other diarrhoeas of unknown aetiology. The diarrhoea is a result of osmotically active bile acids remaining in the GI tract.

Bile acids, synthesized in the liver, are necessary for the absorption of lipids from the small bowel. The distal small bowel (terminal ileum) reabsorbs and returns bile acids to the liver, forming a highly efficient enterohepatic recycling system. Primary, or idiopathic, BAM is thought to be due to dysregulated enterohepatic feedback resulting in increased bile acid secretion which saturates uptake absorption capability. Surgery or diseases affecting the small bowel mucosa (such as Crohn's), or prior cholecystectomy resulting in constant bile acid release, can cause diarrhea (secondary BAM).

If no treatable underlying cause of BAM is identified then a bile acid absorption resin such as colesevelam, colestipol or colestyramine may be given.

Microscopic colitis

This condition presents with diarrhoea; the colonic mucosa is macroscopically normal but histologically shows either lymphocytic infiltration of the mucosa (lymphocytic colitis) or subendothelial fibrosis (collagenous colitis). The condition is benign and spontaneous resolution occurs in a significant proportion. Treatment with aminosalicylates or corticosteroid may hasten this; alternatively, antidiarrhoeals may be attempted to control symptoms.

CONSTIPATION

There are multiple causes of constipation which should be excluded or treated. Symptomatic treatment involves the use of laxatives, which are medicines that promote defaecation, largely by reducing the viscosity of the contents of the lower colon. They are classified as follows:

- Stool bulking agents.
- Osmotic laxatives.
- Faecal softeners.
- Stimulant laxatives.

Stool bulking agents

Dietary fibre comprises the cell walls and supporting structures of vegetables and fruits. Most of the fibre in our diet is in the form of non-starch polysaccharides (NSPs), which are not digestible by human enzymes. Fibre may be soluble (pectins, guar, ispaghula) or insoluble (cellulose, hemicelluloses, lignin). Insoluble fibre has less effect than soluble fibre on the viscosity of gut contents but is a stronger laxative because it resists digestion in the small bowel and so enters the colon intact. In addition it has a vast capacity for retaining water; thus 1 g of carrot fibre can hold 23 g of water. It has been proposed that as humans have refined the carbohydrates in their diet over the centuries, so they have deprived themselves of fibre, the ensuing under-filling of the colon being an important cause of constipation, haemorrhoids and diverticular disease.

Stool bulking agents, which add fibre to the diet, are the treatment of choice for simple constipation. They act by increasing the volume and lowering the viscosity of intestinal contents to produce a soft bulky stool, which encourages normal reflex bowel activity. The mode of action of stool bulking agents is thus more physiological than that of other types of laxative. They should be taken with liberal quantities of fluid (at least 2 L daily).

Individual preparations

Bran is the residue left when flour is made from cereals; it contains between 25% and 50% of fibre. The fibre content of a normal diet can be increased by eating wholemeal bread and bran cereals but overzealous supplementation may cause troublesome flatulence (from bacterial fermentation in the colon).

Viscous (soluble) fibres, e.g. ispaghula, are effective and more palatable than bran. Ispaghula husk contains mucilage and hemicelluloses, which swell rapidly in water. **Methylcellulose** takes up water to swell to a colloid about 25 times its original volume, and sterculia (a tree gum), similarly, swells when mixed with water. These and others are available as a variety of proprietary preparations.

Drugs to stimulate colonic motility

Stimulant laxatives

These drugs increase intestinal motility by various mechanisms; they may cause abdominal cramps, and are contraindicated when intestinal obstruction is suspected.

Bisacodyl stimulates sensory endings in the colon by direct action from the lumen. It is effective orally in 6–10 h and, as a suppository, acts within 1 h. In elderly patients, bisacodyl suppositories reduce the need for regular enemas. There are no important unwanted effects.

Sodium picosulfate is similar and is also used to evacuate the bowel for investigative procedures and surgery.

Glycerol has a mild stimulant effect on the rectum when administered as a suppository.

The anthraquinones includes senna, danthron, rhubarb and aloes. In the small intestine soluble anthraquinone derivates are liberated and absorbed. These are excreted into the colon and act there, along with those that have escaped absorption, probably after being chemically changed by bacterial action.

Senna, available as a biologically standardised preparation, is widely used to relieve constipation and to empty the bowel for investigative procedures and surgery. It acts within 8–12 h.

Danthron is available as a standardised preparation in combination with the faecal softeners poloxamer (co-danthramer) and docusate sodium (as co-danthrusate). It acts within 6–12 h. Evidence from rodent studies indicates a possible carcinogenic risk, and long-term exposure to danthron should be avoided. It can be useful for treating constipation in terminally ill patients.

The 5-HT$_4$ agonist prucalopride has recently

been licensed as second-line therapy for women with chronic constipation.

Osmotic laxatives

These are but little absorbed and increase the bulk and reduce viscosity of intestinal contents to promote a fluid stool.

Some inorganic salts retain water in the intestinal lumen or, if given as hypertonic solution, withdraw it from the body. When constipation is mild, magnesium hydroxide will suffice but magnesium sulphate (Epsom salts) is used when a more powerful effect is needed. Both magnesium salts act within 2–4 h.

Lactulose is a synthetic disaccharide. Taken orally, it is unaffected by small intestinal disaccharidases, is not absorbed and thus acts as an osmotic laxative. Tolerance may develop. Lactulose is also used in the treatment of hepatic encephalopathy. Osmotic laxatives are frequently used to clear the colon for diagnostic procedures or surgery. Enemas containing phosphate or citrate effectively evacuate the distal colon and can be useful for treating obstinate constipation in elderly or debilitated patients. Oral formulations containing magnesium sulphate and citric acid or polyethylene glycol made up with water to create an isotonic solution are used in preparation for colonoscopy; some patients find the necessarily large volumes difficult to tolerate. Excessive use of stimulant and/or osmotic laxatives may lead to severe water and electrolyte depletion, even to hypokalaemic paralysis and renal failure, especially in the elderly[4] or those with diabetes or pre-existing renal impairment. Where bowel cleansing is necessary in these patients (e.g. before surgery or endoscopy), a less aggressive laxative and/or bowel preparation under medical supervision (with electrolyte and fluid balance monitoring) should be considered.

Faecal softeners (emollients)

The softening properties of these agents are useful in the management of anal fissure and haemorrhoids. Docusate sodium (dioctyl sodium sulphosuccinate) softens faeces by lowering the surface tension of fluids in the bowel. This allows more water to remain in the faeces. It appears also to have bowel stimulant properties but these are relatively weak. Docusate sodium acts in 1–2 days. Poloxamers, e.g. poloxalkol (poloxamer 188), act similarly and are used in combination with other agents.

Drastic purgatives (castor oil, cascara and phenolphthalein) are obsolete.

Suppositories and enemas

Suppositories (bisacodyl, glycerin) may be used to obtain a bowel action within about 1 h. Enemas produce defaecation by softening faeces and distending the bowel. They are used in preparation for surgery, radiological examination and endoscopy. Preparations with sodium phosphate, which is poorly absorbed and so retains water in the gut, are generally used. Arachis oil is included in enemas to soften impacted faeces.

Contraindications

Do not give laxatives to patients with undiagnosed abdominal pain, inflammatory bowel disease or obstruction. Likewise, laxatives should not be used to empty the rectum of hardened faeces, for they will fail and cause pain. Initial treatment should be with enemas, but digital removal, traditionally ordered by a senior and performed by a junior doctor, may occasionally be required. A bulking agent or a faecal softener will help to prevent recurrence.

INFLAMMATORY BOWEL DISEASE (IBD)

The inflammatory bowel diseases ulcerative colitis (UC) and Crohn's disease are chronic relapsing/remitting diseases of the GI tract characterised by intestinal mucosal inflammation. The pathogenesis of inflammatory bowel disease (IBD) remains incompletely understood. IBD can be thought of as an inappropriate immunological response to non-pathogenic luminal antigens. This can be either an over enthusiastic damaging pro-inflammatory response to an innocuous stimulus or an underwhelming protective anti-inflammatory response which fails to keep an appropriate inflammatory reaction in check. A combination of genetic predisposition and environmental factors produces either Crohn's disease, which can affect any part of the GI tract, or UC, which is confined to the colon. Classically, UC is thought to result from dysregulation of the Th1/ cell-mediated immune pathway while Crohn's results from disorders of Th2/humoral immunity, but this is almost certainly an oversimplification.

Although Crohn's and UC are different diseases, their medical management shares many similarities. The goal of pharmacological therapy is to induce and then maintain remission. The maintenance of remission is important not only for the patient's general well-being, but also because of the risk of complications such as colorectal cancer, which is directly related to disease activity over a long period of time. There is also increasing evidence that mucosal healing, and not just clinical remission, may be an important factor in determining long-term prognosis.

5-ASA and corticosteroids have been the mainstay of treatment of IBD for decades; indeed, the use of corticosteroids in UC has a particular place in the history of the randomised controlled clinical trial.

More recently, immunosuppressive therapy has found an important role. In the last few years biological therapy has been introduced and this is likely to produce a number of new therapies in the coming years.

Antidiarrhoeals should be used only with extreme caution in active colitis and are contraindicated if the disease is severe. They can lead toxic dilatation of the colon, with perforation.

Drugs to induce remission in UC

Aminosalicylates

5-Aminosalicylate (5-ASA) maintains remission in patients with ulcerative colitis (relapses are reduced by a factor of three), and may also be used for treatment of an acute attack (with or without a corticosteroid, depending on severity). There is increasing evidence that they have a protective effect against colorectal cancer in UC which is independent of its ability to maintain remission.

Its exact mechanism of action remains unclear; putative mechanisms include inhibition of pro-inflammatory prostaglandin synthesis, scavenging of free radicals, inhibition of inflammatory cell recruitment and inhibition of production of pro-inflammatory cytokines and protein mediators such as NFkB, IL1 and TNFa. **Sulfasalazine** has been used to treat rheumatoid arthritis since the 1930s. It was subsequently noted to have activity against ulcerative colitis. It consists of two compounds, sulfapyridine and 5-aminosalicylic acid, joined by an azo bond. Sulfasalazine is available as a tablet, retention enema (for disease extending up to the splenic flexure) or suppository (for treating proctitis). It can be particularly useful in treating patients with enteropathic arthritis associated with IBD, due to its rheumatological activity. Adverse effects are due largely to the sulfonamide moiety and include headache, malaise, anorexia, nausea and vomiting; these are dose related and commoner in slow acetylators (of the sulfonamide). Allergic reactions include rash, fever and lymphadenitis; rarely leucopenia and agranulocytosis occur. Males may suffer from reversible oligospermia and reduced sperm motility. Body secretions may have an orange discoloration.

Mesalazine Patients intolerant of sulfasalazine usually tolerate mesalazine, which is 5-ASA. Mesalazine is absorbed rapidly and completely in the upper jejunum, and is presented in various formulations that delay its release. Asacol tablets are coated in a resin, which dissolves only at pH 7 or higher, favouring its release in the distal ileum and colon. In contrast, Pentasa has a slow-release but pH-independent coating so that 5-ASA is liberated throughout the gastrointestinal tract. Mesalazine preparations are available in oral, enema and suppository forms.

Other 5-ASA. Balsalazide (a 5-ASA prodrug) and olsalazine (a 5-ASA dimer which is cleaved by colonic bacteria yielding active 5-ASA) are the other available aminosalicylates, obtainable in oral forms only. 5-ASA that enters the blood is rapidly cleared by acetylation in the liver and renal excretion. In comparison to sulfasalazine, the newer 5-ASAs are generally well tolerated and very safe. Patients should be counselled about the rare risk of blood dyscrasias and renal impairment, and occasional blood monitoring is required. Patients being initiated on 5-ASAs rarely experience a paradoxical flare in their symptoms.

Corticosteroid

Enemas and suppositories. These can be used in left-sided or distal UC. 5-ASA therapy is more effective in cases not requiring systemic corticosteroid so corticosteroid enemas/suppositories should not be used as first-line treatment. When UC is restricted to the left hemicolon, exacerbations that do not respond to an aminosalicylate alone often benefit from the addition of corticosteroid enemas. Foam-based preparations appear to coat the colonic mucosa more efficiently than the aqueous formulations.

Patients with distal colitis are prone to faecal loading proximal to the inflamed segment and this can lead to overflow diarrhoea and worsening of inflammation.

Systemic corticosteroid. Severe attacks of ulcerative colitis or Crohn's, or flares that are unresponsive to 5-ASA therapy, should be treated with systemic corticosteroid, and oral preparations usually suffice. It is important to start with a dose that will bring the inflammatory process under control, e.g. prednisolone 40 mg/day by mouth. Clinical response should be rapid (within 1 week). Once remission has been attained the dose can be tailed down very slowly over a period of 6–8 weeks. This gradual decrease is important, as stopping treatment too abruptly may result in a further flare.

Very severe attacks of ulcerative colitis necessitate hospital treatment with intravenous corticosteroid; parenteral corticosteroid should also be considered in patients unresponsive to other medical management. The main danger is toxic dilatation of the colon and perforation, which can occur insidiously. Significant clinical improvement should be seen within 72 h. If there is no improvement a trial of ciclosporin or an anti-TNF may induce response. Treatment otherwise is by emergency colectomy.

Ciclosporin

The calcineurin inhibitor ciclosporin will induce remission in some patients with severe ulcerative colitis unresponsive to intravenous corticosteroid. Give 2 mg/kg i.v., titrated to plasma levels, until remission is attained. Available oral preparations have different pharmacokinetic properties such that equivalence between them can not be assumed.

Dose sused in UC are lower than those used in transplant recipients. Renal function and blood pressure must be monitored closely. Ciclosporin is epileptogenic and this effect is enhanced in patients with electrolyte disturbances (particularly calcium and magnesium) and hypocholesterol aemia; it should also be avoided if there is a history of fits. Ciclosporin is ineffective in maintaining remission so maintenance immunosuppressive therapy is generally required.

Biological therapy

There is evidence that the TNFa receptor antagonist infliximab is useful in inducing remission in UC.

Drugs to induce remission in Crohn's disease

5-ASA

These are less effective in Crohn's disease. If they are used, the preparation must be chosen to target the affected part of the GI tract (e.g. Pentasa rather than asacol in small bowel disease).

Antibiotics

These are most useful for controlling perianal or penetrating disease, although anecdotally some patients with ileocolonic disease may also respond. Metronidazole and ciprofloxacin are used most commonly. Adverse effects including alcohol intolerance, peripheral neuropathy and the risk of antibiotic-associated diarrhoea and C. difficile superinfection from such prolonged therapy often limit their use to up to 3 months.

Dietary therapy

There is evidence that liquid diets based on aminoacids (elemental diets) or oligopeptides (semi-elemental diets) for 4–6 weeks are as effective as corticosteroids in controlling Crohn's disease, although relapse is common when the treatment stops. Elemental preparations are notoriously unpalatable even with flavourings and they often have to be administered through a nasogastric tube, which is unpopular with patients. Furthermore, the beneficial effect is lost if non-elemental/semi-elemental dietary components are included. They are worth trying in steroid resistant cases and are particularly favoured by paediatricians, who prefer to avoid systemic steroids because of their adverse effects on growth.

Corticosteroids

Corticosteroids are effective in active Crohn'sdisease. Budesonide, a potent topically active corticosteroid, is an alternative to prednisolone. As a delayed-release formulation it delivers drug to the ileum and ascending colon and is therefore particularly useful in small bowel and ileocaecal Crohn's, where it has comparable (but inferior) efficacy to prednisolone. Extensive first-pass metabolism in the liver limits its systemic availability and potential for adverse effects. Topical steroid preparations are generally not useful in Crohn's disease due to the intermittent nature of mucosal involvement.

Biological therapies

There is much more extensive experience of biological therapies in Crohn's disease, in particular with the use of anti-TNFα therapy. These have been demonstrated to be effective in the induction and maintenance of remission of active Crohn's disease, including perianal and fistulating disease.

Maintenance of remission in IBD

Corticosteroids are ineffective in maintaining remission of UC or Crohn's, largely due to significant adverse effects associated with long-term use.

In UC, maintenance therapy with an aminosalicylate should be started as corticosteroids are being weaned. 5-ASA has limited, if any, efficacy in the maintenance of remission of Crohn's disease.

If the disease is corticosteroid dependent despite adequate 5-ASA therapy, azathioprine or another immunosuppressive agent may be used. Surgery is indicated if medical therapy fails to control the disease or is associated with unacceptable adverse effects.

Azathioprine is effective as a steroid-sparing agent in maintenance therapy in UC and Crohn's, and is used when 5-ASA is insufficient to maintain adequate remission. Azathioprine is converted to 6-mercaptopurine (6-MP) and then to tioguanine, an inhibitor of purine synthesis, which causes a degree of immunosuppression; in this pathway the thiopurine methyltransferase (TPMT) enzyme is rate limiting. TPMT activity assays are now widely available and differentiate between patients with low or absent TPMT activity at high risk of complications, intermediate activity in whom thiopurines may be used with caution, and normal activity. Azathioprine is not an appropriate drug for inducing remission as its onset of action; corticosteroid is used as a 'bridge' to allow its therapeutic action to take effect.

Allopurinol can cause dangerous toxicity at therapeutic doses by inhibiting xanthine oxidase and preventing the conversion of azathioprine to 6-MP.

Adverse effects, in particular myelosuppression, are much more common in TPMT-deficient patients but those with normal enzymatic activity are also at risk. As azathioprine can cause bone marrow suppression and hepatitis, the blood count and liver function should be monitored weekly for the first 2 months of therapy and every 2–3 months thereafter for as long as the drug is taken. Pancreatitis occurs in up to 5% of patients. Intolerance to azathioprine is fairly common, for example malaise, abdominal discomfort and nausea. Mercaptopurine may be better tolerated. But it is not an alternative to azathioprine in patients who have suffered pancreatitis or myelosuppression.

Methotrexate, a folic acid antagonist, can be helpful in controlling relapses of Crohn's disease unresponsive to corticosteroid or azathioprine. It has also been used with benefit in ulcerative colitis. Its short- and long-term use are limited by a wide profile of adverse effects including bone marrow suppression and pulmonary and hepatic fibrosis. It is given once weekly, with folic acid supplements on the days on which it is not taken. It is severely teratogenic and is contraindicated in both men and women trying to conceive.

Biological therapies

TNFα causes activation of immune cells and release of inflammatory mediators by binding surface TNF receptors. Following in vitro demonstration that inhibition of TNFα activity resulted in reduced mucosal inflammation, several anti-TNFα have come to market. Infliximab, adalimumab and certolizumab-PEGol are recombinant monoclonal antiT-NFa-receptor antibodies. Infliximab, the first to come to market, is mouse-human chimaeric antibody and is given as an intravenous infusion of 5 mg/kg at 0, 2 and 6 weeks initially and then at 8-weekly intervals. Adalimumab is a fully human monoclonal antibody and has the advantage of being given subcutaneously at 160 mg at week 0, 80 mg at week 2, and 40 mg every 2 weeks thereafter. Certolizumab-PEGol is also a humanised monoclonal antibody with a PEGylated Fab' fragment. It is also given subcutaneously at a dose of 400 mg at weeks 0, 2 and 4, and at 4-weekly intervals thereafter.

These drugs are effective in inducing and maintaining remission in Crohn's disease. Most experience has been gained with infliximab. Infliximab and adalimumab appear to be effective in penetrating disease.

There is evidence that infliximab is also effective in inducing and maintaining remission in UC. Anti-TNFα are given as a long-term course over at least a year if effective. Adverse effects include hypersensitivity reactions. There is a significant risk of potentially fatal reactivation of TB, which must therefore be excluded before initiating treatment. There is a theoretical risk of increased susceptibility to other atypical infections and cancers, particularly lymphoproliferative disease, but long-term follow-up data are not yet available. Screening for infections such as hepatitis B and C viruses, and HIV is commonplace without as yet definite evidence that TNFα therapy worsens these conditions if coexistent.

Maintenance of remission following surgery for Crohn's disease

An additional difficulty in the medical management of Crohn's disease is prophylaxis against recurrence after surgical resection. Of the drugs studied, antibiotics are effective but cannot be given for longer than3 months because of toxicity and unwanted effects with long-term use. 5-ASA and azathioprine provide some benefit but emerging evidence suggests that infliximab (and potentially other anti-TNFα) are much more effective.

IRRITABLE BOWEL SYNDROME (IBS)

This condition affects 20% of the population and is the commonest reason for referral to a gastroenterologist. It is manifested by a variety of gastrointestinal symptoms including disordered bowel habit (constipation, diarrhoea, or both), abdominal pain and bloating. Upper gastrointestinal symptoms manifest as non-ulcer dyspepsia. All of these symptoms occur in the absence of demonstrable pathology in the gastrointestinal tract, although patients with IBS often have abnormalities of gut motility. Another feature of the condition is visceral hypersensitivity; patients with IBS have lower thresholds for pain from colonic distension induced by inflating balloons placed in the bowel. A proportion of patients develop their IBS symptoms after an episode of gastroenteritis and, in many, emotional stress is an important precipitating factor. Associated psychopathology, with anxiety and sometimes depression, is common.

The mainstay of treatment, after investigation when appropriate, is to reassure the patient of the entirely benign nature of the disorder and the good prognosis. Those with predominant constipation should be encouraged to increase the fluid and fibre content of their diet. Unprocessed bran can lead to trouble some bloating and wind, and a bulking agent such as ispaghula husk is often better tolerated.

Diarrhoea may respond to an antimotility drug such as loperamide, the dose being adjusted to symptoms. Codeine phosphate is effective but may cause sedation.

Low-dose tricyclic antidepressants, i.e. at doses ineffective as antidepressant, and antispasmodics are given for abdominal pain, but there is little objective evidence for their therapeutic efficacy. The generation of evidence is complicated by the variable nature of IBS symptoms, the patients who suffer from them, and the high rate of placebo response in this condition. There are two main classes of antispasmodic, the antimuscarinic drugs and drugs that are direct smooth muscle relaxants.

Antimuscarinic drugs

These drugs block cholinergic transmission at parasympathetic postganglionic nerve endings and cause smooth muscle to relax. The synthetic antimuscarinics dicyclomine and propantheline are probably the most useful in IBS, but therapeutic efficacy is often limited by other anticholinergic effects. The drugs are contraindicated in patients with glaucoma and prostatism, and should be avoided in patients with gastro-oesophageal reflux.

Direct smooth muscle relaxants

Mebeverine is a reserpine derivative that has a direct effect on colonic muscle activity, especially, it appears, on colonic hypermotility. As it does not possess antimuscarinic activity, it does not exhibit the troublesome effects of that group of drugs. Alverine and peppermint oil also have direct smooth muscle relaxing activity. A trial of low dose amitriptyline (10–25 mg by mouth at night) is worthwhile in patients who do not respond to antispasmodics, and associated depression will be helped by conventional doses of this or other antidepressants. Relaxation therapy, and hypnotherapy have a place in selected cases.

GASTROPARESIS

This complication of longstanding diabetes results from diabetic neuropathy affecting the enteric nervous system. Reduced bowel motility results in bloating, nausea, vomiting, impaired gastric emptying and abdominal pain. Prokinetics such as domperidone and metoclopramide are advocated; also erythromycin (250–500 mg four times daily) through a motilin agonist activity. It therefore has synergistic activity when used with domperidone or metoclopramide.

DIVERTICULAR DISEASE

Diverticular disease affects 5%–10% of Western people over the age of 45 years; the incidence rises to 80% in those over 80 years. Colonic dysmotility with increased intracolonic pressure, and diets high in refined carbohydrate and low in fibre, are important pathogenic factors. Some patients experience abdominal pain from dysmotility, whereas others remain asymptomatic. Infection of diverticulae occurs in a minority, giving potential for rupture or abscess formation.

Symptomatic diverticular disease often responds to an increase in dietary fibre and addition of a stool bulking agent. Antispasmodic drugs are helpful in controlling the pain of colon spasm but antimotility drugs encourage stasis of bowel contents, increase intracolonic pressure, and should be avoided. Diverticulitis requires treatment with broad-spectrum antimicrobials for 10 days (e.g. ciprofloxacin and metronidazole, or ampicillin, gentamicin and metronidazole).

ANAL FISSURE

Anal fissures are often intensely painful due to sphincter spasm. Anaesthetic ointments and stool softening agents have been widely used, with surgery (lateral internal sphincterotomy) for severely affected cases, but this procedure can cause incontinence from loss of sphincter control. An alternative is a 4-week course of topical nitrate (0.4%) or diltiazem (2%), which heals two-thirds of fissures by inducing sphincter relaxation, improving blood flow to the relatively ischaemic fissure and so promoting healing. Systemic absorption occurs, usually at insignificant doses to cause haemodynamic problems but which can cause a typical 'nitrate headache'. Use may be complicated by headache; tolerance can develop. Intrasphincteric injection of botulinum toxin has also been shown to be effective.

Part 3 Clinical medication for Liver and biliary tract diseases

SYNOPSIS

The liver is the most important organ for structural alteration and disposal of drugs, generating metabolites which may be biologically active or inactive (toxic). The liver is exposed to drugs at higher concentrations than most organs because most agents are administered orally and absorbed from the gastrointestinal tract, so the whole dose passes through the liver to the systemic circulation, rendering the liver vulnerable to injury from chemicals and drugs. Conversely, disordered hepatic function is an important cause of abnormal drug handling and responses.

- Drugs and the liver.
  - Pharmacodynamic and pharmacokinetic changes
  - Prescribing in liver disease
  - Drug-induced liver injury
  - Aspects of therapy.

EFFECTS OF LIVER DISEASE

PHARMACODYNAMIC CHANGES IN LIVER DISEASE

Patients with advanced liver disease have increased prothrombin time (INR) and serum bilirubin and require particular care when prescribing because they exhibit abnormal end-organ responses to drugs. Sensitivity of the central nervous system (CNS) to opioids, sedatives and antiepilepsy drugs is increased; the effect of oral anticoagulants is increased because synthesis of coagulation factors and thrombotic factors is impaired; fluid and electrolyte balance are altered; sodium retention is induced more readily by non-steroidal anti-inflammatory drugs (NSAIDs) or corticosteroids; ascites and oedema become diuretic resistant.

PHARMACOKINETIC CHANGES IN LIVER DISEASE

The liver has large metabolic reserve and important changes in drug handling occur only with hepatic decompensation. Parenchymal liver disorders, including chronic viral hepatitis or alcohol-related liver disease, have more impact on hepatic drug-metabolising enzyme activity than cholestatic conditions, such as primary biliary cirrhosis, where elimination via biliary excretion may be impaired. Hepatocellular injury leads to decreased activity of drug metabolising enzymes, reflected in diminished plasma clearance of drugs with hepatic metabolism. There is variation between patients and overlap with healthy subjects.

Hepatic blood flow and metabolism

Complex changes in blood flow occur with liver disease. Increased resistance to portal blood flow in cirrhosis and portosystemic/intrahepatic shunts reduce drug delivery to hepatocytes, while increasing delivery direct to the systemic circulation.

- *Drugs metabolised rapidly with high extraction in a single pass through the liver.* Clearance is limited normally by *hepatic blood flow*, but in severe liver disease less drug is extracted from blood passing through the liver because of poor hepatocyte function and portosystemic shunts that allow blood to bypass the liver.
- *Drugs metabolised slowly with poor extraction in a single pass through the liver.* The rate-limiting factor for elimination of this type of drug is *metabolic capacity* and the major effect of liver disease is *prolongation of $t_{1/2}$*. Consequently, the interval between doses may need to be lengthened and the time to reach steady-state concentration in the plasma ($5 \times t_{1/2}$) is increased.

Plasma protein binding of drug

Binding of drugs to albumin is reduced when plasma concentrations of albumin fall with defective synthesis. These changes provide scope to enhance the biological activity of drugs, but assume importance only with extensive protein binding (>90%).

Other considerations

Patients with severe decompensated liver disease develop renal impairment, with consequences for drugs with significant renal elimination. Where possible, dosing should be guided by measuring plasma concentrations (e.g. vancomycin).

PRESCRIBING FOR PATIENTS WITH LIVER DISEASE

Prescribing of most drugs is safe in well-compensated liver disease. If in doubt, check the prothrombin time and serum bilirubin. Take particular care with:

- Impaired hepatic synthetic function (hypoalbuminaemia, increased INR).
- Current/recent hepatic encephalopathy.
- Fluid retention and renal impairment.
- Drugs with:
  - high hepatic extraction
  - high plasma protein binding
  - low therapeutic ratio
  - CNS depressant effect

For drugs with significant hepatic metabolism, a reasonable approach is to reduce the dose to 25%–50% of normal and monitor responses. Specific examples include:

CNS depressants. Sedatives, antidepressants and antiepilepsy drugs should be avoided or used with extreme caution in advanced liver disease, particularly with current/ recent hepatic encephalopathy. Enhanced CNS sensitivity to such drugs is well documented. Treatment of alcohol withdrawal in patients with established liver disease is hazardous; reducing doses of chlordiazepoxide over 5–10 days is recommended (with high-dose thiamine).

Analgesics. Opiates can precipitate hepatic encephalopathy in decompensated liver disease. If required to control postoperative pain, doses should be reduced to 25%–50%. Intravenous infusions risk accidental overdose. Codeine can precipitate hepatic encephalopathy through constipation alone and accumulates with renal impairment. Avoid aspirin and other NSAIDs whenever possible, as they exacerbate impaired renal function and fluid retention by inhibiting prostaglandin synthesis and precipitate gastrointestinal bleeding.

Gastrointestinal system. Antacids that contain large quantities of sodium can precipitate fluid retention and cause ascites. Aluminium- or calcium-based preparations and antimotility drugs cause constipation and may precipitate hepatic encephalopathy.

DRUG-INDUCED LIVER DAMAGE

The spectrum of hepatic abnormalities caused by drugs is broad. Drugs tend to injure specific hepatocyte components, e.g. Plasma membrane, biliary canaliculi, cytochrome P450 enzymes or mitochondria.

Certain drugs interfere with bilirubin metabolism and excretion without causing hepatic injury. Jaundice is induced selectively with minimal or no disturbance of other liver function tests; recovery follows stopping the drug.

Examples are:

- C-17a-substituted steroids impair bilirubin excretion into hepatic canaliculi. These include synthetic anabolic steroids and oestrogens in oral contraceptives; jaundice due to the latter is rare with current formulations. Many have genetic susceptibility with mutations in ABC cassette biliary transporter proteins.
- Rifampicin impairs hepatic uptake and excretion of bilirubin; unconjugated and conjugated bilirubin levels may be raised within 3 weeks.
- Fusidic acid interferes with hepatic bilirubin excretion, causing conjugated hyperbilirubinaemia, particularly with sepsis.

Diagnosis and management of drug-induced liver injury

- Always consider the possibility. Take careful drug histories, including over-the-counter, complementary, illicit and alternative medicines.
- Consider a viral aetiology with hepatitis.
- Consider other causes of cholestatic disease.

- Underlying liver disease can cause diagnostic confusion.
- Liver biopsy is often helpful, but eosinophil infiltration, often thought to be specific for drug reaction, has many causes.
- Diagnostic challenge is dangerous, may precipitate lifethreatening liver disease and is never justified.
- Monitoring liver function in the early weeks of therapy is wise in detecting early reactions to drugs with hepatotoxic potential, e.g. isoniazid. Minor abnormalities (serum transaminase levels less than twice normal) are often self-limiting and progress should be monitored. For increases exceeding three-fold, consider drug withdrawal, even in asymptomatic patients.

ASPECTS OF THERAPY

Complications of cirrhosis

Variceal bleeding

Varices are dilated vessels, linking the portal and systemic venous systems, which return blood from the splanchnic circulation to the systemic circulation, bypassing the liver, decompressing the portal venous system and reducing portal pressure. Varices can be large, and haemorrhage, sometimes catastrophic, occurs from any of these vessels when intravascular pressures reach a threshold. Lower oesophageal or gastric varices, which are thin-walled and submucosal, are most prone to haemorrhage because intravascular pressures rise beyond that threshold.

In cirrhosis, both portal venous resistance and splanchnic blood flow are increased, the latter by a combination of splanchnic vasodilatation and increased cardiac output. Variceal bleeding is more likely once the pressure gradient between the portal and systemic venous systems rises above 12 mmHg (measured as the wedged hepatic venous pressure).

Fifty percent die from hypovolaemia or associated complications after a first oesophageal or gastric variceal haemorrhage, manifest as melaena or haematemesis. Correct hypovolaemia promptly with plasma expanders and blood transfusion. The use

of central venous access and monitoring is recommended; correction of coagulopathy with platelets and clotting factors appears logical. The relation between bacterial infection and haemorrhage is intriguing; bacterial infection is often found at presentation and 60% have evidence of infection within 7 days of haemorrhage. It is unclear whether infection increases the risk of haemorrhage or is a consequence. But bacterial infection should be treated, or anticipated, using broad-spectrum antibiotics with Gram-negative cover. Proton pump inhibitors are also recommended. Many patients cease bleeding spontaneously, but over half re-bleed within 10 days.

Acute variceal haemorrhage

The first step is always resuscitation. If bleeding varices are suspected, give terlipressin, as it reduces splanchnic blood flow, increases systemic blood pressure and reduces haemorrhage, which aids diagnostic endoscopy.

Oesophageal band ligation is the treatment of choice for bleeding varices identified at endoscopy. Varices are obliterated by application of small elastic bands under direct vision by an experienced operative. This has supplanted injection sclerotherapy, which involved injecting sclerosant into and around varices but which carried a higher rate of complications (oesophagitis, oesophageal stricture/perforation and distant sclerosant embolisation). Direct injection of superglue into the varix, the treatment of choice for bleeding gastric varices, requires considerable expertise. Bleeding is controlled in 90% of patients after oesophageal band ligation in conjunction with terlipressin. Obliteration of oesophageal varices requires repeated band ligation over a prolonged period.

Pharmacological reduction of portal pressure

Vasopressin, in addition to its action on renal collecting ducts (through V_2 receptors), constricts smooth muscle (V_1 receptors) in the cardiovascular system and particularly in splanchnic blood vessels, reducing splanchnic blood flow. Systemic, cerebral and coronary artery vasoconstriction are predictable complications necessitating treatment withdrawal in 20% of older patients. In patients with cardiovascular disease and uncontrolled haemorrhage that precludes definitive endoscopic therapy, simultaneous administration of glyceryl trinitrate (transdermally, sublingually or intravenously) allows continued use of vasopressin, reducing cardiac risk, and also reduces portal venous resistance and pressure directly.

Vasopressin is cleared rapidly from the circulation so is given by continuous intravenous infusion; with concerns about distant ischaemia, the short $t_{1/2}$ of vasopressin is advantageous.

The synthetic analogue, terlipressin (triglycyl-lysine vasopressin) has supplanted vasopressin. This prodrug is converted in vivo to vasoactive lysine vasopressin, which has biological activity for 3–4 h, and is effective as bolus injections 4-hourly for 2–5 days, reducing the risk of rebleeding.

Somatostatin and the synthetic analogue octreotide reduce portal pressure by decreasing splanchnic blood flow. Octreotide has the advantage of a longer duration of action and is given as bolus injection. It can be used as an alternative to terlipressin, with similar efficacy and indications, but does not carry a risk of cerebral or cardiac ischaemia.

When endoscopic therapy proves impossible or ineffective and bleeding continues despite pharmacotherapy, the next step is placement of a transjugular intrahepatic portosystemic shunt (TIPS), linking systemic and portal circulations with a covered expandable stent. With this in mind, patients should have early ultrasound assessment of the portal vein after variceal haemorrhage, aspatency is usually a prerequisite for TIPS insertion by interventional radiologists. Covered stents are recommended for long-term patency. Long-term complications of TIPS include loss of patency with recurrent portal hypertension, stent infection and portosystemic encephalopathy.

Direct pressure on varices can be applied with an inflatable triple-lumen tube that abuts the gastro-oesophageal junction providing temporary control of bleeding in 90%. Re-bleeding is common when the tube is withdrawn and use is often complicated by aspiration, oesophageal ulceration or perforation. Advantages of this approach are safer transfer of patients to units with expertise or as a temporary measure before definitive therapy. Patients who continue to bleed or are unsuitable for TIPS have a high mortality and should be considered for surgery.

Prevention of variceal haemorrhage

Endoscopic oesophageal band ligation repeated at regular intervals until varices are obliterated is the treatment of choice for secondary prevention of variceal haemorrhage and substantially reduces the incidence of re-bleeding. Endoscopic band ligation is also the preferred approach for primary prevention of variceal haemorrhage for those at high risk, defined by endoscopic criteria.

Pharmacological therapy

Non-selective β-blockers, e.g. propranolol or nadolol, are also used as primary or secondary prophylaxis against variceal haemorrhage. They reduce cardiac output via β_1-receptor antagonism and induce splanchnic vasoconstriction via β_2-receptor antagonism, allowing unopposed α-adrenergic vasoconstriction. Propranolol is extracted extensively in a single pass through the liver so systemic availability is less predictable in cirrhosis with portal hypertension due to variations in hepatic blood flow and portosystemic shunts. Ideally, the dose of propranolol (given twice daily) should be adjusted by measuring the wedged hepatic venous pressure since haemorrhage is rare if this is below 12 mmHg. Nadolol, with a longer duration of action, is given once daily.

Ascites

Fifty per cent of patients with cirrhosis develop ascites within 10 years. Ascites is an important milestone, since 50% will die within 2 years. The process by which ascites forms in cirrhosis is not understood fully but involves activation of the renin–angiotensin–aldosterone system (causing renal retention of sodium and water) and the production of antidiuretic hormone (causing hyponatraemia due to dilution of plasma sodium). Hypoalbuminaemia and portal hypertension favour formation of ascites.

Management of ascites

Perform an ascitic tap to confirm the presence of a transudate before initiating therapy. Ultrasound assesses portal vein patency and the presence of hepatocellular carcinoma. Treatment targets induction of natriuresis with consequent loss of water. Salt restriction is effective; fluid restriction is unnecessary unless the plasma sodium falls below 125 mmol/L. Measurement of urinary sodium before treatment and changes in therapy is helpful, indicating if dietary restriction of sodium has been achieved, helping time the introduction of diuretics, guiding dose changes and indicating when therapy has ceased to be effective.

Bed rest (reduces plasma renin activity) with dietary sodium restriction is effective, but diuretics are needed eventually. Spironolactone is most useful, although maximum efficacy is seen at 2 weeks, following metabolism to products with long duration of action, e.g. canrenone ($t_{1/2}$ 10–35 h). If renal function is conserved, loop diuretics, e.g. furosemide, may be added, counteracting hyperkalaemia induced by spironolactone. A ratio of spironolactone 100 mg to furosemide 40 mg works well and under careful supervision can be increased weekly to a maximum of spironolactone 400 mg furosemide 160 mg. It is rare for patients to tolerate these doses for long.

Monitor body-weight, as patients with oedema and ascites may exhibit rapid weight loss, which should not exceed 0.5 kg/day; extreme negative fluid balance runs the risk of hypovolaemia, electrolyte disturbance, renal impairment and hepatic encephalopathy.

Patients lose weight if the urinary sodium excretion exceeds intake. Unwanted effects of diuretic use are very common; in addition to electrolyte disturbances and renal impairment, cramps are unpleasant and if spironolactone causes painful gynaecomastia, amiloride is an alternative (10–40 mg/day). Those without natriuresis should have diuretic therapy withdrawn.

Abdominal paracentesis was once shunned because of the risk of circulatory failure, but administration of albumin at the time of paracentesis has led to its safe reintroduction. Drainage leads to prompt relief of discomfort of tense, painful ascites and improves circulatory dynamics; it can be undertaken as other measures to control ascites are introduced. Alternatively, paracentesis is the treatment of choice for patients unresponsive to diuretic therapy or with complications of diuretic treatment, especially renal impairment. Planned procedures at intervals of 2–3 weeks restore a degree of quality of life. It is essential to assess subacute bacterial peritonitis at each paracentesis, limit the duration of paracentesis (6 h) and ensure that each litre of ascites removed is matched by 6–8 g albumin given before or with paracentesis. Paracentesis carries a risk of perforation of abdominal contents and abdominal wall varices.

Patients with ascites should receive prophylaxis against subacute bacterial peritonitis. Quinolones, for example ciprofloxacin or norfloxacin, are effective.

Subacute bacterial peritonitis

This medical emergency has high mortality and should be suspected in any patient with liver disease and ascites who develops pain or clinical deterioration. A white cell count > 500 cells/mL or > 250 neutrophils/mL of ascitic fluid confirms the diagnosis. Culture of ascites is often negative and treatment should be triggered by the leucocyte count. Infection of ascites is a manifestation of severe liver disease and attributed to translocation of Gram-negative organisms across the gut wall. Antibiotic use is guided by local hospital preferences, but quinolones are effective unless the patient has been on antibiotic prophylaxis, when a switch to meropenem is recommended. Treatment is for 7–14 days, with an ascitic tap at completion of therapy.

Hepatorenal syndrome

This occurs in 10% of patients with advanced cirrhosis and ascites and is attributed to intense renal vasoconstriction. Three-month mortality is high. Some patients respond to vasoconstrictor agents, particularly terlipressin, while maintaining volume with albumin, over a 14-day interval. Dopamine is ineffective.

Hepatic encephalopathy

Infection, gastrointestinal bleeding, injudicious use of sedatives and diuretics can precipitate hepatic encephalopathy in cirrhosis. The pathophysiology is complex but ammonia is a key player. Diagnosis is confirmed by elevated plasma ammonia and/or typical EEG appearances. Ammonia is derived from the action of colonic urease-containing bacteria and normally undergoes hepatic extraction from portal blood, but with portal/systemic shunting and impaired hepatic metabolism, it reaches high systemic concentrations, affecting the brain adversely.

Lactulose acts as an osmotic laxative to expedite clearance of potentially toxic substances from the gastrointestinal tract. In addition, colonic bacteria metabolise it to lactic and acetic acids, which inhibit the growth of ammonia producing organisms and by lowering pH, reduce non-ionic diffusion of ammonia from the colon into the bloodstream. The correct dose is that which produces two to four soft acidic stools daily (usually 30–60 mL daily). Exceeding this dose causes dehydration.

Neomycin and metronidazole inhibit urease-producing bacteria, but their use is limited by toxicity. The nonabsorbed antibiotic rifaximin is effective over a prolonged period without significant toxicity.

Dietary restriction of protein reduces ammonia production, but any clinical benefit is outweighed by exacerbating malnutrition characteristic of cirrhosis and it is not recommended.

Hepatocellular carcinoma (HCC)

Patients with cirrhosis face a substantial lifetime risk of HCC, which is higher in men. Surveillance with liver ultrasound and serum α-fetoprotein estimation allows early tumour detection. Liver transplantation is curative for 75% with smaller tumours. Surgical resection, radiofrequency ablation and transarterial embolisation (with or without chemotherapy) have beneficial effects that usually fall short of cure. Recent clinical trials show sorafenib extends life by a few months in patients with compensated cirrhosis, but with significant toxicity.

IMMUNE-MEDIATED LIVER DISEASE

Autoimmune hepatitis (AIH)

This chronic inflammatory disease is associated with circulating antinuclear and smooth muscle antibodies and high serum immunoglobulin concentrations (serum IgG above 20 g/L). The presentations include jaundice with ill-health, relapsing/remitting jaundiceand, less commonly, subacute liver failure. A third of patients have cirrhosis at presentation and untreated cases progress to cirrhosis. Corticosteroids are first-line therapy (prednisolone 20 mg daily). Faced with subacute liver failure (increased INR and hepatic encephalopathy) the choice is between corticosteroids (with a risk of sepsis) or liver transplantation. Rituximab, to deplete B cells, may have a role in this unusual scenario but data are preliminary.

The majority of patients improve substantially with corticosteroids and a fall in serum bilirubin occurs usually within 2 weeks. Azathioprine (1 mg/kg daily) should be introduced when jaundice improves and is an effective steroid-sparing agent. In the long term corticosteroid doses should be adjusted according to liver function. Elevated IgG levels settle with successful therapy; a rise in serum IgG predates relapse. Remission can be maintained in the first 2 years by azathioprine with prednisolone (5–10 mg/day). If there is evidence of biochemical remission with a normal IgG after 2 years then withdrawal of corticosteroids can be considered. A liver biopsy to confirm remission is recommended before reducing the dose of corticosteroids. Long-term remission maintained by azathioprine is the goal. There are no clear criteria to determine whether azathioprine can be stopped safely. Corticosteroids often cause steatosis, increasing liver enzymes, which may be mistaken for active AIH.

Mycophenolate mofetil (500 mg twice daily orally) appears useful when patients are intolerant of azathioprine. Patients intolerant of prednisolone respond to budesonide (3–9 mg daily orally). Budesonide is unproven as induction therapy. Some patients never achieve good control with the prednisolone and azathioprine. Mycophenolate with tacrolimus (trough level 5–10 ng/L) may be effective. All causes of liver injury are associated with accelerated bone loss and the use of calcium, vitamin D and bisphosphonates in AIH is recommended.

Primary biliary cirrhosis (PBC)

PBC is a chronic cholestatic liver disease affecting women predominantly from middle age onwards with a heritable component. Fatigue and pruritus are common, early symptoms that usually predate jaundice. The natural history was thought to be inexorable progress to liver failure over a period of 10 years from presentation, but that view is unduly pessimistic. Once jaundice is present, the course of the illness is predictable.

The aetiology of PBC is unknown but high titres of antimitochondrial antibody in almost all and elevated IgM levels with clustering of 'autoimmune disorders' in many suggest immune involvement. There is no role (yet) for immune modulation. Corticosteroids are ineffective; methotrexate is ineffective; azathioprine has marginal benefit. Curiously, patients with PBC treated with ciclosporin after transplantation are less likely to suffer PBC in the grafted liver than those prescribed tacrolimus.

The pruritus of cholestasis can be debilitating and has been attributed to autotaxin. Cholestyramine, which binds bile salts in the gut, has proved effective, but it is unpleasant to swallow, affecting compliance. Ursodeoxycholic acid 10–15 mg/kg daily, which improves liver function tests and pruritus, is free from unwanted effects other than dose-related diarrhoea. Long-term studies indicate ursodeoxycholic acid is associated with a reduced risk of liver decompensation and need for liver transplantation.

Chronic cholestasis leads to malabsorption of fat-soluble vitamins, particularly vitamin D, and deficiency should be corrected to avoid osteomalacia. The use of calcium, vitamin D and bisphosphonates for bone loss in PBC is recommended.

ALCOHOLIC HEPATITIS

The sudden onset of jaundice in a patient consuming alcohol to excess heralds the onset of alcoholic hepatitis. Men are admitted to hospital more often than women, but the latter develop the syndrome after a lower lifetime consumption of alcohol (corrected for body weight). The biochemistry is characteristic, with conjugated bilirubinaemia but a normal ALT and alkaline phosphatase. Liver ultrasound shows no evidence of biliary tract disease. Several scoring systems based on INR, bilirubin and age predict mortality, which is substantial. Liver biopsy shows intense inflammation with a neutrophil infiltration. The presence of bacterial infection is a poor prognostic sign; serum markers of inflammation suggest bacterial infection, which is not necessarily present and related to elevated plasma cytokine levels.

The inflammatory features led to investigation of immune modulation. Randomised controlled trials of corticosteroids (prednisolone tapered from 40 mg/ day for up to 4 weeks) have rendered diverse results. There may be a role for early corticosteroids in patients without active sepsis or bleeding. High serum levels of tumour necrosis factor-α (TNFα) pointed clinical investigators in the direction of pentoxifylline, which inhibits TNFα production. Limited data suggest significant survival benefit with this agent, which has fewer unwanted effects.

Non-alcohol related fatty liver disease

The triad of hypertension, obesity and diabetes mellitus is found commonly in conjunction with abnormal liver function tests. Liver biopsy is almost always abnormal and patients can be separated into those with steatosis alone or those with steatohepatitis. The latter carries a high risk of progressive liver injury with fibrosis, cirrhosis and eventually HCC, especial in older men. Management is directed at control of weight, hypertension, hyperlipidaemia and diabetes mellitus. Metformin and insulin sensitisers such as piaglitazone and rosiglitazone improve liver function tests and some histological features, but have no effect on fibrosis, progression or survival.

VIRAL HEPATITIS

Hepatitis A virus (HAV)

Changing standards of hygiene and an effective vaccine have altered the pattern of illness associated with HAV infection. Symptomatic infection is uncommon in Western countries but more common than it was in the developing world, because infection now occurs at a later age. Significant disease following HAV infection is confined to those over 40 years. Active immunisation against HAV is recommended before travel; protective antibody takes about 2 weeks to develop and lasts for at least 10 years. Passive immunity, using antibody prepared from pooled plasma from immune donors confers temporary protection, but is no longer recommended.

Hepatitis B virus (HBV)

Exposure to HBV results usually in an acute resolving infection which may be asymptomatic or unrecognised. There is no evidence that intervention in acute infection is helpful, but antiviral therapy (below) should be considered for the tiny proportion that develops acute liver failure with detectable HBV replication. Acute infection in an immune suppressed host, where there is a high risk of serious disease or chronic infection, however, should be treated.

Chronic, usually lifelong, infection follows exposure to HBV in infants; the rate of chronic infection falls throughout childhood, affecting the sexes equally, to 5%–10% in adults and men much more than women. Chronic infection is more common in the immune suppressed and the elderly.

Viral load falls with each decade to low levels and HBV protein production (HBsAg and HBeAg) falls in parallel. Treating all patients is neither practical nor appropriate and careful assessment of the stage of the disease is critical to successful management. Natural history studies reveal that viral replication is associated with progressive liver injury, cirrhosis, liver failure and HCC, all more common in men. Successful antiviral therapy is associated with improved survival, a reduced risk of liver failure, a reduced need for liver transplantation and less HCC.

Interferon-α is available in a pegylated formulation allowing weekly administration by subcutaneous injection. A 6-month course in those with active liver disease, with increased liver enzymes, inflammatory changes on the liver biopsy and a low viral load achieves cure in 25%. Young females fare best. Interferon-α should not be used if there is evidence of hepatic decompensation.

Only a small number of patients are suitable for interferon-α. The majority of patients treated currently receive long-term therapy with an oral *nucleot(s) ide analogue*. Agents include *lamivudine, telbivudine clavudine, emtricitabine, adefovir, tenofovir and entecavir*. Some basic points merit mention. HBV has a high rate of spontaneous mutation and both immune responses to HBV and antiviral therapy select for mutations. Lessons from other infectious diseases (HIV and tuberculosis) suggest that long-term combination therapy reduces the chance of treatment failure. Long-term control rather than cure of HBV replication is the pragmatic goal with oral therapy. The duration of treatment is uncertain. Loss of HBsAg from the blood is one situation when treatment can be curtailed with less concern. Patients on therapy should be monitored to assess viral load. Liver function tests should fall to normal in line with the drop in viral load. A failure to control viral replication may be due to the evolution of mutations, inadequate dosing or poor compliance. Mutations should be sought if HBV-DNA is detected after a reasonable period of treatment and for some agents compliance can be assessed by measurement of drug levels in serum. Because the majority of patients will not develop life-threatening liver disease, treatment needs to be targeted at those with or at risk of fibrosis. Some women are reluctant to embark on antiviral therapy while pregnancy is possible; lamivudine, which has been used for years, appears safe in pregnancy, but newer agents cannot yet be regarded as safe although there is no evidence yet to raise concern. Some patients have a high risk of HCC and should also be considered for treatment. Many patients will have been treated, often with lamivudine and may have developed mutations as a result. Pre-treatment mutation profiles are not undertaken routinely but a strong case can be made that they should. Confirmation that a mutation is present during therapy necessitates a change in strategy. The notion that HBV with mutations is less likely to cause liver injury is incorrect.

Perhaps the most important issue in determining which drugs to use first is the clinical context. Those at greatest immediate risk include those with recrudescent HBV post-chemotherapy or subsequent to immune suppression (when the clinical course is accelerated) and with decompensated liver disease. In these scenarios the drugs with the most rapid and potent antiviral effects should be used (tenofovir and entecavir). Where there is less urgency, a combination of agents such as lamivudine with adefovir/tenofovir can be considered.

Tenofovir (even as monotherapy) is associated with the lowest rate of mutations to date (close to zero in large series) but clinical experience is limited to 5 years so far. Lamivudine and similar agents are associated with the highest rate of mutations, with adefovir in an intermediate position. As first line therapy, entecavir has a low level of breakthrough but mutations are much more likely in those with past use of lamivudine, which may not be recorded.

Hepatitis B vaccination

The hepatitis B vaccine (inactivated HBsAg adsorbed on aluminium hydroxide adjuvant) is effective and provides long-lasting immunity against HBV. Response rates fall with increasing age and are lower in the immune compromised. Protection lasts from years to decades and it is unclear if booster vaccination is ever required.

Targeting and screening mothers for HBV in order to protect their children is effective. Babies born to carrier mothers should be vaccinated at birth and after 1 and 6 months and thereafter tested for evidence of immunity and infection beyond 12 months. Concurrent use of hepatitis B immunoglobulin (pooled plasma from highly selected donors with high titre antibody to HBsAg) as passive pro-

phylaxis is also recommended when the mother has high-level HBV replication, but as a human product, it carries an unquantifiable risk of infection.

Hepatitis B immunoglobulin also has a role in providing passive immunity for post-exposure prophylaxis, e.g. after accidental needle stick injury. Conventional vaccination is also important in such cases.

Hepatitis C virus (HCV)

Exposure to HCV is most often a consequence of injecting drug use; vertical transmission (mother to child) occurs in 5%. Historically, HCV infection was associated with transfusion of blood/blood products, but that risk is close to zero with reliable tests for HCV in donors. Acute HCV infection is usually asymptomatic. Chronic infection follows exposure in 85% of cases and is more likely at extremes of age or with immune suppression. Genetic variation, such as polymorphism of IL28B, underlies spontaneous resolution in some patients. Some 5% develop cirrhosis and 25% of those develop HCC. The rate at which liver disease progresses to cirrhosis varies markedly between individuals, but can be rapid in those acquiring infection over the age of 60 years. Age over 40 years at infection, male sex, a raised body mass index, insulin resistance, immune suppression, HIV infection and alcohol abuse all increase the chance that fibrosis will progress. Significant fibrosis at liver biopsy predicts progression at subsequent biopsy.

Treatment is considered for all with viraemia. Interferon-a was the first agent to show efficacy in chronic HCV infection, with 10% responding with long-term elimination of HCV-RNA from serum. Response rates increased using pegylated interferon-a, given weekly, increasing both compliance and efficacy. Combining the weak antiviral agent ribavirin with interferon-a led to an unexpected but marked increase in permanent loss of HCV-RNA. The mode of action is not known. Successful treatment is defined as HCV-RNA negative at completion of treatment and 6 months after completion. Response rates to combination therapy are influenced by several factors, of which age is the most critical. The chances of long-term elimination of HCV with combination treatment fall with every decade to 10% or less in those over 60 years, an important reason not to delay therapy. Other host factors influencing elimination of HCV with therapy include male sex, elevated body mass index, insulin resistance, excessive alcohol consumption, immune suppression and HIV infection. Ribavirin is a known mutagen and men or women planning to have children should delay conception until 6 months after treatment is completed. The magnitude of change in viral load soon after starting treatment gives an indication of long-term efficacy. Further critical issues are that HCV genotypes influence response rates. Those with genotype 2 or 3 have higher response rates than those with other genotypes; consequently, treatment is for 6 months for those with a favourable genotype and 12 months for those with less favourable genotypes. Unfortunately, the severity of disease also influences the treatment response rates such that those most in need have the lowest response rates; treatment is extended by 6 months in cirrhosis.

Side-effects are frequent and many patients curtail therapy early. A clinical decision may be made to stop treatment early if it appears likely to be ineffective, based on early changes in viral load and marked adverse effects.

Adverse effects of ribavirin include rash and haemolysis, which can be severe. Close monitoring is required and the dose adjusted to maintain the haemoglobin above 10 g/L. The use of serum trough ribavirin levels reduces the risk of anaemia. Blood transfusion may be required and some advocate erythropoietin to maintain the haemoglobin concentration. Interferon-α also causes significant toxicity. Pyrexia, muscle ache and headache are likely. Fatigue and depression are common and often debilitating. Interferon-α must be used with caution and regular supervision be given to those with a history of psychiatric disease, especially depression. Anticipating and/or treating depression with agents such as citalopram is effective. Interferon-α may have profound effects on neutrophil, lymphocyte and platelet counts. Careful supervision is required, with dose reductions when those counts reach critical levels.

Some clinicians use GCSF with neutropenia and eltrombopag in those with thrombocytopenia.

Interferon-α is cleared rapidly, mainly by the kidney ($t_{1/2}$ 4 h) and increasing the molecular weight of the drug by conjugation with polyethylene glycol (pegylation) prolongs the $t_{1/2}$ to 40 h, allowing single weekly injections. Pegylation probably improves compliance. Dose reduction may be needed in renal impairment. Ribavirin is also cleared by the kidney and dose reduction is essential in those with renal impairment (guided by serum ribavirin).

A number of agents that target specific HCV enzymes will be available soon, increasing response rates further.

Hepatitis D virus (HDV)

This virus displaces HBV core replacing it with HDV core, but retaining the outer envelope of HBV. HDV infection is rare in clinical practice and occurs either as a simultaneous infection with HBV or as a superinfection in a patient already HBV-positive. Long-term treatment with pegylated interferon-a, i.e. for more than 1 year, controls HDV replication (measured as HDV-RNA in serum) in about 50% of cases.

GALLSTONES

Ursodeoxycholic acid can dissolve cholesterol gallstones, as it supplements the bile acid pool and improves the solubility of cholesterol in bile. It is used rarely, if at all, for this indication but may have a role in patients with disease due to biliary sludge or microcrystals identified at endoscopic ultrasound of the biliary tree; it is often used in patients with biliary tract disease 'prophylactically' to prevent stone formation within the biliary tree. The dose is 8–12 mg/kg daily orally.

PANCREAS

Digestive enzymes

High fat, calories and protein delay gastric emptying, while gastric acid destroys pancreatic enzymes taken by mouth. Only one-tenth of normal pancreatic output is sufficient to prevent steatorrhoea. Acid suppression by proton pump inhibitors improves the efficacy of pancreatic enzyme supplements.

Preparations are of animal origin and variable potency. *Pancreatin*, as Cotazym, is satisfactory. Start patients on the recommended dose of a reliable formulation and vary this according to clinical need, the size and composition of meals. Enteric-coated formulations (pancreatin granules, tablets) are available.

Acute pancreatitis

- Many drugs have been tested for specific effect, but none has shown convincing benefit. The main requirements of therapy are:
- To provide adequate analgesia. Opioids are generally satisfactory; analgesic efficacy outweighs the potential disadvantage of contracting the sphincter of oddi (and retarding the flow of pancreatic secretion); buprenorphine is often preferred.
- To correct hypovolaemia due to the exudation of large amounts of fluid around the inflamed pancreas. Plasma may be required, or blood if the haematocrit falls; in addition, large volumes of electrolyte solution may be needed to preserve renal function.
- To achieve biliary drainage (by endoscopic retrograde cannulation of the pancreas) early in the illness if gallstones are suspected.
- The value of additional interventions, including nutritional support and antibiotic prophylaxis, is as yet unproven.

Drugs and the pancreas

Adverse effects are most commonly manifest as acute pancreatitis. The strongest association is with alcohol abuse. High plasma calcium concentration, including that caused by hypervitaminosis D and parenteral nutrition, also increases the risk. Corticosteroids, didanosine, azathioprine, diuretics (including thiazides and furosemide), sodium valproate, mesalazine and paracetamol (in overdose) are causally related.

IMPORTANT TERMINOLOGY

oesophagus　食管
duodenum　十二指肠
biliary tract　胆道
acetylcholine　乙酰胆碱
pharmacokinetics　药物代谢动力学
hypoalbuminaemia　低蛋白血症

CHALLENGE YOURSELF

1. Please descript the clinical medication for stomach and duodenum diseases.
2. Please list 3 classes of drugs used in peptic ulcer disease.
3. Please describe the meaning of idiosyncratic drug reactions.
4. Please list the factors involved in pathogenesis of peptic ulcer.

Renbin Huang

Chapter | 19 |

Kidney and genitourinary tract

The kidneys comprise only 0.5% of body-weight, yet they receive 25% of the cardiac output. Drugs that affect renal function have important roles in cardiac failure and hyper-tension. Disease of the kidney must be taken into account when prescribing drugs that are eliminated by it.

- Diuretic drugs: their sites and modes of action, classification, adverse effects and uses in cardiac, hepatic, renal and other conditions.
- Carbonic anhydrase inhibitors.
- Cation-exchange resins and their uses.
- Alteration of urine pH.
- Drugs and the kidney.
- Adverse effects.
- Drug-induced renal disease: by direct and indirect biochemical effects and by immunological effects.
- Prescribing for renal disease: adjusting the dose according to the characteristics of the drug and to the degree of renal impairment.
- Nephrolithiasis and its management.
- Pharmacological aspects of micturition.
- Benign prostatic hyperplasia
- Erectile dysfunction.

DIURETIC DRUGS

Definition. A diuretic is any substance that increases urine and solute excretion. This wide definition includes substances not commonly thought of as diuretics, e.g. water. To be therapeutically useful a diuretic should increase the output of sodium as well as of water, because diuretics are normally required to remove oedema fluid, composed of water and solutes, of which sodium is the most important. Diuretics are among the most commonly used drugs, perhaps because the evolutionary advantages of sodium retention have left an ageing population without salt-losing mechanisms of matching efficiency. Each day the body produces 180 L of glomerular filtrate which is modified in its passage down the renal tubules to appear as 1.5 L of urine. Thus, if reabsorption of tubular fluid falls by 1%, urine output doubles. Most clinically useful diuretics are organic anions, which are transported directly from the blood into tubular fluid. The following brief account of tubular function with particular reference to sodium transport will help to explain where and how diuretic drugs act; it should be read with reference to Figure 19.1.

Sites and modes of action

Proximal convoluted tubule

Some 65% of the filtered sodium is actively transported from the lumen of the proximal tubule by the sodium pump (Na^+, K^+-ATPase). Chloride is absorbed passively, accompanying the sodium; bicarbonate is also absorbed, through an action involving carbonic anhydrase. These solute shifts give rise to the iso-osmotic reabsorption of water, with the result that more than 70% of the glomerular filtrate is returned to the blood from this section of the

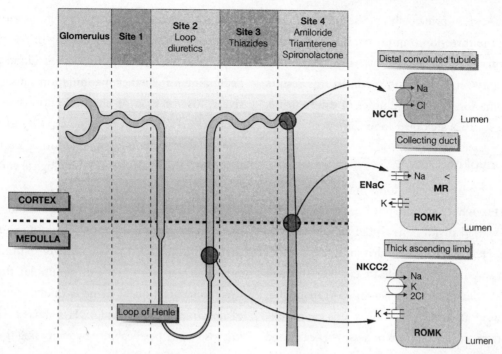

Fig. 19.1 Sites of action of diuretic drugs. Inset cartoons show the transporters and ion channels targeted in tubular cells at these sites. ENaC, epithelial sodium channel; NCCT, thiazide-sensitive Na–Cl co-transporter; NKCC2, Na–K–2Cl co-transporter; ROMK, rectifying outer medullary potassium channel.

nephron. The epithelium of the proximal tubule is described as 'leaky' because of its free permeability to water and a number of solutes.

Osmotic diuretics such as mannitol are non-resorbable solutes which retain water in the tubular fluid (Site 1, Fig. 19.1). Their effect is to increase water rather than sodiumloss, and this is reflected in their special use acutely to reduce intracranial or intraocular pressure and not states associated with sodium overload.

Loop of Henle

The tubular fluid now passes into the loop of Henle where 25% of the filtered sodium is reabsorbed. There are two populations of nephron: those with short loops that are confined to the cortex, and the juxtamedullary nephrons whose long loops penetrate deep into the medulla and are concerned principally with water conservation; the following discussion refers to the latter. The physiological changes are best understood by considering first the ascending limb. In the thick segment (Site 2, Fig. 19.1), sodium and chloride ions are transported from the tubular fluid into the interstitial fluid by the three-ion co-

transporter system (i.e. $Na^+/K^+/2Cl^-$ called NKCC2) driven by the sodium pump. The co-transport of these ions is dependent on potassium returning to the lumen through the rectifying outer medullary potassium (ROMK) channel; otherwise potassium would be rate limiting. As the tubule epithelium is 'tight' here, i.e. impermeable to water, the tubular fluid becomes dilute, the interstitium becomes hypertonic, and fluid in the adjacent descending limb, which is permeable to water, becomes more concentrated as it approaches the tip of the loop, because the hypertonic interstitial fluid sucks water out of this limb of the tubule. The 'hairpin' structure of the loop thus confers on it the property of a countercurrent multiplier, i.e. by active transport of ions a small change in osmolality laterally across the tubular epithelium is converted into a steep vertical osmotic gradient. The high osmotic pressure in themedullary interstitium is sustained by the descending and ascending vasa recta, long blood vessels of capillary thickness that lie close to the loops of Henle and act as countercurrent exchangers, for the incoming blood receives sodium from the outgoing blood. Furosemide, bumetanide, piretanide, torasemide and ethacrynic acid act principally at (Site 2, Fig. 19.1) by inhibiting the three-ion transporter, thus preventing sodium ion reabsorption and lowering the osmotic gradient between cortex and medulla; this results in the formation of large volumes of dilute urine. Hence, these drugs are called 'loop' diuretics.

Distal convoluted tubule

The ascending limb of the loop then re-enters the renal cortex where its morphology changes into the thin-walled distal convoluted tubule (Site 3, Fig. 19.1). Here uptake is still driven by the sodium pump but sodium and chloride are taken up through a different transporter, the Na-Cl co-transporter, called NCC (formerly NCCT). Both ions are rapidly removed from the interstitium because cortical blood flow is high and there are no vasa recta present; the epithelium is also tight at Site 3 and consequently the urine becomes more dilute. Thiazides act principally at this region of the cortical diluting segment by blocking the NCC transporter.

Collecting duct

In the collecting duct (Site 4, Fig. 19.1), sodium ions are exchanged for potassium and hydrogen ions. The sodium ions enter through the epithelial Na channel (called ENaC), which is stimulated by aldosterone. The aldosterone (mineralocorti-coid) receptor is inhibited by the competitive receptor antagonist *spironolactone*, whereas the sodium channel is inhibited by *amiloride and triamterene*. All three of these diuretics are potassium sparing because potassium is normally secreted through the potassium channel, ROMK (Fig. 19.1), down the potential gradient created by sodium reabsorption.

All other diuretics, acting proximal to Site 4, cause potassium loss, because they dump sodium into the collecting duct. Removal of this sodium through ENaC increases the potential gradient for potassium secretion through ROMK. The potassium-sparing diuretics are normally considered weak diuretics because Site 4 is normally responsible for 'only' 2%–3% of sodium reabsorption, and they usually cause less sodium loss than thiazides or loop

diuretics. Nevertheless, patients with genetic abnormalities of ENaC show salt wasting or retention to a degree that significantly affects their blood pressure, depending on whether the mutation causes, respectively, loss or gain of channel activity. Although ENaC clearly does not have the capacity to compensate for large sodium losses, e.g. during loop diuretic usage, it is the main site of physiological control (via aldosterone) over sodium loss.

The collecting duct then travels back through the medulla to reach the papilla; in doing so it passes through a gradient of increasing osmotic pressure which draws water out of tubular fluid. This final concentration of urine is under the influence of *antidiuretic hormone* (ADH) whose action is to increase water permeability by increasing the expression of specific water channels (aquaporins); in its absence water remains in the collecting duct. Ethanol causes diuresis by inhibiting the release of ADH from the posterior pituitary gland.

Diuresis may also be achieved by extrarenal mechanisms, by raising the cardiac output and increasing renal blood flow, e.g. with dobutamine and dopamine.

Classification

The maximum efficacy in removing salt and water that any drug can achieve is dependent on its site of action, and it is appropriate to rank diuretics according to their natriuretic capacity, as set out below. The percentages refer to the highest fractional excretion of filtered sodium under carefully controlled conditions and should not be taken to represent the average fractional sodium loss during clinical use.

High efficacy

Furosemide and the other 'loop' diuretics can cause up to 25% of filtered sodium to be excreted. Their action impairs the powerful urine-concentrating mechanism of the loop of Henle and confers higher efficacy compared with drugs that act in the relatively hypotonic cortex. Progressive increase in dose is matched by increasing diuresis, i.e. they have a high 'ceiling' of effect. In fact, they are so effective that over-treatment can readily dehydrate the patient. Loop diuretics remain effective at a glomerular filtration rate (GFR) below 10 mL/min (normal 120 mL/min).

Moderate efficacy

The thiazide family, including *bendroflumethiazide* and the related *chlortalidone, clopamide, indapamide, mefruside, metolazone* and *xipamide*, cause 5%10% of filtered sodium load to be excreted. Increasing the dose produces relatively little added diuresis compared to loop diuretics, i.e. they have a low 'ceiling' of effect. Such drugs cease to be effective once the GFR has fallen below 20 mL/min (except *metolazone*).

Low efficacy

Triamterene, amiloride and spironolactone cause 2%–3% of the filtered sodium to be excreted. They are potassium sparing and combine usefully with more efficacious diuretics to prevent the potassium loss, which other diuretics cause.

Osmotic diuretics, e.g. *mannitol*, also fall into this category.

INDIVIDUAL DIURETICS

High-efficacy (loop) diuretics

Furosemide

Furosemide acts on the thick portion of the ascending limb of the loop of Henle (Site 2 Fig. 19.1) to produce the effects described above. Because more sodium is delivered to Site 4, exchange with potassium leads to urinary potassium loss and hypokalaemia. Magnesium and calcium loss are increased by furosemide to about the same extent as sodium; the effect on calcium is utilised in the emergency management of hypercalcaemia.

Pharmacokinetics. Absorption of furosemide from the gastrointestinal tract is subject to considerable intra- and inter-individual variation and it is highly bound to plasma proteins. The $t_{1/2}$ is 2 h, but this rises to over 10 h in renal failure.

Uses. Furosemide is very successful for the relief of oedema. Urine production rises progressively with increasing dose. Taken orally it acts within an hour and diuresis lasts up to 6 h. Enormous urine volumes can result and over-treatment may lead to hypovolaemia and circulatory collapse. Given intravenously it acts within 30 min and can relieve acute pulmonary oedema, partly by a venodilator action which precedes the diuresis. An important feature of furosemide is that it retains efficacy even at a low GFR (10 mL/min or less). The dose is 20–120 mg by mouth per day i.m. or i.v. 20–40 mg is given initially. For use in renal failure, special high-dose tablets (500 mg) are available, and a solution of 250 mg in 25 mL, which should be infused intravenously at a rate not greater than 4 mg/min. In patients with heart failure absorption from the gut is prolonged, the dose–response curve for furosemide is shifted to the right and downward, i.e. the response to any given dose is reduced; this should be borne in mind when dosing these patients.

Adverse effects. Adverse effects are uncommon, apart from excess of therapeutic effect (electrolyte disturbance and hypotension due to low plasma volume) and those mentioned in the general account for diuretics (below). They include nausea, pancreatitis and, rarely, deafness, which is usually transient and associated with rapid intravenous injection in renal failure. Non-steroidal anti-inflammatory drugs (NSAIDs), notably indometacin, reduce furosemide-induced diuresis, probably by inhibiting the formation of vasodilator prostaglandins in the kidney.

Bumetanide, piretanide and ethacrynic acid are similar to furosemide. Bumetanide may be preferred over furosemide in heart failure because of its more predictable oral absorption. Ethacrynic acid is less widely used as it is more prone to cause adverse effects, especially nausea and deafness. Torasemide is an effective antihypertensive agent at lower (nonnatriuretic) doses (2.5–5 mg/day) than those used for oedema (5–40 mg/day).

Moderate-efficacy diuretics

Thiazides. Thiazides depress salt reabsorption in the distal convoluted tubule (at Site 3 Fig. 19.1), i.e. upstream of the region of sodium–potassium exchange at Site 4 (Fig. 19.1). Hence these drugs have the important effect of raising potassium excretion. Thiazides lower blood pressure, initially due to a reduction in intravascular volume but chronically by a reduction in peripheral vascular resistance. The latter is accompanied by diminished responsiveness of vascular smooth muscle to noradrenaline/norepinephrine; they may also have a direct action on vascular smooth muscle membranes, acting on an as yet unidentified ion channel.

Uses. Thiazides are given for mild cardiac failure and mild hypertension, or for more severe degrees of hypertension, in combination with other drugs.

Pharmacokinetics. Thiazides are generally well absorbed orally and most begin to act within an hour. Differences among the numerous derivatives lie principally in duration of action. The relatively water-soluble, e.g. *cyclopenthiazide, chlorothiazide, hydrochlorothiazide*, are most rapidly eliminated, their peak effect occurring within 4–6 h and passing off by 10–12 h. They are excreted unchanged in the urine and active secretion by the proximal renal tubule contributes to their high renal clearance and $t_{1/2}$ of less than 4 h.

The relatively lipid-soluble members of the group, e.g. *polythiazide, hydroflumethiazide*, distribute more widely into body tissues and act for >24 h, which can be problematic if the drug is used for diuresis, but there is no evidence this property makes them more effective at controlling hypertension. With the exception of metolazone, thiazides are not effective when renal function is moderately impaired (GFR< 20 mL/min), because they are not filtered in sufficient concentration to inhibit the NCC.

Adverse effects in general are discussed below. Rashes (sometimes photosensitive), thrombocytopenia and agranulocytosis occur. Thiazide-type drugs increase total plasma cholesterol concentration, but in long-term use this is less than 5%, even at high doses. The questions about the appropriateness of thiazides for mild hypertension, of which ischaemic heart disease is a common complication, are laid to rest by their proven success in randomized outcome comparisons.

Bendroflumethiazide is a satisfactory member

for routine use. For a diuretic effect the oral dose is 5–10 mg, which usually lasts less than 12 h, so that it should be given in the morning. As an antihypertensive, 2.5 mg is commonly prescribed. However, this dose does not achieve maximal blood pressure reduction in patients with salt- dependent hypertension (which includes most patients receiving a blocker of the renin–angiotensin system), and has not been shown to prevent strokes or heart attacks. New guidance is likely to recommend some return to higher doses – and/or greater use of the thiazide-like diuretics (below), with or without co-prescribed K^+-sparing diuretic. Important potassium depletion is uncommon, but plasma potassium concentration should be checked in potentially vulnerable groups such as the elderly. If marked hypokalaemia occurs hyperaldosteronism should be excluded.

Hydrochlorothiazide is a satisfactory alternative. Other members of the group include benzthiazide, chlorothiazide, cyclopenthiazide, hydroflumethiazide and polythiazide.

Diuretics related to the thiazides. Several compounds, although not strictly thiazides, share structural similarities with them and probably act at the same site on the nephron; they therefore exhibit moderate therapeutic efficacy. Overall, these substances have a longer duration of action, are used for oedema and hypertension, and their profile of adverse effects is similar to that of the thiazides. They are listed below.

Chlortalidone acts for 48–72 h after a single oral dose.

Indapamide is structurally related to chlortalidone but lowers blood pressure at subdiuretic doses, perhaps by altering calcium flux in vascular smooth muscle. It has less apparent effect on potassium, glucose or uric acid excretion.

Metolazone is effective when renal function is impaired. It potentiates the diuresis produced by furosemide and the combination can be effective in resistant oedema, although the risk of hypokalaemia is very high.

Xipamide is structurally related to chlortalidone and to furosemide. It induces a diuresis for about 12 h that is brisker than with thiazides; this may trouble the elderly.

Low-efficacy diuretics

Spironolactone (Aldactone) is structurally similar to aldosterone and competitively inhibits its action in the distal tubule (Site 4 Fig.19.1; exchange of potassium for sodium); excessive secretion of aldosterone contributes to fluid retention in hepatic cirrhosis, nephrotic syndrome, congestive heart failure and primary hypersecretion (Conn's syndrome). Spironolactone is also useful in the treatment of resistant hypertension, where increased aldosterone sensitivity is increasingly recognised as a contributory factor.

Spironolactone itself has a short $t_{1/2}$ (1.6 h), being extensively metabolised, and its prolonged diuretic effect is due to the most significant active product, canrenone ($t_{1/2}$ 17 h). Spironolactone is relatively ineffective when used alone but is more efficient when combined with a drug that reduces sodium reabsorption proximally in the tubule, i.e. a loop diuretic. Spironolactone (and amiloride and triamterene; see below) usefully reduces the potassium loss caused by loop diuretics, but its combination with another potassium sparing diuretic must be avoided as hyperkalaemia will result. Dangerous potassium retention is particularly likely if spironolactone is given to patients with impaired renal function. It is given orally in one or more doses totaling 100–200 mg/day. Maximum diuresis may not occur for up to 4 days. If after 5 days the response is inadequate, the dose may be increased to 300–400 mg/day. Lower doses (0.5–1 mg/kg) are required to treat hypertension.

Adverse effects. Oestrogenic effects are the major limitation to its long-term use. They are dose dependent, but in the Randomized Aldactone Evaluation Study (RALES) even 25 mg/day caused breast tenderness or enlargement in 10% of men. Women may also report breast discomfort or menstrual irregularities, including amenorrhoea. Minor gastrointestinal upset also occurs and there is increased risk of gastroduodenal ulcer and bleeding. These are reversible on stopping the drug. Spironolactone is reported to be carcinogenic in rodents, but many years of clinical experience suggest that it is safe in humans. Nevertheless, the UK licence for its use in essential hypertension was withdrawn (i.e. possible use long term in a patient group that includes the relatively young), but is retained for other indications.

Eplerenone is a spironolactone analogue licensed for use in heart failure that appears to be free of the oestrogenic effects; probably because of its lower affinity for the oestrogen receptor. It is useful in patients who need an aldosterone-receptor blocking agent, but are intolerant of the endocrine effects of spironolactone.

Amiloride blocks the ENaC sodium channels in the distal tubule. This action complements that of the thiazides with which it is frequently combined to increase sodium loss and limit potassium loss. One such combination, coamilozide (Moduretic; amiloride 2.5–5 mg plus hydrochlorothiazide 25–50 mg) is used for hypertension or oedema. The maximum effect of amiloride occurs about 6 h after an oral dose, with a duration of action greater than 24 h ($t_{1/2}$ 21 h). The oral dose is 5–20 mg daily.

Triamterene (Dytac) is a potassium-sparing diuretic with an action and use similar to that of amiloride. The diuretic effect extends over 10 h. Gastrointestinal upsets occur. Reversible, non-oliguric renal failure may occur when triamterene is used with indometacin (and presumably other NSAIDs). It may also give the urine a blue coloration.

INDICATIONS FOR DIURETICS

- Oedema states associated with sodium overload, e.g. cardiac, renal or hepatic disease, and also without sodium overload, e.g. acute pulmonary oedema following myocardial infarction. Note that oedema may also be localised, e.g. angioedema over the face and neck or around the ankles with some calcium channel blockers, or due to low plasma albumin, or immobility in the elderly; in none of these circumstances is a diuretic indicated.
- Hypertension, by reducing intravascular volume and probably by other mechanisms too, e.g. reduction of sensitivity to noradrenergic vasoconstriction.

- Hypercalcaemia. Furosemide reduces calcium reabsorption in the ascending limb of the loop of Henle, which action may be utilised in the emergency reduction of raised plasma calcium levels in addition to rehydration and other measures.
- Idiopathic hypercalciuria, a common cause of renal stone disease, may be reduced by thiazide diuretics.
- The syndrome of inappropriate secretion of antidiuretic hormone secretion (SIADH) may be treated with furosemide if there is a dangerous degree of volume overload.
- Nephrogenic diabetes insipidus, paradoxically, may respond to diuretics which, by contracting vascular volume, increase salt and water reabsorption in the proximal tubule, and thus reduce urine volume.

Therapy

Congestive cardiac failure

Oral diuretics are easily given repeatedly, and lack of supervision can result in insidious over-treatment. Relief at disappearance of the congestive features can mask exacerbation of the low-output symptoms of heart failure, such as tiredness and postural dizziness due to reduced blood volume. A rising blood urea level is usually evidence of reduced glomerular blood flow consequent on a fall in cardiac output, but does not distinguish whether the cause of the reduced output is over diuresis or worsening of the heart failure itself. The simplest guide to the success or failure of diuretic regimens is to monitor body-weight, which the patient can do equipped with just bathroom scales. Fluid intake and output charts are more demanding of nursing time, and often less accurate.

Renal oedema

The chief therapeutic aims are to reduce dietary sodium intake and to prevent excessive sodium retention using diuretic drugs. Reduction of sodium reabsorption in the renal tubule by diuretics is most effective where glomerular filtration has not been seriously reduced by disease. Furosemide and bumetanide are effective even when the filtration rate is very low; furosemide may usefully be combined with metolazone but the resulting profound diuresis requires careful monitoring. Secondary hyperaldosteronism complicates the nephrotic syndrome because albumin loss causes plasma colloid pressure to fall, and the resulting diversion of intravascular volume to the interstitium activates the renin–angiotensin–aldosterone system; spironolactone may then be added usefully to potentiate a loop diuretic and to conserve potassium, loss of which can be severe.

Hepatic ascites

Ascites and oedema are due to portal venous hypertension together with decreased plasma colloid osmotic pressure causing hyperaldosteronism as with nephrotic oedema (above). Furthermore, diversion of renal blood flow from the cortex to the medulla favours sodium retention. In addition to dietary sodium restriction, spironolactone is the preferred diuretic to produce a gradual diuresis; too vigorous depletion of sodium with added potassium loss and hypochloraemic alkalosis may worsen hepatic encephalopathy. Abdominal paracentesis can be very effective if combined with human albumin infusion to prevent further aggravating hypoproteinaemia.

Adverse effects characteristic of diuretics

Potassium depletion. Diuretics that act at Sites 1, 2 and 3 (Fig. 19.1) cause more sodium to reach the sodium–potassium exchange site in the distal tubule (Site 4) and so increase potassium excretion. This subject warrants discussion because hypokalaemia may cause cardiac arrhythmia in patients at risk (e.g. receiving digoxin). The safe lower limit for plasma potassium concentration is normally quoted as 3.5 mmol/L. Whether or not diuretic therapy causes significant lowering of serum potassium levels depends both on the drug and on the circumstances in which it is used:

- *The loop diuretics* produce a smaller fall in serum potassium concentration than do the thiazides, for equivalent diuretic effect, but have a greater capacity for diuresis, i.e. higher efficacy especially in large dose, and so are associated with greater decline in potassium levels. If diuresis is brisk and continuous, clinically important potassium depletion is likely to occur.

- *Low dietary intake* of potassium predisposes to hypokalaemia; the risk is particularly

- notable in the elderly, many of whom ingest less than 50 mmol per day (the dietary normal is 80 mmol).

- Hypokalaemia may be aggravated by other drugs, e.g. β_2-adrenoceptor agonists, theophylline, corticosteroids, amphotericin.

- Hypokalaemia during diuretic therapy is also more likely in hyperaldosteronism, whether primary or more commonly secondary to severe liver disease, congestive cardiac failure or nephrotic syndrome.

- Potassium loss occurs with diarrhoea, vomiting or small bowel fistula, and may be aggravated by diuretic therapy.

- When a thiazide diuretic is used for hypertension, there is probably no case for routine prescription of a potassium supplement if no predisposing factors are present.

- Potassium depletion can be minimised or corrected by:

- Maintaining a good dietary potassium intake (fruits, fruit juices, vegetables).

- Combining a potassium-depleting with a potassium-sparing drug.

- Intermittent use of potassium-losing drugs, i.e. drug holidays.

- Potassium supplements: KCl is preferred because chloride is the principal anion excreted along with sodium when high-efficacy diuretics are used. Potassium-sparing diuretics generally defend plasma potassium more effectively than potassium supplements. All forms of potassium are irritant to the gastrointestinal tract, and in the oesophagus may even cause ulceration. The elderly, in particular, should be warned never to take such tablets dry but always with a large cupful of liquid and sitting upright or standing.

Hyperkalaemia may occur, especially if a potassium-sparing diuretic is given to a patient with impaired renal function. ACE inhibitors and angiotensin II receptor antagonists can also cause a modest increase in plasma potassium levels. They may cause dangerous hyperkalaemia if combined with KCl supplements or other potassium-sparing drugs, in the presence of impaired renal function. These may not be obvious, for example, to the patient who is using an unprescribed 'low sodium' salt substitute to reduce their salt (NaCl) intake. However, with suitable monitoring the combination can be used safely, as was well illustrated by the RALES trial. Ciclosporin, tacrolimus, indometacin and possibly other NSAIDs may cause hyperkalaemia with the potassium-sparing diuretics.

Hypovolaemia can result from over-treatment. Acute loss of excessive fluid leads to postural hypotension and dizziness. A more insidious state of chronic hypovolaemia can develop, especially in the elderly. After initial benefit, the patient becomes sleepy and lethargic. Blood urea concentration rises and sodium concentration may be low. Renal failure may result.

Urinary retention Sudden vigorous diuresis can cause acute retention of urine in the presence of bladder neck obstruction, e.g. due to prostatic enlargement.

Hyponatraemia may result if sodium loss occurs in patients who drink a large quantity of water when taking a diuretic. Other mechanisms are probably involved, including enhancement of antidiuretic hormone release. Such patients have reduced total body sodium and extracellular fluid and are oedema free. Discontinuing the diuretic and restricting water intake are effective. The condition should be distinguished from hyponatraemia with oedema, which develops in some patients with congestive cardiac failure, cirrhosis or nephrotic syndrome. Here salt and water intake should be restricted because extracellular fluid volume is expanded.

The combination of a potassium-sparing diuretic and ACE inhibitor can also cause severe hyponatraemia – more commonly than life-threatening hyperkalaemia.

Urate retention with hyperuricaemia and, sometimes, clinical gout occurs with thiazides and loop diuretics. The effect is unimportant or negligible with the low-efficacy diuretics, e.g. amiloride and spironolactone. Two mechanisms appear to be responsible. First, diuretics cause volume depletion, reduction in glomerular filtration and increased absorption of almost all solutes in the proximal tubule, including urate. Second, diuretics and uric acid are organic acids and compete for the transport mechanism that pumps such substances from the blood into the tubular fluid. Diuretic-induced hyperuricaemia can be prevented by allopurinol or probenecid (which also antagonizes diuretic efficacy by reducing their transport into the urine).

Magnesium deficiency. Loop and thiazide diuretics cause significant urinary loss of magnesium; potassium-sparing diuretics probably also cause magnesium retention. Magnesium deficiency brought about by diuretics is rarely severe enough to induce the classic picture of neuromuscular irritability and tetany but cardiac arrhythmias, mainly of ventricular origin, do occur and respond to repletion of magnesium (2 g or 8 mmol of Mg^{2+} is given as 4 mL 50% magnesium sulphate infused i.v. over 10–15 min followed by up to 72 mmol infused over the next 24 h).

Carbohydrate intolerance is caused by those diuretics that produce prolonged hypokalaemia, i.e. the loop and thiazide type. This may affect the depolarisation and entry of calcium into islet cells which is necessary to stimulate formation and release of insulin, so glucose intolerance is probably due to secondary insulin deficiency. Insulin requirements thus increase in established diabetics and the disease may become manifest in latent diabetics. The effect is generally reversible over several months.

Calcium homeostasis. Renal calcium loss is increased by the loop diuretics; in the short term this is not a serious disadvantage and indeed furosemide may be used in the management of hypercalcaemia after rehydration has been achieved. In the long term, hypocalcaemia may be harmful, especially in elderly patients, who tend in any case to be in negative calcium balance. Thiazides, by contrast, decrease renal excretion of calcium and this property may influence the choice of diuretic in a potentially calcium-

deficient or osteoporotic individual, as thiazide use is associated with a reduced risk of hip fracture in the elderly. The hypocalciuric effect of the thiazides has also been used effectively in patients with idiopathic hypercalciuria, the commonest metabolic cause of renal stones.

Interactions

Loop diuretics (especially as intravenous boluses) potentiate ototoxicity of aminoglycosides and nephrotoxicity of some cephalosporins. NSAIDs tend to cause sodium retention, which counteracts the effect of diuretics; the mechanism may involve inhibition of renal prostaglandin formation. Diuretic treatment of a patient taking lithium can precipitate toxicity from this drug (the increased sodium loss is accompanied by reduced lithium excretion). Other drugs that may induce hyperkalaemia, hypokalaemia, hyponatraemia or glucose intolerance with diuretics are described above.

Abuse of diuretics

Psychological abnormality sometimes takes the form of abuse of diuretics and/or purgatives. The subject usually desires to slim to become more attractive, or may have anorexia nervosa. There can be severe depletion of sodium and potassium, with renal tubular damage due to chronic hypokalaemia.

Osmotic diuretics

Osmotic diuretics are small molecular weight substances that are filtered by the glomerulus but not reabsorbed by the renal tubule, and thus increase the osmolarity of the tubular fluid. Thus they prevent reabsorption of water (and also, by more complex mechanisms, of sodium) principally in the proximal convoluted tubule and probably also the loop of Henle. The result is that urine volume increases according to the load of osmotic diuretic.

Mannitol, a polyhydric alcohol (mol. wt. 452), is used most commonly; it is given intravenously. In addition to its effect on the kidney, mannitol encourages the movement of water from inside cells to the extracellular fluid, which is thus transiently expanded before diuresis occurs. These properties define its uses, which are for rapid reduction of intracranial or intraocular pressure, and to maintain urine flow to prevent renal tubular necrosis. Because it increases circulatory volume, mannitol is contraindicated in congestive cardiac failure and pulmonary oedema.

Methylxanthines

The general properties of the methylxanthines (theophylline, caffeine) are discussed elsewhere. Their mild diuretic action probably depends in part on smooth muscle relaxation in the afferent arteriolar bed increasing renal blood flow, and in part on a direct inhibitory effect on salt reabsorption in the proximal tubule. Their uses in medicine depend on other properties.

CARBONIC ANHYDRASE INHIBITORS

The enzyme carbonic anhydrase facilitates the reaction between carbon dioxide and water to form carbonic acid (H_2CO_3), which then breaks down to hydrogen (H^+) and bicarbonate (HCO_3^-) ions. This process is fundamental to the production of either acid or alkaline secretions, and high concentrations of carbonic anhydrase are present in the gastric mucosa, pancreas, eye and kidney. Because the number of H^+ ions available to exchange with Na^+ in the proximal tubule is reduced, sodium loss and dieresis occur. But HCO_3^- reabsorption from the tubule is also reduced, and its loss in the urine leads within days to metabolic acidosis, which attenuates the diuretic response to carbonic anhydrase inhibition. Consequently, inhibitors of carbonic anhydrase are obsolete as diuretics, but still have specific uses. Acetazolamide is the most widely used carbonic anhydrase inhibitor.

Reduction of intraocular pressure. This action is not due to diuresis (thiazides actually raise intraocular pressure slightly). The formation of aqueous humour is an active process requiring a supply of bicarbonate ions which depends on carbonic anhydrase. Inhibition of carbonic anhydrase reduces the formation of aqueous humour and lowers intraocular pressure. This is a local action and is not affected

by the development of acid–base changes elsewhere in the body, i.e. tolerance does not develop. In patients with acute glaucoma, acetazolamide can be taken either orally or intravenously. Acetazolamide is not recommended for long-term use because of the risk of hypokalaemia and acidosis, but brinzolamide or dorzolamide are effective as eye drops, well tolerated, and thus suitable for chronic use in glaucoma.

High-altitude (mountain) sickness may affect unacclimatised people at altitudes over 3 000 metres, especially after rapid ascent; symptoms range from nausea, lassitude and headache to pulmonary and cerebral oedema. The initiating cause is hypoxia: at high altitude, the normal hyperventilatory response to falling oxygen tension is inhibited because alkalosis is also induced. Acetazolamide induces metabolic acidosis, increases respiratory drive, notably at night when apnoetic attacks may occur, and thus helps to maintain arterial oxygen tension. The usual dose is 125–250 mg twice daily, given orally on the day before the ascent and continued for 2 days after reaching the intended altitude; 250 mg twice daily is used to treat established high-altitude sickness, combined with a return to a lower altitude. (Note that this is an unlicensed indication in the UK.) As an alternative or in addition to acetazolamide, dexamethasone may be used: 2 mg 6-hourly for prevention, and 4 mg 6-hourly for treatment.

The drug has two other uses. In periodic paralysis, where sudden falls in plasma K^+ concentration occur due to its exchange with Na^+ in cells, the rise in plasma H^+ caused by acetazolamide provides an alternative cation to K^+ for exchange with Na^+. Acetazolamide may be used occasionally as a second-line drug for *tonic–clonic* and *partial epileptic seizures*.

Adverse effects. High doses of acetazolamide may cause drowsiness and fever, rashes (it is a sulfonamide-type drug) and paraesthesiae may occur (from the acidosis). Blood disorders have been reported. Renal calculi may develop, because the urine calcium is in less soluble form, owing to low citrate content of the urine, a consequence of metabolic acidosis.

Dichlorphenamide is a similar, but a more potent, inhibitor of carbonic anhydrase.

413

CATION-EXCHANGE RESINS

Cation-exchange resins are used to treat hyperkalaemia by accelerating potassium loss through the gut, especially in the context of poor urine output or before dialysis (the most effective means of treating hyperkalaemia). The resins consist of aggregations of big insoluble molecules carrying fixed negative charges, which loosely bind positively charged ions (cations); these readily exchange with cations in the fluid environment to an extent that depends on their affinity for the resin and their concentration.

Resins loaded with sodium or calcium exchange these cations preferentially with potassium cations in the intestine (about 1 mmol potassium per g resin); the freed cations (calcium or sodium) are absorbed and the resin plus bound potassium is passed in the faeces. The resin does not merely prevent absorption of ingested potassium, but it also takes up the potassium normally secreted into the intestine and ordinarily reabsorbed.

In hyperkalaemia, oral administration or retention enemas of a polystyrene sulphonate resin may be used. A sodium-phase resin (Resonium A) should obviously not be used in patients with renal or cardiac failure as sodium overload may result. A calcium-phase resin (Calcium Resonium) may cause hypercalcaemia and should be avoided in predisposed patients, e.g. those with multiple myeloma, metastatic carcinoma, hyperparathyroidism and sarcoidosis. Orally they are very unpalatable, and as enemas patients rarely manage to retain them for as long as necessary (at least 9 h) to exchange potassium at all available sites on the resin.

ALTERATION OF URINE pH

Alteration of urine pH by drugs is sometimes desirable. The most common reason is in the treatment of poisoning. A summary of the main indications appears below.

Alkalinisation of urine:

- increases the elimination of salicylate, Phenobarbital and chlorophenoxy herbicides, e.g. 2,4-D, MCPA

- treats crystal nephropathy by increasing drug solubility, e.g. of methotrexate, sulphonamides and triamterene. NB indinavir requires acidification
- reduces irritation of an inflamed urinary tract
- discourages the growth of certain organisms, e.g. *Escherichia coli*.

The urine can be made alkaline by sodium bicarbonate i.v., or by potassium citrate by mouth. Sodium overload may exacerbate cardiac failure, and sodium or potassium excess are dangerous when renal function is impaired.

Acidification of urine:

- is used as a test for renal tubular acidosis
- increases elimination of amfetamine, methylene dioxymethamfetamine (MDMA or 'Ecstasy'), dexfenfluramine, quinine and phencyclidine, although it is very rarely needed.

Oral NH_4Cl, taken with food to avoid vomiting, acidifies the urine. It should not be given to patients with impaired renal or hepatic function. Other means include arginine hydrochloride, ascorbic acid and calcium chloride by mouth.

DRUGS AND THE KIDNEY

Adverse effects

The kidneys comprise only 0.5% of body-weight, yet they receive 25% of the cardiac output. It is hardly surprising that drugs can damage the kidney and that disease of the kidney affects responses to drugs.

Drug-induced renal disease

Drugs and other chemicals damage the kidney by:

1. Direct biochemical effect. Substances that cause such toxicity include:
   - heavy metals, e.g. mercury, gold, iron, lead
   - antimicrobials, e.g. aminoglycosides, amphotericin, cephalosporins
   - iodinated radiological contrast media, e.g. agents for visualising the biliary tract
   - analgesics, e.g. NSAID combinations and paracetamol (actually its metabolite, NABQI, in overdose)

- solvents, e.g. carbon tetrachloride, ethylene glycol

2. Indirect biochemical effect

   - cytotoxic drugs and uricosurics may cause urate to be precipitated in the tubule
   - calciferol may cause renal calcification by inducing hypercalcaemia
   - diuretic and laxative abuse can cause tubular damage secondary to potassium and sodium depletion
   - anticoagulants may cause haemorrhage into the kidney

3. Immunological effect. A wide range of drugs produces a wide range of injuries:

   - drugs include phenytoin, gold, penicillins, hydralazine, isoniazid, rifampicin, penicillamine, probenecid, sulphonamides
   - injuries include arteritis, glomerulitis, interstitial nephritis, systemic lupus erythematosus.

A drug may cause damage by more than one of the above mechanisms, e.g. gold. The sites and pathological types of injury are as follows:

Glomerular damage. The large surface area of the glomerular capillaries renders them susceptible to damage from circulating immune complexes; glomerulonephritis, proteinuria and nephrotic syndrome may result, e.g. following treatment with penicillamine when the patient has made an immune response to the drug. The degree of renal impairment is best reflected in the creatinine clearance, which measures the GFR because creatinine is eliminated entirely by this process.

Tubule damage. By concentrating 180 L glomerular filtrate into 1.5 L urine each day, renal tubule cells are exposed to much greater amounts of solutes and environmental toxins than are other cells in the body. The proximal tubule, through which most water is reabsorbed, experiences the greatest concentration and so suffers most drug-induced injury. Specialised transport processes concentrate acids, e.g. salicylate (aspirin), cephalosporins and bases, e.g. aminoglycosides, in renal tubular cells. Heavy metals and radiographic contrast media also cause damage at this site. Proximal tubular toxicity is manifested by leakage of glucose, phosphate, bicarbonate and amino acids into the urine. The counter-current multiplier and exchange systems of urine concentration cause some drugs to accumulate in the renal medulla. Analgesic nephropathy is often first evident at this site, partly because of high tissue concentration and partly, it is believed, because of ischaemia through inhibition of locally produced vasodilator prostaglandins by NSAIDs. The distal tubule is the site of lithium-induced nephrotoxicity; damage to the medulla and distal nephron is manifested by failure to concentrate the urine after fluid deprivation and by failure to acidify urine after ingestion of ammonium chloride.

Tubule obstruction. Given certain physicochemical conditions, crystals can deposit within the tubular lumen. Methotrexate, for example, is relatively insoluble at low pH and can precipitate in the distal nephron when the urine is acid, typically in high dose for chemotherapy. Similarly the uric acid produced by the metabolism of nucleic acids released during rapid tumour cell lysis can cause a fatal urate nephropathy. This was a particular problem with the introduction of chemotherapy for leukaemias until the introduction of allopurinol, which is now routinely given before the start of chemotherapy to block xanthine oxidase so that the much more soluble uric acid precursor, hypoxanthine, is excreted instead. A recent and highly effective alternative to allopurinol for high-risk patients is recombinant uric acid oxidase (Rasburicase), which catalyses conversion of uric acid to the more soluble allantoin. Crystal nephropathy is also reported with agents as diverse as indinavir, orlistat, ciprofloxacin, aciclovir, sulfadiazine and triamterene.

Other drug-induced lesions of the kidney include:

- Vasculitis, caused by allopurinol, isoniazid, sulphonamides.
- Allergic interstitial nephritis, caused by penicillins (especially), thiazides, allopurinol, phenytoin, sulphonamides.
- Drug-induced lupus erythematosus, caused by hydralazine, procainamide, sulfasalazine. Drugs may thus induce any of the common clinical syndromes of renal injury, namely:
- Acute renal failure, e.g. aminoglycosides, cisplatin.
- Nephrotic syndrome, e.g. penicillamine, gold,

- captopril (only at higher doses than now recommended).
- Chronic renal failure, e.g. NSAIDs.
- Functional impairment, i.e. reduced ability to dilute and concentrate urine (lithium), potassium loss in urine (loop diuretics), acid–base imbalance (acetazolamide).

PRESCRIBING IN RENAL DISEASE

Drugs may:

- exacerbate renal disease (see above)
- be ineffective, e.g. thiazide diuretics in moderate or severe renal failure; uricosurics
- be potentiated by accumulation due to failure of renal excretion

Clearly, the first option is to seek an alternative drug that does not depend on renal elimination. Problems of safety arise for patients with impaired renal function who must be treated with a drug that is potentially toxic and that is wholly or largely eliminated by the kidney.

A knowledge of, or at least access to, sources of pharmacokinetic data is essential for safe therapy for such patients, e.g. manufacturers' data, formularies and specialist journals.

The $t_{1/2}$ of other drugs, where activity is terminated by metabolism, is unaltered by renal impairment, but many such drugs produce pharmacologically active metabolites that are more water soluble than the parent drug, rely on the kidney for their elimination, and accumulate in renal failure, e.g. acebutolol, diazepam, warfarin, pethidine.

The majority of drugs fall into an intermediate class and are partly metabolised and partly eliminated unchanged by the kidney.

Administering the correct dose to a patient with renal disease must therefore take into account both the extent to which the drug normally relies on renal elimination and the degree of renal impairment; the best guide to the latter is the creatinine clearance and not the serum creatinine level itself,6 which can be notoriously misleading in the elderly and at extremes of body mass.

General rules

1. Drugs that are completely or largely excreted by the kidney, or drugs that produce active, renally eliminated metabolites: give a normal or, if there is special cause for caution, a slightly reduced initial dose, and lower the maintenance dose or lengthen the dose interval in proportion to the reduction in creatinine clearance.
2. Drugs that are completely or largely metabolised to inactive products: give normal doses. When the note of special caution applies, a modest reduction of initial dose and the maintenance dose rate are justified while drug effects are assessed.
3. Drugs that are partly eliminated by the kidney and partly metabolised: give a normal initial dose and modify the maintenance dose or dose interval in the light of what is known about the patient's renal function and the drug, its dependence on renal elimination and its inherent toxicity.

Recall that the time to reach steady-state blood concentration is dependent only on drug $t_{1/2}$, and a drug reaches 97% of its ultimate steady-state concentration in $5 \times t_{1/2}$. Thus, if $t_{1/2}$ is prolonged by renal impairment, so also will be the time to reach steady state.

Schemes for modifying drug dosage for patients with renal disease diminish but do not remove their increased risk of adverse effects; such patients should be observed particularly carefully throughout a course of drug therapy. Where the service is available, dosing should be monitored by drug plasma concentration measurements.

Dose adjustment for patients with renal impairment

- Adjustment of the initial dose (or where necessary the priming or loading dose) is generally unnecessary, as the volume into which the drug has to distribute should be the same in the uraemic as in the healthy subject. There are exceptions to this rule of thumb; for example, the volume of distribution of digoxin is contracted in uraemic patients due to altered tissue binding of the drug.
- Adjustment of the maintenance dose involves

either reducing each dose given or lengthening the time between doses.

- Special caution is needed when the patient is hypoproteinaemic and the drug is usually extensively plasma protein bound, or in advanced renal disease when accumulated metabolic products may compete for protein binding sites. Careful observation is required in the early stages of dosing until response to the drug can be gauged.

NEPHROLITHIASIS

Calcareous stones result from hypercalciuria, hyperoxaluria and hypocitraturia. Hypercalciuria and hyperoxaluria render urine supersaturated in respect of calcium salts; citrate makes calcium oxalate more soluble and inhibits its precipitation from solution.

Non-calcareous stones occur most commonly in the presence of urea-splitting organisms, which create conditions in which magnesium ammonium phosphate (struvite) stones form. Urate stones form when urine is unusually acid (pH <5.5). Management. Recurrent stone-formers should maintain a urine output exceeding 2.5 L/day. Some benefit from restricting dietary calcium or reducing the intake of oxalate- rich foods (rhubarb, spinach, tea, chocolate, peanuts).

- Thiazide diuretics reduce the excretion of calcium and oxalate in the urine, and reduce the rate of stone formation.
- Sodium cellulose phosphate (Calcisorb) binds calcium in the gut, reduces urinary calcium excretion and may benefit calcium stone-formers.
- Allopurinol is effective in those who have high excretion of uric acid in the urine.
- Potassium citrate, which alkalinises the urine, should be given to prevent formation of pure uric acid stones.

PHARMACOLOGICAL ASPECTS OF MICTURITION

Some physiology

The detrusor, whose smooth muscle fibres comprise the body of the bladder, is innervated mainly by parasympathetic nerves, which are excitatory and cause the muscle to contract. The internal sphincter, a concentration of smooth muscle at the bladder neck, is well developed only in the male and its principal function is to prevent retrograde flow of semen during ejaculation. It is rich in $\alpha 1$ adrenoceptors, activation of which causes contraction. There is an abundant supply of oestrogen receptors in the distal two-thirds of the female urethral epithelium, which degenerates after the menopause causing loss of urinary control.

When the detrusor relaxes and the sphincters close, urine is stored; this is achieved by central inhibition of parasympathetic tone accompanied by a reflex increase in α-adrenergic activity. Voiding requires contraction of the detrusor, accompanied by relaxation of the sphincters. These acts are coordinated by a micturition centre, probably in the pons.

Functional abnormalities

The main abnormalities that require treatment are:

- *Unstable bladder* or detrusor instability, characterised by uninhibited, unstable contractions of the detrusor which may be of unknown aetiology or secondary to an upper motor neurone lesion or bladder neck obstruction.
- *Decreased bladder activity* or hypotonicity due to a lower motor neurone lesion or over-distension of the bladder, or both.
- Urethral sphincter dysfunction which is due to various causes including weakness of the muscles and ligaments around the bladder neck, descent of the urethrovesical junction and periurethral fibrosis; the result is stress incontinence.
- Atrophic change affecting the distal urethra in females.

Drugs that may be used to alleviate abnormal micturition

Antimuscarinic. drugs such as oxybutynin and flavoxate are used to treat urinary frequency; they increase bladder capacity by diminishing unstable detrusor contractions. Both drugs may cause dry mouth and blurred vision, and may precipitate glaucoma. Oxybutynin has a high level of unwanted effects; the dose needs to be carefully assessed, particularly in the elderly. Flavoxate has less marked side effects but is also less effective. Propiverine, tolterodine and trospium are also antimuscarinic drugs used for urinary frequency, urgency and incontinence. Propantheline was formerly used widely in urinary incontinence but had a low response rate and a high incidence of adverse effects; it is now used mainly for adult enuresis. The need for continuing antimuscarinic drug therapy should be reviewed after 6 months.

Tricyclic antidepressants. Imipramine, amitriptyline and nortriptyline are effective, especially for nocturnal but also for daytime incontinence. Their parasympathetic blocking (antimuscarinic) action is probably in part responsible, but imipramine may also benefit by altering the patient's sleep profile.

Oestrogens, either applied locally to the vagina or taken by mouth, may benefit urinary incontinence due to atrophy of the urethral epithelium in post-menopausal.

Parasympathomimetic drugs, e.g. bethanechol, carbachol and distigmine, may be used to stimulate the detrusor when the bladder is hypotonic, e.g. due to an upper motor neurone lesion. Distigmine, which is an anticholinesterase, is preferred but, as its effect is not sustained, intermittent catheterisation is also needed when the hypotonia is chronic.

BENIGN PROSTATIC HYPERPLASIA (BPH)

One of the commonest problems in men older than 50 years, BPH was for a long time helped only by surgical intervention. The prostate gland is a mixture of capsular and stromal tissue, rich in adrenoceptors, and glandular tissue under the influence of androgens. Both these, the α receptors and androgens, are targets for drug therapy. Because the bladder itself has few α receptors, it is possible to use selective $α_1$-blockade without affecting bladder contraction.

α-Adrenoceptor antagonists. Prazosin, alfuzosin, indoramin, terazosin and doxazosin are all α-adrenoceptor blockers with selectivity for the $α_1$ subtype. They cause significant increases (compared to placebo) in objective measures such as maximal urine flow rate, and drugs also improve semi-objective symptom scores. In normotensive men, falls in blood pressure are generally negligible; in hypertensive patients, the decline in pressure can be regarded as an added bonus (provided concurrent treatment is adjusted). These drugs can cause dizziness and asthenia, even in the absence of marked changes in blood pressure. Nasal stuffiness can be a problem – especially in patients who resort to α-agonists (e.g. pseudoephedrine) for rhinitis.

These adverse events are avoided by using tamsulosin, which selectively blocks the $α_{1A}$ subclass of adrenoceptors and is therefore less likely to affect blood pressure, provided the single 400-microgram daily dose of tamsulosin is not exceeded.

Finasteride. An alternative drug for such prostatic symptoms is the type II 5α-reductase inhibitor, finasteride, which inhibits conversion of testosterone to its more potent metabolite, dihydrotestosterone. Finasteride does not affect serum testosterone, or most non-prostatic responses to testosterone. It reduces prostatic volume by about 20% and increases urinary flow rates by a similar degree. These changes translate into modest clinical benefits, which are generally inferior to those of $α_1$ antagonist.

Finasteride ($t_{1/2}$ 6 h) is taken as a single 5-mg tablet each day. The improvement in urine flow appears over 6 months (as the prostate shrinks in size), and in 5%–10% of patients may be at the cost of some loss of libido. The serum concentration of prostate-specific antigen is approximately halved. Although this may reflect a real reduction in risk of prostatic cancer, in patients receiving finasteride it is safer to regard values of the antigen in the upper half of the usual range as abnormal. Lower doses of finasteride have also been used successfully to halt the development of baldness. *Dutasteride* is an alternative 5α-reductase inhibitor.

Other antiandrogens, such as the gonadorelin agonists, are used in the treatment of prostatic cancer, but the need for parenteral administration makes them less suitable for BPH.

ERECTILE DYSFUNCTION

Erectile dysfunction (ED), the inability to achieve or maintain a penile erection sufficient to permit satisfactory sexual intercourse, is estimated to affect over 100 million men worldwide, with a prevalence of 39% in those aged 40 years.

Its numerous causes include cardiovascular disease, diabetes mellitus and other endocrine disorders, alcohol and substance abuse, and psychological factors (14%). Although the evidence is not conclusive, drug therapy is thought to underlie 25% of cases, reputedly from antidepressants (selective serotonin-reuptake inhibitors (SSRIs) and tricyclics), phenothiazines, cyproterone acetate, fibrates, levodopa, histamine H2-receptor blockers, phenytoin, carbamazepine, allopurinol, indometacin and, possibly, β-adrenoceptor blockers and thiazide diuretics.

Sexual arousal releases from the endothelial cells of penile blood vessels neurotransmitters that relax the smooth muscle of the arteries, arterioles and trabeculae of its erectile tissue, greatly increasing penile blood flow and facilitating rapid filling of the sinusoids and expansion of the corpora cavernosa. The venous plexus that drains the penis thus becomes compressed between the engorged sinusoids and the surrounding and firm tunica albuginea, causing the near-total cessation of venous outflow. The penis becomes erect, with an intracavernous pressure of 100 mmHg. The principal neurotransmitter is nitricoxide, which actsbyraising intracellular concentrations of cyclic guanosinemonophosphate (cGMP) to relax vascular smooth muscle. The isoenzyme phosphodiesterase type 5 (PDE5) is selectively active in penile smooth muscle and terminates the action of cGMP by converting it to the inactive non-cyclic GMP.

Sildenafil (Viagra) is a highly selective inhibitor of PDE5 (70-fold more so than isoenzymes 1, 2, 3 and 4 of PDE), prolonging the action of cGMP, and thus the vasodilator and erectile response to normal sexual stimulation. Its emergence as an agent for erectile dysfunction is an example of serendipity in drug development.

Sildenafil was originally being developed for another indication but when the clinical trials ended the volunteers declined to return surplus tablets for they had discovered that the drug conferred unexpected benefits on their sexual lives. Its development for erectile dysfunction followed.

Sildenafil is well absorbed orally, reaches a peak in the blood after 30–120 min and has a $t_{1/2}$ of 4 h. The drug should be taken 1 h before intercourse in an initial dose of 50 mg (25 mg in the elderly); thereafter 25–100 mg may be taken according to response, with a maximum of one 100-mg dose per 24 h. Food may delay the onset and offset of effect. Sildenafil is effective in 80% of patients with erectile dysfunction.

Adverse effects are short lived, dose related, and comprise headache, flushing, nasal congestion and dyspepsia. High doses can inhibit PDE6, which is needed for phototransduction in the retina, and some patients report a transient blue coloration to their vision. Some patients experience non-arteritic anterior ischaemic optic neuropathy (NAION), consisting of blurred vision and/or visual field loss generally within 24 h of taking sildenafil. Priapism has been reported.

Interactions. Sildenafil is contraindicated in patients who are taking organic nitrates, for their metabolism is blocked and severe and acute hypotension result. Patients with recent stroke or myocardial infarction, or whose blood pressure is known to be less than 90/50 mmHg, should not use it. Sildenafil is a substrate for the P450 isoenzyme CYP 3A4 (and to a lesser extent CYP2C9 which gives scope for drug–drug interactions. The metabolic inhibitors erythromycin, saquinavir and ritonavir (protease inhibitors used for AIDS), and cimetidine produce substantial rises in the plasma level of sildenafil. More selective PDE5 inhibitors now available include vardenafil, which has a kinetic profile similar to that of sildenafil, and taladafil which has a very long $t_{1/2}$ (17 h). This latter could be viewed as a mixed blessing in erectile dysfunction, but is important for the use of this drug class in pulmonary hypertension.

Alprostadil is a stable form of prostaglandin E1, a

powerful vasodilator, and is effective for psychogenic and neuropathic erectile dysfunction. Alprostadil increases arterial inflow and reduces venous outflow by contracting the corporal smooth muscle that occludes draining venules. It can be administered either as a urethral suppository (0.125–1 mg) or injected directly into the dorsolateral aspect of the proximal third of the penis (socalled intracavernosal injection). The duration and grade of erection are dose related. The patient package insert from the manufacturer provides some helpful drawings. The dose (5–20 micrograms) is titrated initially in the doctor's surgery, aiming for an erection lasting for not more than 1 h. Painful erection is the commonest adverse effect.

Papaverine, an alkaloid (originally extracted from opium but devoid of narcotic properties), is also a nonspecific phosphodiesterase inhibitor. It is effective (up to 80%) for psychogenic and neurogenic erectile dysfunction by intracavernosal self-injection shortly before intercourse (efficacy may be increased by also administering the α-adrenoceptor blocker phentolamine), although its use has waned with the availability of orally active selective PDE5 inhibitors such as sildenafil. Papaverine used in this way can cause priapism requiring aspiration of the corpora cavernosa and injection of α-adrenoceptor agonist, e.g. metaraminol.

SUMMARY

- The actions of drugs on the kidney are of an importance disproportionate to the low prevalence of kidney disorders.
- The kidney is the main site of loss, or potential loss, of all body substances. It is among the functions of drugs to help reduce losses of desirable substances and increase losses of undesired substances.
- The kidney is also at increased risk of toxicity from foreign substances because of the high concentrations these can achieve in the renal medulla.
- Diuretics are among the most commonly used drugs, perhaps because the evolutionary advantages of sodium retention have left an ageing

population without salt-losing mechanisms of matching efficiency.

- Loop diuretics, acting on the ascending loop of Henle, are the most effective, and are used mainly to treat the oedema states. Potassium is lost as well as sodium.
- Thiazides, acting on the cortical diluting segment of the tubule, have lower natriuretic efficacy, but slightly greater antihypertensive efficacy than loop diuretics. Potassium loss is rarely a significant problem with thiazides, and thiazides reduce loss of calcium.
- Potassium retention with hyperkalaemia can occur with potassium-sparing diuretics, which block sodium transport in the last part of the distal tubule, either directly (e.g. amiloride) or by blocking aldosterone receptors (spironolactone).
- Drugs have little ability to alter the filtering function of the kidney when this is reduced by nephron loss.
- Prostatic enlargement is the main disease of the lower urinary tract; drugs can be used to postpone, or avoid, surgery. The symptoms of benign prostatic hyperplasia are partially relieved either by α1-adrenoceptor blockade or by inhibiting synthesis of dihydrotestosterone in the prostate.
- Drugs are effective for the relief of erectile dysfunction, notably sildenafil, a highly specific phosphodiesterase inhibitor.

IMPORTANT TERMINOLOGY

congestive cardiac failure　充血性心力衰竭
benign prostatic hyperplasia (BPH)　良性前列腺增生
α-adrenoceptor antagonists　α-受体拮抗剂

CHALLENGE YOURSELF

1. Please descript the clinical application of furosemide.
2. Please descript the adverse effects of the diuretic drugs.
3. Please descript the mechanisms by which high - and medium - acting diuretic drugs induce Low serum potassium.

Jun Li

Chapter 20

Drugs and the skin

DERMAL PHARMACOKINETICS

Human skin is a highly efficient self-repairing barrier that permits terrestrial life by regulating heat and water loss while preventing the ingress of noxious chemicals and microorganisms. A drug applied to the skin may diffuse from the stratum corneum into the epidermis and then into the dermis, to enter the capillary microcirculation and thus the systemic circulation (Fig. 20.1). The features of components of the skin in relation to drug therapy, whether for local or systemic effect, are worthy of examination.

The principal barrier to penetration resides in the multiple-layered lipid-rich stratum corneum. The passage of a drug through this layer is influenced by its:

- *Physicochemical features*: lipophilic drugs can utilise the *intra*cellular route because they readily cross cell walls, whereas hydrophilic drugs principally take the *inter*cellular route, diffusing in fluid-filled spaces between cells.
- *Molecular size*: most therapeutic agents suitable for topical delivery measure 100–500 Da.

Drugs are presented in vehicles (bases), designed to vary in the extent to which they increase hydration of the stratum corneum; e.g. oil-in-water creams promote hydration. Increasing the water content of the stratum corneum via occlusion or hydration generally increases the penetration of both lipophilic and hydrophilic materials. This may be due to an increased fluid content of the lipid bilayers. The stratum corneum and stratum granulosum layers become more similar with hydration and occlusion, thus lowering the partition coefficient of the molecule passing through the interface. Some vehicles also contain substances intended to enhance penetration by reducing the barrier properties of the stratum corneum, e.g. fatty acids, terpenes, surfactants. Encapsulation of drugs into vesicular liposomes may enhance drug delivery to specific compartments of the skin, e.g. hair follicles.

Absorption through normal skin varies with site. From the sole of the foot and the palm of the hand it is relatively low; it increases progressively on the forearm, trunk, head and neck; and on the scrotum and vulva absorption is very high. Where the skin is damaged by inflammation, burn or exfoliation, barrier function is reduced and absorption is further increased.

If an occlusive dressing (impermeable plastic membrane) is used, absorption increases by as much as 10-fold (plastic pants for babies are occlusive, and some ointments are partially occlusive). Systemic toxicity can result from use of occlusive dressing over large areas.

Transdermal delivery systems are now used to administer drugs via the skin for systemic effect.

Vehicles for presenting drugs to the skin

Dermatological formulations tend to be classified by their physical properties. The formulations below

Fig. 20.1 Principal pathways operating during topical drug delivery.

are described in order of decreasing water content. All water-based formulations must contain preservatives, e.g. chlorocresol, but these rarely cause allergic contact dermatitis.

Liquid formulations

Water or a solvent is the most important component. The preparation can be a soak, a bath or a paint. Wet dressings are generally used to cleanse, cool and relieve pruritus in acutely inflamed lesions, especially where there is much exudation, e.g. atopic eczema. The frequent reapplication and the cooling effect of evaporation of the water reduce the inflammatory response by inducing superficial vasoconstriction (an effect enhanced when alcohol is present in the formulation). Sodium chloride solution 0.9%, stringent substances, e.g. aluminium acetate lotion, or potassium permanganate soaks or compresses of approximately 0.01%–0.05% can be used. The use of *lotions* (wet dressings) over very large areas can reduce body temperature dangerously in the old or the very ill.

Two-phase or multiple liquid shake lotions, e.g. calamine lotion, are essentially a convenient way of applying a powder to the skin with additional cooling due to evaporation of the water. They are contraindicated when there is much exudate, because crusts form. Lotions, after evaporation, sometimes produce excessive drying of the skin, but this can be reduced if oils are included, as in oily calamine lotion.

Creams

These are emulsions of either oil in water (washable; cosmetic 'vanishing' creams) or water in oil. The water content allows the cream to rub in well. A cooling effect (cold creams) is obtained with both groups as the water evaporates.

Oil-in-water creams, e.g. aqueous cream, mix with serous discharges and are especially useful as vehicles for water-soluble drugs. They may contain a wetting (surface tension-reducing) agent (cetomacrogol). Various other ingredients, e.g. calamine, zinc, may be added to it.

Water-in-oil creams, e.g. oily cream, zinc cream, behave like oils in that they do not mix with serous discharges, but their chief advantage over ointments (below) is that the water content makes them easier to spread and they give a better cosmetic effect. They act as lubricants and emollients, and can be used on hairy parts. Water-in-oil creams can be used as vehicles for lipid-soluble substances.

Creams, being less occlusive and effective at hydrating the stratum corneum, are not as effective for drug delivery as ointments.

Ointments

Ointments are greasy and thicker than creams. Some are both lipophilic and hydrophilic, i.e. by occlusion they promote dermal hydration, but are also water miscible. Other ointment bases are composed largely of lipid; by preventing water loss they have a hydrating effect on skin and are used in chronic dry conditions. Ointments contain fewer preservatives and are less likely to sensitise. There are two main kinds:

Water-soluble ointments include mixtures of

macrogols and polyethylene glycols; their consistency can be varied readily. They are easily washed off and are used in burn dressings, as lubricants and as vehicles that readily allow passage of drugs into the skin, e.g. hydrocortisone.

Emulsifying ointment is made from emulsifying wax (cetostearyl alcohol and sodium lauryl sulphate) and paraffins. Aqueous cream is an oil-in-water emulsion of emulsifying ointment.

Non-emulsifying ointments do not mix with water. They adhere to the skin to prevent evaporation and heat loss, i.e. they can be considered a form of occlusive dressing (with increased systemic absorption of active ingredients); skin maceration may occur. Non-emulsifying ointments are helpful in chronic dry and scaly conditions, such as atopic eczema, and as vehicles; they are not appropriate where there is significant exudation. They are difficult to remove except with oil or detergents, and are messy and inconvenient, especially on hairy skin. Paraffin ointment contains beeswax, paraffins and cetostearyl alcohol.

Collodions and gels

Collodions are preparations of a thickening agent, e.g. cellulose nitrate (pyroxylin) dissolved in an organic solvent. The solvent evaporates rapidly and the resultant flexible film is used to hold a medicament, e.g. salicylic acid, in contact with the skin. They are irritant and inflammable, and are used to treat only small areas of skin.

Gels or *jellies* are semi-solid colloidal solutions or suspensions used as lubricants and as vehicles for drugs. They are sometimes useful for treating the scalp.

Pastes

Pastes, e.g. zinc compound paste, are stiff, semi-occlusive ointments containing insoluble powders. They are very adhesive and are valuable for treating highly circumscribed lesions while preventing spread of active ingredients on to surrounding skin. Their powder content enables them to absorb a moderate amount of discharge. They can be used as vehicles, e.g. coal tar paste, which is zinc compound paste with 7.5% coal tar. Lassar's paste is used as a vehicle for dithranol in the treatment of well-circumscibed plaque psoriasis.

Solid preparations

Solid preparations such as dusting powders, e.g. zinc starch and talc, may cool by increasing the effective surface area of the skin and they reduce friction between skin surfaces by their lubricating action. Although usefully absorbent, they cause crusting if applied to exudative lesions. They may be used alone or as specialised vehicles for, e.g., fungicides.

Emollients and barrier preparations

Emollients hydrate the skin, and soothe and smooth dry scaly conditions. They need to be applied frequently as their effects are short lived. There is a variety of preparations but aqueous cream, in addition to its use as a vehicle (above), is effective when used as a soap substitute. Various other ingredients may be added to emollients, e.g. menthol, camphor or phenol for its mild antipruritic effect, and zinc and titanium dioxide as astringents.

Barrier preparations. Many different kinds have been devised for use in medicine, in industry and in the home to reduce dermatitis. They rely on water-repellent substances, e.g. silicones (dimethicone cream), and on soaps, as well as on substances that form an impermeable deposit (titanium, zinc, calamine). The barrier preparations are useful in protecting skin from discharges and secretions (colostomies, nappy rash), but are ineffective when used under industrial working conditions. Indeed, the irritant properties of some barrier creams can enhance the percutaneous penetration of noxious substances. A simple after-work emollient is more effective.

Silicone sprays and *occlusives*, e.g. hydrocolloid dressings, may be effective in preventing and treating pressure sores. Masking creams (camouflaging preparations) for obscuring unpleasant blemishes from view are greatly valued by patients. They may consist of titanium oxide in an ointment base with colouring appropriate to the site and the patient.

Topical analgesics

Counterirritants and rubefacients are irritants that stimulate nerve endings in intact skin to relieve pain in skin (e.g. post-herpetic), viscera or muscle supplied by the same nerve root. All produce inflammation of the skin, which becomes flushed – hence the term 'rubefacients'. The best counterirritants are physical agents, especially heat. Many compounds have been used for this purpose and suitable preparations contain salicylates, nicotinates, menthol, camphor and capsaicin. Specific transient receptor potential (TRP) cation channels involved in sensory perception in skin can be stimulated by these drugs. The moderate heat receptor TRPV1 is sensitive to capsaicin as well as moderate heat (42–52℃), whereas TRPM8 is stimulated specifically by temperatures below 26℃ and by menthol.

Topical non-steroidal anti-inflammatory drugs (NSAIDs) can be used to relieve musculoskeletal pain.

Local anaesthetics. Lidocaine and prilocaine are available as gels, ointments and sprays to provide reversible block of conduction along cutaneous nerves. Benzocaine and amethocaine (tetracaine) carry a high risk of sensitisation.

Volatile aerosol sprays, beloved by sports people, produce analgesia by cooling and by placebo effect.

Antipruritics

Mechanisms of itch are both peripheral and central. Itch (at least histamine-induced itch) is not a minor or low-intensity form of pain. Cutaneous histamine injection stimulates a specific group of C fibres with very low conduction speeds and large fields, distinct from those that signal pain. Second-order neurones then ascend via the spinothalamic tract to the thalamus. In the central nervous system, endogenous opioid peptides are released (the opioid antagonist naloxone can relieve some cases of intractable itch). Itch signalling appears to be under tonic inhibition by pain. If pain after histamine injection is reduced by opioid then itch results and, if pain is ablated by lidocaine, itch sensation increases. Prolonged inflam-

mation in the skin may lead to peripheral and central sensitisation, thus leading non-itchy stimuli to be reinterpreted as itch.

Liberation of histamine and other autacoids in the skin also contributes and may be responsible for much of the itch of urticarial allergic reactions. Histamine release by bile salts may explain some, but not all, of the itch of obstructive jaundice. It is likely that other chemical mediators, e.g. serotonin, progesterone metabolites, endogenous opioids and prostaglandins, are involved.

Generalised pruritus

In the absence of a primary dermatosis it is important to search for an underlying cause, e.g. iron deficiency, liver or renal failure, and lymphoma, but there remain patients in whom the cause either cannot be removed or is not known. Antihistamines (H_1-receptor), especially chlorphenamine and hydroxyzine orally, are used for their sedative or anxiolytic effect (except in urticaria); they should not be applied topically over a prolonged period because of risk of allergy. In severe pruritus, a sedative antidepressant may also help.

The itching of obstructive jaundice might be relieved by the anion exchange resin colestyramine, an endoscopically placed nasobiliary drain, or phototherapy with ultraviolet B light. Naltrexone offers short-term relief of the pruritus associated with haemodialysis.

Localised pruritus

Scratching or rubbing seems to give relief by converting the intolerable persistent itch into a more bearable pain. A vicious cycle can be set up in which itching provokes scratching, and scratching leads to infected skin lesions that itch, as in prurigo nodularis. Covering the lesion or enclosing it in a medicated bandage so as to prevent any further scratching or rubbing may help. Multiple intralesional triamcinolone injections and thalidomide may be used in recalcitrant cases of prurigo nodularis.

Topical corticosteroid preparations are used to treat the underlying inflammatory cause of pruritus, e.g. in eczema. A cooling application such as 0.5%–2% menthol in aqueous cream is temporarily antipruritic.

Calamine and *astringents* (aluminium acetate, tannic acid) may help. Local anaesthetics do not offer any long-term solution and, as they are liable to sensitise the skin, they are best avoided. Topical doxepin can be helpful in localised pruritus but extensive use induces sedation and may cause allergic contact dermatitis.

Pruritus ani is managed by attention to any underlying disease, e.g. haemorrhoids, parasites, and hygiene. Emollients, e.g. washing with aqueous cream and a weak corticosteroid with antiseptic/anticandida application, may be used briefly to settle any acute eczema or superinfection. Some cases are a form of neurodermatitis, and an antihistamine with anti-anxiolytic properties, e.g. hydroxyzine, or a low-dose sedative antidepressant, e.g. doxepin, and mirtazapine, may be helpful. Secondary contact sensitivity, e.g. to local anaesthetics, must be considered.

Adrenocortical steroids

Actions. Adrenal steroids possess a range of actions, of which the following are relevant to topical use:

- Inflammation is suppressed, particularly when there is an allergic factor, and immune responses are reduced.
- Antimitotic activity suppresses proliferation of keratinocytes, fibroblasts and lymphocytes (useful in psoriasis, but also causes skin thinning).
- Vasoconstriction reduces ingress of inflammatory cells and humoral factors to the inflamed area; this action (blanching effect on human skin) has been used to measure the potency of individual topical corticosteroids.

Penetration into the skin is governed by the factors outlined at the beginning of the chapter. The vehicle should be appropriate to the condition being treated: an ointment for dry, scaly conditions; a water-based cream for weeping eczema.

Uses. Adrenal corticosteroids should be considered a symptomatic and sometimes curative, but not preventive, treatment. Ideally a potent steroid should

be given only as a short course and reduced as soon as the response allows. Corticosteroids are most useful for eczematous disorders (atopic, discoid, contact), whereas dilute corticosteroids are especially useful for flexural psoriasis (where other therapies are highly irritant). Adrenal corticosteroids of highest potency are reserved for recalcitrant dermatoses, e.g. lichen simplex, lichen planus, nodular prurigo and discoid lupus erythematosus.

Topical corticosteroids should be applied sparingly. The difficulties and dangers of systemic adrenal steroid therapy are sufficient to restrict such use to serious conditions (such as pemphigus and generalised exfoliative dermatitis) not responsive to other forms of therapy.

Guidelines for the use of topical corticosteroids

- Use for symptom relief and not prophylactically.
- Choose the appropriate therapeutic potency, e.g. mild for the face. In cases likely to be resistant, use a very potent preparation, e.g. for 3 weeks, to gain control, after which change to a less potent preparation.
- Choose the appropriate vehicle, e.g. a water-based cream for weeping eczema, an ointment for dry, scaly conditions.
- Prescribe in small but adequate amounts so that serious overuse is unlikely to occur without the doctor knowing, e.g. weekly quantity by group (Table 20.1): very potent 15 g; potent 30 g; other 50 g.
- Occlusive dressing should be used only briefly. Note that babies' plastic pants are an occlusive dressing as well as being a social amenity.
- If it's wet, dry it; if it's dry, wet it. The traditional advice contains enough truth to be worth repeating.
- One or two applications a day are all that is usually necessary.

Choice. Topical corticosteroids are classified according to both drug and potency, i.e. therapeutic efficacy in relation to weight. Their potency is determined by the amount of vasoconstriction a topical corticosteroid produces (McKenzie skin-blanching test) and the degree to which it inhibits inflammation. Choice of preparation relates both to the disease and the site of intended use. High-potency preparations are commonly needed for lichen planus and discoid lupus erythematosus; weaker preparations (hydrocortisone 0.5%–2.5%) are usually adequate for eczema, for use on the face and in childhood.

Table 20.1 Topical corticosteroid formulations conventionally ranked according to therapeutic potency

Potency	Formulations
Very potent	Clobetasol (0.05%); also formulations of diflucortolone (0.3%), halcinonide
Potent	Beclometasone (0.025%); also formulations of betamethasone, budesonide, desoximetasone, diflucortolone (0.1%), fluclorolone, fluocinolone (0.025%), fluocinonide, fluticasone, hydrocortisone butyrate, mometasone (once daily), triamcinolone
Moderately potent	Clobetasone (0.05%); also formulations of alclometasone, clobetasone, desoximetasone, fluocinolone (0.00625%), fluocortolone, fluandrenolone
Mildly potent	Hydrocortisone (0.1%–1.0%); also formulations of alclomethasone, fluocinolone (0.0025%), methylprednisolone

Important note: the ranking is based on agent and its concentration; the same drug appears in more than one rank.

When a skin disorder requiring a corticosteroid is already infected, a preparation containing an antimicrobial is added, e.g. fusidic acid or clotrimazole. When the infection has been eliminated, the corticosteroid may be continued alone. Intralesional injections are used occasionally to provide high local concentrations without systemic effects in chronic dermatoses, e.g. hypertrophic lichen planus and discoid lupus erythematosus.

Adverse effects. Used with restraint, topical corticosteroids are effective and safe. Adverse effects are more likely with formulations ranked therapeutically as very potent or potent.

Short-term use. Infection may spread.

Long-term use. Skin atrophy can occur within 4 weeks and may or may not be fully reversible. It reflects loss of connective tissue, which also causes striae (irreversible) and generally occurs at sites where dermal penetration is high (face, groins, axillae).

Other effects include: local hirsutism; perioral dermatitis (especially in young women), which responds to steroid withdrawal and may be mitigated by tetracycline by mouth for 4–6 weeks; depigmentation (local); monomorphous acne (local). Potent corticosteroids should not be used on the face unless this is unavoidable. Systemic absorption can lead to all the adverse effects of systemic corticosteroid use. Fluticasone propionate and mometasone furoate are rapidly metabolised following cutaneous absorption, which may reduce the risk of systemic toxicity. Suppression of the hypothalamic–pituitary axis occurs readily with overuse of the very potent agents, and when 20% of the body is under an occlusive dressing with mildly potent agents.

Other complications of occlusive dressings include infections (bacterial, candidal) and even heat stroke when large areas are occluded. Antifungal cream containing hydrocortisone and used for vaginal candidiasis may contaminate the urine and misleadingly suggest Cushing's syndrome.

Applications to the eyelids may get into the eye and cause glaucoma.

Rebound exacerbation of the disease can occur after abrupt cessation of therapy. This can lead the patient to reapply the steroid and so create a vicious cycle.

Allergy. Corticosteroids, particularly hydrocortisone and budesonide, or other ingredients in the formulation, may cause allergic contact dermatitis. The possibility of this should be considered when expected benefit fails to occur, e.g. varicose eczema.

Sunscreens (sunburn and photosensitivity)

Ultraviolet (UV) solar radiation (Fig. 20.2) is defined as:
- UVA (320–400 nm), which damages collagen, contributes to skin cancer and drug photosensitivity.
- UVB (280–320 nm), which is 1 000 times more active than UVA, acutely causes sunburn and chronically skin cancer and skin ageing.
- UVC (200–280 nm), which is prevented, at present, from reaching the earth at sea level by the stratospheric ozone layer, although it can cause skin injury at high altitude.

Fig. 20.2 The ultraviolet component of the electro-magnetic spectrum.

Protection of the skin

Protection from UV radiation is effected by: **Absorbent sunscreens.** These organic chemicals absorb UVB and UVA at the surface of the skin (generally more effective for UVB).

UVB protection is provided by aminobenzoic acid and aminobenzoates (padimate-O), cinnamates, salicylates, camphors.

UVA protection is provided by benzophenones (mexenone, oxybenzone), dibenzoylmethanes.

Reflectant sunscreens. Opaque inorganic minerals such as titanium dioxide, zinc oxide and calamine act as a physical barrier to UVB and UVA (especially zinc oxide); they are cosmetically unattractive, but the newer micronised preparations are more acceptable. Because they are able to protect against visible light, they are especially useful in photosensitivity disorders, e.g. porphyria.

The performance of a sunscreen is expressed as the sun protective factor (SPF), which refers to UVB (UVA is more troublesome to measure and the protection is indicated by a star rating system, with four stars providing the greatest). A SPF of 10 means that the dose of UVB required to cause erythema must be 10 times greater on protected than on unprotected skin. The SPF should be interpreted only as a rough guide; consumer use is more haphazard, and less liberal amounts are applied to the skin in practice. The benefits of using active agents including vitamins, antioxidants, osmolytes and DNA repair enzymes in sunscreens and cosmetics to counteract the inherent photochemical processes that can induce DNA damage in skin cells is unproven.

Sunscreens should protect against both UVB and UVA. Absorbent and reflectant components are combined in some preparations. The washability of the preparation (including removal by sweat and swimming) is also relevant to efficacy and frequency of application; some penetrate the stratum corneum (padimate-O) and are more persistent than others.

Uses. Sunscreens are no substitute for light-impermeable clothing and sun avoidance (especially during peak hours of UV light). Daily application of sunscreen appears to protect more against UV-induced skin changes than intermittent use of the product. Methodical use has been demonstrated to reduce the incidence of cutaneous squamous cell carcinoma. Sunscreens are especially beneficial in protecting those who are photosensitive due to drugs (below) or disease, i.e. for photodermatoses such as photosensitivity dermatitis, polymorphic light eruption, cutaneous porphyrias and lupus erythematosus.

Treatment of mild sunburn is usually with a lotion such as oily calamine lotion. Severe cases are helped by topical corticosteroids. NSAIDs, e.g. indometacin, can help if given early, by preventing the formation of prostaglandins.

Drug photosensitivity

Drug photosensitivity means that an adverse effect occurs as a result of drug plus light, usually UVA; sometimes even the amount of UV radiation from fluorescent light tubes is sufficient.

Systemically taken drugs that can induce photosensitivity are many, the most common being the following:

- Antimitotics: dacarbazine, vinblastine, taxanes, methotrexate.
- Antimicrobials: demeclocycline, doxycycline, nalidixic acid, sulfonamides.
- Antipsychotics: chlorpromazine, prochlorperazine.
- Cardiac arrhythmic: amiodarone.
- Diuretics: furosemide, chlorothiazide, hydrochlorothiazide.
- Fibric acid derivatives, e.g. fenofibrate.
- Hypoglycaemics: tolbutamide. NSAIDs: piroxicam.
- Psoralens.

- Antifungals: voriconazole (extreme photoxicity and heightened risk of SCC and melanoma).

Topically applied substances that can produce photosensitivity include:

- Para-aminobenzoic acid and its esters (used as sunscreens).
- Coal tar derivatives.
- Psoralens from juices of various plants, e.g. bergamot oil.
- 6-Methylcoumarin (used in perfumes, shaving lotions, sunscreens).

There are two forms of photosensitivity:

Phototoxicity, like drug toxicity, is a normal effect of too high a dose of UV light in a subject who has been exposed to the drug. The reaction is like severe sunburn. The threshold returns to normal when the drug is withdrawn. Some drugs, notably NSAIDs, induce a 'pseudoporphyria', clinically resembling porphyria cutanea tarda and presenting with skin fragility, blisters and milia on sun-exposed areas, notably the backs of the hands.

Photoallergy, like drug allergy, is a cell-mediated immunological effect that occurs only in some people, and which may be severe with a small dose. Photoallergy due to drugs is the result of a photochemical reaction caused by UVA in which the drug combines with tissue protein to form an antigen. Reactions may persist for years after the drug is withdrawn; they are usually eczematous.

Systemic protection, as opposed to application of drug to exposed areas, should be considered when the topical measures fail.

Antimalarials such as hydroxychloroquine may be effective for short periods in polymorphic light eruption and in cutaneous lupus erythematosus.

Psoralens (obtained from citrus fruits and other plants), e.g. methoxsalen, are used to induce photochemical reactions in the skin. After topical or systemic administration of the psoralen and subsequent exposure to UVA there is an erythematous reaction that goes deeper than ordinary sunburn and may reach its maximum only after 48 h (sunburn maximum is 12–24 h). Melanocytes are activated and pigmentation occurs over the following week. This action is used to repigment areas of disfiguring depigmentation, e.g. vitiligo in black-skinned persons.

In the presence of UVA the psoralen interacts with DNA, forms thymine dimers and inhibits DNA synthesis. Psoralen plus UVA (PUVA) treatment is used chiefly in severe psoriasis (a disease characterised by increased epidermal proliferation) and cutaneous T-cell lymphoma.

Severe *adverse reactions* can occur with psoralens and UV radiation, including sunburn, increased risk of skin cancer (due to mutagenicity inherent in their action), cancer of the male genitalia, cataracts and accelerated skin ageing; the treatment is used only by specialists.

Chronic exposure to sunlight induces wrinkling and yellowing due to the changes in the dermal connective tissue. Topical retinoids are used widely in an attempt to reverse some of these tissue changes. Public pursuit of novel tanning strategies, including the unregulated subcutaneous self-administration of synthetic analogues of alpha-melanocyte-stimulating hormone (alpha-MSH), has been reported. Medical practitioners should be aware that these agents can complicate the clinical presentation of patients with changing moles and suspected melanoma.

Miscellaneous compounds

Keratolytics are used to destroy unwanted tissue, including warts and corns. Great care is obviously necessary to avoid ulceration. They include trichloroacetic acid, salicylic acid and many others. Resorcinol and sulphur are mild keratolytics used in acne. Salicylic acid may enhance the efficacy of a topical steroid in hyperkeratotic disorders.

Tars are mildly antiseptic, antipruritic and inhibit keratinisation in an ill-understood way. They are safe in low concentrations and are used in psoriasis. Photosensitivity occurs and tar–UVB regimens are highly effective therapies for extensive psoriasis. There are very many preparations, which usually contain other substances, e.g. coal tar and salicylic acid ointment.

Ichthammol is a sulphurous, tarry, distillation product of fossilised fish (obtained in the Austrian Tyrol); it has a weaker effect than coal tar.

Zinc oxide provides mild astringent, barrier and occlusive actions. Calamine is basic zinc carbonate that owes its pink colour to added ferric oxide. It has a mild astringent action, and is used as a dusting powder and in shake and oily lotions.

Urea is used topically to assist skin hydration, e.g. in ichthyosis.

Insect repellents, e.g. against mosquitoes, ticks, fleas, such as DEET (diethyl toluamide), dimethyl phthalate. These are applied to the skin and repel insects principally by vaporisation. They must be applied to all exposed skin, and sometimes also to clothes, if their objective is to be achieved (some damage plastic fabrics and spectacle frames). Their duration of effect is limited by the rate at which they vaporise (dependent on skin and ambient temperature), by washing off (sweat, rain, immersion) and by mechanical factors causing rubbing (physical activity). They can cause allergic and toxic effects, especially with prolonged use.

Benzyl benzoate may be used on clothes; it resists one or two washings.

CUTANEOUS DRUG REACTIONS

Drugs applied locally or taken systemically often cause rashes. These take many different forms and the same drug may produce different rashes in different people. Types of drug rash include:

- Exanthems.
- Acute generalised exanthematous pustulosis.
- Fixed drug rash.
- Stevens–Johnson syndrome/erythema multiforme/toxic epidermal necrolysis.
- Hypersensitivity reaction including DRESS (drug rash with eosinophilia and systemic symptoms), e.g. hepatitis. The pathogenesis of DRESS is likely to be multifactorial. The factors include deficient detoxification of a drug metabolite in patients who are genetically susceptible, drug interactions, and direct effects of drug-specific T cells. Recent reports of co-infection with human herpesvirus (HHV)-6 or HHV-7 and a transient hypogammaglobulinaemia may prove important in anti-

convulsant hypersensitivity.

Although drugs may change, the clinical problems remain depressingly the same: a patient develops a rash; he or she is taking many different tablets; which, if any, of these caused the eruption, and what should be done about it? It is no answer simply to stop all drugs, although the fact that this can often be done casts some doubt on the patient's need for them in the first place. All too often, potentially valuable drugs are excluded from further use on totally inadequate grounds. Clearly some guidelines are useful, but no simple set of rules exists that can cover this complex subject:

1. *Can other skin diseases be excluded and are the skin changes compatible with a drug cause?* Clinical features that indicate a drug cause include the type of primary lesion (blisters, pustules), distribution of lesions (acral lesions in erythema multiforme), mucosal involvement and evidence of systemic involvement (fever, lymphadenopathy, visceral involvement).

2. *Which drug is most likely to be responsible?* Document all of the drugs the patient has been exposed to and the date of introduction of each drug. Determine the interval between commencement date and the date of the skin eruption. Chronology is important, with most reactions occurring about 10–12 days after starting a new drug or within 2–3 days in previously exposed patients. A search of standard literature sources of adverse reactions, including the pharmaceutical company data, can be helpful in identifying suspect drugs.

3. *Are any further tests worthwhile?* Excluding infectious causes of skin eruptions is important, e.g. viral exanthems, mycoplasma. A skin biopsy in cases of non-specific dermatitis is helpful, as a predominance of eosinophils would support a drug precipitant.

4. *Is any treatment needed?* Supporting the ill patient and stopping the causative drug is crucial.

Drug-specific rashes

Despite great variability, some hints at drug-specific or characteristic rashes from drugs taken systemically can be discerned; some examples are as follows:

- *Acne and pustular*: corticosteroids, androgens, ciclosporin, penicillins.
- *Allergic vasculitis*: sulfonamides, NSAIDs, thiazides, chlorpropamide, phenytoin, penicillin, retinoids.
- *Anaphylaxis*: X-ray contrast media, penicillins, angiotensin-converting enzyme (ACE) inhibitors.
- *Bullous pemphigoid*: furosemide (and other sulfonamide-related drugs), ACE inhibitors, penicillamine, penicillin, PUVA therapy.
- *Eczema*: penicillins, phenothiazines.
- *Exanthematic/maculopapular* reactions are the most frequent; unlike a viral exanthem, the eruption typically starts on the trunk; the face is relatively spared. Causes include antimicrobials, especially ampicillin, sulfonamides and derivatives (sulfonylureas, furosemide and thiazide diuretics).
- *Morbilliform* (measles-like) eruptions typically recur on rechallenge.
- *Erythema multiforme*: NSAIDs, sulfonamides, barbiturates, phenytoin, paclitaxel.
- *Erythema nodosum*: dermatitis and sulfonamides, oral contraceptives, prazosin.
- *Exfoliative erythroderma*: gold, phenytoin, carbamazepine, allopurinol, penicillins, neuroleptics, isoniazid.
- *Fixed eruptions* are eruptions that recur at the same site, often circumoral, with each administration of the drug: phenolphthalein (laxative self-medication), sulfonamides, quinine (in tonic water), tetracycline, barbiturates, naproxen, nifedipine.
- *Hair loss*: cytotoxic anticancer drugs, acitretin, oral contraceptives, heparin, androgenic steroids (women), sodium valproate, gold.
- *Hypertrichosis*: corticosteroids, ciclosporin, doxasosin, minoxidil.
- *Lichenoid eruption*: β-adrenoceptor blockers, chloroquine, thiazides, furosemide, captopril, gold, phenothiazines.
- *Lupus erythematosus*: hydralazine, isoniazid, procainamide, phenytoin, oral contraceptives, sulfazaline.

- *Purpura*: thiazides, sulfonamides, sulfonylureas, phenylbutazone, quinine. Aspirin induces a capillaritis (pigmented purpuric dermatitis).
- *Photosensitivity*: see above.
- *Pemphigus*: penicillamine, captopril, piroxicam, penicillin, rifampicin.
- *Pruritus* unassociated with rash: oral contraceptives, phenothiazines, rifampicin (cholestatic reaction).
- *Pigmentation*: oral contraceptives (chloasma in photosensitive distribution), phenothiazines, heavy metals, amiodarone, chloroquine (pigmentation of nails and palate, depigmentation of the hair), minocycline.
- *Psoriasis* may be aggravated by β-blockers, lithium and antimalarials.
- *Scleroderma-like*: bleomycin, sodium valproate, tryptophan contaminants (eosinophila–myalgia syndrome).
- *Serum sickness*: immunoglobulins and other immunomodulatory blood products.
- *Stevens–Johnson syndrome and toxic epidermal necrolysis* (TENS): e.g. anticonvulsants, sulfonamides, aminopenicillins, NSAIDs, allopurinol, chlormezanone, corticosteroids.
- *Urticaria and angioedema*: penicillins, ACE inhibitors, gold, NSAIDs, e.g. aspirin, codeine.

Patients with the acquired immunodeficiency syndrome (AIDS) have an increased risk of adverse reactions, which are often severe. Recovery after withdrawal of the causative drug generally begins within a few days, but lichenoid reactions may not improve for weeks.

Diagnosis

The patient's drug history may give clues. Reactions are commoner during early therapy (days) than after the drug has been given for months. Diagnosis by purposeful readministration of the drug (challenge) is not recommended, especially in patients suffering a generalised effect or with mucosal involvement, as it may precipitate toxic epidermal necrolysis.

Patch and photopatch tests are useful in contact dermatitis as they reproduce the causative process, but should be performed only by those with special experience. Fixed drug eruptions can sometimes be reproduced by patch testing with the drug over the previously affected site.

Intradermal tests introduce all the problems of allergy to drugs, e.g. metabolism, combination with protein, fatal anaphylaxis.

Treatment

Treatment involves supportive care and removal of the causative drug. Use cooling applications and antipruritics; use a histamine H_1-receptor blocker systemically for acute urticaria. The use of adrenal corticosteroids is controversial. It may be useful for severe exanthems if the incriminated drug is crucial for other concurrent disease, and is useful for internal organ disease involvement in DRESS. The use of human-derived immunoglobulin infusions is increasingly advocated in the treatment of toxic epidermal necrolysis.

Safety monitoring

Several drugs commonly used in dermatology should be monitored regularly for (principally systemic) adverse effects. These include:

- *Aciclovir* (plasma creatinine).
- *Azathioprine* (blood count and liver function).
- *Colchicine* (blood count, plasma creatinine).
- *Ciclosporin* (plasma creatinine).
- *Dapsone* (liver function, blood count including reticulocytes).
- *Methotrexate* (blood count, liver function).
- *PUVA* (liver function, antinuclear antibodies).
- *Aromatic retinoids* (liver function, plasma lipids).

The patient and doctor must always remain vigilant about drug–drug and drug–food interactions that may result in toxicity, e.g. methotrexate/trimethoprim, ciclosporin/grapefruit juice.

INDIVIDUAL DISORDERS

Secondary infections of ordinarily uninfected lesions may require added topical or systemic antimicrobials. Analgesics, sedatives or tranquilisers may be needed in painful or uncomfortable conditions, or where the disease is intensified by emotion or anxiety.

Psoriasis

In psoriasis there is increased epidermal undifferentiated cell proliferation and inflammation of the epidermis and dermis. The consequence of increased numbers of immature horn cells containing abnormal keratin is that an abnormal stratum corneum is formed. Drugs are used to:

- dissolve keratin (keratolysis)
- inhibit cell division

An emollient such as aqueous cream will reduce the inflammation. The proliferated cells may be eliminated by a *dithranol* (antimitotic) preparation applied accurately to the lesions (but not on the face or scalp) for 1 h and then removed as it is irritant to normal skin and stains skin, blond hair and fabrics. A suitable regimen may begin with 0.1% dithranol, increasing to 1%. Dithranol is available in cream bases or in Lassar's paste (the preparations are not interchangeable). It is used daily until the lesions have disappeared and may produce prolonged remissions of psoriasis. Tar (antimitotic) preparations are used in a similar way, are less irritating to normal skin and are commonly used for psoriasis of the scalp.

Topical adrenal corticosteroids act principally by reducing inflammation. Application, especially under occlusive dressings, can be very effective at suppressing the disease, but increased doses (concentrations) become necessary and rebound, which may be severe, follows withdrawal. For this reason potent corticosteroids should never be used except for lesions on the scalp, palms and soles. Corticosteroids of mild potency may be used for flexural psoriasis where other drugs are too irritating.

Systemic corticosteroid administration should be avoided, for high doses are needed to suppress the disease, which is liable to recur in a more unstable form when treatment is withdrawn, as it must be if complications of long-term steroid therapy are to be avoided.

Calcipotriol and tacalcitol are analogues of calcitriol, the most active natural form of vitamin D. They inhibit cell proliferation and encourage cell differentiation. Although they have less effect on calcium metabolism than does calcitriol, excessive use (more than 100 g/week) can raise the plasma calcium concentration.

Vitamin A (retinols) plays a role in epithelial function, and the retinoic acid derivative acitretin (orally) inhibits psoriatic hyperkeratosis over 4–6 weeks. Acitretin should be used in courses (6–9 months) with intervals (3–4 months). It is teratogenic, like the other vitamin A derivatives. It is not recommended for use in women of childbearing potential because the drug is stored in the liver and in fat, and active metabolites are released many months after cessation of therapy.

UVB light is effective in guttate psoriasis and potentiates the effects of topical agents such as calcipotriol (act by reducing cell division), antimitotic agents like tar (Goeckerman's regimen) and dithranol (Ingram's regimen). Oral psoralen followed by UVA light (PUVA) may be used to clear severe cases of psoriasis, with remissions of more than a year being achievable. Long-term PUVA therapy is associated with an increased risk of cutaneous squamous cell carcinoma and melanoma development (especially in those given maintenance treatment).

Ciclosporin, the systemic calcineurin inhibitor, has been instrumental in shifting the focus of psoriasis research from keratinocyte abnormalities to immune perturbations. It has a rapid onset of action and is useful in achieving remissions in all forms of psoriasis. Monitoring of blood pressure and renal function is mandatory. Severe adverse effects, including renal toxicity, preclude its being used as long-term suppressive therapy.

Since the introduction of ciclosporin for psoriasis, much research has focused on new ways of disrupting T lymphocytes and the cytokines involved in the induction and maintenance of psoriasis. These drugs target specific cellular events, e.g. induction of T-lymphocytic apoptosis, inhibition of tumour necrosis factor. The exact role of these promising therapies is still evolving.

Folic acid antagonists, e.g. methotrexate, can also suppress epidermal activity and inhibit T and B lymphocytes, and are especially useful when psoriasis is severe and remits rapidly with other treatments. Methotrexate is particularly of use if there is associated disabling arthritis. Platelet count, renal and liver function must be monitored regularly. When 1.5 g of the total dose has been taken, liver biopsy should be considered, especially in those with predisposing hepatic steatosis.

The last decade has witnessed a significant advance in the management of refractory moderate-to-severe psoriasis with the introduction of biological therapies to clinical practice. These drugs target specific cellular events, e.g. induction of T-lymphocytic apoptosis, inhibition of tumour necrosis factor. Three classes of biological therapies have been used: T-cell inhibitors, tumour necrosis factor (TNF)-α inhibitors, and interleukin (IL-12 and IL-23) inhibitors. The first of these to be introduced, the T-cell inhibitor efalizumab, was withdrawn because of a rare association with progressive multifocal leukoencephalopathy (PML). In contrast, anti-TNF treatments are now firmly established, offering a high level of efficacy and a good safety record. Ustekinumab, by targeting the p40 subunit common to interleukins 12 and 23, offers a viable alternative to anti-TNFs in the treatment of moderate-to-severe psoriasis. The identification of PML as a serious, but statistically rare risk of efalizumab demonstrates the strengths and weaknesses of the current drug approval and pharmacovigilance processes for fully measuring the safety of a drug. Patients and clinicians need to be aware of the relative completeness and limitations of existing safety data of a drug when selecting a treatment.

It is plain from this brief outline that treatment of psoriasis requires considerable judgement and choice will depend on the patient's sex, age and the severity of the condition. Topical therapies such as calcipotriol, tar or dithranol-containing compounds should be the mainstay of limited mild psoriasis. Topical corticosteroids can be used for psoriasis inversus under close supervision, as overuse can lead to cutaneous atrophy. Phototherapy is useful for widespread psoriasis where compliance with topical treatments is difficult. Resistant disease is best managed by the specialist who may utilise a rotation of treatments, including retinoids, methotrexate, ciclosporin, UVB plus dithranol and PUVA + acitretin, to reduce the unwanted effects of any single therapy. Fumaric acid compounds, hydroxyurea and specific biological agents are useful for severe cases.

Acne

Acne vulgaris results from disordered function of the pilosebaceous follicle whereby abnormal keratin and sebum (the production of which is androgen driven) form debris that plugs the mouth of the follicle. *Propionibacterium acnes* colonises the debris. Bacterial action releases inflammatory fatty acids from the sebum, resulting in inflammation. Acne is a chronic disorder and if uncontrolled can lead to irreversible scarring.

The following measures are used progressively and selectively as the disease becomes more severe; they may need to be applied for up to 3–6 months:

- *Mild keratolytic* (exfoliating, peeling) formulations unblock pilosebaceous ducts, e.g. benzoyl peroxide, sulphur, salicylic acid, azelaic acid.
- *Systemic or topical antimicrobial therapy* (tetracycline, erythromycin, lymecycline) is used over months (expect 30% improvement after 3 months). Bacterial resistance is not a problem; benefit is due to suppression of bacterial lipolysis of sebum, which generates inflammatory fatty acids. (Avoid minocycline because of adverse effects, including raised intracranial pressure and drug-induced lupus.)
- *Vitamin A (retinoic acid) derivatives* reduce sebum production and keratinisation. Vitamin A is a teratogen. *Tretinoin* (Retin-A) is applied topically (but not in combination with other keratolytics). Tretinoin should be avoided in sunny weather and in pregnancy. Benefit is seen in about 10 weeks. *Adapalene*, a synthetic retinoid, may be better tolerated as it is less irritant. *Isotretinoin* (Roaccutane) orally is highly effective (a single course of treatment to a cumulative dose of 100 mg/kg is curative

in 94% of patients), but is known to be a *serious teratogen*; its use should generally be confined to the more severe cystic and conglobate cases, where other measures have failed. Fasting blood lipids should be measured before and during therapy (levels of cholesterol and triglycerides may rise). Women of childbearing potential should be fully informed of this risk, pregnancy-tested before commencement and use contraception for 4 weeks before, during and for 4 weeks after cessation. Other adverse effects are described, including mood change and severe depression.

- *Hormone therapy.* The objective is to reduce androgen production or effect by using ① oestrogen, to suppress hypothalamic–pituitary gonadotrophin production, or ② an antiandrogen (cyproterone). An oestrogen alone as initial therapy to get the acne under control or, in women, the cyclical use of an oral contraceptive containing 50 micrograms of oestrogen diminishes sebum secretion by 40%. A combination of ethinylestradiol and cyproterone (Dianette) orally is also effective in women (it has a contraceptive effect, which is desirable as the cyproterone may feminise a male fetus).

Urticaria

Acute urticaria (named after its similarity to the sting of a nettle, *Urtica*) and *angioedema* usually respond well to H$_1$-receptor antihistamines, although severe cases are relieved more quickly with use of adrenaline/epinephrine (adrenaline injection 1 mg/mL: 0.1–0.3 mL s.c.). A systemic corticosteroid may be needed in severe cases, e.g. urticarial vasculitis.

In some individuals, urticarial weals are provoked by physical stimuli, e.g. friction (dermographism), heat or cold. Exercise may induce weals, particularly on the upper trunk (cholinergic urticaria). Physical urticarias are particularly challenging to treat.

Chronic urticaria usually responds to an H$_1$-receptor antihistamine with low sedating properties, e.g. cetirizine or loratidine. Terfenadine is also effective, but may cause dangerous cardiac arrhythmias if the recommended dose is exceeded or if it is administered with drugs (grapefruit juice) that inhibit its metabolism. But lack of sleep increases the intensity of itch (similar to pain), and a sedating antihistamine may be useful at night. H_2-receptor antihistamines may be added for particularly resistant cases. In some patients with antibodies against the Fc receptor on mast cells, immunosuppressive therapies (e.g. ciclosporin, methotrexate or intravenous immunoglobulin) may be required.

Hereditary angioedema, with deficiency of C_1-esterase inhibitor (a complement inhibitor), may not respond to antihistamines or corticosteroid but only to fresh frozen plasma or, preferably, C_1-inhibitor concentrate. Delay in initiating the treatment may lead to death from laryngeal oedema (try adrenaline/epinephrine i.m. in severe cases). Icatibant is a selective and specific antagonist of bradykinin B2 receptors. It has been approved in Europe for the symptomatic treatment of acute attacks of hereditary angioedema (HAE) in adults (with C1-esterase-inhibitor deficiency). For long-term prophylaxis an androgen (stanozolol, danazol) can be effective. Hereditary angioedema does not manifest as simple urticaria.

Atopic dermatitis

Atopic dermatitis is a chronic condition, and treatment must be individualised and centred around preventive measures. Successful management includes the elimination of precipitating and exacerbating factors, and maintaining the skin barrier function by use of topical or systemic agents.

Immunological triggers of atopic dermatitis vary and can include aeroallergens, detergents (including soaps), irritants, climate and microorganisms. Identification and modification of these factors is useful.

Antiseptic-containing soap substitutes are useful in reducing pro-inflammatory *Staphylococcus aureus* colonies.

In *acute* weeping dermatitis, lotions, wet dressing or soaks (sodium chloride, potassium permanganate) are used.

In *subacute* and *chronic* disease, skin care with occlusive emollients helps to offset the xerosis (dryness) that creates microfissures in the skin and disturbs its normal barrier function. Topical corticosteroids form the cornerstone of pharmacological therapy. In general, the lowest-potency topical steroid should be used initially and higher-potency agents considered only if these fail, the aim being to switch to intermittent steroid use protocols once the disease has been controlled. Higher potency agents are usually inappropriate for young children and highly permeable areas. Very potent steroids should not be used for longer than 2 consecutive weeks to minimise the likelihood of unwanted effects.

The calcineurin inhibitors, tacrolimus and pimecrolimus, are effective topically. Local irritation may result but they do not cause skin atrophy and so are especially useful on the face. Long-term safety data are still lacking and the FDA cautions against long-term use in children on the grounds of cutaneous carcinogenesis.

Sedating H_1-receptor antihistamines with anxiolytic properties may assist with sleep and nocturnal itch. A 2-week course of systemic corticosteroid is useful, especially in cases of acute allergic contact dermatitis. Long-term oral immunosuppression with ciclosporin, mycophenylate or azathioprine should be undertaken only in specialist centres. Although there is minimal objective improvement in atopic dermatitis with UVB phototherapy, patients have consistently reported subjective improvement in itch.

Skin infections

Superficial bacterial infections, e.g. impetigo, eczema, are commonly staphylococcal or streptococcal. They are treated with a topical antimicrobial for less than 2 weeks, applied twice daily after removal of crusts that prevent access of the drug, e.g. with a povidone–iodine preparation. Very extensive cases need systemic treatment.

Topical *sodium fusidate* and *mupirocin* are preferred (as they are not used ordinarily for systemic infections and therefore development of drug-resistant strains is less likely to have any serious consequences). Framycetin and polymyxins are also used. Absorption of neomycin from all topical preparations can cause serious injury to the eighth cranial nerve. It is also a contact sensitiser.

When prolonged treatment is required, topical antiseptics (e.g. chlorhexidine) are preferred and bacterial resistance is less of a problem.

Combination of an antimicrobial drug with a corticosteroid (to suppress inflammation) can be useful for secondarily infected eczema.

The *disadvantages* of antimicrobials are contact allergy and developments of resistant organisms (which may cause systemic, as well as local, infection). Failure to respond may be due to the development of a contact allergy (which may be masked by corticosteroid).

Infected leg ulcers generally do not benefit from long-term antimicrobials, although topical metronidazole is useful when the ulcer is malodorous due to colonisation with Gram-negative organisms. An antiseptic (plus a protective dressing with compression) is preferred if antimicrobial therapy is needed.

Nasal carriers of staphylococci may be cured (often temporarily) by topical mupirocin or neomycin plus chlorhexidine.

Deep bacterial infections, e.g. boils, generally do not require antimicrobial therapy, but if they do it should be systemic. Cellulitis requires systemic chemotherapy initially with benzylpenicillin and flucloxacillin.

Infected burns are treated with a variety of antimicrobials, including silver sulfadiazine and mupirocin.

Fungal infections. Superficial dermatophyte or Candida infections purely involving the skin can be treated with a topical imidazole, e.g. clotrimazole, miconazole. Pityriasis versicolor, a yeast infection, primarily involves the trunk in young adults. It responds to topical antifungals or selenium sulfide preparations; severe infection may require systemic itraconazole. It tends to recur and regular treatments are frequently necessary. Invasion of hair or nails by a dermatophyte or a deep mycosis requires systemic therapy; terbinafine is the most effective drug. Terbinafine and griseofulvin are ineffective against yeasts, for which itraconazole is an alternative. Itraconazole can be used in weekly pulses each month for 3–4 months; it is less effective against dermatophytes than terbinafine.

Viral infections. Topical antivirals, e.g. aciclovir, penetrate the stratum corneum poorly. Aciclovir is used systemically for severe infections, e.g. eczema herpeticum.

SUMMARY

Human skin is a highly efficient self-repairing barrier that permits terrestrial life by regulating heat and water loss while preventing the ingress of noxious chemicals and microorganisms. When physiological function of skin is damaged, skin diseases will occur.

Common skin diseases include infectious skin diseases (e.g., viral, bacterial and fungal diseases), allergies (e.g., dermatitis, eczema, psoriasis and lichen planus) and autoimmune diseases (e.g., lupus erythematosus, dermatomyositis and scleroderma). The pharmacological managements of skin diseases are mainly classified into oral and topical treatments. In addition, there are physical therapy, including phototherapy, laser and cryotherapy, radiotherapy, surgery and adjuvant therapy.

Dermatology drug therapy, can be divided into two major categories: systemic medication and topical administration. Dermatological formulations are also classified by their physical properties into water-based formulations (e.g., liquid formulations, creams, ointments, collodions and gels) and solid preparations (e.g. dusting powders, fungicides).

This chapter focuses on dermatological medications, such as topical analgesics and adrenocortical steroids, and treatment of psoriasis, acne, urticarial, atopic dermatitis, skin infections and other drugs. External medication is a major treatment of skin diseases. According to the cause of skin diseases and skin lesions characteristics, selection of suitable topical medications and appropriate dosage is the key for successful treatment.

IMPORTANT TERMINOLOGY

drug photosensitivity   药物光敏性

psoriasis 牛皮癣

acne 痤疮

urticaria 荨麻疹

atopic dermatitis 过敏性皮肤炎

CHALLENGE YOURSELF

1. What kinds of drugs can be absorbed through the skin?

What are the principal pathways of transdermal drug delivery?

2. What are the commonly used dermatological formulations? What are the characteristics and indications of various drug formulations?

3. What are the main therapeutic strategies for skin diseases?

4. What are the common skin diseases and what's the treatment strategy for these skin diseases?

Jinhan He

Chapter | **21** |

Clinical application of antibacterial drugs

Part 1. antibacterial drugs

CLASSIFICATION OF ANTIMICROBI-ALDRUGS

Antimicrobial agents may be classified according to the type of organism against which they are active:

- Antibacterial drugs.
- Antiviral drugs.
- Antifungal drugs.
- Antiprotozoal drugs.
- Anthelminthic drugs.

A few antimicrobials have useful activity across several of these groups. For example, metronidazole inhibits obligate anaerobic bacteria as well as some protozoa that rely on anaerobic metabolic pathways (such as *Trichomonas vaginalis*).

Antimicrobial drugs have also been classified broadly into:

- Bacteriostatic, i.e. those that act primarily by arresting bacterial multiplication, such as sulfonamides, tetracyclines and chloramphenicol.
- Bactericidal, i.e. those which act primarily by killing bacteria, such as penicillins, aminoglycosides andrifampicin.

Bactericidal drugs act most effectively on rapidly dividing organisms. Thus a bacteriostatic drug, by reducing multiplication, may protect the organism from the killing effect of a bactericidal drug.

More important is whether its antimicrobial effect is concentration-dependent or time-dependent.

Examples of the former include the quinolones and aminoglycosides in which the outcome is related to the peak antibiotic concentration achieved at the site of infectionin relation to the minimum concentration necessary to inhibit multiplication of the organism (the minimum inhibitory concentration, or MIC). These antimicrobials produce a prolonged inhibitory effect on bacterial multiplication (the post-antibiotic effect, or PAE) which suppresses growth until the next dose is given. In contrast, agents such as the β-lactams and macrolides have more modest PAEs and exhibit time-dependent killing; their concentrations should be kept above the MIC for a high proportion of the time between each dose (Fig. 21.1).

HOW ANTIMICROBIALS ACT – SITES OF ACTION

It should always be remembered that drugs are seldom the sole instruments of cure but act together with the natural defences of the body. Antimicrobials may act at different sites in the target organism, and these are characteristically structures or metabolic pathways that differ from those in the human host – this allows for 'selective toxicity':

The cell wall. Bacterial multiplication involves breakdown and extension of the cell wall; interference with these processes prevents the organism from resisting osmotic pressures, so that it bursts. Obviously, the drugs are effective principally against

437

Fig. 21.1 Efficacy of antimicrobials: examples of concentration- dependent and time-dependent killing (see text) (cfu= colony-forming units).

growing cells. They include: penicillins, cephalosporins, vancomycin, bacitracin, cycloserine.

The cytoplasmic membrane. Drugs that interfere with its structure include: polyenes (nystatin, amphotericin), azoles (fluconazole, itraconazole), polymyxins (colistin, polymyxin B) and daptomycin.

Protein synthesis. Drugs that interfere at various points with the build-up of peptide chains on microbial ribosomes include: chloramphenicol, erythromycin, fusidic acid, tetracyclines, aminoglycosides, quinupristin/dalfopristin, linezolid.

Figure 21.1 shows the results of an experiment in which a culture broth initially containing 10^6 bacteria per mL is exposed to various concentrations of two antibiotics, one of which exhibits concentration-dependent and the other time-dependent killing. The 'control' series contains no antibiotic, and the other series contain progressively higher antibiotic concentrations from 0.5× to 64× the MIC. Over 6 h incubation, the time-dependent antibiotic exhibit skilling, but there is no difference between the 1×MIC and 64×MIC. The additional cidal effect of rising concentrations of the antibiotic which has concentrationdependent killing can be clearly seen.

Nucleic acid metabolism. Drugs may interfere:

- directly with microbial DNA or its replication or repair, e.g. quinolones, metronidazole, or with RNA, e.g.rifampicin.
- indirectly on nucleic acid synthesis, e.g. sulfonamides, trimethoprim.

PROBLEMS WITH ANTIMICROBIAL DRUGS

Resistance

Microbial resistance to antimicrobials is a matter of great importance; if sensitive strains are supplanted by resistant ones, then a valuable drug may become useless. Just as 'some are born great, some achieve greatness, and some have greatness thrust upon them, so microorganisms may be naturally ('born') resistant, 'achieve' resistance by mutation or have resistance, 'thrust upon them' by transfer of plasmids and other mobile genetic elements.

Mechanisms of resistance act as follows:

- *Naturally resistant strains.* Some bacteria are innately resistant to certain classes of antimicrobial agent, e.g. coliforms and many other Gramnegative bacteria possess outer cell membranes which protect their cell walls from the action of certain penicillins and cephalosporins. Facultatively anaerobic bacteria (such as *Escherichia coli*) lack the ability to reduce the nitro group of metronidazole which therefore remains in an inactive form.

- *Spontaneous mutation brings* about organisms with novel antibiotic resistance mechanisms. If these cells are viable, in the presence of the antimicrobial agent selective multiplication of the resistant strain occurs sothat it eventually dominates.

- *Transmission of genes from other organisms is the* commonest and most important mechanism. Genetic material may be transferred, e.g. in the *form of plasmids which* are circular strands of DNA that lie out with the chromosomes and contain genes capable of controlling various metabolic processes including formation of β-lactamases (that destroy some penicillins and cephalosporins), and enzymes that inactivate aminoglycosides. Alternatively, genetic transfer may occur through *bacteriophages* (viruses which infect bacteria), particularly in the case of staphylococci.

Resistance is mediated most commonly by the production of enzymes that modify the drug, e.g. aminoglycosides are phosphorylated, β-lactamases hydrolysepenicillins. Other mechanisms include decreasing the passage into or increasing the efflux of drug from the bacterial cell (e.g. meropenem resistance in *Pseudomonas aeruginosa*), modification of the target site so that the antimicrobial binds less effectively (e.g. methicillin resistance in *Staphylococci*), and by passing of inhibited metabolic pathways (e.g. resistance to trimethoprim in many bacteria). More is becoming known of the complex molecular systems which control expression of antimicrobial resistance, and this knowledge should soonlead to novel compounds that inhibit resistance mechanisms at the genetic and phenotypic levels.

Limitation of resistance to antimicrobials may beachieved by 'antibiotic stewardship' which includes:

- Avoidance of indiscriminate use by ensuring that the indication for, and the dose and duration of treatment are appropriate; Performing ward rounds on areas of the hospital with high rates of antibiotic use (e.g. intensive care units, acute surgical wards) to assess the justification for treatment of individual patients and to educate other doctors in limiting unnecessary courses of antibiotics has recently become an important role for clinical microbiologists.
- Restricting use of antimicrobial combinations to appropriate circumstances, e.g. tuberculosis.
- Constant monitoring of resistance patterns in a hospital or community (changing recommendedantibiotics used for empirical treatment when the prevalence of resistance becomes high), and good infection control in hospitals (e.g. isolation of carriers, hand hygiene practices for ward staff) to prevent the spread of resistant bacteria.
- Restricting drug use, e.g. delaying the emergence

of resistance by limiting the use of the newest member of a group of antimicrobials so long as the currently used drugs are effective; restricting use of a drug may become necessary where it promotes the proliferation of resistant strains.

- Avoiding transmission of multiply resistant bacteria among patients and staff in hospital, by healthcare workers performing careful hand hygiene between each patient contact, and through identification and isolation of carriers.

'The over-riding principle of medicine is "do no harm", yet, in the case of antibiotics, harm is inevitable, for use (even appropriate usage) selects for resistance, complicating the treatment of future patients.

Antibiotic policies are agreed among clinicians, microbiologists and pharmacists which guide prescribing towards a limited range of agents which provide adequate choice to cover therapy of important infections while limiting confusion and maximising the opportunities for economical purchase in bulk. Analysis of the many trials of 'antibiotic cycling', where first-choice antibiotics for commonly treated infections in a hospital or ward are formally rotated with a periodicity of several months or years, has shown that this strategy does not reduce overall resistance rates or total antibiotic usage. Use of 'delayed prescriptions' in primary health care management of less serious infections, where a prescription is given to patients for them to taketo the pharmacy only if their symptoms fail to improve in 24–48 h, has been shown to reduce antibiotic usage and not impair outcomes in upper and lower respiratory tract infection.

Recent prospective studies have shown that initial broad spectrum empirical therapy given to acutely ill patients in hospital can be safely 'de-escalated' to narrower spectrum and cheaper antimicrobial agents as soon as the results of initial cultures have been obtained (i.e. usually after 48 h).

Evidence is accumulating that resistance rates do not rise inevitably and irreversibly. In both hospital and domiciliary practice, reductions in antibiotic usage are often shown to be followed by reductions in the prevalence of microbial resistance, although there can be a 'lag' of months or years. The situation is sometimes complicated by the phenomenon of 'linked multiple resistance' whereby the genes coding resistance mechanisms to several antibiotics are carried on the same genetic elements (e.g.plasmid). In this case, use of any of these antibiotics will select for increased resistance via all the mechanisms carried by the plasmid.

Although clinical microbiology laboratories report microbialsusceptibility test results as 'sensitive/susceptible'or 'resistant' to a particular antibiotic, this is not an absolute predictor of clinical response. In a given patient's infection, variables such as absorption of the drug, its penetration to the site of infection, and its activity once there (influenced, for example, by protein binding, pH, concentration of oxygen, metabolic state of the pathogen, intracellular location and concentration of microbes) profoundly alter the likelihood that effective therapy will result.

Superinfection

When any antimicrobial drug is used, there is usually suppression of part of the normal bacterial flora of the patient which is susceptible to the drug. Often, this causes no ill effects, but sometimes a drug-resistant organism, freed from competition, proliferates to an extent which allows an infection to be established. The principal organisms responsible are *Candida albicans* and *pseudomonads*. But careful clinical assessment of the patient is essential, as the mere presence of such organisms in diagnostic specimens taken from a site in which they may be present as commensals does not necessarily mean they are causing disease.

Antibiotic-associated (*Clostridium difficile-associated*) colitis is an example of a superinfection. It is caused by alteration of the normal bowel flora, which allowsmultiplication of *Clostridium difficile* which releases several toxins that damage the mucosa of the bowel and promote excretion of fluid. Almost any antimicrobial may initiate this condition, but the drugs most commonly reported today are cephalosporins and quinolones (e.g.ciprofloxacin). It takes the form of an acute colitis (pseudomembranous-

colitis) with diarrhoeal stools containing blood or mucus, abdominal pain, leucocytosis and dehydration. A history of antibiotic use in the previous 3 weeks, even if the drug therapy has been stopped, should alert the physician to the diagnosis which is confirmed by detection of *C. difficile* toxin in the stools and typical appearances onproctosigmoidoscopy. Mild cases usually respond to discontinuation of the offending antimicrobial, allowingre-establishment of the patient's normal bowel flora, but more severe cases merit treatment with oral metronidazole.

Opportunistic infection arises in patients whose immune systems are compromised or whose phagocytic cellular defences have been reduced by disease (e.g. AIDS, hypogammaglobulinaemia, leukaemia) or drugs (e.g. cytotoxics). Such infections may involve organisms that rarely or never cause clinical disease in normal hosts. Treatment of possible infections in such patients should be prompt, initiated before the results of bacteriological tests are known, and usually involve combinations of bactericidal drugs administered parenterally. Infections of this type include *Pneumocystis carinii* pneumonia, and 'primary' septicaemia in neutropenic patients with gut organisms such as *Escherichia coli* and *Klebsiella* spp.which cross the mucosa of the gut and invade the bloodstream directly.

Masking of infections

Masking of infections by chemotherapy is an important possibility. For example, a course of penicillin adequate to cure gonorrhoea may prevent simultaneously contracted syphilis from showing primary and secondary stages without effecting a cure, and a serological test for syphilis should therefore be done 3 months after treatment for gonorrhoea.

PRINCIPLES OF ANTIMICROBIAL CHEMOTHERAPY

The following principles, many of which apply to drug therapy in general, are a guide to good practice with antimicrobial agents.

Make a diagnosis as precisely as is possible and

define the site of infection, the organism(s) responsible and their susceptibility to a range of antimicrobial agents (to give several therapeutic options to cater for different sites of infection and the possibility of allergies or other drug sensitivities in the infected individual). This objective will be more readily achieved if all relevant samples for laboratory culture are taken before treatment is begun. Once antimicrobials have been administered, isolation of the underlying organism by culture may be inhibited and its place in diagnostic samples may be taken by resistant, colonizing bacteria which obscure the true causative pathogen. New diagnostic methods that rely on detecting specific microbial nucleic acids (e.g. the polymerase chain reaction, PCR), lipids or proteins allow detection of the causative pathogen in patients who have already received antimicrobial-therapy, although it is currently usually not possible simultaneously to determine the antimicrobial susceptibilitypatterns of these microbes.

It is inconsistent that the assessment of new antibiotics for therapeutic use is very much more rigorously controlled than is the introduction of diagnostic tests that direct their use – Gluud and Gluud propose a harmonised approach to the assessment and regulation of new diagnostic procedures in clinical microbiology.

Remove barriers to cure, e.g. drain abscesses, remove obstruction in the urinary tract and infected intravenous catheters.

Decide whether chemotherapy is really necessary. Chronic abscesses or empyemata respond poorly to antibiotics alone and require surgical drainage, although chemotherapeutic cover may be essential if surgery is undertaken in order to avoid dissemination of infection during the operation. Even some acute infections are better managedsymptomatically than by antimicrobials; thus the risks of adverse drug reactions for previously healthy individuals might outweigh the modest clinical benefits that follow antibiotic therapy of *salmonella* gastroenteritis and streptococcal sore throat.

Select the best drug. This involves consideration of the following factors:

- Specificity: indiscriminate use of broad-spectrum drugs promotes antimicrobial resistance and encourages opportunistic infections, e.g. with yeasts. At the beginning of treatment, empirical 'best guess' chemotherapy of reasonably broad spectrum must often be given because the susceptibility and identity of the responsible microbe is uncertain. The spectrum may be narrowed once these are microbiologically confirmed.
- Pharmacokinetic factors: to ensure that the chosen drug is capable of reaching the site of infection in adequate amounts, e.g. by crossing the blood–brain barrier.
- The patient: who may previously have exhibited allergy to a group of antimicrobials or whose routes of elimination may be impaired, e.g. by renal disease.

Administer the drug in optimum dose and frequency and by the most appropriate route(s). Inadequate doses may encourage the development of microbial resistance. In general, on grounds of practicability, intermittent dosing is preferred to continuous infusion. Plasma concentration monitoring can be performed to optimise therapy and reduce adverse drug reactions (e.g. aminoglycosides, vancomycin).

Continue therapy until apparent cure has been achieved; most acute infections are treated for 5–10 days. There are many exceptions to this, such as typhoid fever, tuberculosis and infective endocarditis, in which relapse is possible long after apparent clinical cure and so the drugs are continued for a longer period determined by comparative or observational trials. Otherwise, prolonged therapy is to be avoided because it increases costs and the risks of adverse drug reactions.

Test for cure. In some infections, microbiological proof of cure is desirable because disappearance of symptoms and signs occurs before the organisms are eradicated. This is generally restricted to especially susceptible hosts, e.g. urinary tract infection in pregnancy. Confirmatory culture must be done, of course, after withdrawal of chemotherapy.

USE OF ANTIMICROBIAL DRUGS

Choice

Identification of the microbe and performing susceptibility tests take time, and therapy at least of the more serious infections must usually be started on the basis of the informed 'best guess' (i.e. 'empirical' therapy). Especially in critically ill patients, choosing initial therapy to which the infecting microbes are susceptible has been shown to improve the outcome – with the worldwide rise in prevalence of multiply resistant bacteria during the past decade, knowledge of local antimicrobial resistance rates is therefore an essentialprerequisite. Publication of these rates (and corresponding guidelines for choice of empirical therapy for common infections) is now an important role for clinical diagnostic microbiology laboratories. Such guidelines must be reviewed regularly to keep pace with changing resistance patterns.

When considering 'best guess' therapy, infections may be categorised as those in which:

1. Choice of antimicrobial follows automatically from the clinical diagnosis because the causative organism is always the same, and is virtually always sensitive to the same drug, e.g. meningococcal septicaemia (benzylpenicillin), some haemolytic streptococcal infections, e.g. scarlet fever, erysipelas (benzylpenicillin), typhus (tetracycline), leprosy (dapsone with rifampicin).

2. The infecting organism is identified by the clinical diagnosis, but no safe assumption can be made as to its sensitivity to any one antimicrobial, e.g. tuberculosis.

3. A single infecting organism is not identified by the clinical diagnosis, e.g. in urinary tract infection or abdominal surgical wound infection.

Particularly in the second and third categories, choice of an antimicrobial may be guided by:

Knowledge of the likely pathogens (and their current local susceptibility rates to antimicrobials) in the clinical situation.

Rapid diagnostic tests. Rapid detection of markers of infection such as C-reactive protein (CRP) and procalcitonin assays are now available, and evidence is accruing as to how they should best be used. Both CRP and procalcitonin concentrations rise in the serum within a few hours of the commencement of serious bacterial infections, and it appears that clinical decisions on antimicrobial use based on algorithms that include the results of such assays may be more accurate, and may spare some patients from antibiotic exposure.

Route of administration. Parenteral therapy (which maybe i.m. or i.v.) is preferred for therapy of serious infections because high therapeutic concentrations are achieved reliably and rapidly. Initial parenteral therapy should be switched to the oral route whenever possible once the patient has improved clinically and as long as a suitable oral antibiotic is available and they are able to absorb it (i.e. not with vomiting, ileus or diarrhoea). Many antibiotics are well absorbed orally, and the long-held assumption that prolonged parenteral therapy is necessary for adequate therapy of serious infections (such as osteomyelitis) is often not supported by the results of clinical trials.

Combinations

Treatment with a single antimicrobial is sufficient for most infections. The indications for use of two or more antimicrobials are:

* To avoid the development of drug resistance, especially in chronic infections where many bacteria are present (hence the chance of a resistant mutant emerging is high), e.g. tuberculosis.

* To broaden the spectrum of antibacterial activity: ① in a known mixed infection, e.g. peritonitis following gut perforation, or ② where the infecting organism cannot be predicted but treatment is essential before adiagnos is has been reached, e.g. septicaemia complicating neutropenia or severe community acquired pneumonia.

* To obtain potentiation (or 'synergy'), i.e. an effect unobtainable with either drug alone, e.g. penicillin plus gentamicin for enterococcal endocarditis.

* To enable reduction of the dose of one component and hence reduce the risks of adverse drug reactions, e.g. flucytosine plus amphotericin B for *Cryptococcus neoformans* meningitis.

Chemoprophylaxis and pre-emptive suppressive therapy

It is sometimes assumed that what a drug can cure it will also prevent, but this is not necessarily so. The basis of effective chemoprophylaxis is the use of a drug in a healthy person to prevent infection by one organism of reliable and predictable susceptibility, e.g. benzylpenicillin against a Group Astreptococcus. However, the term chemoprophylaxis is commonly extended to include suppression of existing infection.

It is essential to know the organisms causing infection and their local resistance patterns, and the period of time the patient is at risk. A narrow-spectrum antibiotic regimen should be administered only during this period – ideally for a few minutes before until a few hours after the risk period. It is therefore much easier to define chemotherapeutic regimens for short-term exposures (e.g. surgical operations) than it is for longer-term and less well-defined risks. The main categories of chemoprophylaxis may be summarised as follows:

- True prevention of primary infection: rheumatic fever, recurrent urinary tract infection.
- Prevention of opportunistic infections, e.g. due to commensals getting into the wrong place (coagulase-negative staphylococcal prosthetic joint infection from the patient's skin during the operation, and peritonitis after bowel surgery).
- Suppression of existing infection before it causes overt disease, e.g. tuberculosis, malaria.
- Prevention of acute exacerbations of a chronic infection, e.g. bronchitis, cystic fibrosis.
- Prevention of spread among contacts (in epidemics and/or sporadic cases).
- Chemoprophylaxis in surgery
- When the risk of infection is high because of large numbers of bacteria at the operative site, e.g. in operations on the large bowel.
- When the risk of infection is low but the consequences of infection would be disastrous, e.g. infection of prosthetic joints or prosthetic heart valves.
- When the risks of infection are low but randomized controlled trials have shown the benefits of prophylaxis to outweigh the risks, e.g. single-dose antistaphylococcal prophylaxis for uncomplicated hernia and breast surgery.

Antimicrobials should be selected in the light of knowledge of the likely pathogens at the sites of surgery and their locally prevalent antimicrobial susceptibility.

Antimicrobials should be given i.v., i.m. or occasionallyrectally at the beginning of anaesthesia and for no more than 48 h. A single preoperative dose, given at the time of induction of anaesthesia, has been shown to give optimal cover for most operations. Vancomycin is often included in prophylactic regimens when the patient is known to be a carrier of MRSA or its local prevalence is high (ask microbiological advice).

CLASSIFICATION, MODES OF ACTION AND RESISTANCE MECHANISMS OF β-LACTAMS

Classification

β-lactams, the structure of which contains a β-lactam ring. The major subdivisions are:

- Penicillins, whose official names usually include, or end in, 'cillin'.
- Cephalosporins and cephamycins, which are recognized by the inclusion of 'cef' or 'ceph' in their official names.
- Other subcategories of β-lactams include: Carbapenems (e.g. meropenem). Monobactams (e.g. aztreonam). β-lactamase inhibitors (e.g. clavulanic acid).

Other inhibitors of cell wall synthesis include vancomycin and teicoplanin.

Penicillins

Benzylpenicillin (1942) is produced by growing one of thepenicilliummoulds in deep tanks. In 1957 the penicillin nucleus (6-amino-penicillanic acid) was synthesised and it became possible to add various side-chains and so to make semi-synthetic penicillins with different properties. Penicillins differ widely in antibacterial spectrum. A general account of the penicillins follows and then of the individual drugs in so far as they differ.

Mode of action. Penicillins act by inhibiting the enzymes (penicillin binding proteins, PBPs) involved in the cross-linking of the peptidoglycan layer of the cell wall, which is weakened, and this leads to osmotic rupture. Penicillins are thus bactericidal and are ineffective against resting organisms which are not making new cell wall. The main defence of bacteria against penicillins is to produce enzymes, β-lactamases, which hydrolyse the blactam ring. Other mechanisms that have been described include modifications to PBPs to render them unable to bind β-lactams, reduced permeability of the outer cell membrane of Gram-negative bacteria, and pumps in the outer membrane which remove β-lactam molecules. Some particularly resistant bacteria may possess several mechanisms that act in concert. The remarkable safety and high therapeutic index of the penicillins is due to the fact that human cells, while bounded by a cell membrane, lack a cell wall. They exhibit time-dependent bacterial killing.

Pharmacokinetics. Benzylpenicillin is destroyed by gastric acid and is unsuitable for oral use. Others, e.g. phenoxymethylpenicillin, resist acid and are absorbed in the upper small bowel. The plasma $t_{1/2}$ of penicillins is usually <2 h. They are distributed mainly in the body water and enter well into the CSF if the meninges are inflamed. Penicillins are organic acids and their rapid clearance from plasma is due to secretion into renal tubular fluid by the anion transport mechanism in the kidney. Renal clearance therefore greatly exceeds the glomerular filtration rate (127 mL/min). The excretion of penicillin can be usefully delayed by concurrently giving probenecid which competes successfully for the transport mechanism. Dosage of penicillins may need to be reduced for patients with severely impaired renal function

Adverse effects. The main hazard with the penicillins is allergic reactions. These include itching, rashes (eczematous or urticarial), fever and angioedema. Rarely (about 1 in10 000) there is anaphylactic shock, which can be fatal (about 1 in 50 000–100 000 treatment courses). Allergies are least likely when penicillins are given orally and most likely with topical application. The anaphylactic reaction involves specific IgE antibodies which can be detected in the plasma of susceptible persons.

Narrow-spectrum penicillins

Benzylpenicillin

Benzylpenicillin ($t_{1/2}$ 0.5 h) (penicillin G) has to be given with spaced doses that have to be large to maintain a therapeutic concentration, but the large therapeutic ratio of penicillin allows the resulting fluctuations to be tolerable. Benzylpenicillin is eliminated by the kidney, with about 80% being actively secreted by the renal tubule and this can be blocked by probenecid.

Uses. Benzylpenicillin is highly active against Streptococcus pneumoniae and the Lancefield Group A, β-haemolyticstreptococcus (*Streptococcus pyogenes*). Viridans streptococci are usually sensitive unless the patient has recently received penicillin. *Enterococcus faecalis* is less susceptible and, especially for endocarditis, penicillin should be combined with an aminoglycoside, usually gentamicin. This combination is synergistic unless the enterococcus is highly resistant to the aminoglycoside (minimal inhibitory concentration (MIC) of 128 mg/L or above); such strains are becoming more frequent in hospital patients and present major difficulties in therapy. Over 90% of *Staphylococcus aureus* are now resistant in hospital and domiciliary practice. Benzylpenicillin is a drug of choice for infections due to *Neisseria meningitidis* (meningococcalmeningitis and septicaemia), *Bacillus anthracis* (anthrax), *Clostridium perfringens* (gas gangrene) and *tetani* (tetanus), *Corynebacterium diphtheriae* (diphtheria), *Treponemapallidum* (syphilis), *Leptospira* spp. (leptospirosis), *Actinomycesisraelii* (actinomycosis) and for *Borrelia burgdorferi* (Lyme disease) in children. Penicillin resitance rates in *Neisseria gonorrhoeae* are high in many parts of the world.

Adverse effects are in general uncommon, apart

from allergy (above). It is salutary to reflect that the first clinically useful true antibiotic (1942) is still in use and remains among the least toxic.

Preparations and dosage for injection. Benzylpenicillin may be given i.m. or i.v. (by bolus injection or by continuous infusion). For a sensitive infection, benzylpenicillin 600 mg 6-hourly is enough.

For relatively insensitive infections and where sensitive organisms are sequestered within avascular tissue (e.g. infective endocarditis) 7.2 g is given daily i.v. in divided doses. When an infection is controlled, a change may be made to the oral route with phenoxymethylpenicillin (amoxicillin is more reliably absorbed in adults).

Procaine penicillin, given i.m. only, liberates benzylpenicillinover 12–24 h, but it will not give therapeutic blood concentrations for some hours after injection, and peak concentrations are low.

Preparations and dosage for oral use. Phenoxymethylpenicillin (penicillin V), is resistant to gastric acid and so is moderately well absorbed, sometimes erratically in adults. It is less active than benzylpenicillin against *Neisseriagonorrhoeae* and *meningitidis*, and so is unsuitable for use in gonorrhoeaandmeningococcal meningitis, although satisfactory against *Streptococcus pneumoniae* and *Streptococcuspyogenes*, especially after the acute infection has been controlled by intravenous therapy. The dose is 500 mg 6-hourly.

All oral penicillins are best given on an empty stomach to avoid the absorption delay caused by food.

Broad-spectrum penicillins

The activity of these semi-synthetic penicillins extends to include many Gram-negative bacilli. They do not resist β-blactamases, and their usefulness has reduced markedly in recent years because of the increased prevalence of organism sthat produce these enzymes.

These agents are less active than benzylpenicillin against Gram-positive cocci, but more active than the β-lactamase resistant penicillins (above). They have useful activity against *Enterococcus faecalis* and many strains of *Haemophilus influenzae*. *Enterobacteriaceae* are unreliably susceptible. Members of this group

differ more pharmacologically than antibacterially.

Amoxicillin ($t_{½}$ 1 h; previously known as amoxycillin) is a structural analogue of ampicillin (below) and is better absorbed from the gut (especially after food), and for the same dose achieves approximately double the plasma concentration. Diarrhoea is less frequent with amoxicillin than with ampicillin. The oral dose is 250 mg 8-hourly; a parenteral form is available but offers no advantage over ampicillin.

Co-amoxiclav (Augmentin). Clavulanic acid is a β-lactam molecule which has little intrinsic antibacterial activity but binds irreversibly to β-lactamases. Thereby it competitively protects the penicillin against bacterial β-lactamases, acting as a 'suicide' inhibitor. It is formulated in tablets as its potassium salt (equivalent to 125 mg of clavulanic acid) in combination with amoxicillin (250 or 500 mg), as coamoxiclav, and is a satisfactory oral treatment for infections due to β-lactamase-producing organisms, notably in the respiratory or urogenital tracts. These include many strains of *Staphylococcus aureus*, *Escherichia coli* and an increasing proportion of *Haemophilus influenzae*. It also has useful activity against β-lactamase-producing *Bacteroides* spp. The $t_{½}$ is 1 hand the dose one tablet 8-hourly.

Ampicillin ($t_{½}$ 1 h) is acid-stable and is moderately well absorbed when swallowed. The oral dose is 250 mg–1 g 6–8-hourly; or i.m. or i.v. 500 mg 4–6-hourly. Approximatelyone-third of a dose appears unchanged in the urine. The drug is concentrated in the bile.

Adverse effects. Ampicillin may cause diarrhoea but the incidence (12%) is less with amoxicillin. Ampicillin and amoxicillin are commonly associated with *Clostridium difficile* diarrhoea, related to the frequency of their use rather than to high innate risk of causing the disease. Ampicillin and its analogues may cause a macular rash resembling measles or rubella, usually unaccompanied by other signs of allergy, and seen in patients with disease of the lymphoid system, notably *infectious mononucleosis* and lymphoid leukaemia.

Antipseudomonal penicillins

Ticarcillin ($t_{½}$ 1 h) is presented in combination with clavulanic acid (as Timentin), so to provide greater activity against β-lactamase-producing organisms. It is given by i.m. or slow i.v. injection or by rapid i.v. infusion.

Piperacillin ($t_{1/2}$ 1 h) is available as a combination with the β-lactamase inhibitor tazobactam (as Tazocin).

CEPHALOPORINS

Cephalosporins were first obtained from a filamentous fungus Cephalosporium cultured from the sea near a Sardinian sewage outfall in 1945; their molecular structure is closely related to that of penicillin, and many semisynthetic forms have been introduced. They now comprise a group of antibiotics having a wide range of activity and low toxicity. The term cephalosporins will be used here in a general sense although some are strictly cephamycins, e.g. cefoxitin and cefotetan.

Mode of action is that of the β-lactams, i.e. cephalosporins impair bacterial cell wall synthesis and hence are bactericidal. They exhibit time-dependent bacterial killing.

Addition of various side-chains on the cephalosporin molecule confers variety in pharmacokinetic and antibacterial activities. The β-lactam ring can be protected by such structural manoeuvring, which results in compounds with improved activity against Gram-negative organisms, but less anti-Gram-positive activity. The cephalosporins resist attack by some β-lactamases, but resistance is mediated by other means.

Pharmacokinetics. Usually, cephalosporins are excreted unchanged in the urine, but some, including cefotaxime, form a desacetyl metabolite which possesses some antibacterial activity. Many are actively secreted by the renal tubule, a process which can be blocked with probenecid. As a rule, the dose of cephalosporins should be reduced in patients with poor renal function. Cephalosporins in general have a $t_{1/2}$ of 1–4 h although there are exceptions (e.g. ceftriaxone, $t_{1/2}$ 8 h). Wide distribution in the body allow streatment of infection at most sites, including bone, soft tissue, muscle and (in some cases) CSF.

Classification and uses. The cephalosporins are conventionally categorised by 'generations' sharing broadly similar antibacterial and pharmacokinetic properties; newer agents have rendered this classification less precise but it retains sufficient usefulness.

Adverse effects. Cephalosporins are well tolerated. The most usual unwanted effects are allergic reactions of the penicillin type, and gastrointestinal upset. Overall the rate of cephalosporin skin reactions such as urticarial rashes and pruritis lies between 1% and 3%. There is cross-allergy between penicillins and cephalosporins involving up to 10% of patients; if a patient has had a severe or immediate allergic reaction or if serum or skin testing for penicillin allergy is positive, then a cephalosporin should not be used. Pain may be experienced at the sites of i.v. or i.m. injection. If cephalosporins are continued for more than 2 weeks, reversible thrombocytopenia, haemolytic anaemia, neutropenia, interstitialnephritis or abnormal liver function tests may occur. The broad spectrum of activity of the third generation cephalosporins may predispose to opportunist infection with resistant bacteria or *Candida albicans* and to *Clostridium difficile* diarrhoea.

Ceftobiprole is an interesting new investigational parenteral cephalosporin which binds avidly to the mutated penicillin binding protein 20 responsible for methicillin resistance in staphylococci. It has good activity in vitro and in animal models against MRSA and vancomycin resistant strains and better activity than ceftriaxone against penicillin-resistant pneumococci. Clinical trials are underway in skin and soft tissue infection and pneumonia.

OTHER β-LACTAM ANTIBACTERIALS

Carbapenems

Members of this group have the widest spectrum of all currently available antimicrobials, being bactericidal against most Gram-positive and Gram-negative aerobic and anaerobic pathogenic bacteria. They are resistant to hydrolysis by most β-lactamases, including ESBLs. Only occasional pseudomonas relatives are naturally resistant, and acquired resistance is uncommon in all species.

Imipenem

Imipenem ($t_{1/2}$ 1 h) is inactivated by metabolism in the kidney to products that are potentially toxic to renal tubules; combining imipenem with cilastatin (as Primaxin), a specific inhibitor of dihydropeptidase – the enzyme responsible for its renal metabolism – prevents both inactivation and toxicity.

Imipenem is used to treat septicaemia, intra-abdominal infection and nosocomial pneumonia. In terms of imipenem,1–2 g/day is given by i.v. infusion in 3–4 doses.

Adverse effects. It may cause gastrointestinal upset including nausea, blood disorders, allergic reactions, confusion and convulsions.

Meropenem ($t_{1/2}$ 1 h) is similar to imipenem, but is stable to renal dihydropeptidase and can therefore be given without cilastatin. It penetrates into the CSF and is not associated with nausea or convulsions.

Ertapenem ($t_{1/2}$ 4 h) is given as a single daily injection; because of this it has found a niche indication for parenteral therapy of multiply resistant Gram-negative bacteria out of hospital, such as ESBL-producing coliforms. It is, however, much less active against *Pseudomonas aeruginosa*, *Acinetobacter* and their relatives. Adverse events are uncommon, but include diarrhoea (4.8%), infusion vein phlebitis (4.5%) and nausea (2.8%).

Penems

Faropenem ($t_{1/2}$ approximately 1 h) is the first of this group to reach the clinical trial stage. Penems are hybrids of penicillins and cephalosporins, and faropenem is well absorbed by mouth, and is active against a wide range of Gram-positive and Gram-negative pathogens. It will probably be marketed first for upper and lower respiratory tract infection.

Monobactam

Aztreonam ($t_{1/2}$ 2 h) is the first member of this class of β-lactam antibiotic. It is active against Gram-negative organisms including *Pseudomonas aeruginosa*,

Haemophilus influenzae and *Neisseria meningitidis* and *gonorrhoeae*. Aztreonam is used to treat septicaemia and complicated urinary tract infections, lower urinary tract infections and gonorrhoea.

Adverse effects include reactions at the site of infusion, rashes, gastrointestinal upset, hepatitis, thrombocytopenia and neutropenia. It may be used with caution in penicillin allergic patients.

MACROLIDES

Erythromycin

Erythromycin ($t_{1/2}$ 2–4 h) binds to bacterial ribosomes and interferes with protein synthesis; it is bacteriostatic and exhibitstime-dependent killing. It is effective against Gram-positive organisms because these accumulate the drug more efficiently, and its antibacterial spectrum is similar to that of penicillin.

Absorption after oral administration is best with erythromycinestolate, even if there is food in the stomach. Hydrolysis of the estolate in the body releases the active erythromycin which diffuses readily into most tissues;the $t_{1/2}$ is dose-dependent and elimination is almost exclusively in the bile and faeces.

Uses. Erythromycin is the drug of choice for:

- *Mycoplasma pneumoniae* in children, although in adults a tetracycline may be preferred.
- *Legionella* spp., with or without rifampicin, although some authorities prefer a quinolone.
- Diphtheria (including carriers), pertussis and for some chlamydial infections.

In gastroenteritis caused by *Campylobacter jejuni*, erythromycin is effective in eliminating the organism from the faeces, although it does not reduce the duration of the symptoms unless given very early in the illness.

Erythromycin is an effective alternative choice for penicillin-allergic patients infected with *Staphylococcus aureus*, *Streptococcus pyogenes*, *Streptococcus pneumoniae* or *Treponema pallidum*.

Dose is 250 mg 6-hourly or twice this in serious infection and four times for legionnaires' disease.

Adverse reactions. Erythromycin is remarkably

nontoxic, but the estolate can cause cholestatic hepatitis. This is probably an allergy, and recovery is usual, but the estolate should not be given to a patient with liver disease. Other allergies are rare. Gastrointestinal disturbances occur frequently (up to 28%), particularly diarrhoea and nausea, but opportunistic infection is uncommon.

Interactions. Erythromycin and the other macrolides are enzyme inhibitors and interfere with the cytochrome P450 metabolic inactivation of some drugs, e.g. warfarin, cyclosporin, tacrolimus, digoxin, carbamazepine, theophylline, disopyramide, increasing their effects. Reduced inactivation of terfenadine may lead to serious cardiac arrhythmias, and of ergot alkaloids may cause ergotism. Increased serum erythromycin concentrations are seen with coadministration of azole antifungal agents, some calcium channel blockers and anti-HIV protease inhibitors (ritonavir, saquinavir). Combination of erythromycin with strong inhibitors of P450 enzymes has been associated with an increased risk of sudden cardiac death (azole antifungal agents, diltiazem, verapamil and troleandomycin).

Clarithromycin acts like erythromycin and has a similar spectrum of antibacterial activity, i.e. mainly against Gram-positive organisms, although it is usefully more active against *Haemophilus influenzae*. The usual dose is 250 mg 12-hourly or twice that for serious infections. It is rapidly and completely absorbed from the gastrointestinal tract, 60% of a dose is inactivated by metabolism which is saturable (note that the $t_{1/2}$ increases with dose: 3 h after 250 mg, 9 h after 1 200 mg) and the remainder is eliminated in the urine. Clarithromycin is used for respiratory tract infections including atypical pneumonias and soft tissue infections. It is concentrated intracellularly, achieving concentrations which allow effective therapy in combination for mycobacterial infections such as *Mycobacterium avium-intracellulare* inpatients with AIDS. Gastrointestinal tract adverse effects are uncommon (7%). **Interactions:** see erythromycin (above).

Azithromycin has additional activity against a number of important Gram-negative organisms including *Haemophilus influenzae* and *Neisseria* gonorrhoeae, and also *Chlamydiae*, but is a little less effective than erythromycin against Gram-positive organisms. Azithromycin achieves high concentrations in tissues relative to those in plasma. It remains largely unmetabolised and is excreted in the bile and faeces ($t_{1/2}$ 50 h). Azithromycin is used to treat respiratory tract and soft tissue infections and sexually transmitted diseases, especially genital *Chlamydia* infections, and is effective for travellers' diarrhoea, especially when combined with loperamide. It has been used in patients with cystic fibrosis who are colonised with *Pseudomonas aeruginosa*: azithromycin may have synergistic activity with other anti-pseudomonal agents, and its modestanti-inflammatory effects may also reduce the intensity of symptoms. Gastrointestinal effects (9%) are less than with erythromycin but diarrhoea, nausea, dyspepsia and abdominal pain occur. In view of its high hepatic excretion, use in patients with liver disease should be avoided. Interactions: see erythromycin (above).

Telithromycin ($t_{1/2}$ 10 h) is the first of the ketolides, semisynthetic relatives of the macrolides which bind to the 50S bacterial ribosomal subunit, preventing translation and ribosome assembly. Its molecular differences from erythromycin make it more acid stable and less susceptible to bacterial export pumps, while increasing its ribosomal binding. Its spectrum of activity includes most erythromycin-resistant strains of *Streptococcus pneumoniae*, but it is not active against erythromycin-resistant staphylococci, including most MRSA.

It is licensed for once-daily oral therapy of upper and lower respiratory tract infections and good efficacy has been demonstrated with relatively short courses (e.g.5 days). Bioavailability is approximately 57% and is unaffected by food intake. It is generally well tolerated, although it causes diarrhoea more commonly than the newer macrolides and some patients experience transient visual disturbance (blurred or double vision). Rare cases of serious hepatotoxicity have been reported although dose adjustment is not required in hepatic failure. Some authoritiesrecommend halving the daily dose with severe renal failure, and it is a potent inhibitor of cytochrome P450 liver enzymes, resulting in interactions with, for example, itraconazole, rifampicin, midazolam and atorvastatin.

Clindamycin, structurally a lincosamide rather than a macrolide, binds to bacterial ribosomes to inhibit protein synthesis. Its antibacterial spectrum is similar to that of erythromycin (with which there is partial cross-resistance– so-called 'inducible MLS resistance') and benzylpenicillin; inducible resistance is variable in prevalence in common pathogens in different parts of the world, with the result that clindamycin can be a useful second-line agent for oral treatment of some difficult infections (e.g. MRSA osteomyelitis) as long as susceptibility testing is correctly performed. Clindamycin is well absorbed from the gut and distributes to most body tissues including bone. The drug is metabolized by the liver and enterohepatic cycling occurs with bile concentrations 2–5 times those of plasma ($t_{\frac{1}{2}}$ 3 h). Significant excretion of metabolites occurs via the gut.

Clindamycin is used for staphylococcal bone and joint infections, dental infections and serious intra-abdominal sepsis (in the last, it is usually combined with an agent active against Gram-negative pathogens such as gentamicin). Because of its ability to inhibit production of bacterial protein toxins, it is the antibiotic of choice for serious invasive *Streptococcus pyogenes* infections (although surgical resection of affected tissue plays a prime role) and it is also an alternative to linezolid for treatment of Panton-Valentine leukocidin-producing strains of *Staphylococcus aureus*. It is a second choice in combination for some *Toxoplasma* infections. Topical preparations are used for therapy of severe acne and non-sexually transmitted infection of the genital tract in women.

The most serious **adverse effect** is antibiotic-associated (pseudomembranous) colitis; clindamycin should be stopped if any diarrhoea occurs.

POLYPEPTIDE ANTIBIOTICS

Vancomycins

Vancomycin ($t_{\frac{1}{2}}$ 8 h), a 'glycopeptide' or 'peptolide', acts on multiplying organisms by inhibiting cell wall formation at a site different from the β-lactam antibacterials. It is bactericidal against most strains of clostridia (including *Clostridium difficile*), almost all strains of *Staphylococcus aureus* (including those that produce β-lactamase and methicillin-resistant strains), coagulase-negative staphylococci, viridans group streptococci and enterococci. Frankly resistant *Staphylococcus aureus* strains have been exceptionally rarely reported, although isolates with raised (but still formally susceptible) vancomycin MICs around 2–3 mg/L have been increasingly recognised and have a somewhat poorer outcome when the drug is used to treat serious, systemic infections such as endocarditis and bacteraemia. Detecting these borderline-susceptible strains reliably in the microbiology laboratory can be technically challenging. Combining vancomycin with linezolid, daptomycin or rifampicin may give better results in such cases, and therapeutic drug monitoring is important to keep trough concentrations at the upper end of the acceptable scale.

Vancomycin is poorly absorbed from the gut and is given i.v. for systemic infections as there is no satisfactory i.m. preparation. It distributes effectively into body tissues and is eliminated by the kidney.

Uses. Vancomycin is effective in cases of antibioticassociated pseudomembranous colitis (caused by *Clostridium difficile* or, less commonly, staphylococci) in a dose of 125 mg 6-hourly by mouth. Combined with an aminoglycoside, it may be given i.v. for streptococcal endocarditis in patients who are allergic to benzylpenicillin and for serious infection with multiply resisant staphylococci. It is not as effective as flucloxacillin for serious infections caused by methicillin-susceptible *S. aureus*. Dosing is guided by plasma concentration monitoring with the aim of achieving trough concentrations between 10 and 20 mg/L (15–20 mg/L in patients being treated for infective endocarditis). Trough concentrations of up to 25 mg/L of recent vancomycin formulations have not been associated with significant toxicity, and may give better outcomes for the most severe infections and those with less-susceptible strains. There is actually no strong evidence that monitoring peak and/or trough serum vancomycin concentrations reduces the incidence of renal or ototoxicity. However, achieving adequate serum concentrations clearly correlates with both outcome and avoidance of rises in isolates' vancomycin MICs, so initial doses should be calculated on total body-weight even in obese subjects, and dose adjustments should be based on measured serum concentrations performed at least weekly in subjects with stable renal function (and more often in those with reduced or varying renal function).

Adverse effects. Tinnitus and deafness may occur, but may improve if the drug is stopped. Nephrotoxicity and allergic reactions also occur. Rapid i.v. infusion may cause amaculopapular rash, possibly due to histamine release (the'red person' syndrome).

Teicoplanin is structurally related to vancomycin and is active against Gram-positive bacteria. The $t_{1/2}$ of 50 h allows once daily i.v. or i.m. administration. It is less likely than vancomycin to cause oto- or nephrotoxicity, but serum monitoring is required to assure adequate serum concentrations for severely ill patients and those with changing renal function.

Daptomycin ($t_{1/2}$ 9 h) is a recently released lipopeptide antibiotic, naturally produced by the bacterium *Streptomyces roseosporus* which was first isolated from a soil sample from Mount Ararat in Turkey. It has activity against virtually all Gram-positive bacteria, including penicillin resistant *Streptococcus pneumoniae* and MRSA, regardless of vancomycin resistance phenotype. It is unable to cross the Gram-negative outer membrane, rendering these bacteria resistant.

It is administered by single daily intravenous injection, and is over 90% protein bound. Virtually no metabolism occurs and excretion is predominantly renal, with about 60% of a dose being recoverable unchanged from the urine. The standard dosage is 4 mg/kg per dose, with the frequency of dosing reduced to 48-hourly for patients with creatinine clearances below 30 mL/min. A higher dose of 6 mg/kg everyday is being assessed for infective endocarditis. CSF penetration is only about 5%, but sufficient concentrations may be achieved to be useful, for example, for penicillin-resistant pneumococcal meningitis.

Adverse drug reactions have been reported at similar rates to vancomycin. Use of a longer dose interval has avoided the problems of skeletal muscle pain and rises in serum creatinine phosphokinase that were reported when daptomycin was first introduced in the 1980s in a twice daily regimen.

Oritavancin, dalbavancin and telavancin are semisynthetic lipoglycopeptides with high, concentration dependent bactericidal activity *in vitro* against most Gram-positive pathogens. Their modes of action probably resemble that of vancomycin, inhibiting the late stages of cell wall peptidoglycan synthesis. The large molecular size of these compounds impairs their diffusion in laboratory agars, creating technical difficulties in some antimicrobial susceptibility tests. The drugs are currently under assessment for clinical use in resistant and difficult Gram-positive infections, initially of skin and the soft tissues. Dalbavancin may be of particular use in outpatient antibiotic therapy clinics since it has a prolonged half-life ($t_{1/2}$ 5 –7 days) and re-dosing may be required only weekly, and excretion occurs via both urine and faeces.

Polymyxins

Colistin ($t_{1/2}$ 6 h) is a polypeptide effective against Gram-negative organisms. It is sometimes used orally for bowel decontamination, by inhalation via a saline nebuliser inpatients with cystic fibrosis who are infected with *Pseudomonas aeruginosa*, and is applied to skin, including external ear infections. It is currently undergoing a renaissance with systemic use for severe infections with multiply resistant Gram-negative pathogens such as pseudomonads and *Acinetobacter* when no alternative agents are available. The usual dose is 1–2 million units 8-hourly. Inhalational use is also being assessed for adjunctive therapy of Gram-negative ventilator associated pneumonia (usually in combination with intravenous colistin therapy), and it can be administered intrathecally. Adverse effects of systemic administration include nephrotoxicity, neurological symptoms and neuromuscular blockade; renal function should be monitored daily and the dose reduced to 12–18-hourly in patients with creatinine clearance <10–20 mL/min. Recently published case series of parenteral use have reported few problems of serious toxicity even in patients who received over 4 weeks of therapy.

Polymyxin B is also active against Gram-negative organisms, particularly *Pseudomonas aeruginosa*. Its principal use now is topical application for skin, eye and external ear infections.

AMINOGLYCOSIDES

In the purposeful search that followed the demonstration of the clinical efficacy of penicillin, streptomycin was obtained from *Streptomyces griseus* in 1944, cultured from a heavily manured field, and also from a chicken's throat. Aminoglycosides resemble each other in their mode of action and pharmacokinetic, therapeutic and toxic properties.

Mode of action. The aminoglycosides act inside the cell by binding to the ribosomes in such a way that incorrect amino acid sequences are entered into peptide chains. Aminoglycosides are bactericidal and exhibit concentration dependent bacterial killing.

Pharmacokinetics. Aminoglycosides are water-soluble and do not readily cross cell membranes. Poor absorption from the intestine necessitates their administration i.v. or i.m. for systemic use and they distribute mainly to the extracellular fluid; transfer to the cerebrospinal fluid is poor even when the meninges are inflamed. Their $t_{1/2}$ is 2–5 h.

Aminoglycosides are eliminated unchanged mainly by glomerular filtration, and attain high concentrations in the urine. Significant accumulation occurs in the renal cortex. Plasma concentration should be measured regularly (and frequently in renally impaired patients). With prolonged therapy, e.g. endocarditis (gentamicin), monitoring must be meticulous.

Current practice is to administer aminoglycosides as a single daily dose rather than as twice- or thrice-daily doses. Algorithms are available to guide such dosing according to patients' weight and renal function, and in this case only trough concentrations

need to be assayed. Lean body-weight should be used because aminoglycosides distribute poorly in adipose tissue. Single daily dose therapy is probably less oto- and nephrotoxic than divided-dose regimens, and appears to be as effective. The immediate high plasma concentrations that result from single daily dosing are advantageous, e.g. for acutely ill septicaemic patients, as aminoglycosides exhibit concentration-dependent killing.

Antibacterial activity. Aminoglycosides are in general active against staphylococci and aerobic Gram-negative organisms including almost all the Enterobacteriaceae. Bacterial resistance to aminoglycosides is an increasing but patchily distributed problem, notably by acquisition of plasmids which carry genes coding for the formation of drug-destroying enzymes. Gentamicin resistance is rare in community-acquired pathogens in many hospitals in the UK.

Uses include:

- Gram-negative bacillary infection, particularly-septicaemia, renal, pelvic and abdominal sepsis. Gentamicin remains the drug of choice, but tobramycin may be preferred for *Pseudomonas aeruginosa*. Amikacin has the widest antibacterial spectrum of the aminoglycosides but is best reserved for infection caused by gentamicin-resistant organisms. If local resistance rates are low, an aminoglycoside may be included in the initial best-guess regimen for treatment of serious septicaemia. A potentially less toxic antibiotic may be substituted when culture results are known (48–72 h), and toxicity is very rare after such a short course.

- Bacterial endocarditis. An aminoglycoside, usually gentamicin, usually comprises part of the antimicrobial combination for enterococcal, streptococcal or staphylococcal infection of the heart valves.

- Other infections: tuberculosis, tularaemia, plague, brucellosis.

- Topical uses. Neomycin and framycetin, too toxic for systemic use, are effective for topical treatment of infections of the conjunctiva or external ear. Tobramycin is given by inhalation for therapy of infective exacerbations of cystic fibrosis: sufficient systemic absorption may occur to recommend assay of serum concentrations in such patients.

Adverse effects. Aminoglycoside toxicity is a risk when the dose administered is high or of long duration, and the risk is higher if renal clearance is inefficient (because of disease or age), other potentially nephrotoxic drug sare co-administered (e.g. loop diuretics, amphotericin B) or the patient is dehydrated. It may take the following forms:

- Ototoxicity. Both vestibular (especially with gentamicin and streptomycin) and auditory (amikacin, neomycin) damage may occur, causing hearing loss, vertigo, nystagmus and tinnitus which may be permanent (see above). Tinnitus may give warning of auditory nerve damage. Early signs of vestibular toxicity include motion-related headache, dizziness or nausea. Serious ototoxicity can occur with topical application, including ear drops. At least five mutations in the mitochondrial gene encoding 12S rRNA have been found that predispose patients to irreversible aminoglycoside hearing loss, and the possibility of screening individuals before commencing therapy is being investigated. Anti-free radical agents such as salicylate may reduce aminoglycoside toxicity.

- Nephrotoxicity. Dose-related changes, which are usually reversible, occur in renal tubular cells, where aminoglycosides accumulate. Low blood pressure, loop diuretics and advanced age are recognised as added risk factors.

- Neuromuscular blockade. Aminoglycosides may impair neuromuscular transmission and aggravate (reveal) myasthenia gravis, or cause a transient myasthenic syndrome in patients whose neuromuscular transmission is normal.

- Other reactions include rashes and haematological abnormalities, including marrow depression, haemolytic anaemia and bleeding due to antagonism of factor V.

For gentamicin and tobramycin, oto- and nephrotoxicity are increased if peak concentrations exceed 12–14 mg/L consistently, or troughs exceed 2 mg/L. For amikacin the corresponding concentrations are 32–34 mg/L and 10 mg/L.

Individual aminoglycosides

Gentamicin is active against aerobic Gram-negative bacilli including *Escherichia coli*, *Enterobacter*, *Klebsiella*, *Proteus* and *Pseudomonas*. In streptococcal and enterococcal endocarditis gentamicin is combined with benzylpenicillin, in staphylococcal endocarditis with an antistaphylococcal penicillin, and in enterococcal endocarditis with ampicillin (true synergy is seen provided the enterococcus is not highly resistant to gentamicin).

Dose is 3–5 mg/kg body-weight per day (the highest dose for more serious infections) either as a single dose or in three equally divided doses. The rationale behind single-dose administration is to achieve high peak plasma concentrations (10–14 mg/L, which correlate with therapeutic efficacy) and more time at lower trough concentrations (16 h at <1 mg/L, which are associated with reduced risk of toxicity). Therapy should rarely exceed7 days. Patients with cystic fibrosis eliminate gentamicin rapidly and require higher doses. Gentamicin applied to the eye gives effective corneal and aqueous humour concentrations.

Tobramycin is similar to gentamicin; it is more active against most strains of *Pseudomonas aeruginosa* and maybe less nephrotoxic.

Amikacin is mainly of value because it is more resistant to aminoglycoside-inactivating bacterial enzymes than gentamicin. It is finding new application in the initial management of multiply resistant Gram-negative sepsis, especially in areas with high rates of ESBL-producing coliforms. Peak plasma concentrations should be kept between 20–30 mg/L and trough concentrations below 10 mg/L.

Netilmicin is active against some strains of bacteria that resist gentamicin and tobramycin; it may be less oto- and nephrotoxic.

TETRACYCLINES

Tetracyclines have a broad range of antimicrobial activity and differences between the individual members have traditionally been small, but new tetracyclines and tetracycline relatives are now being developed with even wider spectra of activity that include some bacteria with acquired resistance to other classes of antibiotic.

Mode of action. Tetracyclines interfere with protein synthesis by binding to bacterial ribosomes and their selective action is due to higher uptake by bacterial than by human cells. They are bacteriostatic.

Pharmacokinetics. Most tetracyclines are only partially absorbed from the alimentary tract, enough remaining in the intestine to alter the flora and cause diarrhoea. They are distributed throughout the body and cross the placenta. Tetracyclines in general are excreted mainly unchanged in the urine and should be avoided when renal function is severely impaired, although doxycycline and minocycline are eliminated by non-renal routes and are preferred for patients with impaired renal function.

Uses. Tetracyclines are active against nearly all Gram-positive and Gram-negative pathogenic bacteria, but increasing bacterial resistance and low innate activity limit the clinical use of most members of the class. Although 4-quinolone usage has replaced them especially in the developed world, they remain drugs of first choice for infection with chlamydiae (psittacosis, trachoma, pelvic inflammatory disease, lymphogranuloma venereum), mycoplasma (pneumonia), rickettsiae (Q fever, typhus), *Bartonella* spp., and borreliae (Lyme disease, relapsing fever).

Doxycycline is used in therapeutic and prophylactic regimens for malaria and is active against amoebae and a variety of other protozoa. Their most common other uses are as second-line therapy of minor skin and soft tissue infections especially in β-lactam allergic patients; surprisingly, many MRSA strains currently remain susceptible to tetracyclines in the UK.

An unexpected use for a tetracycline is in the treatment of chronic hyponatraemia due to the syndrome of inappropriate antidiuretic hormone secretion (SIADH) when water restriction has failed. Demeclocycline produces a state of unresponsiveness to ADH, probably by inhibiting the formation and action of cyclic AMP in the renal tubule. It is effec-

tive and convenient to use in SIADH because this action is both dose-dependent and reversible.

Adverse reactions. Heartburn, nausea and vomiting due to gastric irritation are common, and attempts to reduce this with milk or antacids impair absorption of tetracyclines. Diarrhoea and opportunistic infection may supervene. Disorders of epithelial surfaces, perhaps due partly to vitamin B complex deficiency and partly to mild opportunistic infection with yeasts and moulds, lead to sore mouth and throat, black hairy tongue, dysphagia and perianal soreness. Vitamin B preparations may prevent or arrest alimentary tract symptoms.

Due to their chelating properties with calcium phosphate, tetracyclines are selectively taken up in the teeth and growing bones of the fetus and of children. This causes hypoplasia of dental enamel with pitting, cusp malformation, yellow or brown pigmentation and increased susceptibility to caries. After the 14th week of pregnancy and in the first few months of life even short courses can be damaging. Prolonged tetracycline therapy can also stain the finger nails at all ages.

Tetracyclines induce photosensitisation and other rashes. Liver and pancreatic damage can occur, especially in pregnancy and with renal disease, when the drugs have been given i.v.

Interactions. Dairy products reduce absorption to a degree but antacids and iron preparations do so much more, by chelation to calcium, aluminium and iron.

Individual tetracyclines

Tetracycline is eliminated by the kidney and in the bile ($t_{1/2}$ 6 h). Because of incomplete absorption from the gut i.v. doses need be less than half of the oral dose to be similarly effective. The dose is 250–500 mg 6-hourly by mouth.

Doxycycline is well absorbed from the gut, even after food. It is excreted in the bile, in the faeces which it reenters by diffusing across the small intestinal wall and, to some extent, in the urine ($t_{1/2}$ 16 h). These non-renal mechanisms compensate effectively when renal function is impaired and no reduction of dose is necessary; 200 mg is given on the first day, then 100 mg/day.

Minocycline differs from other tetracyclines in that its antibacterial spectrum includes *Neisseria meningitidis* and it has been used for meningococcal prophylaxis. It is well absorbed from the gut, even after a meal, partly metabolized in the liver and partly excreted in the bile and urine ($t_{1/2}$ 15 h). Dose reduction is not necessary when renal function is impaired; 200 mg initially is followed by 100 mg 12-hourly. Minocycline, but not other tetracyclines, may cause a reversible vestibular disturbance with dizziness, tinnitus and impaired balance, especially in women.

Tigecycline ($t_{1/2}$ 42 h) is the first of the glycylcyclines to be licensed. These are close relatives of the tetracyclines – tigecycline shares the same molecular structure as minocycline with the addition of a 9-glycylamide group as a side chain on the tetracycline ring. The molecule binds to the 30S bacterial ribosomal subunit, blocking entry of amino-acyl tRNA molecules to the A site and preventing amino acid chain elongation. Probably because of stearic hindrance from the 9-glycylamide structure and avid ribosomal binding, tigecycline is unaffected by the two commonest tetracycline resistance mechanisms – ribosomal alteration and efflux pumps. Consequently the compound displays useful bacteriostatic activity against a wide range of pathogens including streptococci and staphylococci (including vancomycin resistant enterococci (VRE) and MRSA), Gram-negative bacilli (including *Legionella* spp., although not *Proteus* spp. or *Pseudomonas* spp. and their relatives) and anaerobes.

It is licensed for skin and soft tissue infection, complicated intra-abdominal infections and community-acquired pneumonia, in which trial outcomes have shown equivalent efficacy to carbapenems and other similar agents. Resistance has emerged during treatment of a variety of serious infections. A somewhat higher mortality rate than comparator agents (4% vs. 3%) has been reported by post-marketing surveillance during treatment of a range of serious infections: this observation requires scientific inves-

tigation before tigecycline's use is re-evaluated, but caution is warranted.

It is only available for parenteral use and is administered as a 100 mg first dose followed by 50 mg twice daily. Distribution is widespread throughout the body, although little crosses the blood–brain barrier and concentrations achieved in the urine are below the tigecycline MIC of many pathogens. Limited metabolism occurs, with about 60% of a dose eliminated via the gut and bile and 33% in the urine (only 22% as unchanged tigecycline). No dosage adjustment is required in renal failure or dialysis, and a dose reduction is required only in severe hepatic failure. A similar range and rate of side-effects to the tetracyclines has been reported.

CHLORAMPHENICOLS

Chloramphenicol

Chloramphenicol has a broad spectrum of activity and is primarily bacteriostatic, but may be bactericidal against *Haemophilus influenzae*, *Neisseria meningitidis* and *Streptococcus pneumoniae*.

Pharmacokinetics. Chloramphenicol succinate is hydrolysed to active chloramphenicol and there is much individual variation in the capacity to perform this reaction. Chloramphenicol is inactivated by conjugation with glucuronic acid in the liver ($t_{1/2}$ 5 h in adults). In the neonate, the process of glucuronidation is slow, and plasma concentrations are extremely variable, especially in premature neonates in whom monitoring of plasma concentration is essential. Chloramphenicol penetrates well into all tissues, including the CSF and brain even in the absence of meningeal inflammation.

Uses. Chloramphenicol's role in meningitis and brain abscess has largely been superseded, but it is a second-line agent for these indications. Chloramphenicol may be used for *salmonella* infections (typhoid fever, *salmonella* septicaemia) but ciprofloxacin is now preferred. Topical administration is effective for bacterial conjunctivitis.

Adverse effects. Systemic use of chloramphenicol is dominated by the fact that it can cause rare (between 1:18 000 and 1:100 000 courses) though serious bone marrow damage which may be a dose-dependent, reversible depression of erythrocyte, platelet and leucocyte formation that occurs early in treatment (type A adverse drug reaction), or an idiosyncratic (probably geneticallydetermined), non-dose-related, and usually fatal aplastic anaemia which may develop during, or even weeks after, prolonged treatment, and sometimes on re-exposure to the drug (type B adverse reaction). This has also occurred, very rarely, with eye drops. Marrow depression may be detected at an early and recoverable stage by frequent checking of the full blood count.

The 'grey baby' syndrome occurs in neonates as circulatory collapse in which the skin develops a cyanotic grey colour.

Sodium fusidate

Sodium fusidate is a steroid antimicrobial which is used almost exclusively against β-lactamase-producing staphylococci. Because staphylococci may rapidly become resistant via a one-step genetic mutation, the drug should be combined with another antistaphylococcal drug, e.g. flucloxacillin. Sodium fusidate is readily absorbed from the gut and distributes widely in body tissues including bone. It is metabolised and very little is excreted unchanged in the urine; the $t_{1/2}$ is 5 h.

Uses. Sodium fusidate is a valuable drug for treating severe staphylococcal infections, including osteomyelitis, and is available as i.v. and oral preparations. In an ointment or gel, sodium fusidate is used topically for staphylococcal skin infection. Another gel preparation is used for topical application to the eye: this contains such a high fusidic acid concentration that it possesses useful activity against most bacteria that cause conjunctivitis.

Adverse effects. It is well tolerated, but mild gastrointestinal upset is frequent. Jaundice may develop, particularly with high doses given intravenously, and liver function should be monitored.

SYNTHESIZED ANTIBIOTICS

Quinolones

(4-quinolones, fluoroquinolones)

The first widely used quinolone, nalidixic acid, was discovered serendipitously as a by-product of chloroquinesynthesis. It is effective for urinary tract infections because it is concentrated in the urine, but it has little systemic activity. Fluorination of the quinolone structure was subsequently found to produce compounds that were up to 60 times more active than nalidixic acid and killed a wider range of organisms. These newer '4-quinolones' act principally by inhibiting bacterial (but not human) DNA gyrase (topoisomerase II and IV), thus preventing the supercoiling of DNA, a process that is necessary for compacting chromosomes in the bacterial cell; they are bactericidal and exhibit concentration-dependent bacterial killing. In general quinolones are extremely active against Gram-negative organisms and most have useful activity against *Pseudomonas aeruginosa*, mycobacteria and *Legionella pneumophila*. Most are less active against Gram-positive organisms (resistance commonly emerges) and anaerobes.

Pharmacokinetics. Quinolones are well absorbed from the gut, and widely distributed in tissue. Mechanisms of inactivation (hepatic metabolism, renal and biliary excretion) are detailed below for individual members. There is substantial excretion and re-absorption via the colonic mucosa, and patients with renal failure or intestinal malfunction, e.g. ileus, are prone to accumulate quinolones.

Uses vary between individual drugs.

Adverse effects include gastrointestinal upset and allergic reactions (rash, pruritus, arthralgia, photosensitivity andanaphylaxis). CNS effects may develop with dizziness, headache and confusion. Convulsions have occurred during treatment (avoid or use with caution where there is a history of epilepsy or concurrent use of NSAIDs, which potentiate this effect). Rupture of tendons, notably the Achilles, has occurred, more commonly in the elderly and those takingcorticosteroids concurrently.

Some are potent liver enzyme inhibitors and impair the metabolic inactivation of other drugs including warfarin, theophylline and sulphonylureas, increasing their effect. Magnesium- and aluminium-containing antacids impair absorption of quinolones from the gastrointestinal tract, probably through forming a chelate complex; ferrous sulphate and sucralfate also reduce absorption.

Individual members of the group include the following:

Ciprofloxacin ($t_{1/2}$ 3 h) is effective against a range of bacteria but particularly the Gram-negative organisms. Ciprofloxacinis indicated for use in infections of the urinary, gastrointestinal and respiratory tracts, tissue infections, gonorrhoea and septicaemia. It has proven especially useful for oral therapy of chronic Gram-negative infections such as osteomyelitis, and for acute exacerbations of *Pseudomonas* infection in cystic fibrosis. It has been used for the prophylaxis and therapy of anthrax, including cases resulting from bioterrorism. Ciprofloxacin impairs metabolism of theophylline and of warfarin, both of which should be monitored carefully when co-administered.

Norfloxacin ($t_{1/2}$ 3 h) is used for acute or chronic recurrent urinary tract infections.

Ofloxacin ($t_{1/2}$ 4 h) has modestly greater Gram-positive, but less Gram-negative activity than ciprofloxacin. It is used for urinary and respiratory tract infections, gonorrhoea, and topically for eye infection.

Others Levofloxacin ($t_{1/2}$ 7 h) has greater activity against *Streptococcus pneumoniae* than ciprofloxacin and is used for respiratory and urinary tract infection. Moxifloxacin ($t_{1/2}$ 9 –12 h) has strong anti-Gram-positive activity and is also effective against many anaerobes, but it is only weakly active against *Pseudomonas*. It is recommended as a second-line agent for upper and lower respiratory tract infections including those caused by 'atypical' pathogens and penicillin-resistant *Streptococcus pneumoniae*. QT prolongation occurs, and moxifloxacinis contra-indicated in patients with cardiac failure orrhythm disorders. It has balanced renal and hepatic excretion so dose modification in renal failure is not necessary.

SULFONAMIDES AND SULFONAMIDE COMBINATIONS

Sulfonamides now have their place in medicine mainly in combination with trimethoprim. Because of the risks of adverse drug reactions associated with their use, this is generally restricted to specific indications where other therapeutic agents have clearly inferior efficacy.

The enzyme dihydrofolic acid (DHF) synthase converts p-aminobenzoic acid (PABA) to DHF which is subsequently converted to tetrahydric folic acid (THF), purines and DNA. The sulfonamides are structurally similar to PABA, successfully compete with it for DHF synthase, and thus ultimately impair DNA formation.

Pharmacokinetics. Sulfonamides for systemic use are absorbed rapidly from the gut. The principal metabolic path is acetylation and the capacity to acetylate is genetically determined in a bimodal form, i.e. there are slow and fast acetylators, but the differences are of limited practical importance in therapy. The kidney is the principal route of excretion of drug and acetylate.

Systemic use

Sulfonamide-trimethoprim combination. Co-trimoxazole (sulfamethoxazole plus trimethoprim); the optimum synergistic in vitro effect against most susceptible bacteria is achieved with 5:1 ratio of sulfamethoxazole to trimethoprim, although concentrations achieved in the tissues vary considerably. Each drug is well absorbed from the gut, has a $t_{1/2}$ of 10 h and is 80% excreted by the kidney; consequently, the dose of co-trimoxazole should be reduced when renal function is impaired.

Trimethoprim on its own is now used in many conditions for which the combination was originally recommended, and it may cause fewer adverse reactions (see below). The combination is, however, retained for the following:

- Prevention and treatment of pneumonia due to *Pneumocystis carinii* infection in immunosuppressed patients (for therapy, high doses of 120 mg/kg·day in 2–4 divided doses are used and therapeutic drug monitoring is essential).

- Prevention and treatment of toxoplasmosis, and treatment of nocardiasis and *Stenotrophomonas maltophilia* infection (90–120 mg/kg·day dosing).

Sulfadiazine ($t_{\frac{1}{2}}$ 10 h), sulfametopyrazine ($t_{\frac{1}{2}}$ 38 h) and sulfadimidine (sulfamethazine) ($t_{\frac{1}{2}}$ approximately 6 h, dose dependent) are available in some countries for urinary tract infections, meningococcal meningitis and other indications, but resistance rates are high.

Silver sulfadiazine is used topically for prophylaxis and treatment of infected burns, leg ulcers and pressure sores because of its wide antibacterial spectrum (which includes pseudomonads).

AZOLES

This group includes:

- Metronidazole and tinidazole (antibacterial and antiprotozoal) which are described here.
- Fluconazole, itraconazole, clotrimazole, econazole, ketoconazole, isoconazole and miconazole which are described under Antifungal drugs.

Metronidazole

In obligate anaerobic microorganisms (but not in aerobes) metronidazole is converted into an active form by reduction of its nitro group: this binds to DNA and prevents nucleic acid formation; it is bacteriostatic.

Pharmacokinetics. Metronidazole is well absorbed after oral or rectal administration and distributed widely. It is eliminated in the urine, partly unchanged and partly as metabolites. The $t_{\frac{1}{2}}$ is 8 h.

Uses. Metronidazole's clinical indications are:

- Treatment of sepsis to which anaerobic organisms, e.g. *Bacteroides* spp. and anaerobic cocci, are contributing, including post-surgical infection, intra-abdominal infection and septicaemia, osteomyelitis and abscesses of brain or lung.
- Antibiotic-associated pseudomembraneous colitis (caused by *Clostridium difficile*).
- Trichomoniasis of the urogenital tract in both sexes.
- Amoebiasis (*Entamoeba histolytica*), including both intestinal and extra-intestinal infection.
- Giardiasis (*Giardia lamblia*).
- Acute ulcerative gingivitis and dental infections (*Fusobacterium* spp. and other oral anaerobic flora).
- Anaerobic vaginosis (*Gardnerella vaginalis* and vaginal anaerobes).

Dose. Established anaerobic infection is treated with metronidazole by mouth 400 mg 8-hourly; by rectum 1 g 8-hourly for 3 days followed by 1 g 12-hourly; or by i.v. infusion 500 mg 8-hourly. A topical gel preparation is useful for reducing the odour associated with anaerobic infection of fungating tumours.

Adverse effects include nausea, vomiting, diarrhoea, furred tongue and an unpleasant metallic taste in the mouth; also headache, dizziness and ataxia. Rashes, urticaria and angioedema occur. Peripheral neuropathy occurs if treatment is prolonged and epileptiform seizures if the dose is high. Large doses of metronidazole are carcinogenic in rodents and the drug is mutagenic in bacteria; long-term studies have failed to discover oncogenic effects in humans.

A disulfiram-like effect occurs with alcohol because metronidazole inhibits alcohol and aldehydedehydrogenase; patients should be warned appropriately.

Tinidazole is similar to metronidazole in use and adverse effects, but has a longer $t_{\frac{1}{2}}$ (13 h). It is excreted mainly unchanged in the urine. The longer duration of action of tinidazole may be an advantage, e.g. in giardiasis, trichomoniasis and acute ulcerative gingivitis, in which tinidazole 2 g by mouth in a single dose is as effective as a course of metronidazole.

MINOR ANTIMICROBIALS

These are included because they are effective topically without serious risk of allergy, while toxicity or chemical instability limits or precludes their systemic use.

RESISTANCE TO ANTIMICROBIALS: LINEZOLID, QUINUPRISTIN-DALFOPRISTIN AND FOSFOMYCIN

Linezolid and quinupristin-dalfopristin (Synercid) were developed in response to the emergence of multiply resistant Gram-positive pathogens during the 1990s. Both have clinically useful activity against MRSA (including vancomycin intermediate and resistant strains), vancomycin-resistant enterococci and penicillin-resistant *Streptococcus pneumoniae*. They are currently reserved for treatment of infections caused by such bacteria and for use in patients who are allergic to more established antibiotics. These agents are inactive against most Gram-negative bacteria.

Linezolid, a synthetic oxazolidinone, is the first member of the first totally new class of antibacterial agents to be released to the market for 20 years, the first new agent approved for therapy of MRSA for over 40 years, and the first oral antibiotic active against VRE. It has a unique mode of action, binding to domain V of the 23S component of the 50S ribosomal subunit and inhibiting formation of the initiation complex between transfer-RNA, messenger-RNA and the ribosomal subunits. It is bacteriostatic against most Gram-positive bacteria, but is bactericidal against pneumococci.

Resistance has been reported so far in occasional enterococcus and *Staphylococcus aureus* isolates from immunocompromised patients and others with chronic infections who had been treated with linezolid for long periods; a handful of examples from other species have also been found. Linezolid-resistant isolates possess modified 23S ribosomal RNA genes, and the level of resistance correlates with the number of gene copies the organisms carry. Most Gram-negative bacteria are resistant by virtue of possessing membrane efflux pumps, although many obligate anaerobes are susceptible.

It is eliminated via both renal and hepatic routes ($t_{1/2}$ 6 h) with 30%–55% excreted in the urine as the active drug. Oral and parenteral formulations are available, and the usual dose is 600 mg 12-hourly by both routes; absorption after oral administration is rapid, little affected by food, and approaches 100%. Dose modification in hepatic or renal impairment is not necessary. Distribution includes to the CSF, eye and respiratory tract, although variability in concentrations achieved is seen with systemic sepsis, cystic fibrosis and burn injuries and also in neonates, and it is note worthy that linezolid resistance has developed during treatment of patients with low serum concentrations.

Linezolid is licensed in the UK for skin, soft tissue and respiratory tract infections, and it is usually restricted on grounds of cost to those caused by multiply resistant pathogens. The oral formulation has proven useful for follow-on therapy of severe and chronic infections caused by bacteria resistant to other agents, e.g. MRSA osteomyelitis, although its drug cost is high for both oral and parenteral preparations.

Quinupristin-dalfopristin is a 30%:70% combination of two streptogramin molecules: the dalfopristin component binds first to the 50S bacterial ribosome, inducing a conformational change which allows the additional binding of quinupristin. The combination results in inhibition of both aminoacyl-tRNA attachment and the peptidyltransferase elongation step of protein synthesis, resulting in premature release of polypeptide chains from the ribosome. The summative effect is bactericidal. Acquired resistance is currently rare, but a variety of possible mechanisms of resistance have been reported including methylation of the 23S RNA molecule (also involved in erythromycin resistance), enzymatic hydrolysis and phosphorylation and efflux pumps. Most strains of *Enterococcus faecalis* are naturally resistant, but *E. faecium* is susceptible, as are the respiratory pathogens *Legionella pneumophila*, *Moraxella catarrhalis* and *Mycoplasma pneumoniae*. Other Gram-negative bacteria have impermeable membranes and hence are resistant. The $t_{1/2}$ is 1.5 h. Quinupristin-dalfopristin is available for administration only by i.v. injection; the usual dose is 7.5 mg/kg every 8 h.

Injection to peripheral veins frequently causes phlebitis, so a central line is required. Arthralgia and myalgia are seen in about 10% of patients. No dosage reduction is recommended in renal impairment, but the dose should be reduced in moderate hepatic impairment and it should generally be avoided if the impairment is severe.

Fosfomycin, a phosphonic acid derivative, was

originally extracted from a *Streptomyces* sp. bacterium in 1969, but is now fully synthetic. Oral preparations have been used in a number of countries for over 20 years mainly for urinary tract infection, and a disodium derivative is available for intravenous and intramuscular use.

Fosfomycin is bactericidal against many Gram-positive and Gram-negative bacteria via inhibition of uridinediphosphate-GlcNAc enol-pyruvyltransferase (MurA). It enters bacterial and mammalian cells via an active transport system. Susceptible bacteria include most coliforms, *Staphylococcus aureus* and *epidermidis*, *Streptococcus pneumonia* and *Enterococcus faecalis*. In some cases synergy has been demonstrated with β-lactam antibiotics. Predictably resistant species include *Acinetobacter* spp., *Listeria monocytogenes* and anaerobes, while few *Pseudomonas aeruginosa* or *Enterococcus faecium* are inhibited. Fosfomycin has a small molecular size and relatively long half life ($t_{1/2}$ 5.7 h) and so penetrates most tissues, including the CSF and eye. Few data are available on drug interactions, although reported adverse events are uncommon, mainly including mild gastrointestinal disturbance (in 5%–6%) and rashes (4%), and pain and inflammation at the infusion and injection site of the parenteral preparation (3%).

Most published experience is with single 3 g oral doses for lower urinary tract infection, where fosfomycin activity persists in the urine for 48 h and is as effective as 3–5 day courses of conventional agents: it is one convenient choice for ESBL-producing coliforms. A 3 g once-daily regimen for 3 days may be used for complicated urinary tract infection. Prolonged and successful use is reported for a wide variety of serious infections where treat menthad been complicated by bacterial resistance and host allergy to other agents, including infections with penicillin resistant pneumococci, MRSA, ESBL coliforms and vancomycin-resistant *E. faecalis*. Resistance can emerge during therapy of the individual, mediated by conjugation of glutathione to the antibiotic molecule by bacterial metalloglutathione transferase, but surveys in countries where the drug has been used for two decades have shown a consistently low (3%)

primary resistance rate in urinary tract pathogens and there is no cross-resistance to other antimicrobial classes. Fosfomycin is currently not licensed in the UK but is available via the European license on a named patient basis.

Part 2. Chemotherapy Of Bacterial Infections

INFECTION OF THE BLOOD

Septicaemia is a medical emergency that moves clinically from sepsis (systemic inflammatory response syndrome, 'SIRS') via organ dysfunction ('severe sepsis') to septicshock as the associated mortality rates progress from16% to 46%. In a shocked patient (i.e. with low blood pressure that does not promptly respond to circulatory volume enhancement) survival rates fall by over 7% for each hour of delay in commencing effective antibiotics. Urgent support of the circulation and other organs is necessary for survival, and rapid assessment by senior medical staff and early involvement of infection specialists have also been associated with an improved outcome and lowest antibiotic costs during treatment.

Usually, the infecting organism(s) is not known at the time of presentation and treatment must be instituted onthe basis of a 'best guess' (i.e. 'empirical therapy'). The clinical circumstances and knowledge of local resistance patterns may provide clues. Examples of suitable choices are given in the list below: patients who have been in hospital for some time before presenting with septicaemia need antibiotic regimens that provide more reliable cover for multiply resistant pathogens, and examples of these are given in square brackets:

- Septicaemia accompanied by a spreading rash that doesnot blanch with pressure should be assumed to be meningococcal, and the patient must be referred to hospital urgently (after an immediate parenteral dose of benzylpenicillin): ceftriaxone.
- Community-acquired pneumonia: co-amoxiclav + clarithromycin.

- When septicaemia follows gastrointestinal or genital tract surgery, *Escherichia coli* (or other coliforms), anaerobic bacteria, e.g. *Bacteroides*, streptococci or enterococci are likely pathogens: piperacillin tazobactam or gentamicin plus benzylpenicillin plus metronidazole [meropenem, plus vancomycin if MRSA is a risk].

- Septicaemia related to urinary tract infection usually involves *Escherichia coli* (or other Gram-negativebacteria), enterococci: gentamicin plus benzylpenicillin or piperacillin-tazobactam alone [meropenem plus vancomycin].

- Staphylococcal septicaemia may be suspected where there is an abscess, e.g. of bone or lung, or with acute infective endocarditis or infection of intravenous catheters: high-dose flucloxacillin [vancomycin]. Uncomplicated *Staphylococcus aureus* bacteraemia should be treated for 14 days to reduce the risk of metastatic infection: patients with prolonged bacteraemia or who fail to settle promptly should be considered for treatment as for staphylococcal endocarditis.

- Severe cellulitis, bites and necrotising fasciitisac companied by septicaemia should be treated with optimal cover for Lancefield Group A streptococcus, anaerobes and coliforms: piperacillin-tazobactam + clindamycin [meropenemt clindamycin].

- Septicaemia in patients rendered neutropenic by cytotoxic drugs frequently involves coliforms and *Pseudomonas* spp. translocating to the circulation directly from the bowel, while coagulase-negative staphylococci also commonly arise from central venous catheter infection: piperacillin-tazobactam, sometimes plus vancomycin.

Patients who have had a splenectomy are at risk of fulminant septicaemia especially from capsulate bacteria, e.g. *Streptococcus pneumoniae, Neisseria meningitidis*. The risk is greatest in the first 2 years after splenectomy (but is lifelong), in children, and in those with splenectomy for haematological malignancy. Patients must be immunised against appropriate pathogens and receive continuous low-dose oral prophylaxis with phenoxymethylpenicillin (penicillin V), or erythromycin in those allergic to penicillin.

INFECTION OF PARANASAL SINUSES AND EARS

Sinusitis

As oedema of the mucous membrane hinders the drainage of pus, a logical first step is to open the obstructed passage with a sympathomimetic vaso-constrictor, e.g. ephedrine nasal drops. Antibiotic therapy produces limited additional clinical benefit, but the common infecting organism(s) –*Streptococcus pneumoniae, Haemophilus influenzae, Streptococcus pyogenes, Moraxella (Branhamella) catarrhalis* – usually respond to oral amoxicillin (with or without clavulanic acid) or doxycycline if serious.

Otitis media

Mild cases are normally viral and often resolve spontaneously, needing only analgesia and observation. A bulging, inflamed eardrum indicates bacterial otitis media usually due to *Streptococcus pneumoniae, Haemophilus influenzae, Moraxella (Branhamella) catarrhalis, Streptococcus pyogenes* (Group A) or *Staphylococcus aureus*. Amoxicillin or coamoxiclav is satisfactory, but the clinical benefit of antibiotic therapy is small in controlled trials and good outcomes with reduced use of antibiotics have been demonstrated if patients are given a prescription which they only fill if they worsen or fail to improve after 48 h (sometimes known as a 'WASP' – a 'wait and see' prescription).

INFECTION OF THE THROAT

Pharyngitis is usually viral but the more serious cases maybe due to *Streptococcus pyogenes* (Group A) (always sensitive to benzylpenicillin), which cannot be differentiated clinically from virus infection with any certainty. Prevention of complications is more important than relief of the symptoms, which seldom last long and corticosteroids are much more effective than antibiotics at shortening the period of pain.

Chemoprophylaxis

Chemoprophylaxis of streptococcal (Group A) infection with phenoxymethylpenicillin is necessary for patients who have had one attack of rheumatic fever. Continue for at least 5 years or until aged 20 years, whichever is the longer period (although some hold that it should continue for life). Chemoprophylaxis should be continued for life after a second attack of rheumatic fever. A single attack of acute nephritis is not an indication for chemoprophylaxis. Ideally, chemoprophylaxis should continue throughout the year but, if the patient is unwilling to submit to this, cover at least the colder months.

Adverse effects are uncommon. Patients taking penicillin prophylaxis are liable to have penicillin-resistant viridians type *streptococci* in the mouth, so that during even minor dentistry, e.g. scaling, there is a risk of bacteraemia and thus of infective endocarditis with a penicillin-resistant organism in those with any residual rheumatic heart lesion. Patients taking penicillins are also liable to be carrying resistant staphylococci and pneumococci.

INFECTION OF THE BRONCHI, LUNGS AND PLEURA

Bronchitis

Most cases of acute bronchitis are viral; where bacteria are responsible, the usual pathogens are *Streptococcus pneumoniae* and/or *Haemophilus influenzae*. It is questionable whether there is a role for antimicrobials in uncomplicated acute bronchitis, but amoxicillin, a tetracycline or trimethoprim is appropriate if treatment is considered necessary. Whether newer antimicrobials, e.g. moxifloxacin, confer significant outcome advantages to justify their expense is debatable.

In chronic bronchitis, suppressive chemotherapy with amoxicillin or trimethoprim may be considered during the colder months (in temperate, colder regions), for patients with symptoms of pulmonary insufficiency, recurrent acute exacerbations or permanently purulent sputum.

For intermittent therapy, the patient is given a supply of the drug and told to take it in full dose at the first sign of a 'chest' cold, e.g. purulent sputum, and to stop the drug after 3 days if there is rapid improvement. Otherwise, the patient should continue the drug until recovery takes place. If the exacerbation lasts for more than 10 days, there is a need for clinical reassessment.

Pneumonias

The clinical setting is a useful guide to the causal organism and hence to the 'best guess' early choice of antimicrobial. It is not possible reliably to differentiate between pneumonias caused by 'typical' and 'atypical' pathogens on clinical grounds alone and most experts advise initial cover for both types of pathogen in seriously ill patients. However, there is no strong evidence that adding 'atypical' cover to empirical parenteral treatment with a β-lactam antibiotic improves the outcome. Published guidelines often recommend hospital admission and parenteral and broader-spectrum therapy for the most severely affected patients as assessed by the 'CUR -65' score (one point is scored for each of Confusion, elevated serum Urea, Respiratory rate >30 breaths per minute, low Blood pressure, and age of 65 or above). Delay of 4 hours or more in commencing effective antibiotics in the most seriously ill patients is associated with increased mortality.

Pneumonia in previously healthy people (community acquired)

Disease that is segmental or lobar in its distribution is usually due to *Streptococcus pneumoniae* (pneumococcus). *Haemophilus influenzae* is a rare cause in this group, although it more often leads to exacerbations of chronic bronchitis and does cause pneumonia in patients infected with HIV. Benzylpenicillin i.v. or amoxicillin or clarithromycin p.o. are the treatments of choice if pneumococcal pneumonia is very likely; use clarithromycin, doxycycline or moxifloxacin in a penicillin-allergic patient. Seriously ill patients should receive benzylpenicillin (to cover the pneumococcus) plus ciprofloxacin (to cover *Haemophilus* and 'atypical' pathogens), and co-amoxiclav plus clarithromycin is an alternative that may have a lower propensity to promote *Clostridium difficile* diarrhoea. Where penicillin-resistant pneumococci are common, i.v. cefotaxime is a reasonable 'best guess' choice pending confirmation of susceptibilities from the laboratory, with vancomycin as an alternative. A wide variety of new antibiotics is under investigation for use in penicillin resistant pneumococcal infections, including cephalosporins, e.g. ceftobiprole, penicillin relatives, e.g faropenem, quinolones, glycopeptides, e.g. oritavancin, and ketolides, e.g. cethromycin.

Pneumonia following influenza is often caused by *Staphylococcus aureus*, and 'best guess' therapy usually involves adding flucloxacillin to one of the regimens above. When staphylococcal pneumonia is proven, sodium fusidate or rifampicin p.o. plus flucloxacillin i.v. should be used in combination. Staphylococcal pneumonia that involves strains producing Panton-Valentine leucocidin toxin is frequently necrotising in nature, and linezolid or clindamycin have been shown to reduce toxin production at the ribosomal level so are recommended for inclusion when this condition is suspected.

'Atypical' cases of pneumonia may be caused by *Mycoplasma pneumoniae* or more rarely *Chlamydia pneumonia* or *psittaci* (psittacosis/ornithosis), *Legionella pneumophila* or *Coxiellaburnetii* (Q fever), and doxycycline or clarithromycin should be given by mouth. Treatment of ornithosis should continue for 10 days after the fever has settled, and that of mycoplasma pneumonia and Q fever for 3 weeks to prevent relapse.

Pneumonia acquired in hospital

Pneumonia is usually defined as being nosocomial (Greek: *nosokomeian*, hospital) if it presents after at least 48 h in hospital. It occurs primarily among patients admitted with medical problems or recovering from abdominal or thoracic surgery and those who are on mechanical ventilators. The common pathogens are *Staphylococcus aureus*, Enterobacteriaceae, *Streptococcus pneumoniae*, *Pseudomonas aeruginosa* and *Haemophilus influenzae*, and anaerobes after aspiration. Mild cases can be given co-amoxiclav

unless they are known to be colonised with resistant bacteria, but for severe cases it is reasonable to initiate therapy with piperacillin-tazobactam (plus vancomycin if the local prevalence of MRSA is high) pending the results of sputum culture and susceptibility tests. Vancomycin or teicoplanin are equally effective for MRSA pneumonia as linezolid, and have an overall lower rate of adverse reactions.

Pneumonia in people with chroniclung disease

Normal commensals of the upper respiratory tract proliferate in damaged lungs especially following virus infections, pulmonary congestion or pulmonary infarction. Antibiotics should not be given to patients who do not demonstrate two or more of increased dyspnoea, sputum volumeand sputum purulence. Mixed infection is common, and as *Haemophilus influenzae* and *Streptococcus pneumonia* are often the pathogens, amoxicillin or trimethoprim is a reasonable choice in domiciliary practice; if response is inadequate, co-amoxiclav or a quinolone should be substituted, but there is no evidence that they are superior first line to the older choices.

Klebsiella pneumoniae is a rare cause of lung infection (Friedlander's pneumonia) in the alcoholic and debilitated elderly. Cefotaxime or piperacillin-tazobactam, possibly plus an aminoglycoside, is recommended.

Pneumonia in immunocompromised patients

Pneumonia is common, e.g. in acquired immune deficiency syndrome (AIDS) or in those who are receiving immunosuppressive drugs.

Common pathogenic bacteria may be responsible (*Staphylococcus aureus*, *Streptococcus pneumoniae*), but often organisms of lower natural virulence (Enterobacteriaceae, viruses, fungi) are causal and necessitate strenuous efforts to identify the microbe including, if feasible, bronchial washings or lung biopsy.

- Until the pathogen is known the patient should receive broad-spectrum antimicrobial treatment, such as an aminoglycoside plus ceftazidime.
- Aerobic Gram-negative bacilli, e.g. Enterobacte-

riaceae, *Klebsiella* spp., are pathogens in half of the cases, especially in neutropenic patients, and respond topiperacillin-tazobactam or ceftazidime. These and *Pseudomonas aeruginosa* may respond better with addition of an aminoglycoside.

- The fungus *Pneumocystis carinii* is an important respiratory pathogen in patients with deficient cell mediated immunity; treat with co-trimoxazole 120 mg/kg daily by mouth or i.v. in two to four divided doses for 14 days, as modified by serum assay, or with pentamidine.

Pneumonia due to anaerobic microorganisms

Pneumonia often follows aspiration of material from the oropharynx, or accompanies other lung pathology such as pulmonary infarction or bronchogenic carcinoma. In addition to conventional microbial causes, pathogens include anaerobic and aerobic streptococci, *Bacteroides* spp. And *Fusobacterium*. Co-amoxiclav or piperacillin-tazobactam may be needed for several weeks to prevent relapse.

Pulmonary abscess: treat the identified organism and employ aspiration or formal surgical drainage if necessary.

Empyema: aspiration or drainage is essential, followed by antibiotic treatment of the isolated organism.

ENDOCARDITIS

When there is suspicion, two or three blood cultures should be taken over a few hours and antimicrobial treatment commenced, to be adjusted later in the light of the results. Delay in treating only exposes the patient to the risk of grave cardiac damage or systemic embolism. Streptococci, enterococci and staphylococci are causal in 80% of cases, with viridans group streptococci having recently been overtaken by *Staphylococcus aureus* as the most common pathogens. In intravenous drug users, *Staphylococcus aureus* is particularly likely, although the potential list of pathogensis extensive in this group. Culture-negative endocarditis (in 8%–10% of cases in contemporary practice) is usually due to previous antimicrobial therapy or to special culture requirements of the microbe; it is best regarded as being due to *streptococci* and treated accordingly.

Principles for treatment

- Use high doses of bactericidal drugs because the organisms are difficult to access in avascular vegetations on valves.
- Give drugs parenterally and preferably by i.v. bolus injection to achieve the necessary high peak concentration to penetrate the vegetations.
- Examine the infusion site daily and change it regularly to prevent opportunistic infection, which is usually with coagulase-negative staphylococci or fungi. Alternatively, use a central subclavian venous catheter.
- Continue therapy, usually for 2–4 weeks, and, in the case of infected prosthetic valves, 6 weeks. Prolonged courses may also be indicated for patients infected with enterococci or other strains with penicillin minimum inhibitory concentrations (MICs) above 0.5mg/L, whose presenting symptoms have been present for over 6 weeks, for those with large vegetations, and those whose clinical symptoms and signs are slow to settle after treatment has started. Highly susceptible streptococcal endocarditis (penicillin MIC of 0.1mg/L or below) can be treated successfully with 2 week courses.
- Valve replacement may be needed at any time during and after antibiotic therapy if cardiovascular function deteriorates or the infection proves impossible to control.
- Adjust the dose according to the sensitivity of the infecting organism – use the minimum inhibitory concentration test.

Dose regimens

The following regimens are commonly recommended (the reader is referred to the British Society for Antimicrobial Chemotherapy treatment guidelines 2006; currently under review, the European Society of Cardiology (2009) or to other published references for detailed advice):

1. Initial ('best guess') treatment should comprise benzylpenicillin (7.2 g i.v. daily in six divided doses), plus gentamicin (1 mg/kg body-weight 8-hourly-synergy allows this dose of gentamicin and minimizes risk of adverse effects). Regular serum gentamicin assay is vital: trough concentrations should be below 1 mg/Land peak concentrations 3–5 mg/L; if *Staphylococcus aureus* is suspected, high-dose flucloxacillin plus rifampicin should be used. Patients allergic to penicillin and those with intracardiac prostheses or suspected MRSA infection should receive vancomycin plus rifampicin plus gentamicin. Patients presenting acutely (suggesting infection with *Staphylococcus aureus*) should receive flucloxacillin (8–12 g/day in four to six divided doses) plus gentamicin.

2. When an organism is identified and its sensitivity determined:

   - *Viridans group streptococci*: the susceptibility of the organism determines the antimicrobial(s) and its duration of use, ranging from benzylpenicillin plus gentamicin for 2 weeks, to vancomycin plus gentamicin for 6 weeks. Patients with uncomplicated endocarditis caused by very sensitive strains may be managed as outpatients;for these patients ceftriaxone 2 g/day for 4 weeks may be suitable.

   - *Enterococcus faecalis* (Group D): ampicillin 2 g 4-hourly or benzylpenicillin 2.4 g 4-hourly plus gentamicin 1 mg/kg 8–12-hourly i.v. for 4–6 weeks. The prolonged gentamicin administration carries a significant risk of adverse drug reactions, but is essential to assure eradication of the infection. *Streptococci* from endocarditis are checked for high-level gentamicin resistance (MIC above 128 mg/L) because cidal synergy is not seen with β-lactams in such strains. Alternative regimens for such infections include ampicillin plus streptomycin (if not similarly high-level resistant) or high-dose ampicillin alone.

   - *Staphylococcus aureus*: flucloxacillin 2 g 4–6-hourly i.v. for at least 4 weeks. In the presence of intracardiac prostheses, flucloxacillin is combined with rifampicin orally (or fusidic acid) for at least he first 2 weeks, and MRSA may be treated with vancomycin plus rifampicin plus fusidic acid (or gentamicin) for 4–6 weeks.

   - *Staphylococcus epidermidis* infecting native heart valves is managed as for *Staphylococcus aureus* if the organism is sensitive.

   - *Coxiella* or *Chlamydia*: give doxycycline 100 mg once daily orally, plus ciprofloxacin 500 mg8-hourly for at least 3 years. Valve replacement is advised in many cases.

   - Fungal endocarditis: amphotericin plus flucytosine has been used, although experience is growing with the new azoles and echinocandins, and specialist advice should be sought. Valve replacement is usually essential.

   - Culture-negative endocarditis: benzylpenicillin plus gentamicin i.v. are given for 4–6 weeks.

MENINGITIS

Speed of initiating treatment and accurate bacteriological diagnosis are the major factors determining the fate of the patient, especially with invasive meningococcal disease where fulminant meningococcal septicaemia still carries a 20%–50% mortality rate (and supporting the circulation in the intensive care unit is as important a determinant of outcome as the rapid commencement of antibiotic therapy). With suspected meningococcal disease, unless the patient has a history of penicillin anaphylaxis, benzylpenicillin should be started by the general practitioner before transfer to hospital; the benefit of rapid treatment outweighs the reduced chance of identifying the causative organism.

Drugs must be given i.v. in high dose. The regimens below provide the recommended therapy, with alternatives for patients allergic to first choices, and septic shock requires appropriate management. Intrathecal therapy is now considered unnecessary (except for neurosurgical infections in association with indwelling CSF drains and shunts) and can be dangerous, e.g. encephalopathy with penicillin.

Initial therapy

Initial therapy should be sufficient to kill all pathogens.

All ages over 5 years

For *Neisseria meningitidis* and *Streptococcus pneumoniae*, give benzylpenicillin 2.4 g 4-hourly followed, in the case of *Neisseria meningitidis*, by rifampicin for 2 days prior to discharge from hospital (to eradicate persisting organisms). Some prefer cefotaxime 2–3 g 6–8-hourly or ceftriaxone 2 g i.v. 12-hourly in all cases pending the results of susceptibility tests, and this may be generally preferred depending upon the local prevalence of penicillin resistance. In such cases, in elderly, pregnant or immunocompromised patientsit is prudent to add amoxicillin initially to cover the possibility of listeria involvement. Optimal therapy for known or suspected penicillin-resistant pneumococcal meningitis comprises ceftriaxone 2 g i.v. 12-hourly plus vancomycin 15 mg/kg i.v. 12-hourly plus rifampicin 300 mg i.v. 12-hourly.

Children under 5 years

Neisseria meningitidis is now commonest and *Haemophilus influenzae*, formerly a frequent pathogen, is much less often isolated following immunisation programmes. *Streptococcus pneumoniae* is also less common than in older patients. Give a cephalosporin, e.g. ceftriaxone.

Neonates

For *Escherichia coli*, give cefotaxime or ceftazidime perhaps with gentamicin. For Group B *streptococci*, give benzylpenicillin plus gentamicin. Consult a specialist text for details of doses. Add ampicillin if *Listeria monocytogenes* issuspected.

Dexamethasone given i.v. (0.15 mg/kg 6-hourly for 4 days) and early appears to reduce long-term neurological sequelae, especially sensorineural deafness, in infants and children. In adults there is evidence to support dexamethasone therapy in pneumococcal meningitis, but outcome is not affected in meningitis caused by other pathogens.

Subsequent therapy

Necessarily, i.v. administration should continue until the patient can take drugs by mouth, but whether or when continuation therapy should be oral or i.v. is a matter of debate. Antimicrobials (except aminoglycosides) enter well into the CSF when the meninges are inflamed; relapse may be due to restoration of the blood–CSF barrier as inflammation reduces. The following are recommended (adult doses).

Neisseria meningitidis. Give benzylpenicillin 2.4 g4-hourly or ceftriaxone 2 g i.v. 12-hourly for a minimum of 5 days.

Streptococcus pneumoniae. Give ceftriaxone 2 g i.v. 12-hourly or benzylpenicillin 2.4 g 4-hourly if the organism is penicillin-sensitive and continue for 10 days after the patient has become afebrile.

Haemophilus influenzae. Give ceftriaxone 2 g i.v. 12-hourly or chloramphenicol 100 mg/kg daily for 10 days after the temperature has settled. Subdural empyema, often presenting as persistent fever, is relatively common after haemophilus meningitis and may require surgical drainage.

Chemoprophylaxis

The three common pathogens (below) are spread by respiratory secretions. Asymptomatic nasopharyngeal carriers seldom develop meningitis but may transmit the pathogens to close personal contacts. Rifampicin by mouth is effective at reducing carriage rates.

Meningococcal meningitis often occurs in epidemics in closed communities, but also in isolated cases. Patients and close personal contacts should receive rifampicin 600 mg 12-hourly by mouth for 2 days. Single doses of ciprofloxacin (500 mg by mouth) or ceftriaxone (2 g i.m.) are alternatives, the latter of particular value for pregnant women.

Haemophilus influenzae type b has similar infectivity to that of the meningococcus; give rifampicin 600 mg by mouth daily for 4 days to unimmunised contacts.

Pneumococcal meningitis tends to occur in isolated cases and contacts do not need chemoprophylaxis.

INFECTION OF THE URINARY TRACT

Common pathogens include *Escherichia coli* (commonest in all patient groups), *Proteus* spp., *Klebsiella* spp., other Enterobacteriaceae, *Pseudomonas aeruginosa*, *Enterococcus* spp. and *Staphylococcus saprophyticus*.

For infection of the lower urinary tract a low dose maybe effective, as many antimicrobials are concentrated inthe urine. Infections of the substance of the kidney require the doses needed for any systemic infection. A large urine volume (over 1.5 L/day) and frequent micturition hasten elimination of infection.

Drug treatment of urinary tract infection falls into several categories:

Lower urinary tract infection

This is most commonly seen in young women with normal urinary tracts. Antibiotic treatment shortens the duration of symptoms but may cause adverse reactions, and 20%–30% are free of symptoms at 5–7 days even without antibiotics. Initial treatment with co-amoxiclav, an oral cephalosporin (e.g.cefalexin) or trimethoprim, is usually satisfactory. Current resistance rates of 20%–50% among common pathogens for trimethoprim and amoxicillin threaten their value for empirical therapy in many parts of the world. Therapy should normally last for 3 days and may need to be altered once the results of bacterial sensitivity are known.

Upper urinary tract infection

Acute pyelonephritis may be accompanied by septicaemia and is usually marked by fever and loin pain. In such patients it is advisable to start with co-amoxiclavi.v. or alternatively gentamicin (perhaps plus amoxicillin) i.v. If oral therapy is considered suitable, co-amoxiclav or ciprofloxacinis recommended for 2 weeks. This is an infection of the kidney substance and so needs adequate blood as well as urine concentrations, although a switch to an oral agent (guided by the results of susceptibility testing) to complete the course is recommended after the patient has clinically improved. Upper or lower tract infection with extended-spectrum β-lactamase (ESBL) coliform strains has become more common in some locales, even in patients with no prior hospital contact. Such bacteria are usually resistant also to ciprofloxacin, parenteral cephalosporins and gentamicin. Parenteral meropenem, ertapenem or amikacin, or oral pivmecillinam or fosfomycin may be effective.

Recurrent urinary tract infection

Attacks following rapidly with the same organism may be relapses and indicate a failure to eliminate the original infection. Attacks with a longer interval between them and produced by differing bacterial types may be regarded as due to reinfection, most often by ascending infection from the perineal skin. Repeated short courses of antimicrobials should overcome most recurrent infections but, if these fail,7–14 days of high-dose treatment may be given, following which continuous low-dose prophylaxis may be needed with trimethoprim, nitrofurantoin or an oral cephalosporin.

Asymptomatic infection ('asymptomaticbacteriuria')

This may be found by routine urine testing of pregnant women or patients with known structural abnormalities of the urinary tract. Such infection may explain micturition frequency or incontinence in the elderly. Appropriate antimicrobial therapy should be given, chosen on the basis of susceptibility tests, and normally for 7–10 days. Amoxicillin or a cephalosporin is preferred in pregnancy, although nitrofurantoin may be used if imminent delivery is not likely.

Prostatitis

The commonest pathogens here are Gram-negative aerobicbacilli, although chlamydia may also be involved. A quinolone such as ciprofloxacin is commonly used, although trimethoprim, doxycycline or erythromycin are also effective. Being lipid soluble, these drugs penetrate the prostatein adequate concentration; they may usefully be combined. Response to a single, short course is often good, but recurrence is common and a patient can be regarded as cured only if he has been symptom-free without resort to antimicrobials for a year. Four weeks of oral therapy is often given for recurrent attacks.

Chemoprophylaxis

Chemoprophylaxis is sometimes undertaken in patients liable to recurrent attacks or acute exacerbations of ineradicable infection. It may prevent progressive renal damage in children who are found to have asymptomatic bacteriuria on routine screening. Nitrofurantoin (50–100 mg/day), nalidixic acid (0.5–1.0 g/day) or trimethoprim (100 mg/day) is satisfactory. The drugs are best given as a single oral dose at night.

Tuberculosis of the genitourinary tract is treated on the principles described for pulmonary infection.

Special drugs for urinary tract infections

General antimicrobials used for urinary tract infections are described elsewhere. A few agents find use solely for infection of the urinary tract:

Nitrofurantoin, a synthetic antimicrobial, is active against the majority of urinary pathogens except pseudomonas, and has increased in importance recently because it has retained activity against a useful proportion of urinary tract coliforms that have acquired resistance to trimethoprim, oral β-lactams and quinolones. It is well absorbed from the gastrointestinal tract and is concentrated in the urine ($t_{1/2}$ 1 h), but plasma concentrations are too low to treat infection of kidney tissue. Excretion is reduced when there is renal insufficiency, rendering the drug both more toxic and less effective. Adverse effects include nausea and vomiting (much reduced with the macrocrystalline preparation) and diarrhoea.

Fosfomycin trometamol 3 g p.o. in a single dose.

GENITAL TRACT INFECTIONS

A general account of orthodox literature is given below, but treatment is increasingly the prerogative of specialists, who, as is so often the case, get the best results. Interested readers are referred to specialist texts. Sexually transmitted infections are commonly multiple. Tracing and screening of contacts plays a vital part in controlling spread and reducing re-infection. Recommended treatment regimens vary to some extent among countries, and this is in response to differences in antimicrobial susceptibility of the relevant pathogens and availability of antimicrobial agents.

Gonorrhoea

The problems of β-lactam and quinolone resistance in *Neisseria gonorrhoeae* infection are increasing (ciprofloxacin resistance rates rose from 2.1% in 2 000 to 9.8% in 2002 in England and Wales, reaching over 60% in ethnic white patients in 2009), and selection of a particular drug will depend on sensitivity testing and a knowledge of resistance patterns in different locations. Cefixime and ceftriaxone resistance on testing *in vitro* are increasing, but not yet to levels that compromise therapeutic efficacy. Effective treatment requires exposure of the organism briefly to a high concentration of the drug. Single-dose regimens are practicable and improve compliance. The following schedules are effective:

Uncomplicated anogenital infections. High-dose cefixime 400 mg by mouth; spectinomycin i.v., or ceftriaxone 250 mg i.m. UK resistance rates for oral ciprofloxacin orofloxacin are now considered too high for recommendation unless the isolate is known to be susceptible.

Pharyngeal gonorrhoea responds less reliably, and i.m. ceftriaxone is recommended.

Coexistent infection. *Chlamydia trachomatis* is frequently present with *Neisseria gonorrhoeae*; tetracycline by mouth for 7 days or a single oral dose of azithromycin 1 g or ofloxacin 400 mg will treat the chlamydial urethritis.

Non-gonococcal urethritis

The vast majority of cases of urethritis with pus in which gonococci cannot be identified are due to sexually transmitted organisms, usually *Chlamydia trachomatis* (the most common bacterial sexually-transmitted infection world wide) and sometimes *Ureaplasma urealyticum*. Tetracycline for 1 week, or single-dose azithromycin by mouth are effective.

Pelvic inflammatory disease

Several pathogens are usually involved, including *Chlamydia trachomatis*, *Neisseria gonorrhoeae* and *Mycoplasma hominis*, and there may be superinfection with bowel and other urogenital tract bacteria. A combination of antimicrobials is usually required, e.g. ceftriaxone plus doxycycline plus metronidazole i.v. for severe, acute infection where chlamydia involvement is likely, or co-amoxiclav alone for post-partum chorioamnionitis.

Syphilis

Primary and secondary syphilis are effectively treated by a single dose of 2.4 million units (MU) benzathine penicillin i.m. Doxycycline or erythromycin orally for 2 weeks maybe used for penicillin-allergic patients, and a single oral dose of 2 g azithromycin appears to have equivalent efficacy. *Treponema pallidum* is invariably sensitive to penicillin but macrolide resistance has been reported worldwide rarely except in infections in men who have sex with men.

Tertiary syphilis responds to doxycycline for 28 days or to 3 weekly doses of 2.4 MU benzathine penicillin i.m. Neurosyphilis requires higher serum concentrations for cure and should be treated with procaine penicillin 2.4 megaunits i.m. once daily for 17 days with oral probenecid 500 mg four times a day.

Results of treatment of syphilis with penicillin are excellent. Follow-up of all cases is essential, for 5 years if possible.

The Herxheimer (Jarisch–Herxheimer) reaction is probably caused by cytokine (mainly tumour necrosis factor) release following massive slaughter of spirochaetes. Presenting as pyrexia, it is common during the few hours after the first penicillin injection; other features include tachycardia, headache, myalgia and malaise, which last for up to a day. It cannot be avoided by giving graduated doses of penicillin. Prednisolone may prevent it and should probably be given if a reaction is specially to be feared, e.g. in a patient with syphilitic aortitis.

Bacterial vaginosis (bacterialvaginitis, anaerobic vaginosis)

Bacterial vaginosis is a common form of vaginal discharge in which neither *Trichomonas vaginalis* nor *Candida albicans* can be isolated and inflammatory cells are not present: it is diagnosed from the characteristic Gram's stain appearances of a vaginal swab. The condition is associated with overgrowth of several normal commensals of the vagina including *Gardnerella vaginalis*, Gram-negative curved bacilli and anaerobic organisms, the latter being responsible for the characteristic fishy odour of the vaginal discharge. The condition responds well to a single dose of metronidazole 2 g or 400 mg thrice daily for a week by mouth, with 7 days of topical clindamycin cream offering an alternative.

INFECTION OF BONES AND JOINTS

Causative bacteria of **osteomyelitis** may arrive via the bloodstream or be implanted directly (through a compound fracture, chronic local infection of local tissue, or surgical operation). *Staphylococcus aureus* is the commonest isolate in all patient groups, and *Salmonella* species in the tropics. Chronic osteomyelitis of the lower limbs (especially when underlying chronic skin infection in the elderly) frequently involves obligate anaerobes (such as *Bacteroides* spp.) and coliforms.

Strenuous efforts should be made to obtain bone for culture because superficial and sinus cultures are poorly predictive of the underlying flora, and prolonged therapy is required for chronic osteomyelitis (usually 6–8 weeks, sometimes longer). Surgical removal of dead bone improves the outcome of chronic osteomyelitis.

Definitive therapy is guided by the results of culture but commonly used regimens include co-amoxiclav (community-acquired cases in adults), flucloxacillin with or without fusidic acid (for *Staphylococcus aureus*), cefotaxime or co-amoxiclav (in children), and ciprofloxacin (for coliforms). Short courses of therapy (3–6 weeks) may suffice for acute osteomyelitis, but vertebral body osteomyelitisrequires at least 8 weeks' treatment.

Septic arthritis is a medical emergency if good joint function is to be retained. *Staphylococcus aureus* is the commonest pathogen, but a very wide range of bacteria may be involved including streptococci, coliforms and Neisseria spp. Aspiration of the joint allows specific microbiological diagnosis, differentiation from non-infectious causes such as crystal synovitis, and has therapeutic benefit, e.g. for the hip joint, where formal drainage is recommended. Initial therapy is as for chronic osteomyelitis, and continuation guided by culture results for 4–6 weeks is usually required. Switching to oral therapy is often possible with satisfactory progress.

Infection of prosthetic joints may also involve a range of bacteria, but is most commonly staphylococcal. Debridement of the prosthesis and culture of adjacent bone biopsy samples fulfils both therapeutic and diagnostic needs, and prolonged antibiotic therapy guided by cultureis successful (with retention of the prosthesis in situ) in 60% of cases or more as long as it is commenced within a few weeks of first presentation of the infection and the prosthesis is stable.

EYE INFECTIONS

Superficial infections, caused by a variety of organisms, are treated by chloramphenicol, fusidic acid, framycetin, gentamicin, ciprofloxacin, levofloxacin, ofloxacin or neomycin in drops or ointments. Ciprofloxacin, ofloxacin, levofloxacin, gentamicin or tobramycin is used for *Pseudomonas aeruginosa*, and fusidic acid principally for *Staphylococcus aureus*. Preparations often contain hydrocortisone or prednisolone, but the steroid masks the progress of the infection, and should it be applied with an antimicrobial to which the organism is resistant (bacterium or virus) it may aggravate the disease by suppressing protective inflammation. Local chemoprophylaxis without corticosteroid is used to prevent secondary

bacterial infection in viral conjunctivitis. A variety of antibiotics may be given by direct injection to the chambers of the eye for treatment of bacterial endophthalmitis.

Chlamydial conjunctivitis. In the developed world, the genital (D–K) serotypes of the organism are responsible, and the reservoir and transmission is maintained by sexual contact. Endemic trachoma in developing countries is usually caused by serotypes A, B and C. In either case, oral tetracycline is effective. Pregnant or lactating women may receive systemic erythromycin. Neonatal ophthalmia responds to systemic erythromycin and topical tetracycline.

MYCOBACTERIAL INFECTIONS

Pulmonary tuberculosis

Nearly one-third of the world's population is infected with *Mycobacterium tuberculosis*, and it is the second leading cause of death due to an identified pathogen, after HIV infection. Drug therapy has transformed tuberculosis from adisabling and often fatal disease into one in which almost 100% cure is obtainable, although the recent emergence of multiple drug-resistant tuberculosis (MDR-TB) and extensively-drug-resistant tuberculosis (XDR-TB) strains and their interaction with HIV infection has disturbed this optimistic view. Chemotherapy was formerly protracted, but a better understanding of the mode of action of antituberculosis drugs and of effective immune reconstitution in HIV infection has allowed the development of shorter-course regimens.

Principles of antituberculosis therapy

- Kill a large number of actively multiplying bacilli: isoniazid achieves this.
- Treat persisters, i.e. semi-dormant bacilli that metabolise slowly or intermittently: rifampicin and pyrazinamide are the most efficacious.
- Prevent the emergence of drug resistance by multiple therapy to suppress single-drug-resistant mutants that may exist de novo or emerge during therapy: isoniazid and rifampicin are best.

- Combined formulations are used to ensure that poor compliance does not result in monotherapy with consequent drug resistance.

Most contemporary regimens employ an initial intensive phase with rifampicin, isoniazid, pyrazinamide with or without ethambutol, to reduce the bacterial load as rapidly as possible (usually for 2 months), followed by a continuation phase with rifampicin and isoniazid given for at least 4 months (Fig. 21.2).

All short-course regimens include isoniazid, pyrazinamide and rifampicin. After extensive clinical trials, the following have been found satisfactory:

1. An unsupervised regimen of daily dosing comprising isoniazid and rifampicin for 6 months, plus pyrazinamide for the first 2 months.

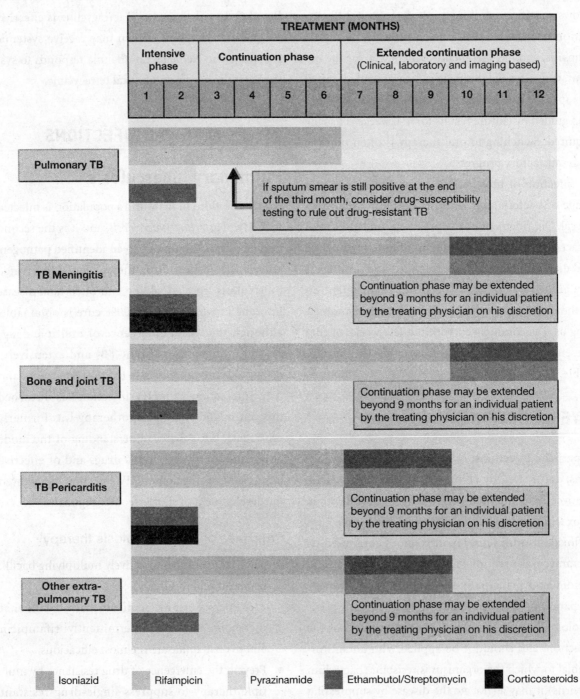

Fig. 21.2 Treatment of drug-sensitive pulmonary and extrapulmonary tuberculosis. Daily supervised treatment is preferred. Intermittent, thrice-weekly treatment administered under direct observation equally effective. Monitor adverse effects (hepatic functions, serum uric acid) periodically.

2. A supervised (directly observed therapy, DOT) regimen for patients who cannot be relied upon to comply with treatment, comprising thrice-weekly dosing with isoniazid and rifampicin for6 months, plus pyrazinamide for the first 2 months (isoniazid and pyrazinamide are given in higher dose than in the unsupervised regimen). With both of the above regimens, ethambutol by mouth or streptomycin i.m. should be added for the first 2 months if there is a likelihood of drug-resistant organisms, or if the patient is severely ill with extensive active lesions. Ethambutol should not be administered in small children as they are unable to report visual side-effects.

All of the regimens are highly effective, with relapse rates of 1%–2% in those who continue for 6 months; even if patients default after, say, 4 months, tuberculosis can be expected to recur in only 10%–15%. Drug resistance seldom develops with any of these regimens.

Compliance is often a concern with multiple drug therapy given for long periods, especially in the developing world, and (surprisingly) DOT did improve relapse rates in many trials. Fixed-dose combination therapy is assumed to improve compliance; however, bio-availability of rifampicin remains a matter of concern in fixed-dose combinations; some commonly used fixed-dose combinations include Rifater (rifampicin, isoniazid plus pyrazinamide), and Rifinah or Rimactazid (rifampicin plus isoniazid). In all cases, effective control of tuberculosis in a population requires optimal therapy of index cases combined with careful screening and case finding among their contacts.

Special problems

Drug resistant organisms. Patients with multiply drug-resistant tuberculosis, i.e. resistant to rifampicin and isoniazid at least, should be treated with three or four drugs to which the organisms are sensitive, and treatment should extend for 12–24 months after cultures become negative (Fig. 21.3). Treatment of such cases requires expert management.

Non-tuberculous mycobacteria are often resistant to standard drugs; their virulence is low but they can produce serious infection in immunocompromised patients which may respond, e.g. to macrolide (clarithromycin), ethambutolor rifabutin, often in combination.

Chemoprophylaxis may be either:

- primary, i.e. the giving of antituberculous drugs to uninfected but exposed individuals, which is seldom justified, or
- secondary, which is the treatment of infected but

Fig. 21.3 Treatment of MDR-TB. The number and category of drugs in the intensive phase may vary according to country's national programme. Monitor adverse effects (neuropsychiatric, renal, hepatic and thyroid functions) periodically. MDR-TB, multidrugresistant tuberculosis.

symptom-free individuals, e.g. those known to be incontact with the disease and who develop a positive tuberculin reaction. Secondary chemoprophylaxis may be justified in children under the age of 3 years because they have a high risk of disseminated disease; isoniazid alone for 6–9 months may be used as there is little risk of resistant organisms emerging because the organism load is low. Shorter treatment regimens with an alternative drug (rifampicin for4 months or 3 months) or drug combinations (rifampicin plus isoniazid for 3 months) have better adherence rates. Combined use of rifampicin and pyrazinamide for 2 months in HIV-negative contacts is not recommended as it produces severe drug induced hepatitis.

Pregnancy. Drug treatment should never be interrupted or postponed during pregnancy. On the general principle of limiting exposure of the fetus, the standard three-drug,6-month course (no. 1 above) is best. Exclude streptomycin from any regimen (danger of fetal eighth cranial nervedamage). Treatment of MDR-TB is not contraindicated during pregnancy. While treating MDR-TB, risks and benefits should be discussed with the mother. Treatment should be started in the second trimester or earlier if the disease is severe; to avoid teratogenic effects drugs should not be administered in the first trimester. Injectables should be avoided. Capreomycin is the injectable of choice in an unavoidable situation but carries the risk of ototoxicity. Ethionamide should be avoided as it aggravates nausea and vomiting and also has teratogenic effects.

Extrapulmonary tuberculosis. The principles of treatment, i.e. multiple therapy and prolonged follow-up, are the same as for pulmonary tuberculosis (Fig. 21.2). Many chronic tuberculosis lesions may be relatively inaccessible to drugs as a result of avascularity, so treatment frequently has to be prolonged and dosage high, especially if damaged tissue cannot be removed by surgery, e.g. tuberculosis of bones.

Meningeal tuberculosis. It is essential to use isoniazid and pyrazinamide, which penetrate well into the CSF. Rifampicin and streptomycin enter inflamed meninges well, but non-inflamed meninges less so, whereas ethambutol has poor penetration. An effective regimen is isoniazid, rifampicin, pyrazinamide and streptomycin. Treatment may need to continue for much longer (9–12 months) than modern short-course chemotherapy for pulmonary tuberculosis.

Bone and joint tuberculosis. Six to nine months drug regimens containing rifampicin are effective (Fig. 21.2). Surgery is indicated when chemotherapy fails with evidence of ongoing infection and for relief of cord compression with persistent or recurrent neurological deficits or instability of the spine

Lymph node tuberculosis. In drug-susceptible lymphnode tuberculosis a 6-month regimen is adequate. Affected lymph nodes may enlarge while the patient is on treatment or after the end of treatment without any evidence of mycobacterial relapse (immune reconstitution inflammatory syndrome (IRIS)). Cold abscesses of lymph nodes require needle drainage.

Adrenal steroid and tuberculosis. Corticosteroids are administered in adrenal gland involvement with Addison's disease, in meningeal and pericardial tuberculosis (Fig. 21.2).

Tuberculosis in the immunocompromised. Such patients require special measures because they may be infected more readily when exposed; their infections usually involve large numbers of tubercle bacilli (multibacillary disease), and patients with AIDS are more likely to be infected with multiply antibiotic-resistant strains.

While treating patients co-infected with HIV and tuberculosis, antituberculosis treatment (ATT) is started first and antiretroviralt reatment (ART) is started subsequently. ART-naïve HIV/AIDS patients should be started on ART between 2 weeks and 2 months after anti-TB drugs, depending on CD4 cell counts. Patients already on ART require some modification in treatment; efavirenz should be used in place of nevirapine. Rifabutin should be preferred over rifampicin while using protease inhibitors. Patients while on ART and ATT may develop IRIS (within 3 months of treatment). In this paradoxical reaction, patients initially show some improvement and subsequently reveal either aggravation of existing lesions or appearance of fresh lesions. Development of IRIS does not require stopping of ART and usually non-steroidal anti-inflammatory drugs (NSAIDs) are sufficient. Drug-resistant TB should be ruled out. Usually at least four drugs are started, and patients are isolated until bacteriological results have been obtained and they have shown clinical improvement. If infections are proved to involve antibiotic-susceptible mycobacteria, therapy can continue with a conventional 6-month regimen with careful follow-up. Particular problems may occur with multiple drug interactions during antituberculous treatment of patients receiving antiretroviral therapy.

Antituberculosis drugs

Isoniazid

Isoniazid (INH, INAH, isonicotinic acid hydrazide) is selectively effective against *Mycobacterium tuberculosis* because it prevents the synthesis of components that are unique to mycobacterial cell walls. Hence it is bactericidal against actively multiplying bacilli (whether within macrophages or at extracellular sites) but is bacteriostatic against nondividing bacilli; it has little or no activity against other bacteria. Isoniazid is well absorbed from the alimentary tract and is distributed throughout the body water, including CSF. It should always be given in cases where there is special risk of meningitis (miliary tuberculosis and primary infection). Isoniazid is inactivated by conjugation with an acetyl group and the rate of the reaction is bimodally distributed. The $t_{1/2}$ is 1 h in fast and 4 h in slow acetylators; fast acetylators achieve less than half the steady-state plasma concentration of slow acetylators but standard oral doses (300 mg/day) on daily regimens give adequate tuberculocidal concentrations in both groups.

Adverse effects. Isoniazid is in general well tolerated. The most severe adverse effect is liver damage, ranging from a moderate rise in hepatic enzymes to severe hepatitis and death. Liver histology in isoniazid hepatitis is indistinguishable from acute viral hepatitis. It is probably caused by a chemically reactive metabolite(s), e.g. acetylhydrazine. Most cases are in patients aged over 35 years, and develop within the first 8 weeks of therapy; liver functions hould be monitored monthly during this period at least. High-dose isoniazid (16–20 mg/kg·day) may be useful in DR-TB.

Isoniazid is a structural analogue of pyridoxine and accelerates its excretion, the principal result of which is peripheral neuropathy with numbness and tingling of the feet, motor involvement being less common. Neuropathy is more frequent in slow acetylators, malnourished people, the elderly and those with HIV infection, liver disease, diabetes mellitus and alcoholism, chronic renal failure, malnutrition, pregnant and breast-feeding women. Such patients should receive pyridoxine 10 mg/day by mouth, which prevents neuropathy and does not interfere with the therapeutic effect; some prefer simply to give pyridoxine to all patients. Other adverse effects include mental disturbances, incoordination, optic neuritis and convulsions.

Isoniazid inhibits the metabolism of phenytoin, carbamazepine and ethosuximide, increasing their effect. Ideally, blood levels of these drugs should be monitored (therapeutic drug monitoring).

Rifampicin

Rifampicin has bactericidal activity against the tubercle bacillus, comparable to that of isoniazid. It is also used in leprosy.

It acts by inhibiting RNA synthesis, bacteria being sensitive to this effect at much lower concentrations than mammalian cells; it is particularly effective against mycobacteria that lie semi-dormant within cells. Rifampicin has a wide range of antimicrobial activity. Other uses include leprosy, severe legionnaires' disease (with erythromycin or ciprofloxacin), the chemoprophylaxis of meningococcal meningitis, and severe staphylococcal infection (with flucloxacillin or vancomycin).

Rifampicin is well absorbed from the gastrointestinal tract. It penetrates most tissues. Entry into the CSF when meninges are inflamed is sufficient to maintain therapeutic concentrations at normal oral doses but transfer is reduced as inflammation subsides in 1–2 months.

Enterohepatic recycling takes place, and eventually about 60% of a single dose is eliminated in the faeces; urinary excretion of unchanged drug also occurs. The $t_{1/2}$ is 4 h after initial doses, but shortens on repeated dosing because rifampicin is a very effective enzyme inducer and increases its own metabolism (as well as that of several other drugs; see below).

Adverse reactions. Rifampicin rarely causes any serious toxicity. Adverse reactions include flushing and itching with or without a rash, and thrombocytopenia. Rises in plasma levels of bilirubin and hepatic enzymes may occur when treatment starts, but are often transient and are not necessarily an indication for stopping the drug; fatal hepatitis, however, has occurred. Hepatic function should be checked before starting treatment and at least for the first few months of therapy. Intermittent dosing, i.e. less than twice weekly, eitheras part of a regimen or through poor compliance, promotes an influenza-like syndrome (malaise, headache and fever, shortness of breath and wheezing), acute haemolytic anaemia and thrombocytopenia, and acute renal failure sometimes with haemolysis.

Interactions. Rifampicin is a powerful enzyme inducer and speeds the metabolism of numerous drugs, including warfarin, steroid contraceptives, narcotic analgesics, oral antidiabetic agents, phenytoin and dapsone. Appropriate increase in dosage, and alternative methods of contraception, are required to compensate for increased drug metabolism.

Rifabutin ($t_{1/2}$ 36 h) has similar activity and adverse reactions, and is used for prophylaxis of *Mycobacterium avium* infection in patients with AIDS, and for treatment of tuberculous and non-tuberculous mycobacterial infection in combination with other drugs. All rifamycins have high levels of cross-resistance. It is preferred over rifampicin when protease inhibitors are used for treating HIV-TB coinfection. Rifabutin and saquinavir should not be used together.

Pyrazinamide

Pyrazinamide is a derivative of nicotinamide and is included in first-choice combination regimens because of its particular ability to kill intracellular persisters, i.e. mycobacteria that are dividing or semi-dormant, often with incells. Its action is dependent on the activity of intrabacterial pyrazinamidase, which converts pyrazinamide to the active pyrazinoic acid; this enzyme is most effective in an acidic environment such as the interior of cells. In drug-sensitive tuberculosis it should not be administered beyond 2 months. It is inactive against *Mycobacterium bovis*. Pyrazinamide is well absorbed from the gastrointestinal tract and metabolised in the liver, very little unchanged drug appearing in the urine ($t_{1/2}$ 9 h). CSF concentrations are almost identical to those in the blood. Pyrazinamide is safe touse in pregnancy.

Adverse effects include hyperuricaemia and arthralgia, which is relatively frequent with daily but less so with intermittent dosing and, unlike gout, affects both large and small joints. Pyrazinoic acid, the principal metabolite of pyrazinamide, inhibits renal tubular secretion of urate. Symptomatic treatment with a non-steroidal anti-inflammatory drug is usually sufficient and it is rarely necessary to discontinue pyrazinamide because of arthralgia. Incidence of hepatitis which occurred with high doses has decreased with modern short-course schedules, but still requires close clinical and laboratory monitoring. Sideroblastic anaemia and urticaria also occur.

Ethambutol

Ethambutol, being bacteriostatic, is used in conjunction with other antituberculous drugs to delay or prevent the emergence of resistant bacilli. It is well absorbed from the gastrointestinal tract and effective concentrations occur in most body tissues including the lung; in tuberculous meningitis, sufficient may reach the CSF to inhibit mycobacterial growth but insignificant amounts enter CSF if the meninges are not inflamed. Excretion is mainly by the kidney, by tubular secretion as well as by glomerular filtration ($t_{1/2}$ 4 h); the dose should be reduced when renal function is impaired.

Adverse effects. In recommended oral doses (15 mg/kg·day), with dose adjustment for reduced renal function, ethambutol is relatively non-toxic.

The main problem is rare optic neuritis (unilateral or bilateral) causing loss of visual acuity, central scotomata, occasionally also peripheral vision loss and red–green colour blindness. The changes reverse if treatment is stopped promptly; if not, the patient may go blind. It is prudent to note any history of eye disease and to get baseline tests of vision before starting treatment with ethambutol. The drug should not be given to a patient with reduced vision who may not notice further deterioration. Patients should be told to read small print in newspapers regularly (with each eye separately) and, if there is any deterioration, to stop the drug immediately and seek advice. Patients who cannot understand and comply (especially children) should be given alternative therapy if possible. The need for repeated specialist ophthalmological monitoring is controversial. Peripheral neuritis occurs but is rare.

Antituberculosis drug-induced hepatitis

Among the first-line antituberculosis drugs, rifampicin, isoniazid and pyrazinamide are potentially hepatotoxic drugs. Additionally, rifampicin can cause asymptomatic jaundice without evidence of hepatitis. Rifampicin rarely causes hepatitis when administered alone and rifampicin and isoniazid are ~3 times less toxic in the absence of pyrazinamide. It is essential to rule out acute viral hepatitis by performing markers for viral hepatitis before diagnosing antituberculosis drug-induced hepatitis in developing nations. Drug-induced hepatitis can be life-threatening if drugs are continued despite its occurrence. All hepatotoxic drugs should be immediately stopped until complete biochemical recovery occurs. In the interim period, ethambutol, streptomycin and one of the fluoroquinolones should be administered. The best approach to reintroducing antituberculosis drugs is still debatable. The approach could be sequential or simultaneous. Some advocate re introduction of all three drugs one by one as it allows identification of the culprit drug, while others prefer to use rifampicin first followed by isoniazid and if the patient tolerates both drugs avoid pyrazinamide.

Thiacetazone

Thiacetazone is tuberculostatic and is used with isoniazidto inhibit the emergence of resistance to the latter drug. It is absorbed from the gastrointestinal tract, partly metabolized and partly excreted in the urine ($t_{1/2}$ 13 h). Usual adult dose is 150 mg/day. It is not used in HIV-TBco-infection because of severe cutaneous reactions; Asian patients may have higher incidence of Stevens–Johnson syndrome.

Adverse reactions include gastrointestinal symptoms, conjunctivitis and vertigo. More serious effects are erythema multiforme, haemolytic anaemia, agranulocytosis, cerebral oedema and hepatitis.

Second-line antituberculosis drugs

Kanamycin and amikacin

Both kanamycin ($t_{1/2}$ 2–4 h) and amikacin ($t_{1/2}$ 2–4 h) are bactericidal drugs of the aminoglycoside class, valuable in patients with resistance to streptomycin. Cross-resistance between kanamycin and amikacin is usual. The optimal dose is 15 mg/kg body-weight; usually 0.75–1.0 g/day i.m. Adverse effects are similar to streptomycin.

Capreomycin

Capreomycin ($t_{1/2}$ 4–6 h) is a bactericidal aminoglycoside derived from *Streptomyces capreolus*. There is no cross-resistance with other aminoglycosides. The usual dose is 20 mg/kg·day up to 1 g in a single dose daily i.m. for 40–120 days; the dose is then reduced to 2–3 times weekly as the risk of adverse effects increases sharply. Adverse effects are similar to streptomycin. Hypokalaemia, hypocalcaemia and hypomagnesaemia have been reported. Rarely, hepatitis and general cutaneous reactions may occur.

Thioamides

Ethionamide and prothionamide. Ethionamide ($t_{1/2}$ 2–3 h) and prothionamide ($t_{1/2}$ 2–3h) are bactericidal drugs. Their chemical structure resembles thioacetazone and there is frequent partial cross-resistance. The maximum optimum dose is 15–20 mg/kg·day up to 1 g/day and the usual dose is 750 mg/day in patients weighing 50 kg or more (can be split in two doses: 500 mg in the morning and 250 in the evening) and 500 mg/day in patients weighing<50 kg. These drugs are more acceptable when administered with orange juice or milk. Adverse reactions include gastrointestinal side-effects, depression, hallucinations, hepatitis, hypothyroidism and peripheral neuropathy. The drugs should be avoided during pregnancy.

Cycloserine and terizidone

Cycloserine ($t_{1/2}$ 10 h) is bacteriostatic at the usual dosage and terizidone is a combination of two molecules of cycloserine. The maximum daily dose is 15–20 mg/kg; the usual dose of cycloserine and terizidone is 500–750 mg/day (250 mg in the morning and 500 mg 12 hours later). Main adverse effects are related to the central nervous system (less with terizidone) and include headache, tremors, insomnia, depression, convulsions, altered behaviour and suicidal tendencies. Addition of pyridoxine (50 mg/250 mg of cycloserine and terizidone is recommended) decreases these adverse effects.

Fluoroquinolones

Ciprofloxacin ($t_{1/2}$ 3–5 h) is no longer recommended to treat drug-susceptible or drug-resistant tuberculosis. The most potent available fluoroquinolones, in descending order, include: moxifloxacin ($t_{1/2}$ 9–10 h) (400 mg/day) or gatifloxacin ($t_{1/2}$ 8 h) (400 mg/day) > levofloxacin ($t_{1/2}$ 6–8 h) (750 mg/day) > ofloxacin ($t_{1/2}$ biphasic: 4–5 h) and 20–25 h (accounts for <5%) (800 mg/day). Though moxifloxacin and gatifloxacin have equal potency, the latter is not favoured in those with diabetes mellitus because of the risk of hyperglycaemia, hypoglycaemia and new onset diabetes mellitus. Later-generation fluoroquinolone shave some efficacy against ofloxacin-resistant strains and are recommended for the treatment of XDR-TB. Close monitoring is required as safety data on long-term use are limited. Prolonged QT interval occurs with moxifloxacin.

Para-aminosalicylic acid (PAS)

Usual dose of para-aminosalicylic acid (PAS) ($t_{1/2}$ 1 h) is 8–12 g/day in divided doses. Commonly observed adverse effects include gastrointestinal upset, hepatic dysfunction, hypothyroidism; it should be administered cautiously inpatients with cardiac and renal insufficiency because of the sodium load.

Other bacterial infections

Burns. Use of systemic antibiotics for days 4 to 14 in patients with large burns has been shown to reduce mortality by nearly 50% at the expense of a significant rise in the prevalence of antibiotic resistance.

Gas gangrene. The skin between the waist and the knees is normally contaminated with anaerobic faecal organisms. Surgery done for vascular insufficiency where tissue oxygenation may be poor is likely to be followed by infection. Gas gangrene (*Clostridium perfringens*) may occur; prophylaxis with benzylpenicillin or metronidazole is used.

Cellulitis (inflammation of the skin) is most commonly a haemolytic streptococcal infection, although *Staphylococcus aureus* may also be implicated, and a wide range of bacteria including obligate anaerobes may be involved in cases associated with arterial insufficiency (e.g. lower limb infections in diabetes mellitus). Mild streptococcal/staphylococcal cases will usually respond to flucloxacillin, although more clinically severe infections may require the addition of high-dose parenteral benzylpenicillin.

Health-care-associated infections (HCAIs) comprising ventilator-associated pneumonia, surgical wound infection, intravenous catheter-associated bacteraemia, meningitis following neurosurgery, and infection of prosthetic devices such as joint replacements and heart valves may involve conventional pathogens such as *Staphylococcus aureus* and Lancefield Group A beta-haemolytic streptococcus, but a number of antibiotic-resistant pathogens are also commonly involved. These isolates can pose difficult therapeutic problems, especially because the infections often present inpatients with multiple pre-existing pathologies, including liver and renal impairment. The causative bacteria include MRSA and multiply resistant coagulase-negative staphylococci, ESBL-producing coliforms, and a number of normally weakly pathogenic Gram-negative bacteria such as *Stenotrophomonas maltophilia* and *Acinetobacter* spp. These bacteria can be resistant to all conventional antimicrobial agents, and discussion with a microbiologist or infectious diseases physician is recommended before treatment is attempted. A number of unusual combinations of antibiotics have been recommended and previously outdated agents have been resurrected for treatment of infections with these pathogens: for example, colistin.

Community-acquired MRSA (CA-MRSA) has caused large outbreaks of infection in North American cities, and clusters in other parts of the world. Many reported strains produce a white-cell toxin, the Panton–Valentine leucocidin, and affected patients may suffer cutaneous abscesses and necrotizing fasciitis and pneumonia. Recommended treatment regimens include antibiotics active at the ribosome to reduce toxin production –especially linezolid and clindamycin – and topical mupirocin and fucidin, although these strains are often more susceptible to non-β-lactam antibiotics than traditional health-care-associated MRSA.

SUMMARY

The mechanisms of antibacterial action include the inhibition of cell wall synthesis, inhibition of protein synthesis, inhibition of synthesis or metabolism of nucleic acids, decrease of the cytoplasm membrane,

The mechanisms of bacterial resistance include enzymic inactivation, alteration or protection of drug target site, decreased drug uptake and other mechanisms.

All of β-lactam, glycopeptides and fosfomycin play their bactericidal effect via inhibition of synthesis of cell wall. Penicillins, cephalosporins, monobactams, cephamycins and oxacephems are classified as β-lactam drugs because of their unique lactam ring. They inhibit bacterial growth by inhibiting

transpeptidase activity in bacterial cell wall synthesis. Resistance to β-lactams is mainly due to inactivation by β-lactamases and other mechanisms.

Penicillin is active against nearly all staphylococci and gram-positive bacilli. Semisynthesizedpenicillins are not only against gram-positive organisms but also to gram-negative organisms. The penicillins are markably nontoxic, but more attention should be paid on allergic shock.

Cephalosporins have broad antimicrobial spectrum. They can be classified into four generations, depending mainly on the spectrum of antimicrobial activity. The antibacterial spectrum is gradually extended from gram-positive to gram-negative organisms. Carbapenems also posses very broad antimicrobial spectrum except mycoplasm, Chlamydia and legionella. Cephamycins and oxacephems have unique effects against anaerobes.

Glycopeptide antibiotics, such as vancomycin, teicoplanin and telavancin, are used as last-resort antibiotics for the treatment of notoriously resistant gram-positive pathogens, in particular enterococci and staphylococci (e.g. MRSA). The antibiotic activity of vancomycin relies on binding to the D-Ala-D-Ala terminus of the peptide side chain.

Daptomycin is a lipopeptide antibiotic used clinically to treat infections caused by gram-positive bacteria. It has rapid bactericidal activity via penetrating into the bacterial cell wall with consecutive formation of pores, loss of electrical membrane potential and inhibition of peptidoglycan synthesis.

Aminoglycoside antibiotics have same characteristics in chemical properties, pharmacokinetics, antibacterial spectrum, antibacterial mechanism, adverse reaction and drug resistance. They are quiescent bactericidal drugs which can inhibit the synthesis of bacterial proteins. There are two kinds of them: natural and semi-artificial synthesized ones. They can both produce ototoxicity and nephrotoxicity.

All of macrolides, clindamycin, tetracyclines, chloramphenicol, linezolid, and quinupristin play their antibacterial effects via inhibiting microbial protein synthesis.

Macrolides inhibit microbial protein synthesis by

binding reversibly to the 50S ribosome subunit.

Lindamycin targets 50S subunit of the bacterial ribosome to interfere with protein synthesis of gram-positive bacteria. It is effective in treating severe anaerobic infections and against other anaerobes that participate in mixed infections.

Tetracyclines inhibit protein synthesis thus blocking growth of microorganisms. Tetracyclines also have serious adverse reactions.

Chloramphenicol inhibits protein synthesis in both aerobic and anaerobic gram-positive and gram-negative organisms. Chloramphenicol is seldom used in clinic due to its toxicity such as bone marrow disturbances. Linezolid binds to the 50S subunit of the prokaryotic ribosome, preventing it from complexing with the 30S subunit, mRNA, initiation factors and formylmethionyl-tRNA.

Linezolid is equally active against methicillin-susceptible and-resistant *staphylococcus aureus* (MRSA), against vancomycin-susceptible *enterococci* and those with VanA, VanB or VanC determinants, and against pneumococci with susceptibility or resistance to penicillins and/or macrolides.

Quinolones are chemical synthetic fluorinated antibacterial agents. They are active against a variety of bacteria and have strong antibacterial activity. Quinolones block bacterial DNA synthesis by inhibiting bacterial topoisomerase II (DNA gyrase) and topoisomerase IV. Based on developmental time scale and antimicrobial spectrum, the type of drugs are divided into four generations. They are relatively nontoxic, well tolerated agents. Their excellent oral bioavailability permits their use for treatment of a variety of serious bacterial infections.

IMPORTANT TERMINOLOGY

bacteriostatic antibiotic　抑菌性抗生素
bactericidal antibiotic　杀菌性抗生素
minimum inhibitory concentration　最低抑菌浓度
post-antibiotic effect, PAE　抗生素后效应
time-dependent antibiotic　时间依赖性抗生素
concentration-dependent antibiotic　浓度依赖性
　抗生素
multidrug-resistant (MDR) bacteria　多重耐药细菌
extensively drug-resistant (XDR) bacteria　广泛耐
　药细菌
pan-drug resistant (PDR) bacteria　全耐药细菌

CHALLENGE YOURSELF

1. What is the main cause for the prevalence of antibiotic resistance? How do we control or slow down the antibiotic resistance development?

2. What is the structure characteristic of beta-lactam antibiotics? What is the bactericidal mechanism and resistance mechanism?

3. How to select the optimal dose and optimal therapy duration for antibiotics?

4. What is the synergy? Take an example to explain the synergy mechanism.

Jing Zhang

Chapter | 22 |

Viral, fungal, protozoal and helminthic infections

Part 1. Viral Infections

Antiviral agents are most active when viruses are replicating. The earlier that treatment is given, therefore, the better the result. Apart from primary infection, viral illness is often the consequence of reactivation of latent virus in the body. Patients whose immune systems are compromised may suffer particularly severe illness. Viruses are capable of developing resistance to antimicrobial drugs.

HERPES SIMPLEX AND VARICELLA ZOSTER

Aciclovir

Aciclovir ($t_{1/2}$ 3 h) is a nucleoside analogue that is selectively phosphorylated by virus-specific thymidine kinase. Phosphorylated aciclovir inhibits viral replication by acting as a substrate for viral DNA polymerase, thus accounting for its high therapeutic index. It is effective against susceptible herpes viruses if started early in the course of infection, but it does not eradicate persistent infection because viral DNA is integrated in the host genome. About 20% is absorbed from the gut, but this is sufficient for oral systemic treatment of some infections. It distributes widely in the body; the concentration in CSF is approximately half that of plasma, and the brain concentration may be even lower. These differences are taken into account in dosing for viral encephalitis (for which aciclovir must be given i.v.). Dose adjustment is required for patients with impaired renal function, as the drug is predominantly excreted in the urine. For oral and topical use the drug is given five times daily. It can be given twice daily orally for suppressive therapy.

Indications for aciclovir include:

Herpes simplex virus:

- Skin infections, including initial and recurrent labial and genital herpes, most effective when new lesions are forming; skin and mucous membrane infections (as tablets or oral suspension).
- Ocular keratitis (topical treatment with ophthalmic ointment is standard, oral treatment is also effective).
- Prophylaxis and treatment in the immunocompromised (oral, as tablets or suspension).
- Encephalitis and disseminated disease (i.v.).

Aciclovir-resistant herpes simplex virus has been reported in patients with AIDS but remains rare in immunocompetent patients. Foscarnet) and cidofovir have been used in these cases.

Varicella-zoster virus:

- Chickenpox, particularly in the immunocompromised (i.v.) or in the immunocompetent with pneumonitis or hepatitis (i.v.).
- Shingles in immunocompetent persons (as tablets or suspension, and best started within 48 h of the appearance of the rash). Immunocompromised persons will often have more severe symptoms and require i.v. administration.

Adverse reactions are remarkably few. The ophthalmic ointment causes a mild transient stinging sensation and a diffuse superficial punctate keratopathy which clears when the drug is stopped. Oral or i.v. use may cause gastrointestinal symptoms, headache and neuropsychiatric reactions. Extravasation with i.v. use causes severe local inflammation. Crystal-induced acute renal failure is an important complication of i.v. therapy that can be avoided by ensuring good hydration during treatment.

Valaciclovir is a prodrug (ester) of aciclovir, i.e. after oral administration the parent aciclovir is released. It has an improved bio-availability (about 60%) due to the addition of an ester side chain, thus allowing for a less frequent, 8-hourly, dosing. It is used for treating herpes zoster infections and herpes simplex infections of the skin and mucous membranes.

Famciclovir ($t_{1/2}$ 2 h) is a prodrug of penciclovir, which is similar to aciclovir; it is used for herpes zoster and genital herpes simplex infections, and a single dose is effective at reducing the time to healing of labial herpes simplex. It need be given only 8-hourly. Penciclovir is also available as a cream for treatment of labial herpes simplex.

Idoxuridine was the first widely used antiviral drug; it is variably effective topically for ocular and cutaneous herpes simplex, with few adverse reactions. It has been superseded by aciclovir.

HUMAN IMMUNODEFICIENCY VIRUS (HIV)

According to World Health Organization data, 33 million people worldwide were living with human immunodeficiency virus (HIV) in 2008, with close to 3 million new infections yearly; almost 10 million were in need of antiretroviral therapy but more than half of these had no access to treatment.

General comments

- The aims of antiretroviral therapy are to delay disease progression and prolong survival by suppressing the replication of the virus. Optimal suppression also prevents the emergence of drug resistance and reduces the risks of onward transmission to sexual partners and the unborn children of HIV-infected mothers. Virological failure may be defined as primary where there is inability to reduce plasma HIV viral load to fewer than 50 copies per microlitre despite 6 months of antiretroviral therapy, or secondary if there is failure to maintain viral load suppression at less than 50 copies per microlitre.

- No current antiviral agents or combinations eliminate HIV infection, but the most effective combinations (socalled 'highly active antiretroviral therapy', HAART) produce profound suppression of viral replication in many patients and allow useful reconstitution of the immune system, measured by a fall in the plasma viral load and an increase in the numbers of cytotoxic T cells (CD4 count). Rates of opportunistic infections such as Pneumocystis carinii pneumonia and cytomegalovirus (CMV) retinitis are reduced when CD4 counts are restored, and life expectancy is markedly increased.

- Combination therapy reduces the risks of emergence of resistance to antiretroviral drugs, which is increasing in incidence even in patients newly diagnosed with HIV. Mutations in the viral genome either prevent binding of the drug to the active site of the protease or reverse transcriptase enzymes, or lead to removal of the drug from the reverse transcriptase active site. The potential for rapid development of resistance is immense because untreated HIV replicates rapidly (50% of circulating virus is replaced daily), the spontaneous mutation rate is high, the genome is small, the virus will develop single mutations at every codon every day, and for many antiretroviral agents a single mutation will render the virus fully resistant.

- The decision to begin antiretroviral therapy is based primarily on the CD4 cell count (most current recommendations are to start in patients with counts below 350 cells per microlitre). Early initiation of antiretroviral therapy should also be considered for patients with CD4 cell count above 350 cells per microlitre but a low CD4 percentage (e.g <14%), those with an AIDS diagnosis (e.g. Kaposi sarcoma), hepatitis B and HIV co-infection where treatment is indicated, and in conditions where achieving a suppressed viral load is desired in order to prevent transmission (e.g. in pregnancy).

- There are currently more than 20 approved antiretroviral agents in four classes, plus various fixed drug combinations.

- Current HAART regimens use a combination of drugs that act at different phases of the viral life cycle. The most frequently used combinations employ a backbone of two nucleoside analogue reverse transcriptase inhibitors (NRTIs) plus either a non-nucleoside reverse transcriptase inhibitor (NNRTI) or a ritonavir-boosted protease inhibitor (rPI). The choice for the individual patient is best made after reference to contemporary, expert advice.

- Alternative combinations are used if these variables deteriorate or unwanted drug effects occur. Antiretroviral resistance testing, both genetic (by searching viral RNA for sequences coding for resistance) and phenotypic (by testing antiretroviral agents against the patient's virus in cell culture), also guide the choice of drug regimen, especially after virological failure.

- Pregnancy and breast feeding pose special problems. The objectives of therapy are to minimise drug toxicity to the fetus while reducing the maternal viral load and the catastrophic results of HIV transmission to the neonate. Prevention of maternal–fetal and maternal–infant spread is the most cost-effective way of using antiretroviral drugs in less developed countries. Maternal–fetal transmission rates are related to maternal viral load, with rates of 0.1% reported when maternal viral load is less than 50 copies per microlitre while on HAART. Where resources permit, access to safe alternatives to breast feeding should be provided to infected mothers.

- Combination antiretroviral therapy, especially the thymidine nucleoside analogue reverse transcriptase inhibitors zidovudine and stavudine, causes

redistribution of body fat in some patients – the 'lipodystrophy syndrome'. Protease inhibitors can disturb lipid and glucose metabolism to a degree that warrants a change to drugs with limited effects on lipid metabolism, e.g. ritonavir-boosted atazanavir, and the introduction of lipid-lowering agents.

- Impaired cell-mediated immunity leaves the host prey to opportunistic infections including: candidiasis, coccidioidomycosis, cryptosporidiosis, CMV disease, herpes simplex, histoplasmosis, Pneumocystis carinii pneumonia, toxoplasmosis and tuberculosis (often with multiply resistant organisms). Treatment of these conditions is referred to elsewhere in this text.

- Improvement in immune function as a result of antiretroviral treatment may provoke an inflammatory reaction against residual opportunistic organisms (immune reconstitution inflammatory syndrome, IRIS). Although infrequent, this may present with development of new infections or worsening opportunistic infections, e.g. tuberculosis and cryptococcal disease.

- Antiretroviral drugs may also be used in combination to reduce the risks of infection with HIV from injuries, e.g. from HIV-contaminated needles and following sexual exposure to a high-risk partner. The decision to offer such post-exposure prophylaxis (PEP), and the optimal combination of drugs used, is a matter for experts; administration must begin within a few hours of exposure and continue for 28 days.

- Some drugs described here have found additional indications, or are used only, for therapy of non-HIV infections, e.g. adefovir for chronic hepatitis B infection.

Nucleoside and nucleotide reverse transcriptase inhibitors

The HIV replicates by converting its single-stranded RNA into double-stranded DNA, which is incorporated into host DNA; this crucial conversion, the reverse of the normal cellular transcription of nucleic acids, is accomplished by the enzyme reverse transcriptase. Nucleoside reverse transcriptase inhibitors have a high affinity for the reverse transcriptase enzyme and are integrated by it into the viral DNA chain, causing premature chain termination. While all nucleoside reverse transcriptase inhibitors require activation by host enzymes to triphosphates prior to incorporation into the DNA chain, tenofovir (as the only nucleotide analogue) is unique in requiring only two phosphorylations for activation.

Zidovudine (AZT, Retrovir)

Zidovudine, a thymidine analogue, is the first antiretroviral licensed for the treatment of HIV-1. Resistance develops rapidly when used as monotherapy through the sequential accumulation of thymidine analogue mutations (TAMs) at codon 41, 67, 70, 215 and 219; conversely, point mutations at codon 184 selected by lamivudine and emtricitabine therapy enhance susceptibility to zidovudine (and stavudine) by delaying the emergence of TAMs.

Uses. Zidovudine is indicated for the treatment of HIV infection as part of a combination regimen. It is an established choice for the prevention of maternal–fetal transmission, both as part of a combination regimen antenatally in the mother and as monotherapy in the newborn. The enhanced CNS penetration of zidovudine makes it an important option for the treatment of HIV-associated neurocognitive disease (HAND). The drug is available as part of a fixed drug combination with lamivudine (as Combivir), and with abacavir and lamivudine (as Trizivir).

Adverse reactions early in treatment may include anorexia, nausea, vomiting, headache, dizziness, malaise and myalgia, but tolerance develops to these and usually the dose does not need to be altered. More serious are anaemia and neutropenia, which develop more commonly when the dose is high, with advanced disease, and in combination with ganciclovir, interferon-α and other marrow suppressive agents. A toxic myopathy (not easily distinguishable from HIV-associated myopathy) may develop with long-term use. Rarely, a syndrome of hepatic necrosis with lactic acidosis may occur with zidovudine (and with other reverse transcriptase inhibitors).

Didanosine

Didanosine (ddI) is a thymidine analogue with similar activity to zidovudine. It has a short plasma half-life ($t_{1/2}$ 1 h) but a much longer intracellular duration than zidovudine, and thus prolonged antiretroviral activity. Didanosine is rapidly but incompletely absorbed from the gastrointestinal tract (30%–40%) and is widely distributed in body water; 30%–65% is recovered unchanged in the urine. Drug absorption is affected by food and therefore it has to be taken on an empty stomach or at least 2 h after a meal. Didanosine may cause pancreatitis, lactic acidosis, hepatomegaly with steatosis and peripheral neuropathy. Other adverse effects include hyperuricaemia and diarrhoea, any of which may give reason to reduce the dose or discontinue the drug. Retinal changes and optic neuritis have also been reported. The combination of stavudine and didanosine is associated with a high risk of toxicity and should be avoided. Dose adjustment of didanosine is required when used in combination with tenofovir and in patients with renal insufficiency.

Lamivudine and emtricitabine

Lamivudine (3TC) is a reverse transcriptase inhibitor with a relatively long intracellular half-life (14 h; plasma $t_{1/2}$ 6 h). Lamivudine is the most common nucleoside analogue used in HAART regimens due to its excellent tolerance profile. A nucleoside backbone of lamivudine with zidovudine (Combivir), abacavir (Kivexa) or emtricitabine and tenofovir (Truvada) as fixed drug combinations, appears to reduce viral load effectively and to be well tolerated. The drug is well absorbed from the gastrointestinal tract (86%) and excreted mainly by the kidney with minimal metabolism; dose modification is necessary in renal impairment.

Lamivudine was the first nucleoside analogue to be licensed for therapy of chronic hepatitis B infection, for which it should be used in combination with tenofovir (as part of a HAART regimen) in HIV co-infected patients. Emergence of resistant mutants of hepatitis B is troublesome (due to mutations of the viral reverse transcriptase/DNA polymerase), occurring in up to about 30% of patients after 1 year and 70% after 5 years of therapy. The most common unwanted effects include headache and gastrointestinal upset. Lactic acidosis and severe hepatomegaly with steatosis, including fatal cases, have been reported. A higher dose of lamivudine is required for the treatment of HIV than for hepatitis B infection; patients with co-infection should receive doses appropriate for treatment of HIV.

Emtricitabine

Emtricitabine has a similar structure, tolerability, efficacy and resistance profile. It should not be used in combination with lamivudine, as it contains the same active constituent.

Abacavir

Abacavir ($t_{1/2}$ 2 h) has high therapeutic efficacy; it is usually well tolerated, but adverse effects include hypersensitivity reactions especially during the first 6 weeks of therapy, affecting about 8% of patients; the drug must be stopped immediately and avoided in future if hypersensitivity is suspected. The presence of the HLA-B*5701 allele predicts increased risk of hypersensitivity reaction in the Caucasian population; patients should be tested for the presence of this allele prior to starting therapy.

Tenofovir

Tenofovir ($t_{1/2}$ 17 h), administered orally as the prodrug tenofovir disoproxil fumarate, is also effective against hepatitis B virus. Some 80% is excreted renally and dose adjustment is recommended in patients with a creatinine clearance of less than 50 mL/min. Monitor closely for signs of new onset or acute renal impairment, electrolyte and renal tubular disturbance (Fanconi syndrome); avoid concomitant nephrotoxic drugs while on tenofovir.

Tenofovir competes with didanosine for renal tubular excretion, raising didanosine plasma concentrations with associated risk of pancreatitis, peripheral neuropathy and lactic acidosis. Severe acute exacerbation of hepatitis has been described following cessation of therapy for hepatitis B infection.

Stavudine

Stavudine (d4T) inhibits reverse transcriptase by competing with the natural substrate deoxythymidine triphosphate, and additionally is incorporated into viral DNA, causing termination of chain elongation ($t_{1/2}$ 1.5 h). Troublesome lipoatrophy has limited its use by most authorities outside the developing world. Hepatic toxicity and pancreatitis are reported, and a dose-related peripheral neuropathy may occur, all probably related to mitochondrial toxicity. Stavudine is more frequently associated with lactic acidosis than other nucleoside analogues.

Adefovir

Adefovir dipivoxil is a nucleoside analogue used for chronic hepatitis B infection, including against lamivudine-resistant strains. It is administered as the oral prodrug (plasma $t_{1/2}$ 8 h, intracellular $t_{1/2}$ of active metabolite 17 h). Adverse effects are uncommon, but include headache, abdominal pain and diarrhoea. Resistance emerges over time (30% after 5 years), but much less commonly than with lamivudine therapy, possibly due to the flexibility of the adefovir molecule, which allows it to conform to mutated binding sites. Dose adjustment is required for patients with renal impairment. Adefovir should not be co-prescribed with tenofovir. The recommended adefovir dose for hepatitis B therapy will not suppress HIV infection; HIV status should therefore be confirmed prior to commencing adefovir for hepatitis B infection, as unrecognized co-infection may lead to the emergence of HIV resistance.

Protease inhibitors

In its process of replication, HIV produces precursor proteins, which are subsequently cleaved by the protease enzyme into component parts and reassembled into virus particles; protease inhibitors disrupt this essential process.

Protease inhibitors reduce viral RNA concentration ('viral load'), increase the CD4 count and improve survival when used in combination with other agents. They are metabolised extensively by isoenzymes of the cytochrome P450 system, notably by CYP 3A4, and most protease inhibitors inhibit these enzymes. They have a plasma $t_{1/2}$ of 2–4 h, except for fosamprenavir (8 h) and atazanavir (7 h with food). The drugs have broadly similar therapeutic effects. Members of the group include:

- amprenavir, atazanavir, fosamprenavir (a prodrug of amprenavir), lopinavir, ritonavir, saquinavir, tipranavir, indinavir and darunavir.

Adverse effects include gastrointestinal disturbance, headache, dizziness, sleep disturbance, raised liver enzymes, neutropenia, pancreatitis and rashes. Unique side-effects include asymptomatic reversible unconjugated hyperbilirubinaemia with atazanavir and nephrolithiasis with indinavir.

Interactions. Involvement with the cytochrome P450 system provides scope for numerous drug–drug interactions. Agents that induce P450 enzymes, e.g. rifampicin, St John's wort, accelerate their metabolism, reducing plasma concentration and therapeutic efficacy; enzyme inhibitors, e.g. ketoconazole, cimetidine, raise their plasma concentration with risk of toxicity.

The powerful inhibiting effect of ritonavir on CYP 3A4 and CYP 2D6 is harnessed usefully by its combination in low (subtherapeutic) dose with other protease inhibitors; the result is to decrease the metabolism and increase the therapeutic efficacy of the concurrently administered protease inhibitors (called ritonavir 'boosting' or 'potentiation'), i.e. a beneficial drug–drug interaction. Ritonavir boosting is particularly advantageous in patients infected with low level resistant virus where the high drug levels help improve efficacy, but this may be at the detriment of increased gastrointestinal side-effects and metabolic disturbances. Ritonavir boosting is now a recommended treatment standard for all protease inhibitor containing regimens.

Non-nucleoside reverse transcriptase inhibitors

This group is structurally different from the reverse transcriptase inhibitors; members are active against the subtype HIV-1 but not HIV-2, a subtype encountered mainly in West Africa. Non-nucleoside reverse transcriptase inhibitors are metabolised by CYP 450 enzymes and hence the potential for significant drug–drug interactions. The drugs have considerably longer half-lives when compared to nucleoside reverse transcriptase inhibitors.

Efavirenz is taken once per day ($t_{1/2}$ 52 h). Rash is relatively common during the first 2 weeks of therapy, but resolution usually occurs within a further 2 weeks; the drug should be stopped if the rash is severe or if there is blistering, desquamation, mucosal involvement or fever. Neurological adverse reactions occur in about 50% of patients, usually insomnia, depression and abnormal dreams; this may be reduced by taking the drug before retiring at night; gastrointestinal side-effects and occasional hepatitis and pancreatitis have also been reported. Efavirenz is teratogenic, so should be avoided in pregnancy. Resistance is associated with mutations at codon 103 and 181, which also confers cross-resistance to nevirapine.

Nevirapine is used in combination with at least two other antiretroviral drugs. It is commonly prescribed in the developing world and is relatively safe in pregnancy. It penetrates the CSF well, and undergoes hepatic metabolism ($t_{1/2}$ 28 h); it induces its own metabolism and the dose should be increased gradually. Nevirapine is initially commenced as a once-daily regimen, with a 2-week lead-in period to twice daily if tolerated. Rash (including Stevens–Johnson syndrome) is seen in up to 20% of patients and, occasionally, fatal hepatitis. The risk of an adverse drug event is closely related to the CD4 count; nevirapine is contraindicated in females with CD4 counts above 250 per microlitre and males with CD4 counts above 400 per microlitre.

Etravirine ($t_{1/2}$ 41 h) is administered twice daily after meals; rash is the commonest adverse effect, generally appearing within the first 6 weeks of therapy, and peripheral neuropathy. Etravirine has activity againt NNRTI resistant HIV strains and should be used in combination with other antiretroviral agents. Due to potentially significant drug interactions, etravirine should not be co-administered with other NNRTIs, unboosted protease inhibitors and ritonavir-boosted tipranavir, fosamprenavir and atazanavir.

Entry inhibitors

Enfuvirtide is the first antiretroviral agent to target the host cell attachment/entry stage in the HIV replication cycle; the linear 36-amino acid synthetic peptide inhibits fusion of the cellular and viral membranes. It is given by subcutaneous injection ($t_{1/2}$ 4 h). The drug seems most effective when combined with several antiretroviral agents to which the virus is susceptible and is licensed for use in treatment-experienced patients with extensive drug resistance. Enfuvirtide does not inhibit cytochrome P450 enzymes and therefore has limited drug interactions.

Adverse effects are usually limited to mild injection-site reactions, although hypersensitivity, peripheral neuropathy and other adverse reactions are reported rarely. HIV isolates with decreased susceptibility have been recovered from enfuvirtide-treated patients; these exhibit mutations in the gp41 outer envelope glycoprotein of the virus (which plays a key role in infection of CD4 cells by fusing the HIV envelope with the host cell membrane).

Maraviroc is an entry inhibitor that specifically targets and blocks the chemokine co-receptor CCR5, which is used by HIV for fusion and cell entry. Maraviroc has no activity against HIV virions that preferentially bind to another surface chemokine co-receptor (CXCR4), found in about 60% of antiretroviral experienced patients. Hence a 'Trofile assay' is required to determine if a susceptible (CCR5 tropic) strain is present as the dominant quasispecies in a patient prior to commencing maraviroc therapy. It is recommended as part of a combination regimen in treatment-experienced patients with multidrug-resistant strains.

Integrase inhibitors

Raltegravir ($t_{1/2}$ 41 h) targets the HIV integrase enzyme, which is essential in integrating viral genetic material into the DNA of the host target cell. It is generally well tolerated and metabolised by glucuronidation. It has a low genetic barrier to resistance (arising from mutations in the integrase gene) and should be used with caution in patients at increased risk of myopathy or rhabdomyolysis.

Fixed-dose combinations of antiretroviral drugs are convenient, help to lessen pill burden and may improve compliance, but the components of the combination may differ in their dependence on metabolic inactivation or renal excretion; particular attention to these is necessary when use in patients with renal or hepatic impairment is proposed.

Fixed-dose combination antiretrovirals	
Combivir	zidovudine and lamivudine
Kivexa (Europe), Epzicom (USA)	abacavir and lamivudine
Truvada	tenofovir and emtricitabine
Trizivir	zidovudine and lamivudine and abacavir
Atripla	tenofovir and emtricitabine and efavirenz
Kaletra	lopinavir and ritonavir

INFLUENZA A

Neuraminidase inhibitors are highlighted by the emergence of avian influenza viruses with the potential for mutation to cause pandemic spread in the human population, although their clinical effectiveness is not high. The two antiviral drugs oseltamivir and zanamivir were widely used for the public health control of the 2009 influenza A (H1N1) pandemic.

Amantadine

Amantadine is effective only against influenza A; it acts by interfering with the uncoating and release of viral genome into the host cell. It is well absorbed from the gastrointestinal tract and is eliminated in the urine ($t_{1/2}$ 3 h). Following the emergence of the 2009 influenza A (H1N1) virus as the predominant circulating strain, resistance to amantadine is now almost universal; for this reason amantidine is no longer recommended for the treatment of influenza.

Adverse reactions include dizziness, nervousness, lightheadedness and insomnia. Drowsiness, hallucinations, delirium and coma may occur in patients with impaired renal function. Convulsions may be induced, and amantadine should be avoided in epileptic patients.

Zanamivir (Relenza)

Zanamivir is a viral neuraminidase inhibitor that blocks both entry of influenza A and B viruses to target cells and the release of their progeny. It is administered as a dry powder twice daily in a 5-day course by a special inhaler. The limited bio-availability (2%) of zanamivir has made it the preferred antiviral in pregnancy. The duration of symptoms is reduced from about 6 to 5 days, with a smaller reduction in the mean time taken to return to normal activities. In high-risk groups the reduction in duration of symptoms is a little greater, and fewer patients need antibiotics. It is also effective for prophylaxis given as a once-daily inhalation.

The UK National Institute for Health and Clinical Excellence (NICE) recommends that zanamivir be reserved for:

- At-risk patients (those with chronic respiratory or cardiovascular disease, immunosuppression or diabetes mellitus, or over the age of 65 years).
- When virological surveillance in the community indicates that influenza virus is circulating.
- Only those presenting within 48 h of the onset of influenza-like symptoms.

Zanamivir retains activity against amantadine-resistant and some oseltamivir-resistant strains.

Unwanted effects are uncommon, but bronchospasm may be precipitated in asthmatics, and gastrointestinal disturbance and rash are occasionally seen.

Oseltamivir (Tamiflu)

Oseltamivir is an oral prodrug of a viral neuraminidase inhibitor. It reduces the severity and duration of symptoms caused by influenza A or B in adults and children if commenced within 36 h of the onset of symptoms. More specifically, the risk of respiratory complications such as secondary pneumonia, antibiotic use and hospital admission are reduced. It is effective for post-exposure prophylaxis, where it should be started within 48 h of contact with the index case and continued daily for 10 days, a usage that might be appropriate for health-care workers and those especially likely to suffer serious complications from pre-existing illness. Prophylaxis may be given for 2 weeks after influenza immunisation while protective antibodies are being produced.

Oseltamivir is one option for treatment and prophylaxis of avian H5N1 and 2009 influenza A (H1N1) virus. In the event of a pandemic, treatment for 5 days and prophylactic use for up to 6 weeks (or until 48 h after last exposure) are suggested.

Unwanted effects are uncommon; some people experience gastrointestinal symptoms that are reduced by taking the drug with food.

Resistance to oseltamivir emerged in late 2007 among seasonal influenza A H1N1 viruses as a result of a spontaneous mutation at position 274 (His274Tyr) in the neuraminidase enzyme. So far, this mutation appears to be confined mostly to seasonal influenza A H1N1 strains, with the majority of 2009 influenza A (H1N1) viruses still susceptible to oseltamivir; the mutation also does not appear to confer resistance to zanamivir.

Peramivir is the third neuraminidase inhibitor approved by the FDA to treat flu infection, but the first approved as an IV formulation. The drug was granted temporary emergency use for hospitalised patients with severe suspected or confirmed influenza A (H1N1) infection where oseltamivir or zanamivir therapy has failed or the inhalational or oral routes are considered unreliable. Peramivir is the first neuraminidase inhibitor that has shown to be safe and effective as a single-dose, i.v. therapy for patients with acute, uncomplicated influenza. Peramivir is intended for certain groups of patients, such as those who have vomiting and diarrhea, for whom a 5-day course of oral capsules would be inappropriate, or those who would have trouble taking an inhaled drug because of upper respiratory symptoms. The most common adverse reaction to peramvir has been diarrhea, in less than 2% of patients. Rare side effects have included serious skin reactions, such as Stevens-Johnson syndrome and erythema multiforme.

CYTOMEGALOVIRUS

Ganciclovir

Ganciclovir resembles aciclovir in its mode of action, but is much more toxic. An acyclic analogue of guanosine, the drug is converted to a triphosphate form which competitively inhibits virion DNA polymerase, leading to chain termination. It is given i.v. and is eliminated in the urine, mainly unchanged ($t_{1/2}$ 4 h). Ganciclovir is active against several types of virus but toxicity limits its i.v. use to life- and sight-threatening CMV infection in immunocompromised patients, including CMV retinitis, pneumonitis, colitis and disseminated disease.

Valganciclovir is an oral prodrug of ganciclovir that provides systemic concentrations almost as high as those following i.v. therapy. It is used for treatment of CMV retinitis (acute treatment of peripheral retinal lesions and maintenance suppressive therapy) in patients with AIDS, and to prevent CMV disease in patients receiving immunosuppressive therapy following organ transplantation (especially liver transplants). A combined approach of ganciclovir-releasing intraocular implant plus oral valganciclovir is sometimes considered in patients with immediate sight-threatening CMV retinitis. Ganciclovir-resistant CMV isolates have been reported, and require treatment with foscarnet or cidofovir.

Adverse reactions include neutropenia and thrombocytopenia, which are usually but not always reversible. Concomitant use of potential marrow-depressant drugs, e.g. co-trimoxazole, amphotericin B, azathioprine, zidovudine, should be avoided, and co-administration of granulocyte colony-stimulating factor may ameliorate the myelosuppressive effects. Other reactions are fever, rash, gastrointestinal symptoms, confusion and seizure (the last especially when imipenem is co-administered).

Foscarnet

Foscarnet finds use i.v. for CMV retinitis in patients with HIV infection when ganciclovir is contraindicated, and for aciclovir-resistant herpes simplex virus infection. It is generally less well tolerated than ganciclovir; adverse effects include renal toxicity (usually reversible), nausea and vomiting, neurological reactions and marrow suppression. Hypocalcaemia is seen especially when foscarnet is given with pentamidine, e.g. during treatment of multiple infections in patients with AIDS. Renal toxicity can beminimised with good hydration and dose modification. Foscarnet causes a contact dermatitis which can lead to unpleasant genital ulcerations due to high urine drug concentrations; this is potentially preventable with good urinary hygiene.

Cidofovir

Cidofovir is given by i.v. infusion (usually every 1 –2 weeks) for CMV retinitis in patients with AIDS when other drugs are unsuitable or resistance is a problem. It has also been used i.v. and topically to produce resolution of molluscum contagiosum skin lesions in immunosuppressed patients, and it may be effective in other poxvirus infections. Nephrotoxicity is common with i.v. use, but is reduced by hydration with i.v. fluids before each dose and co-administration with probenecid. Other unwanted effects include bone marrow suppression, nausea and vomiting, and iritis and uveitis, and cause about 25% of patients to discontinue therapy.

RESPIRATORY SYNCYTIAL VIRUS (RSV)

Ribavirin is a synthetic nucleoside used for RSV bronchiolitis in infants and children, inhaled by a special ventilator. As therapeutic efficacy for this indication is controversial, it is usually reserved for the most severe cases and those with coexisting illnesses, such as immunosuppression. Systemic absorption by the inhalational route is negligible.

Ribavirin is effective by mouth ($t_{1/2}$ 45 h) for reducing mortality from Lassa fever and hantavirus infection (possibly also other viral haemorrhagic fevers and West Nile virus) and, when combined with interferon α-2b or peginterferon, for chronic hepatitis C infection. It does not cross the blood–brain barrier, so is unlikely to be effective in viral encephalitides. Systemic ribavirin is an important teratogen, and it may cause cardiac, gastrointestinal and neurological adverse effects. It may also cause haemolytic anaemia, for which close monitoring is required.

Palivizumab is a humanised monoclonal antibody directed against the F glycoprotein on the surface of RSV. It is given by monthly i.m. injection in the winter and early spring to infants and children less than 2 years old at high risk of RSV infection. Transient fever and local injection site reactions are seen and rarely, gastrointestinal disturbance, rash, leucopenia or disturbed liver function occur. Anaphylaxis has occurred rarely (1 in 10 000).

DRUGS THAT MODULATE THE HOST IMMUNE SYSTEM

Interferons

Virus infection stimulates the production of protective glycoproteins (interferons) which act:

- directly on uninfected cells to induce enzymes that degrade viral RNA
- indirectly by stimulating the immune system
- to modify cell regulatory mechanisms and inhibit neoplastic growth.

Interferons are classified as α, β or γ according to their antigenic and physical properties. α-Interferons (subclassified -2a, -2b and -N1) are effective against conditions that include hairy cell leukaemia, chronic myelogenous leukaemia, recurrent or metastatic renal cell carcinoma, Kaposi's sarcoma in patients with AIDS (an effect that may be due partly to its activity against HIV) and condylomata acuminata (genital warts).

Interferonα-2a and -2b also improve the manifestations of viral hepatitis, but responses differ according to the infecting agent. Therapy with interferonα-2b

leads in about a third of patients with chronic hepatitis B to loss of circulating 'e' antigen, a return to normal liver enzyme levels, histological improvement in liver architecture, and a lowered rate of progression of liver disease. It is contraindicated in patients with decompensated liver disease.

Pegylated (bound to polyethylene glycol) interferon α-2a is more effective than standard interferon α and is now the standard of care for patients with chronic hepatitis C infection. Over 50% of patients with hepatitis C respond to the combination of pegylated interferon plus ribavirin, and 30–40% to peg-interferon alone. Successful treatment results in the serum concentration of viral RNA becoming undetectable by polymerase chain reaction (PCR). Hepatitis D (δ agent co-infection with hepatitis B) requires a much larger dose of interferon to obtain a response, and relapse may yet occur when the drug is withdrawn. Interferon α-2b may be effective in West Nile virus encephalitis.

See also p. 553 for lamivudine and adefovir, use in chronic hepatitis B infection.

Adverse reactions are common and include an influenzalike syndrome (naturally produced interferon may be responsible for symptoms in natural influenza infection), fatigue and depression, which respond to lowering the dose but tend to improve after the first week. Other effects are anorexia (sufficient to induce weight loss), alopecia, convulsions, hypotension, hypertension, cardiac arrhythmias and bone marrow depression (which may respond to granulocyte colony-stimulating factors and erythropoietin). Interferons inhibit the metabolism of theophylline, increasing its effect, and autoimmune diseases such as thyroiditis may be induced or exacerbated.

Imiquimod is used topically for genital warts (caused by papillomaviruses). Treatment for 2–3 months results in gradual clearance of warts in about 50% of patients, and recurrence is less common than after physical removal, e.g. with liquid nitrogen.

Inosine pranobex is reported to stimulate the host immune response to virus infection and has been used for mucocutaneous herpes simplex, genital warts and subacute sclerosing panencephalitis. It is administered by mouth and metabolised to uric acid, so should be used with caution in patients with hyperuricaemia or gout.

Part 2. Fungal infections

Widespread use of immunosuppressive chemotherapy and the emergence of AIDS have contributed to a rise in the incidence of opportunistic infection ranging from comparatively trivial cutaneous infections to systemic diseases that demand prolonged treatment with potentially toxic agents.

SUPERFICIAL MYCOSES

Dermatophyte infections (ringworm, tinea)

Longstanding remedies such as Compound Benzoic Acid Ointment (Whitfield's ointment) are still acceptable for mild infections, but a topical imidazole (clotrimazole, econazole, miconazole, sulconazole), which is also effective against candida, is now usually preferred. Tioconazole is effective topically for nail infections. When multiple areas are severely affected, especially if the scalp or nails are included, and when topical therapy fails, oral itraconazole or terbinafine are used.

Candida infections

Cutaneous infection is generally treated with topical ketoconazole, clotrimazole, econazole, miconazole or nystatin. Local hygiene is also important. An underlying explanation should be sought when a patient fails to respond to these measures, e.g. diabetes, the use of a broad-spectrum antibiotic or of immunosuppressive drugs.

Candidiasis of the alimentary tract mucosa responds to fluconazole, ketoconazole, miconazole or nystatin as lozenges (to suck, for oral infection), gel (held in the mouth before swallowing), suspension or tablets.

Vaginal candidiasis is treated by clotrimazole, econazole, isoconazole, ketoconazole, miconazole or nystatin as pessaries or vaginal tablets or cream inserted once or twice a day with cream or ointment on surrounding skin. Failure may be due to a concurrent intestinal infection causing re-infection, and nystatin tablets may be given by mouth 8-hourly with the local treatment. Alternatively, oral fluconazole may be used, now available without prescription ('over the counter') in the UK. The male sexual partner may use a similar antifungal ointment for his benefit and for the patient's (re-infection).

Fluconazole is often given orally or i.v. to heavily immunocompromised patients, e.g. during periods of profound granulocytopenia, and to severely ill patients on intensive care units to reduce the incidence of systemic candidiasis. Candida albicans is increasingly resistant to fluconazole, other Candida species may also be commonly resistant in hospitals where prophylactic fluconazole use is extensive.

Isolation of candida from the bloodstream or intravenous catheter tips of patients with predisposing factors for systemic candidasis, e.g. prolonged intravenous access, neutropenia, is associated with a significant risk of serious sequelae, e.g. retinal or renal deposits, and should be treated with an effective antifungal for at least 3 weeks; fluconazole, echinocandins or the amphotericin will be appropriate.

SYSTEMIC MYCOSES

Classification of antifungal agents
- Drugs that disrupt the fungal cell membrane: polyenes, e.g. amphotericin
  azoles: imidazoles, e.g. ketoconazole, triazoles, e.g. fluconazoleallylamine: terbinafine
- Drugs that disrupt the fungal cell wall: echinocandins, e.g. caspofungin, anidulafungin, micafungin
- Drugs that inhibit mitosis: griseofulvin.
- Drugs that inhibit DNA synthesis: flucytosine.

Pneumocystosis, caused by Pneumocystis jirovecii, is an important cause of potentially fatal pneumonia in the immunosuppressed, especially HIV-positive patients. It is treated with high dose co-trimoxazole at 120 mg/kg daily in two to four divided doses for 21 days by mouth or i.v. infusion; monitoring of plasma concentrations is recommended. Patients with more severe illness should also receive corticosteroid. Although co-trimoxazole resistance is rare, patients who fail to respond or are intolerant may benefit from pentamidine or primaquine plus clindamycin. Other options include atovaquone for mild disease. Co-trimoxazole, dapsone (with pyrimethamine if toxoplasma prophylaxis is indicated) or atovaquone by mouth, or intermittent inhaled pentamidine, are used for primary and secondary prophylaxis in patients with AIDS.

DRUGS THAT DISRUPT THE FUNGAL CELL MEMBRANE

Polyenes

These act by binding tightly to sterols present in cell membranes. The resulting deformity of the membrane allows leakage of intracellular ions and enzymes, causing cell death. Those polyenes that have useful antifungal activity bind selectively to ergosterol, the most important sterol in fungal (but not mammalian) cell walls.

Amphotericin (amphotericin B)

Amphotericin is absorbed negligibly from the gut and must be given by i.v. infusion for systemic infection; about 10% remains in the blood and the fate of the remainder is not known but is probably bound to tissues. The $t_{1/2}$ is 15 days and, after stopping treatment, drug persists in the body for several weeks.

Amphotericin is at present the drug of choice for most systemic fungal infections. The diagnosis of systemic infection should, whenever possible, be firmly established; tissue biopsy and culture may be necessary, and methods using the PCR to detect aspergillus DNA may revolutionise management of invasive infection.

A conventional course of treatment for filamentous fungal infection lasts 6–12 weeks, during which at least 2 g amphotericin is given (usually 0.7–1 mg/kg daily, and up to 10 mg/kg daily of lipid-associated formulations for the most severe, invasive infections), but lower total and daily doses (e.g. 0.6 mg/kg daily) are used for candida infections, with correspondingly better tolerance. Antifungal drugs may be combined with immune-stimulating agents, e.g. granulocyte colony-stimulating factor, and clinical response in neutropenic episodes is closely related to return of normal neutrophil counts.

Lipid-associated formulations of amphotericin offer the prospect of reduced risk of toxicity while retaining therapeutic efficacy. In an aqueous medium, a lipid with hydrophilic and hydrophobic properties will form vesicles (liposomes) comprising an outer lipid bilayer surrounding an aqueous centre. The AmBisome formulation incorporates amphotericin in a lipid bilayer (55–75 nm diameter) from which the drug is released. Other lipid-associated complexes include Abelcet ('amphotericin B lipid complex') and Amphocil ('amphotericin B colloidal dispersion'). Lipid-associated formulations may be more effective for some indications because higher doses (3 mg/kg daily) may be given rapidly and safely. They are the first choice when renal function is impaired. Treatment often begins with the conventional formulation in those with normal kidneys, resorting to lipid-associated formulations if the patient's renal function deteriorates.

Adverse reactions. Gradual escalation of the dose limits toxic effects, which may be deemed justifiable in lifethreatening infection if conventional amphotericin is used. A strategy of continuous i.v. infusion appears to combine therapeutic efficacy with tolerability. Renal impairment is invariable, although reduced by adequate hydration; nephrotoxicity is reversible, at least in its early stages. Hypokalaemia and hypomagnesaemia (due to distal renal tubular acidosis) may necessitate replacement therapy. Other adverse effects include anorexia, nausea, vomiting, malaise, abdominal, muscle and joint pains, loss of weight, anaemia, and fever. Aspirin, an antihistamine (H_1-receptor) or an antiemetic may alleviate symptoms. Severe febrile reactions are mitigated by hydrocortisone 25–50 mg before each infusion. Lipid-formulated preparations are associated with adverse reactions much less often, but fever, chills, nausea, vomiting, nephrotoxicity, electrolyte disturbance and occasional nephrotoxicity and hepatotoxicity are reported.

Azoles

The antibacterial, antiprotozoal and anthelminthic members of this group are described in the appropriate sections. Antifungal azoles comprise the following:

- Imidazoles (ketoconazole, miconazole, fenticonazole, clotrimazole, isoconazole, tioconazole) interfere with fungal oxidative enzymes to cause lethal accumulation of hydrogen peroxide; they also reduce the formation of ergosterol, an important constituent of the fungal cell membrane which thus becomes permeable to intracellular constituents. Lack of selectivity in these actions results in important adverse effects.
- Triazoles (fluconazole, itraconazole, voriconazole, posaconazole) damage the fungal cell membrane by inhibiting lanosterol 14-α-demethylase, an enzyme crucial to ergosterol synthesis, resulting in accumulation of toxic sterol precursors. Triazoles have greater selectivity against fungi, better penetration of the CNS, resistance to degradation and cause less endocrine disturbance than do the imidazoles.

Ketoconazole

Ketoconazole is well absorbed from the gut (poorly where there is gastric hypoacidity; see below); it is widely distributed in tissues but concentrations in CSF and urine are low; its action is terminated by metabolism by cytochrome P450 3A ($t_{1/2}$ 8 h). For systemic mycoses, ketoconazole has been superseded by fluconazole and itraconazole on grounds of improved pharmacokinetics, tolerability and efficacy. Impairment of steroid synthesis by ketoconazole has been put to other uses, e.g. inhibition of testosterone synthesis lessens bone pain in patients with advanced androgen-dependent prostatic cancer.

Adverse reactions include nausea, giddiness, headache, pruritus and photophobia. Impairment of testosterone synthesis may cause gynaecomastia and decreased libido in men. Of particular concern is impairment of liver function, ranging from a transient increase in levels of hepatic transaminases and alkaline phosphatase to severe injury and death.

Other imidazoles. Miconazole is an alternative. Clotrimazole is widely used as an effective topical agent for dermatophyte, yeast and other fungal infections (intertrigo, athlete's foot, ringworm, pityriasis versicolor, fungal nappy rash). Econazole and sulconazole are similar. Tioconazole is used for fungal nail infections, and isoconazole and fenticonazole for vaginal candidiasis.

Fluconazole

Fluconazole is absorbed from the gastrointestinal tract and is excreted largely unchanged by the kidney ($t_{1/2}$ 30 h). It is effective by mouth for oropharyngeal and oesophageal candidiasis, and i.v. for systemic candidiasis and cryptococcosis (including cryptococcal meningitis; it penetrates the CSF well). It is used prophylactically in a variety of conditions predisposing to systemic candida infections, including at times of profound neutropenia after bone marrow transplantation, and in patients in intensive care units who have intravenous lines in situ, are receiving antibiotic therapy and have undergone bowel surgery. It may cause gastrointestinal discomfort, headaches, reversible alopecia, increased levels of liver enzymes and allergic rash, but is generally well tolerated. Animal studies demonstrate embryotoxicity and there have been reports of multiple congenital abnormalities in women treated with long-term high-dose fluconazole, therefore fluconazole should be avoided in pregnant women. High doses increase the effects of phenytoin, ciclosporin, zidovudine and warfarin.

Itraconazole

Itraconazole is available for oral (suspension and capsule) and i.v. administration ($t_{1/2}$ 25 h, increasing to 40 h with continuous treatment). The intravenous preparation is not available in many countries. Absorption from the gut is about 55%, but variable. It is improved by ingestion with food, but decreased by fatty meals and therapies that reduce gastric acidity. Plasma concentrations should be monitored during prolonged use for critical indications. The oral suspension formulation has significantly improved bioavailability compared to the capsule formulation and is much less affected by gastric hypoacidity. Itraconazole is heavily protein bound and virtually none is found within the CSF. It is almost completely oxidised in the liver (by CYP 3A) and excreted in the bile; little unchanged drug enters the urine.

Itraconazole is used for a variety of superficial mycoses, as a prophylactic agent for aspergillosis and candidiasis in the immunocompromised, and i.v. for treatment of histoplasmosis. It is licensed in the UK as a second-line agent for Candida, Aspergillus and Cryptococcus infections, and it may be convenient as 'follow-on' therapy after systemic aspergillosis has been brought under control by an amphotericin preparation. It appears to be an effective adjunct treatment for allergic bronchopulmonary aspergillosis.

Adverse effects are uncommon, but include transient hepatitis and hypokalaemia. Prolonged use may lead to cardiac failure, especially in those with pre-existing cardiac disease. Co-administration of a calcium channel blocker adds to the risk. Cyclodextrin (used as a vehicle for the i.v. formulation) accumulates and causes sodium overload in renally impaired patients, but the oral formulation avoids this problem.

Interactions. Enzyme induction of CYP 3A, e.g. by rifampicin, reduces the plasma concentration of itraconazole. Additionally, its affinity for several P450 isoforms, notably CYP3A4, causes it to inhibit the oxidation of a number of drugs, including phenytoin, warfarin, ciclosporin, tacrolimus, midazolam, triazolam, cisapride and terfenadine, increasing their intensity and/or duration of effect.

Voriconazole

Voriconazole ($t_{1/2}$ 7 h) is more active in vitro than itraconazole against Aspergillus because of more avid binding of the sterol synthetic enzymes of filamentous fungi; it also appears to have synergistic activity against Aspergillus in combination with amphotericin. It is as active as the other triazoles against yeasts and is more reliably and rapidly absorbed than itraconazole by mouth, but cross-resistance between these agents is usual. It is more effective than conventional amphotericin in invasive aspergillosis, and probably equivalent to lipid-associated formulations. Oral absorption is not significantly reduced by gastric hypoacidity. CSF and brain tissue concentrations are at least 50% of those in the plasma, and are sufficient for effective therapy of fungal infections of the eye and CNS.

Adverse effects. Administration i.v. gives rise rapidly to transient visual disturbance in 30% of patients (blurring, alerted visual perception such as reversal of light and dark, visual hallucinations and photophobia). These often resolve after the first week of therapy, and almost all of those affected are able to continue with the course of treatment.

Accumulation of the cyclodextrin vehicle may cause sodium retention in renally impaired patients with i.v. use. Patients with hepatic cirrhosis should receive a standard loading, but only half of the daily maintenance dose. Transiently raised liver enzyme levels are seen in up to 20% of patients, but serious liver impairment is rare. Rashes and photosensitivity appear to be more common than with the other triazoles.

Extensive metabolism of voriconazole by the cytochrome P450 system (predominantly CYP 2C19) may lead to unwanted interaction with patients receiving rifampicin, ciclosporin or tacrolimus.

Posaconazole

Posaconazole ($t_{1/2}$ 20 h) is structurally related to itraconazole and has similar in vitro antifungal activity to voriconazole. It is fungistatic against Candida spp. but fungicidal against Aspergillus spp., and is also active against a range of other filamentous fungi. It provides effective prophylaxis against invasive fungal infection in leukaemia and bone marrow transplant patients. The oral bio-availabilty is high (90%), especially when taken with a fatty meal. More than 75% of the dose is excreted in the faeces.

Adverse effects are uncommon, but include gastrointestinal disturbance, dizziness and fatigue, neutropenia (7% of patients) and transient disturbance of liver function. Dose adjustment is not required for renal or hepatic impairment.

Allylamine

Terbinafine

Terbinafine interferes with ergosterol biosynthesis, and thereby with the formation of the fungal cell membrane. It is absorbed from the gastrointestinal tract and undergoes extensive metabolism in the liver ($t_{1/2}$ 14 h). Terbinafine is used topically for dermatophyte infections of the skin and orally for infections of hair and nails where the site, e.g. hair, severity or extent of the infection renders topical use inappropriate. Treatment may need to continue for several weeks. Terbinafine may cause nausea, diarrhoea, dyspepsia, abdominal pain, headaches and cutaneous reactions.

DRUGS THAT DISRUPT THE FUNGAL CELL WALL

Echinocandins

The echinocandins are large lipopeptide molecules that inhibit synthesis of β-(1,3)-d-glucan, a vital component of the cell walls of many fungi (excepting Cryptococcus neoformans, against which they have no useful activity). In vitro and in vivo, the echinocandins are rapidly fungicidal against most Candida spp. and fungistatic against Aspergillus spp. Echinocandins have no activity against emerging pathogens such as Fusarium sp., Scedosporium sp. and zygomycetes. They are available as i.v. preparations only.

Caspofungin ($t_{1/2}$ 10 h) is the first member of this group. It is licensed for i.v. treatment of invasive candidiasis, suspected fungal infections in febrile neutropenic patients, and Aspergillus infections in patients who have not responded to amphotericin or itraconazole. Caspofungin retains activity against most triazole- and polyene-resistant yeasts, and is also active against Pneumocystis jirovecii. It is widely distributed through body tissues and highly protein bound. It penetrates the CSF poorly, but

clinical responses in fungal CNS infection have been reported.

Caspofungin is generally well tolerated, but headache, fever, raised liver function tests and hypokalaemia occur. Patients with significant liver impairment should receive a reduced dose. Patients might experience histamine induced reactions when the drug is infused too rapidly.

Micafungin has similar activity to caspofungin and is licensed for the treatment of invasive candida infections (oesophagitis, peritonitis and candidaemia) and for prophylaxis of Candida spp. and Aspergillus infection in patients undergoing haemopoetic stem cell transplantation. It is highly protein bound and, unlike caspofungin and anidulafungin, does not require a loading dose. Micafungin was found to induce the development of liver tumours in rats after treatment for 3 months and longer; close monitoring of patients for liver damage is advised.

Anidulafungin is a semi-synthetic echinocandin derived from Aspergillus nidulans. It has a much longer elimination half-life than the other echinocandins (27 h) and is not metabolised by the liver, but undergoes slow chemical degradation to inactive metabolites. It has no significant drug–drug interactions, with no dose adjustment required in renal or hepatic impairment. Anidulafungin is approved for the treatment of invasive candidiasis in adult non-neutropenic patients.

OTHER ANTIFUNGAL DRUGS

Griseofulvin

Griseofulvin prevents fungal growth by binding to microtubular proteins and inhibiting mitosis. The therapeutic efficacy of griseofulvin depends on its capacity to bind to keratin as it is being formed in the cells of the nail bed, hair follicles and skin, for dermatophytes specifically infect keratinous tissues. Griseofulvin does not kill fungus already established; it merely prevents infection of new keratin so that the duration of treatment is governed by the time that it takes for infected keratin to be shed. On average, hair and skin infection should be treated for 4–6 weeks, although toenails may need a year or more. Treatment must continue for a few weeks after both visual and microscopic evidence has disappeared. Fat in a meal enhances absorption of griseofulvin; it is metabolised in the liver and induces hepatic enzymes ($t_{1/2}$ 15 h).

Griseofulvin is effective against all superficial ringworm (dermatophyte) infections, but ineffective against pityriasis versicolor, superficial candidiasis and all systemic mycoses. Adverse reactions include gastrointestinal upset, rashes, photosensitivity, headache and various CNS disturbances.

Flucytosine

Flucytosine (5-fluorocytosine) is metabolised in the fungal cell to 5-fluorouracil, which inhibits nucleic acid synthesis. It is well absorbed from the gut, penetrates effectively into tissues, and almost all is excreted unchanged in the urine ($t_{1/2}$ 4 h). The dose should be reduced for patients with impaired renal function, and the plasma concentration monitored. The drug is well tolerated when renal function is normal. Candida albicans rapidly becomes resistant to flucytosine, which ought not to be used alone; it may be combined with amphotericin, but this increases the risk of adverse effects (leucopenia, thrombocytopenia, enterocolitis) and it is reserved for serious infections where the risk: benefit balance is favourable, e.g. Cryptococcus neoformans meningitis.

Part 3. Protozoal infections

MALARIA

About half of the world's population is exposed to malaria, with an estimated 250 million cases and 1 million deaths annually, mainly in sub-Saharan African children (where a child dies from malaria on average every 30 seconds). In terms of socioeconomic impact, malaria is the most important of the transmissible parasitic diseases.

Quinine as cinchona bark was introduced into Europe from South America in 1631 (by Agostino

Salumbrino, a Jesuit priest and trained apothecary, who sent a small quantity of bark to Rome where much of the terrain was swampy and fevers were common – hence the term 'Jesuit's bark'). It was used for all fevers, among them malaria, the occurrence of which was associated with damp places with bad air ('mal aria').

Quinine, mefloquine, chloroquine, artesunate, artemether and primaquine (gametocytocides) act on sexual forms and prevent transmission of the infection because the patient becomes non-infective and the parasite fails to develop in the mosquito (.

In summary,. drugs may be selected for:

- treatment of clinical attacks
- prevention of clinical attacks
- radical cure

Drug-resistant malaria

Drug-resistant parasites constitute a persistent problem. Plasmodium falciparum is now resistant to chloroquine and sulfadoxine-pyrimethamine in many parts of the world. Areas of high risk for resistant parasites include sub-Saharan Africa, Latin America, Oceania (Papua New Guinea, Solomon Islands, Vanuatu) and some parts of South-East Asia. Mefloquine resistance is rare outside South-East Asia. There are concerns with emerging artesunate resistance in western Cambodia due to monotherapy. Chloroquine-resistant Plasmodium vivax is also reported. Hyperparasitaemia and inappropriate or low dosing of antimalarials are important drivers of resistance.

Resistance can be reduced by combining antimalarials with different mechanisms of action, usually in the form of artemisinin-based combination therapies (ACTs). ACTs are often more effective than single-agent therapy or non-artemisinin-based combinations and are now recommended by the World Health Organization for the treatment of Plasmodium falciparum malaria globally.

Any physician who is unfamiliar with the resistance pattern in the locality from which patients have come, or to which they are going, is well advised to check the current position. Because prevalence and resistance rates are so variable, advice on therapy and prophylaxis in this section is given for general guidance only and readers are referred to specialist sources for up-to-date information.

Chemotherapy of an acute attack of malaria

Successful management demands attention to the following points of principle:

- Whenever possible, the diagnosis should be confirmed before treatment by examination of blood smears; this is not often possible in the developing world, where clinically diagnosed illnesses may receive unnecessary courses of antimalarials, thus increasing the risks of plasmodial resistance.
- When the infecting organism is not known or infection is mixed, treatment should begin as for Plasmodium falciparum (below).
- Drugs used to treat Plasmodium falciparum malaria must always be selected with regard to the prevalence of local patterns of drug resistance.
- Patients not at risk of re-infection should be reexamined several weeks after treatment for signs of recrudescence, which may result from inadequate chemotherapy or survival of persistent hepatic forms.

Falciparum ('malignant') malaria

Falciparum malaria in the non-immune is a medical emergency, and malaria of unknown infecting species should be treated as though it were falciparum. The regimen depends on the condition of the patient; the doses quoted are for adults. Chloroquine resistance is now widespread; therefore this drug should not be used for the treatment of falciparum malaria.

If the patient can swallow and there are no serious complications such as impairment of consciousness, treatment options are as follows:

- A quinine salt: 600 mg 8-hourly by mouth for 5–7 days, followed by doxycycline 200 mg daily for at least 7 days. This additional therapy is necessary as quinine alone tends to be associated with a higher rate of relapse. Clindamycin (450 mg four times daily for 7 days) maybe given as an alterna-

tive follow-on therapy instead of doxycycline, and is particularly suitable for pregnant women. If the parasite is likely to be sensitive, Fansidar (pyrimethamine plus sulfadoxine) 3 tablets as a single dose is an alternative.

- Malarone (atovaquone and proguanil hydrochloride): 4 tablets once daily for 3 days. Riamet (artemether plus lumefantrine): if weight >35 kg, 4 tablets initially, followed by five further doses of 4 tablets given at 8, 24, 36, 48 and 60 h.
- Mefloquine is also effective, but resistance has been reported in several regions, including South-East Asia. It is not necessary to use follow-on therapy after Riamet, mefloquine or Malarone.

Seriously ill patients. should be treated with:

- A quinine salt: 20 mg/kg as a loading dose5 (maximum 1.4 g) infused i.v. over 4 h, followed 8 h later by a maintenance infusion of 10 mg/kg (maximum 700 mg) infused over 4 h, repeated every 8 h until the patient can swallow tablets to complete the 7-day course. Patients at increased risk of arrhythmias and the elderly should have ECG monitoring while on the infusion.
- Doxycycline or clindamycin should be given subsequently, as above (mefloquine is an alternative, but this must begin at least 12 h after parenteral quinine has ceased). Intravenous artesunate showed a clear benefit when compared to quinine in patients with severe falciparum malaria. A large randomised trial showed a 34% reduction in mortality with intravenous artesunate when compared to quinine; the number needed to treat to prevent one death was 13. Intravenous artesunate is not licensed in the European Union, but should be considered on a 'named patient' basis for severe cases not responsive to quinine or if quinine resistance is suspected, or there is a high parasite count (>20%). Intravenous artesunate should be accompanied by a 7-day course of doxycycline.

Treatment in pregnancy should always be based on expert advice.

Non-falciparum ('benign') malarias

These are usually due to Plasmodium vivax or less

commonly to Plasmodium ovale or Plasmodium malariae. The drug of choice is chloroquine, which should be given by mouth as follows:

- Initial dose: 620 mg (base), then 310 mg as a single dose 6–8 h later.
- Second day: 310 mg as a single dose.
- Third day: 310 mg as a single dose.

The total dose of chloroquine base over 3 days should be approximately 25 mg/kg base. This is sufficient for Plasmodium malariae infection, but for Plasmodium vivax and Plasmodium ovale eradication of the hepatic parasites is necessary to prevent relapse, by giving:

- Primaquine, 15 mg/day for 14 days started after the chloroquine course has been completed. Plasmodium vivax infections require 30 mg/day for 14 days. Primaquine can lead to haemolysis in patients with G6PD deficiency (if mild G6PD deficiency, lower dosing of 45 mg once-weekly for 8 weeks may suffice without undue risk of haemolysis).

Chemoprophylaxis of malaria

Geographically variable plasmodial drug resistance has become a major factor. The World Health Organization gives advice in its annually revised booklet Vaccination Certificate Requirements and Health Advice for International Travel, and national bodies publish recommendations, e.g. British National Formulary, that apply particularly to their own residents.

General principles

- Chemoprophylaxis aims to prevent deaths from falciparum malaria, but only ever gives relative protection; travellers should guard against bites by using mosquito nets and repellents, and wearing well-covering clothing especially during high-risk times of day (after dusk).
- Mefloquine, doxycycline and atovaquone-proguanil (Malarone) are the most commonly advised prophylactic regimens, and are particularly recommended for areas of chloroquine-resistant falciparum malaria. Chloroquine, alone or in combination with proguanil, may be considered in areas of the world where the risk of acquiring chloroquine resistant falciparum malaria is low, although there is considerable concern regarding the protective efficacy of this regimen. Due to widespread P. falciparum resistance to proguanil, single-agent prophylaxis with this agent is rarely appropriate for most regions of the world.

- Effective chemoprophylaxis requires that there be a plasmodicidal concentration of drug in the blood when the first infected mosquito bites, and that it be sustained safely for long periods.
- The progressive rise in plasma concentration to steady state (after $t_{1/2} \times 5$), sometimes attained only after weeks (consider mefloquine $t_{1/2}$ 21 days, chloroquine $t_{1/2}$ 50 days), allows unwanted effects (which can impair compliance or be unsafe) to be delayed, in some instances until after a subject has entered a malarial area. Thus, it is advised that prophylaxis begin long enough before travel to reveal acute intolerance and to impress on the subject the importance of compliance (to relate drug-taking to a specific daily or weekly event).
- Prompt achievement of efficacy and safety, i.e. plasmodicidal concentrations, by one (or two) doses is plainly important for travellers who cannot wait on dosage schedules to deliver both only when steadystate blood concentrations are attained; the schedules must reflect this need.
- Prophylaxis should continue for at least 4 weeks after leaving an endemic area to kill parasites that are acquired about the time of departure, are still incubating in the liver and will develop into the erythrocyte phase. Malarone, however, only needs to be taken for a week after return. The traveller should be aware that any illness occurring within a year, and especially within 3 months, of return, may be malaria.
- Chloroquine and proguanil may be used for periods of up to 5 years, and mefloquine for up to 1–2 years; expert advice should be taken by long-term travellers, especially those going to areas for which other prophylactic drugs are recommended.
- Naturally acquired immunity offers the most

reliable protection for people living permanently in endemic areas (below). Repeated attacks of malaria confer partial immunity and the disease often becomes no more than an occasional inconvenience. Vaccines to confer active immunity are under development.

- A short course of prophylaxis (4–6 weeks) may be considered for pregnant women and young children returning to their permanent homes in malarious areas after a prolonged period of stay in a non-endemic area, pending suitable arrangements for health care.

- As a rule, the partially immune should not take a prophylactic. The reasoning is that immunity is sustained by the red cell cycle, loss of which through prophylaxis diminishes their resistance and leaves them highly vulnerable to the disease. There are, however, exceptions to this general advice, and the partially immune may or should use a prophylactic:
  - if it is virtually certain that they will never abandon its use
  - if they go to another malarial area where the strains of parasite may differ
  - during the last few months of pregnancy in areas where Plasmodium falciparum is prevalent (to avert the risk of miscarriage)

Examples of standard prophylactic regimens

- Chloroquine: 300 mg (base) once weekly (start 1 week before travel).
- Proguanil: 200 mg once daily (start 1 week before travel).
- Chloroquine plus proguanil in the above doses.
- Malarone: 1 tablet daily (start 1–2 days before travel).
- Mefloquine: 250 mg once weekly (start 1 week, preferably 2–3 weeks, before travel).
- Doxycycline: 100 mg once daily (start 1–2 days before travel).

For 'last minute' travellers. The standard regimens normally provide immediate protection, but it will be sensible to avoid mefloquine (if an alternative antimalarial is available) in the last minute traveller

with no history of previous mefloquine exposure or who is intolerant of the drug. Current UK national guidelines do not recommend giving a loading dose of prophylactic antimalarials for the purpose of rapidly achieving steady-state plasma concentration.

Drug interactions. Where subjects are already taking other drugs, e.g. antiepileptics and cardiovascular drugs, it is desirable to start prophylaxis as much as 2–3 weeks in advance to establish safety.

Antimalarial drugs and pregnancy

Women living in endemic areas in which Plasmodium falciparum remains sensitive to chloroquine should take chloroquine prophylactically throughout pregnancy. Proguanil (an 'antifol', see below) may be taken for prophylaxis provided it is accompanied by folic acid 5 mg/day. Chloroquine may be used in full dose to treat chloroquinesensitive infections. Quinine is the only widely available drug that is acceptable as suitable for treating chloroquine-resistant infections during pregnancy. Mefloquine is teratogenic in animals and a woman should avoid pregnancy while taking it, and for 3 months afterwards (although evidence is accruing that it may be safe for use in chloroquine-resistant areas). Doxycycline is contraindicated throughout pregnancy, and Malarone (proguanil plus atovaquone) should be avoided unless there is no suitable alternative.

AMOEBIASIS

Infection occurs when mature cysts are ingested and pass into the colon, where they divide into trophozoites; these forms either enter the tissues or form cysts. Amoebiasis occurs in two forms, both of which need treatment:

- Bowel lumen amoebiasis is asymptomatic, and trophozoites (non-infective) and cysts (infective) are passed into the faeces. Treatment is directed at eradicating cysts with a luminal amoebicide; diloxanide furoate is the drug of choice; iodoquinol or paromomycin are alternatives.

- Tissue-invading amoebiasis gives rise to dysentery, hepatic amoebiasis and liver abscess. A systemically active drug (tissue amoebicide) effective against trophozoites must be used, e.g. metronidazole, tinidazole, ornidazole. Parenteral forms of these are available for patients too ill to take drugs by mouth. In severe cases of amoebic dysentery with suspected or confirmed peritonitis, broad-spectrum antibiotics should be administered and surgical intervention considered.

Treatment with tissue amoebicides should always be followed by a course of a luminal amoebicide to eradicate the source of the infection.

Dehydroemetine (from ipecacuanha), less toxic than the parent emetine, is claimed by some authorities to be the most effective tissue amoebicide. It is reserved for the treatment of metronidazole-resistant amoebiasis and in dangerously ill patients, but these are more likely to be vulnerable to its cardiotoxic effects. When dehydroemetine is used to treat amoebic liver abscess, chloroquine should also be given.

Notes on drugs for protozoal infections

Atovaquone is a quinone; it may cause gastrointestinal and mild neurological side-effects, and rare hepatotoxicity and blood dyscrasias.

Benznidazole is a nitroimidazole that may occasionally cause peripheral neuritis but is generally well tolerated, including by infants.

Dehydroemetine inhibits protein synthesis; it may cause pain at the site of injection, weakness and muscular pain, hypotension, precordial pain and cardiac arrhythmias.

Diloxanide furoate may cause troublesome flatulence, and pruritus and urticaria may occur.

Eflornithine inhibits protozoal DNA synthesis; it may cause anaemia, leucopenia and thrombocytopenia, and seizures.

Iodoquinol may cause abdominal cramps, nausea and diarrhoea. Skin eruptions, pruritus ani and thyroid gland enlargement have been attributed to its iodine content. The recognition of severe neurotoxicity with the related drug, clioquinol, in Japan in the 1960s must give cause for caution in its use.

Meglumine antimonate is a pentavalent antimony compound, similar to sodium stibogluconate (below).

Melarsoprol, a trivalent organic arsenical, acts through its high affinity for sulphydryl groups of enzymes. Adverse effects include encephalopathy, myocardial damage, proteinuria and hypertension.

Mepacrine (quinacrine) was formerly used as an antimalarial but is now an alternative to metronidazole or tinidazole for giardiasis. It may cause gastrointestinal upset, occasional acute toxic psychosis, hepatitis and aplastic anaemia.

Nifurtimox is a nitrofuran derivative. Adverse effects include anorexia, nausea, vomiting, gastric pain, insomnia, headache, vertigo, excitability, myalgia, arthralgia and convulsions. Peripheral neuropathy may necessitate stopping treatment.

Paromomycin, an aminoglycoside, is not absorbed from the gut; it is similar to neomycin.

Pentamidine is a synthetic aromatic amidine; it must be administered parenterally or by inhalation as it is absorbed unreliably from the gastrointestinal tract; it does not enter the CSF. Given systemically it frequently causes nephrotoxicity, which is reversible; acute hypotension and syncope are common especially after rapid i.v. injection. Pancreatic damage may cause hypoglycaemia due to insulin release.

Sodium stibogluconate (Pentostam) is an organic pentavalent antimony compound; it may cause anorexia, vomiting, coughing and substernal pain. Used in mucocutaneous leishmaniasis, it may lead to severe inflammation around pharyngeal or tracheal lesions which may require control with corticosteroid. Meglumine antimoniate is similar.

Suramin forms stable complexes with plasma protein and is detectable in urine for up to 3 months after the last injection; it does not cross the blood–brain barrier. It may cause tiredness, anorexia, malaise, polyuria, thirst, and tenderness of the palms and soles.

Miltefosine is a phosphocholine analogue that was originally developed as an oral antineoplastic. It is the only effective oral treatment for cutaneous and visceral leishmaniasis. The main adverse effects are vomiting, diarrhoea and raised transaminases. The drug is teratogenic in animals, and therefore should be avoided in pregnancy and used with caution in women of reproductive age.

Part 4. Helminthic infections

Helminths have complex life cycles, special knowledge of which is required by those who treat infections. Drug resistance has not so far proved to be a clinical problem, though it has occurred in animals on continuous chemoprophylaxis.

Drugs for helminthic infections

Albendazole is similar to mebendazole (below).

Diethylcarbamazine kills both microfilariae and adult worms. Fever, headache, anorexia, malaise, urticaria, vomiting and asthmatic attacks following the first dose are due to products of destructionof the parasite, and reactions areminimised by slow increase in dosage over the first 3 days. Ivermectin may cause immediate reactions due to the death of the microfilaria. It can be effective in a single dose, but is best repeated at intervals of 6–12 months.

Levamisole paralyses the musculature of sensitive nematodes which, unable to maintain their anchorage, are expelled by normal peristalsis. It is well tolerated, but may cause abdominal pain, nausea, vomiting, headache and dizziness.

Mebendazole blocks glucose uptake by nematodes. Mild gastrointestinal discomfort may be caused, and it should not be used in pregnancy or in children under the age of 2 years.

Metriphonate is an organophosphorus anticholinesterase compound that was originally used as an insecticide. Adverse effects include abdominal pain, nausea, vomiting, diarrhoea, headache and vertigo.

Niclosamide blocks glucose uptake by intestinal tapeworms. It may cause some mild gastrointestinal symptoms.

Piperazine may cause hypersensitivity reactions, neurological symptoms (including 'worm wobble') and may precipitate epilepsy.

Praziquantel paralyses both adult worms and larvae. It is metabolised extensively. Praziquantel may cause nausea, headache, dizziness and drowsiness; it cures with a single dose (or divided doses in 1 day).

Pyrantel depolarises neuromuscular junctions of susceptible nematodes, which are expelled in the faeces. It cures with a single dose. It may induce gastrointestinal disturbance, headache, dizziness, drowsiness and insomnia.

Tiabendazole inhibits cellular enzymes of susceptible helminths. Gastrointestinal, neurological and hypersensitivity reactions, liver damage and crystalluria may be induced.

SUMMARY

Viruses present a more difficult problem of chemotherapy than do other microorganisms, e.g. bacteria, for they are intracellular parasites that use the metabolism of host cells. In the past 15 years, identification of the molecular differences between viral and human metabolism has led to the development of many effective antiviral agents; Only four were available in 1990, now there are over 40. Fungal infections range from inconvenient skin conditions to life-threatening systemic diseases; the latter have become more frequent as opportunistic infections in patients immunocompromised by drugs or AIDS, or in those receiving intensive medical and surgical interventions in intensive care units. Protozoal infections such as Malaria is the major transmissible parasitic disease in the world. Drug resistance is an increasing problem and differs with geographical location, and species of plasmodium. Helminthic infestations cause considerable morbidity. The drugs that are effective against these organisms are also summarised.

IMPORTANT TERMINOLOGY

antiviral agents　抗病毒药物

antiretroviral drugs　抗逆转录病毒药物

reverse transcriptase inhibitors　逆转录酶抑制剂

protease inhibitors　蛋白酶抑制剂

entry inhibitors　进入抑制剂

integrase inhibitors　整合酶抑制剂

viral neuraminidase inhibitor 病毒神经氨酸酶抑制剂

highly active antiretroviral therapy (HAART) 高效抗逆转录病毒治疗

immunosuppressive drugs 免疫抑制药物

Echinocandins 棘球白素类

Polyenes 多烯类

Azoles 氮唑类

Allylamine 烯丙胺类

Radical cure 根治法

Artemisinin-based combination therapies (ACTs) 基于青蒿素的联合疗法

CHALLENGE YOURSELF

1. What are the targets and mechanisms of antiviral drugs?
2. Application of drugs against systemic fungal infections should pay attention to what matters?
3. What are the measures for the treatment and prevention of Malaria, including 'malignant' and 'benign' Malaria?

Yuanying Jiang

Chapter | 23 |

Anticancer Drugs

CANCER TREATMENTS AND OUTCOMES

Cancers share some common characteristics:

- Growth that is not subject to normal spatial restrictions for that tissue and fails to respond to apoptotic signals or in which a high proportion of cells are dividing, i.e. there is a high 'growth fraction'.
- Local invasiveness.
- Tendency to spread to other parts of the body (metastasis).
- Less differentiated cell morphology.
- Tendency to retain some characteristics of the tissue of origin, at least initially.

Cancer treatment employs six established principal modalities:

1. Surgery.
2. Radiotherapy.
3. Cytotoxic chemotherapy.
4. Endocrine therapy.
5. Immunotherapy.
6. Biological (or targeted) therapy.

This account describes the main groups of drugs but it is important to understand the overall context in which systemic therapy is offered to patients.

Systemic cancer therapy

Cancers originating from different organs of the body differ in their initial behaviour and in their response to treatments. Primary surgery and/or radiotherapy to a *localised* cancer offer the best chance of *cure* for patients. Drug treatments offer cure only for certain types of cancer, often characterised by their high proliferative rate, e.g. lymphoma, testicular cancer, Wilms' tumour. More often, systemic therapy offers prolongation of life from months to many years and associated improvements in quality of life, even if patients ultimately die from their disease.

Use of drugs as *adjuvant therapy* attempts to eradicate residual microscopic cancer by treating patients after their primary surgery. This strategy has improved overall survival for patients after surgical resection of primary breast, colorectal and gastric cancer. In some situations, drugs are administered prior to surgery (*neoadjuvant therapy*), primarily to shrink large, locally advanced disease to subsequently enable surgical resection. Many patients with cancer are not cured by their primary treatment due to the presence of micrometastatic disease; the disease often returns months or years later even though at the time of completing their initial treatment there was no visible evidence of cancer. Clearly, this is a limitation of current standard techniques used to identify residual disease. Currently, radiological techniques cannot clearly visualise lesions smaller than 5 mm in most organs, which equates to over many million cancer cells.

Palliative therapy, offered to patients with advanced, incurable cancer, aims both to increase survival and to improve quality of life by symptom control. Despite significant improvements in cancer outcomes in the last 5–10 years, there remain a number of types of cancer that are poorly responsive to currently available drugs. Patients with *chemoresistant* cancers who are fit enough and willing may be offered experimental treatments within Phase 1 or 2 clinical trials.

Most treatments currently available are associated with unwanted effects of varying degrees of severity. The risk of causing harm must be weighed against the potential to do good in each individual case. *Systemic therapy* aims to kill malignant cells or modify their growth but leave the normal cells of the host unharmed or, more usually, temporarily harmed but capable of recovery. When there is realistic expectation of cure or extensive life prolongation, then to risk more severe drug toxicity is justified. For example, the treatment of testicular cancer with potentially life-threatening platinum-based combination chemotherapy regimens offers a greater than 85% chance of cure, even for those with extensive, metastatic disease.

Where expectation is confined to palliation in terms of modest life prolongation of less certain quality, then the benefits and risks of treatment must be judged carefully. Palliative treatments should involve low risk of adverse effects, e.g. 5-fluorouracil-based chemotherapy for advanced colorectal cancer is well tolerated by most patients, while improving survival by around 1–2 years. A modern prerequisite of cancer chemotherapy Phase 3 trials is concomitantly and objectively to assess patient quality of life while on drug therapy. This helps clinicians and nurses to explain the potential benefits and harm of treatment to patients and their families, who may themselves hold strong views about the quality and quantity of life.

RATIONALE FOR CYTOTOXIC CHEMOTHERAPY

The narrow therapeutic index of cytotoxic agents means that escalation of drug doses is constrained by damage to normal cells and the maximum doses that patients can tolerate are often suboptimal to achieve total cancer cell killing. Even so, cytotoxic chemo-

therapy agents remain the mainstay of systemic anticancer treatment, as an understanding of their pharmacology has enabled clinicians to exploit the benefits of these drugs.

The very real limitations of cytotoxic chemotherapy have forced a concentration of cancer research on trying to understand the carcinogenic process, the aim being to identify specific molecular targets that can be exploited to develop novel therapeutic approaches. So-called *targeted* therapies are now well-established groups of anticancer drugs.

CLASSES OF CYTOTOXIC CHEMOTHERAPY DRUGS ON CELL CYCLE

Cytotoxic chemotherapy drugs exert their effect by inhibiting cell proliferation. All proliferating cells, whether normal and malignant, cycle through a series of phases of: *synthesis* of DNA (S phase), *mitosis* (M phase) and *rest* (G_1 phase, or G_2 phase). Non-cycling cells are quiescent in G_0 phase (Fig. 23.1).

Fig.23.1 The cell cycle. Most cytotoxic drugs inhibit the processes of DNA replication or mitosis.

Cytotoxic drugs interfere with cell division at various points of the cell cycle, in particular G_1/S phase (e.g. synthesis of nucleotides from purines and pyrimidines), S phase (preventing DNA replication) and M phase (e.g. blocking the process of mitosis).

They are thus all potentially mutagenic. Cytotoxic drugs ultimately induce cell death by *apoptosis*, a process by which single cells are removed from living tissue by being fragmented into membrane-bound particles and phagocytosed by other cells. This occurs without disturbing the architecture or function of the tissue, or eliciting an inflammatory response. The instructions for apoptosis are built into the cell's genetic material, i.e. 'programmed cell death'.

In general, cytotoxics are most effective against actively cycling cells and least effective against resting or quiescent cells. The latter are particularly problematic in that, although inactive, they retain the capacity to proliferate and may start cycling again after a completed course of chemotherapy, often leading later to rapid regrowth of the cancer.

Cytotoxic drugs can be classified as either:

- *cell cycle non-specific*: these kill cells whether they are resting or actively cycling (as in a low growth fraction cancer such as solid tumours), e.g. alkylating agents, doxorubicin and allied anthracyclines, or

- *cell cycle (phase) specific*: these kill only cells that are actively cycling, often because their site of action is confined to one phase of the cell cycle, e.g. antimetabolite drugs.

CLASSES OF CYTOTOXIC AGENTS

Alkylating agents

Alkylating agents (nitrogen mustards and ethylenimines) act by transferring alkyl groups to DNA in the N-7 position of guanine during cell division. Normal synthesis is prevented because of either DNA strand breakage or cross-linking of the two strands. Examples include: busulfan, carmustine, chlorambucil, cyclophosphamide, ifosfamide, lomustine, melphalan, mustine (mechlorethamine), thiotepa, treosulfan.

Antimetabolites

Antimetabolites are synthetic analogues of normal metabolites and act by competition to 'deceive' or 'defraud' bodily processes.

Methotrexate, a folic acid antagonist, competitively inhibits dihydrofolate reductase, preventing the synthesis of tetrahydrofolic acid (the coenzyme that is important in synthesis of amino and nucleic acids). The drug also provides a cogent illustration of the need to exploit every possible means of enhancing selectivity. Where the desire is to maximise the effect of methotrexate, a potentially fatal dose is given, followed 24 h later by a dose of tetrahydrofolic (folinic) acid as calcium folinate (Ca Leucovorin) to bypass and terminate its action. This is called folinic acid 'rescue', because, if it is not given, the patient will die. The therapeutic justification for this manoeuvre is the cell kill obtained with very high plasma concentrations of methotrexate, allied to the fact that the bone marrow cells recover better than the tumour cells. The outcome is a useful degree of selectivity.

Pyrimidine antagonists: 5-fluorouracil (5FU) is metabolised intracellularly and its metabolite binds covalently with thymidilate synthase, thereby inhibiting DNA (and RNA) synthesis. 5FU has a short duration of action and addition of folinic acid in 5FU therapy improves its antitumour activity; protracted infusion can achieve the same outcome. Oral prodrugs of 5FU include capecitabine and UFT (a mixture of tegafur and uracil). These prodrugs have a cytotoxic action equivalent to that of 5FU but cause less myelosuppression and stomatitis; the risk of hand–foot syndrome (damage to the palmar and plantar surfaces of the hands and feet causing reddening, soreness and blistering) is considerably higher.

Arabinosides (cytosine arabinoside, gemcitabine) and the *purine antagonists* (deoxycoformycin, fludarabine, 2-chloroadenisine) azathioprine, mercaptopurine and tioguanine are also converted intracellularly to active metabolites that inhibit DNA synthesis.

Antimetabolites find extensive use in anticancer therapy, either alone or in combination with other drugs. They remain the mainstay of treatment for haematological as well as common solid tumours such as breast and gastrointestinal tract cancers.

Anthracyclines and related compounds

The original anthracyclines were antibiotics pro-

503

duced by microorganisms such as *Streptomycetes* spp. Daunorubicin and doxorubicin were the first compounds to be isolated and appear to interfere with both DNA and RNA synthesis. Other examples include bleomycin, dactinomycin, epirubicin, mitoxantrone, idarubicin, plicamycin (mithramycin), mitomycin and streptozotocin (most often used to treat the rare islet-cell pancreatic tumours).

Topoisomerase inhibitors

These inhibit enzymes essential for spatial conformation ('unwinding') prior to DNA replication. The epipodophyllotoxins (etoposide, teniposide) are major inhibitors of topoisomerase II. Topotecan and irinotecan selectively inhibit topoisomerase I and are effective in relapsed ovarian and colorectal cancer respectively. Bone marrow depression is dose limiting as, in the case of irinotecan, is delayed diarrhoea (which relates to a specific polymorphism in a drug metabolising gene). Administration of irinotecan is often complicated by an acute cholinergic reaction, reversible by prophylactic subcutaneous atropine. Doxorubicin is a non-specific inhibitor of topoisomerase I and II.

Spindle poisons

The plant alkaloids (vincristine, vinblastine, vindesine and vinorelbine) and taxoids (paclitaxel, docetaxel) inhibit microtubule assembly and cause cell cycle arrest in mitosis. They particularly cause bone marrow depression and alopecia. Vincristine causes neuropathy.

Platinum drugs

This family of drugs (which include cisplatin, carboplatin and oxaliplatin) act by cross-linking DNA in a similar manner to alkylating agents. The parent drug, cisplatin, is associated with a variety of adverse effects, including severe emesis, nephrotoxicity and ototoxicity. Renal damage is ameliorated by carefully pre-hydrating patients, and emetogenicity is effectively controlled with $5HT_3$ receptor (serotonin) antagonists. Second- (carboplatin) and third- (oxaliplatin; no nephrotoxicity) generation platinum agents have improved toxicity profiles, by small alterations to the basic molecular structure, and offer effective treatment for germ cell, ovarian and colorectal cancers.

Miscellaneous agents

Asparaginase starves tumour cells dependent upon a supply of the amino acid, asparagine (except those able to synthesise it for themselves); its use is largely confined to acute lymphoblastic leukaemia.

Adverse effects of cytotoxic chemotherapy

Principal adverse effects are manifest as, or follow damage to, the following:

Nausea and vomiting may occur within hours of treatment or be delayed, and last for several days, depending on the agent. As emetogenicity is largely predictable, preventive action can be taken. The most effective drugs are competitive antagonists of serotonin (5-hydroxytryptamine type 3, $5HT_3$) receptors, e.g. ondansetron, and corticosteroids such as dexamethasone, which benefit by unknown, multifactorial mechanisms. Other effective antiemetics include domperidone, metoclopramide, cyclizine and prochlorperazine. Combinations of drugs are frequently used and routes of administration selected as commonsense counsels, e.g. prophylaxis may be oral, but when vomiting occurs the parenteral route and suppositories are available.

Suppression of bone marrow and the lymphoreticular system

Myelosuppression with depression of both antibody- and cell-mediated immunity is the single most important dose-limiting factor with cytotoxic agents, and carries life-threatening consequences. Repeated blood monitoring is essential and transfusion of red cells and platelets may be necessary. Cell growth factors, e.g. the natural granulocyte colony-stimulating factor (filgrastim), are available to protect against or to resolve severe neutropenia.

Opportunistic infection by Gram-negative bacteria from the patient's own flora, e.g. from the gut that has been damaged by chemotherapy, may occur. Infections with virus (herpes zoster), fungus (candida) and protozoa (pneumocystis) are also increased. Fever in a patient receiving chemotherapy usually requires immediate hospitalisation, collection of samples for microbiological studies and urgent empirical initiation of antibiotic treatment. Where risk of neutropenia is high, antimicrobial prophylaxis may be used. High-dose chemoradiotherapy and allogeneic bone marrow transplant produce profound immunosuppression with significant risk of opportunistic infection and third-party graft-versus-host disease following unirradiated blood transfusion. Live vaccines are *contraindicated* in these patients.

Diarrhoea and mouth ulcers usually arise from drug damage to gut epithelium and other mucosal surfaces with a naturally rapid cell turnover.

Alopecia is due to an effect on the hair bulb but is not invariable; it recovers 2–6 months after ceasing treatment. Scalp cooling may prevent or limit this with certain drugs, e.g. vinca alkaloids.

Urate nephropathy is due to rapid destruction of malignant cells releasing purines and pyrimidines, which are metabolised to uric acid that may crystallise in and block the renal tubule (urate nephropathy). In practice this occurs only when there is a large cell mass or a tumour is very sensitive to drugs, e.g. acute leukaemias and high-grade lymphomas. High fluid intake, alkalinisation of the urine and use of allopurinol or rasburicas during the early stages of chemotherapy avert this outcome.

Local extravasation may damage surrounding tissues; it is a problem with certain vesicant cytotoxics, e.g. doxorubicin, dacarbazine. This is a medical emergency and policies for management (which may include debridement by a plastic surgeon) should be in place in every centre.

Hypersensitivity reactions may occur with susceptible patients. These are more problematic with certain cytotoxic agents, e.g. paclitaxel, carboplatin and the newer hybrid targeted monoclonal antibodies, for which prophylactic corticosteroid and antihistamine are offered routinely.

Specific organ damage may result, e.g. lung toxicity with bleomycin, cardiotoxicity with anthracyclines, nephrotoxicity with platinum agents.

Delayed wound healing can be expected. Surgical wounds should be healed prior to commencing chemotherapy, wherever possible.

Germ cells and reproduction deserve special attention as chemotherapy may cause infertility. In addition, the theoretical mutagenic effects of cytotoxic drugs mean that reproduction is to be avoided during and for several months after therapy (although both men and women have reproduced normally while undergoing chemotherapy). When treatment may cause permanent sterility, men are offered the facility for prior storage of sperm. Cryopreservation of ovarian tissue is now also feasible. Prior contraceptive advice is necessary, as most cytotoxic drugs are teratogenic and are contraindicated during pregnancy.

Carcinogenicity may result in delayed second malignancies, a potentially serious issue where treatment improves life expectancy. Many cytotoxic drugs are themselves carcinogenic, and a patient may be cured of the primary disease only to succumb to a second, treatment-induced, cancer 5–20 years later. Examples include patients with Hodgkin's lymphoma who are often young with high cure rates. Whether this is due to a mutagenic effect, to chronic immunosuppression, or to both, remains unclear. Alkylating agents and radiotherapy are particularly incriminated, as are some antimetabolites (mercaptopurine) and anthracyclines (doxorubicin). The relative risk can be as high as 10 to 20 times the normal risk. The second cancers caused include leukaemia, lymphoma and squamous carcinoma.

CHEMOTHERAPY IN CLINICAL PRACTICE

Drug use and tumour cell kinetics

Evidence from leukaemia in laboratory animals shows that:

- Survival time is inversely related to the initial number of leukaemia cells, or to the number remaining after treatment.

- A single leukaemia cell is capable of multiplying and eventually killing the host.

Cytotoxic drugs act against all multiplying cells. Bone marrow, mucosal surfaces (gut), hair follicles, reticuloendothelial system and germ cells all divide more rapidly than many cancer cells and are damaged by cytotoxic drugs, leading to the particular adverse effects of chemotherapy. In contrast to haematological cancers, most solid tumours in humans divide slowly and recovery from cytotoxic agents is slow, whereas normal marrow and gut recover rapidly. This speed of recovery of normal tissues is exploited in devising intermittent courses of chemotherapy.

In cancer, the normal feedback mechanisms that mediate cell growth are defective and cell proliferation continues unchecked, cancer cells multiplying, at first exponentially. Cancers with high growth fractions, e.g. acute leukaemias, high-grade lymphomas, may visibly enlarge at an alarming rate, but are frequently highly sensitive to cytotoxic chemotherapy. In later stages, the growth rate of these cancers often slows and the volume-doubling time lengthens due to several factors, most of which conspire to render the advanced cancer less susceptible to drugs, namely:

- Increased cell cycle (division) time.
- Decrease in the number of cells actively dividing, with more in the resting state (decrease in growth fraction), but with the potential to switch back to a fast growth state.
- Increased cell death within the tumour as it ages.
- Overcrowding of cells leading to necrotic, avascular and hypoxic areas that cannot easily be penetrated by drugs. These are fertile areas for clonal selection of the most robust cancer cells.

Selectivity of drugs for cancer cells is generally low compared with the selectivity shown by antimicrobial agents but it can be substantial, e.g. in lymphoma, where tumour cell kill with some drugs is 10 000 times greater than that of marrow cells. Cell destruction by cytotoxic drugs follows first-order kinetics, i.e. a given dose of drug kills a constant *fraction* of cells (not a constant *number*) regardless of the number of cells present. Thus a treatment that reduces a cell population from 1 000 000 to 10 000 (a two-log cell kill) will reduce a cell population of 1000 to 10. Furthermore, cell chemosensitivity within a cancer is not homogeneous owing to random mutations (clonal selection) as the tumour grows, the cells remaining after initial doses being more likely to resist further treatment. Therefore, combining several drugs may be more effective than a single agent given repeatedly to the limit of tolerance.

The selection of drugs in combination chemotherapy is influenced by:

- Choosing drugs that act at different biochemical sites in the cell.
- Using drugs that attack cells at different phases of the growth cycle (Fig. 23.1). 'CHOP' (cyclophosphamide, doxorubicin (previously known as hydroxydoxorubicin) vincristine (previously called oncovin) and prednisolone), is a standard combination chemotherapy regimen for non-Hodgkin's lymphoma. The first three cytotoxic drugs exert their antitumour effect on different aspects of cell proliferation. The antitumour effect of corticosteroid remains unclear.
- The desirability of attaining synchronisation of cell cycling to achieve maximum cell kill. Cells are killed or are arrested in mitosis by vincristine, which is then withdrawn. Cells then enter a new reproductive cycle more or less synchronously, and when most are judged to be in a phase sensitive to a particular phase-specific drug, e.g. methotrexate or cytarabine, it is given.
- Avoidance of cross-resistance between drugs. In some instances, use of one drug regimen *followed* by another rather than using them simultaneously in combination avoids drug resistance and improves therapeutic efficacy. For example, epirubicin given for four cycles followed by CMF (concomitant cyclophosphamide, methotrexate and 5-fluorouracil) for four cycles has largely replaced CMF alone as standard adjuvant chemotherapy for breast cancer, because the outcome is better.
- Non-overlapping toxicity profiles. Before establishing a combination regimen, Phase 1 trials are undertaken, frequently fixing the dose of one

drug while escalating the dose of another, in small cohorts of carefully monitored patients, so that toxicity and patient safety can be monitored.

- Empirical evidence of efficacy against a particular tumour type. The antitumour activity of platinum complexes was a chance finding.
- Enhanced cell killing in preclinical models when drugs are combined. Oxaliplatin on its own has limited cytotoxicity against colorectal cancer cell lines in vitro and in mouse xenograft models, but its combination with 5FU confers a more than additive, i.e. synergistic, killing effect on tumour cells.

Considerations of pharmacokinetics in relation to cell kinetics are of great importance, as drug treatment alters the behaviour of both malignant and normal cells.

Drug resistance

Resistance to a cytotoxic chemotherapy agent may be present at the outset (primary resistance), or may develop with repeated drug exposure (acquired resistance). Increasing dosage is limited by toxicity, e.g. to bone marrow, which does not become tolerant. Combination chemotherapy is a strategy commonly used to address the problems of tumour resistance.

Multiple drug resistance (MDR) of a cancer is not uncommon. MDR is most frequently due to increased expression of an ATP-dependent membrane efflux pump called P-glycoprotein (Pgp), which is a member of a class of membrane proteins called the ATP-binding cassette superfamily. Pgp is an important protective mechanism possessed by many normal cells against environmental toxins and has broad specificity for hydrophobic compounds. Long-lived cells such as the haemopoietic stem cell, cells on excretory surfaces such as biliary hepatocytes, proximal renal tubule and intestinal cells, and the cells of the blood–brain barrier all have high expression of Pgp. A number of agents including immunosuppressants (ciclosporin) and calcium channel blockers (verapamil and nifedipine) block Pgp in theory.

The MDR phenomenon illustrates how tumour cells adapt and enhance normal cell mechanisms

to deal with the effects of chemotherapy, and how repeated cycles of chemotherapy select out a population of cells that have developed adaptive survival mechanisms, e.g. in myeloma where MDR proteins are rare at diagnosis but common at progression.

In those tumours for which cures can be achieved by chemotherapy (childhood acute lymphoblastic leukaemia,, Hodgkin's lymphoma, choriocarcinoma) it is essential that optimal doses of initial chemotherapy be administered and dose intensity maintained in order to avoid the emergence of chemoresistance.

Improving efficacy of chemotherapy

Methods that potentially widen the narrow therapeutic index of cytotoxic agents include:

- Regional (as opposed to systemic) administration of drugs: intrathecal, intra-arterial into liver and isolated limb perfusion.
- Selective organ delivery of drug by altered formulation e.g. Caelyx is a formulation comprising high concentrations of doxorubicin encased in liposomes. This also alters toxicity profiles (e.g. less renal but more mucosal toxicity).
- High-dose (bone marrow ablative) chemotherapy is feasible by harvesting stem cells prior to drug exposure, and returning the cells to the patient on completion of treatment. This is a successful strategy in haematological malignancies but failed trials in almost all solid tumours.
- Circadian rhythms exist in cell metabolism and proliferation, and those of leukaemic cells differ from normal leucocytes. The time of day at which therapy is administered can theoretically influence the outcome (chronomodulation).
- In large solid tumours, the fraction of cells multiplying rapidly is often relatively small. In ovarian cancer, for example, patients benefit from debulking surgery (cytoreduction) prior to cytotoxic drug therapy.

Interactions of anticancer agents with other drugs

The diverse modes of action of cytotoxic drugs offer ample scope for serious *unwanted drug–drug interac-*

tions, and by different mechanisms. There is general cause for alertness. Drugs that inhibit enzymes and thus delay normal metabolic breakdown may cause harmful reactions to standard doses of cytotoxics, e.g. allopurinol (xanthine oxidase inhibitor) with mercaptopurine or cyclophosphamide. Enzyme-inducing drugs can reduce the therapeutic efficacy of anticancer drugs by accelerating metabolism. Competition with non-steroidal anti-inflammatory drugs (NSAIDs) reduces the renal tubular excretion of methotrexate, leading to methotrexate toxicity. A combination of cytotoxics causing a dangerous degree of immunosuppression represents an adverse pharmacodynamic reaction.

Therapeutic drug–drug interactions are an essential part of treatment, as witnessed by the many drug combinations used to treat cancer.

ENDOCRINE THERAPY

The growth of some cancers is hormone dependent and is inhibited by surgical removal of gonads, adrenals and/or pituitary. The same effect is achievable, at less cost to the patient, by administering hormones, or hormone antagonists, of oestrogens, androgens or progestogens and inhibitors of hormone synthesis.

Breast cancer cells may have receptors for oestrogen, progesterone and androgen, and hormonal manipulation benefits some 30% of patients with metastatic disease; when a patient's tumour is oestrogen-receptor positive the response is about 60%, and when negative it is only 10%. After treatment of the primary cancer, endocrine therapy with the *anti-oestrogen, tamoxifen,* is the adjuvant therapy of choice for postmenopausal women who have disease in the lymph nodes; both the interval before the development of metastases and overall survival are increased. Adjuvant therapy with cytotoxic drugs and/or tamoxifen is recommended for node-negative patients with large tumours or other adverse prognostic factors. Cytotoxic chemotherapy is more useful in younger women, with tamoxifen, increasingly, as adjuvant therapy. The optimal duration of dosing

with tamoxifen is not yet established, but is likely to be 5 years or more.

Aromatase inhibitors cause 'medical adrenalectomy' in postmenopausal women by blocking conversion of adrenal androgens to oestrogens in peripheral fat by the enzyme aromatase. The first drug in this class, *aminoglutethimide,* causes significant adverse effects. More selective and less toxic aromatase inhibitors now include *anastrozole, letrozole* and *exemestane,* and find use after treatment with tamoxifen fails. Clinical trial data suggest that these drugs rival tamoxifen in efficacy for both advanced and early breast cancer. *Progestogens,* e.g. *megestrol* or *medroxyprogesterone,* are third-line agents in postmenopausal women.

Prostatic cancer is androgen dependent and metastatic disease can be helped by *orchidectomy,* or by pituitary suppression of androgen secretion with a gonadorelin (LHRH) analogue, e.g. *buserelin, goserelin, leuprorelin* or *triptorelin.* These cause a transient stimulation of luteinising hormone and thus testosterone release, before inhibition occurs; some patients may experience exacerbation of tumour effects, e.g. bone pain, spinal cord compression. Where this can be anticipated, prior orchidectomy or *anti-androgen* treatment, e.g. with *cyproterone* or *flutamide,* is protective.

Benign prostatic hypertrophy is also androgen dependent, and drug therapy includes use of *finasteride,* an inhibitor of the enzyme (5α-reductase) that activates testosterone.

Adrenocortical steroids are used for their action on specific cancers and also to treat some of the complications of cancer, e.g. hypercalcaemia, raised intracranial pressure. In leukaemias, corticosteroid may reduce the incidence of complications, e.g. haemolytic anaemia and thrombocytopenia. A glucocorticoid is preferred, e.g. prednisolone, as doses are high, and the mineralocorticoid actions are not needed and cause fluid retention.

In general, endocrine therapy carries less acute serious consequences for normal tissues than do cytotoxic agents. In a sense, they represent the first generation of mechanism-driven targeted agents used to treat cancer. As cancer patients live longer, the chronic effects of hormonal therapies are becoming more evident, such as a higher incidence of endometrial cancer with chronic use of tamoxifen in a minority of patients and osteoporosis in breast and prostate cancer patients who have had anti-oestrogens and/or anti-androgens including gonadorelin (LHRH) analogues.

IMMUNOTHERAPY

Immunotherapy (immunostimulation) derives from an observation in the 19th century that cancer sometimes regressed after acute bacterial infections, i.e. in response to non-specific immunostimulant effect. In general, it appears that the immune response is attenuated in cancer. Strategies to stimulate the host's own immune system to kill cancer cells more effectively are:

- *Non-specific stimulation* of active immunity with vaccines, e.g. BCG (bacille Calmette–Guérin) instilled into the urinary bladder for bladder cancer. Other approaches involve the injection of tumour cells or tumour cell extracts combined with an immune stimulant such as BCG.
- *Specific immunisation strategies*, where tumour-specific and tumour-associated antigens have been identified. Melanomas, for example, possess melanoma differentiation antigens (tyrosinase, gp100, MART1) as well as tumour-associated antigens (MAGE, BAGE, GAGE series of major histocompatibility complex (MHC)-associated peptides and a family of lipoproteins known as gangliosides). Both DNA and whole-protein vaccines derived from these antigens are being evaluated in melanoma, but results to date have been clinically disappointing.

Naturally occurring substances are increasingly used to treat cancer. Cytokines are produced in response to various stimuli, such as antigens, e.g. viruses. These peptides regulate cell growth, activation and differentiation, and immune responses and can be synthesised by recombinant DNA technology. Examples include:

- *Interleukins* that stimulate proliferation of T lymphocytes and activate natural killer cells; interleukin-2 is used in metastatic renal cell carcinoma with marginal effectiveness.
- *Interferons*. Interferon-α is used for chronic granulocytic leukaemia, hairy cell leukaemia, renal cell carcinoma and Kaposi's sarcoma.

Thalidomide was withdrawn in the 1960s following evidence of its teratogenic effects, including some on fetal limb development. These very effects prompted the notion that suppression of cell proliferation might actually provide benefit. Investigation revealed that thalidomide possessed immunomodulatory properties, anti-inflammatory actions, direct effects on tumour cells and their microenvironment, and actions on angiogenesis. Thalidomide and analogues designed to reduce toxicity (immunomodulatory drugs: lenalidomide) have a therapeutic role in myeloma and are synergistic with dexamethasone and chemotherapeutic agents.

ATRA

All-trans-retinoic acid (ATRA) induces remission in newly diagnosed patients with promyelocytic leukaemia (APL), by leukaemic cell differentiation. APL is due to reciprocal translocation between chromosomes 15 and 17 producing a fusion gene PML–RARa. The fusion protein blocks differentiation but is overcome by ATRA. Subsequent administration of anthracycline improves cure rates.

DEVELOPMENT OF ANTICANCER DRUG THERAPY

In general, anticancer drugs develop from:
- *Chance discovery*: cisplatin. In the 1960s, scientists studying the effect of an electric current on bacteria cultured in a Petri dish noted that the cells stopped dividing, instead forming long filamentous structures. Further investigation revealed that the inhibitor of cell division was in fact an ion formed in solution from the platinum electrodes used in the experiment. The platinum complex, *cis*-diammine-dichloroplatinum (II),

later known as cisplatin, was isolated and subsequently developed for its potential to kill cancer cells. When given to patients with a variety of different types of cancer, germ cell tumours in particular were found to possess remarkable sensitivity to cisplatin treatment, and this drug remains in use for treating such patients today.

- *Analogues.* Severe vomiting, renal and nerve damage, and deafness limit the therapeutic efficacy of cisplatin. Carboplatin and oxaliplatin, second- and third-generation compounds derived from cisplatin, combine enhanced toxicity towards cancer cells with improved tolerance.

- *Mass screening programmes.*

- *Rational drug design.* Academic institutions and commercial biotechnology companies involved in experimental therapeutics study the cancer process to identify key ('target') genes or gene products that regulate aspects of carcinogenesis and then try to find ways of blocking the function of these targets. Unlike conventional cytotoxic chemotherapy, many of these agents are thus more cancer-cell selective and thus *cytostatic*. In other words, a targeted biological agent may prevent tumour growth or progression and delay recurrence, but may not induce rapid tumour shrinkage, hitherto the key conventional endpoint for evaluating cytotoxic drugs. Some examples follow to illustrate the opportunities created by this type of approach.

TARGETED BIOLOGICAL THERAPIES

Passive immunotherapy using monoclonal antibodies raised against specific tumour-associated antigens on the cell surface

Targeted antibodies have the advantage of high cancer specificity and relatively low host toxicity.

- *Rituximab,* an anti-CD20 monoclonal antibody, for the treatment of low-grade follicular lymphomas and for use in combination with CHOP for high-grade lymphoma, as these tumours carry the antigen CD20 on the cell surface.

- Significant over-expression of the Her2/neu (erbB2) cell surface growth factor receptor occurs in approximately 20% of breast cancers and gastric cancers and is associated with a far more aggressive form of breast cancer compared with non-Her2-expressing tumours. *Trastuzumab* (Herceptin), a humanised monocolonal antibody, binds specifically to the Her2/neu receptor, blocking its function in regulating intracellular processes, including cell proliferation. In combination with conventional cytotoxic chemotherapy, trastuzumab significantly improves the survival of patients with advanced or early breast cancer, compared with cytotoxic chemotherapy alone. A series of key adjuvant trials conducted across Europe and the USA showed that trastuzumab combined with chemotherapy provided the biggest survival gains ever recorded for this disease. Potential cumulative cardiac dysfunction with trastuzumab is dose limiting.

- Her2 is a member of the epidermal growth factor receptor (EGFR) family. EGFRs are highly expressed by about 85% of colorectal cancers and are important in regulating cell proliferation. Another monoclonal antibody, *cetuximab* (Erbitux), blocks EGFR function and is used for selected colorectal cancers. It was subsequently found that this drug had no benefit in approximately 40% of all colorectal cancers with a mutation in the *K-RAS* oncogene. The mutation constitutively activates the cell pathway downstream of the EGFR receptor, so blocking it with cetuximab has no effect. This is an important example of personalising medicine to the individual cancer type and selecting which agents are suitable in individual cancers. It is also crucial in the design and selection of patients for future evolutions of this therapy in colorectal cancer, as patients with *K-RAS* mutations would only get the unwanted effects and absolutely no benefit if treated with EGFR inhibitors. Limiting toxicities for this class of drugs are fatigue, rash, mucositis and hypomagnesaemia.

- *Vasculoendothelial growth factor* (VEGF) is a major angiogenic signal regulator for new blood vessel formation (angiogenesis). Angiogenesis, a process that is common to all cancers, is vital for the growth and establishment of secondary tumours to grow beyond 1–2 mm when diffusion of nutrients becomes insufficient to maintain tumour growth. Blockade of VEGF and its receptor is a successful strategy for treating several types of neoplasm. The monoclonal antibody *bevacizumab* (Avastin) improves survival or slows tumour growth significantly, when combined with cytotoxic chemotherapy for advanced colorectal, lung and breast cancers. This novel approach evokes a range of adverse drug reactions that differ from those of conventional cytotoxics: hypertension, proteinuria, bleeding, and increased risk of thromboembolic events.

Similar drugs that block effects of VEGF are now used to treat neovascular age-related wet macular degeneration, a condition that causes loss of central vision in 2.3% of people > 65 years.

Radioimmunotherapy

Monoclonal antibodies targeted against epitopes on tumour cells, e.g. rituximab against CD20 in lymphoma, are conjugated to radionuclides such as yttrium-90 (ibritumomab) or iodine-131 (tositumomab) to deliver radiation directly to the cellular target; they produce durable responses in patients resistant to chemotherapy and unconjugated antibody.

Chemo-immunotherapy

Monoclonal antibodies conjugated to toxins deliver high concentrations of agents that are too toxic to give systemically, e.g. CD33 plus calicheamicin (Gemtuzumab ozogamicin) in AML.

Most therapeutic antibodies are monoclonal immunoglobulin (Ig) G antibodies produced in mammalian cell lines by recombinant DNA technology. Genetic engineering alters the molecular structure of key immunogenic portions of the antibody to generate 'humanised' chimeric antibodies that avoid rejection by the human immune system (but hypersensitivity reactions may occur).

Signal transduction inhibitors

Tyrosine kinase activation of cell surface receptors and their downstream proteins is an important mechanism by which messages are translated to the nucleus to affect cell function. A family of small molecules called *tyrosine kinase inhibitors* (TKIs) is now showing significant promise as anticancer agents. These small molecules are often orally administered. Multitargeted kinase inhibitors are also attractive, as they may possess a wide spectrum of antitumour activity, but their potential for toxicity is a real concern.

- Imatinib (Glivec, Gleevec) blocks the dysregulated tyrosine kinase hyperactivity produced by the Philadelphia chromosome (bcr-abl) that occurs in chronic myeloid leukaemia and some cases of acute lymphoblastic leukaemia; clinical trials support its therapeutic efficacy. This is an important example of a drug designed precisely to address the biological abnormality that causes a disease. By serendipity, ii imatinib also blocks an oncogenelled c-kit (CD-117) and has now revolutionised treatment of a rare cancer called GIST (gastrointestinal stromal tumour) that hitherto had no known systemic treatment options (both chemo- and radiotherapy primary resistant), and frequently carries a c-kit mutation.

- Tyrosine kinase inhibitors of VEGF receptor and its downstream effector pathways are also in clinical trial (Fig. 23.2).

- The EGFR tyrosine kinase inhibitors, gefitinib (Iressa) and erlotinib (Tarceva), now find use for a variety of EGFR-expressing tumours, specifically in lung cancer, that have a mutation in the EGFR gene, with marked benefit, although cure remains elusive.

Targeting the cell cycle

Recent advances in molecular biology have shown that the cell cycle is regulated by a series of proteins that include *cyclins, cyclin-dependent kinases* and *cyclin-dependent kinase inhibitors* (Fig. 23.3). Aberra-

Fig.23.2 Many new drugs target the vasculoendothelial growth factor (VEGF) pathway.

tions in these proteins are implicated in uncontrolled progression through the cell cycle (and hence in carcinogenesis), but also represent a new set of therapeutic targets for anticancer therapy, e.g. flavopiridol, which has cyclin-dependent kinase inhibitor activity, and rapamycin, which inhibits mTOR (mammalian target of rapamycin), another key regulator of cell cycle progression. Arsenic trioxide modulates cell growth and differentiation, and induces remission in relapsed refractory acute promyelocytic leukaemia in part through apoptosis induction and down-regulation of *Bcl-2*.

Protease inhibition

The ubiquitin–proteasome pathway is an intracellular proteolytic system that degrades cyclins and

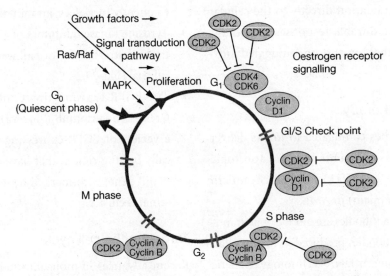

Fig. 23.3 The cell cycle is regulated by a series of proteins called cyclins, cyclin-dependent kinases (CDKs) and cyclin-dependent kinase inhibitors (CDKIs). Many CDKIs appear to be tumour-suppressing genes. These moieties are potential targets for anticancer therapy. MAPK, mitogen-activated protein kinase.

cyclin-dependent kinase inhibitors which regulate cell cycle progression. Bortezomib inhibits proteasome activity and, in myeloma, prevents degradation of nuclear factor κB inhibitor (IκB), resulting in a directly apoptotic effect, antiangiogenesis and inhibition of myeloma–stromal cell interaction. It has single-agent activity and restores chemosensitivity in resistant cells.

CHEMOPREVENTION OF CANCER

Because many cancers are currently incurable once metastasised, cancer prevention is a logical objective. Individuals can change aspects of their lifestyle significantly to influence their risk of developing particular cancers. Ceasing to smoke tobacco is an obvious health benefit. The individual benefits attributable to other changes are more difficult to quantify. The connection between environment and cancer risk is complex and as yet poorly understood, as genetic susceptibilities may obviate or accentuate certain risks.

Chemical interventions to reduce cancer risk may be an option for the population as a whole, or for groups at high risk of a specific cancer. Retrospective epidemiological and association studies suggest large effects of certain dietary manipulation but prospective interventional studies have rarely been confirmatory and have even shown harm. The best example is supplemental vitamins, derivatives and dietary micronutrients that may inhibit the development of cancers in the laboratory, e.g. β-carotene, isotretinoin, folic acid, ascorbic acid, α-tocopherol. In a trial of antioxidant supplementation with ascorbic acid, vitamin E, β-carotene, selenium and zinc over 7.5 years, the total cancer incidence was lower in men (who had a lower baseline antioxidant status) than in women. Subsequent large-scale randomised trials with supplementation have demonstrated the opposite effect with an unexpectedly higher incidence of new cancers.

The anti-oestrogen tamoxifen, used as an adjuvant therapy in women undergoing surgery for primary breast cancer, reduced the risk of cancer occurring in the contralateral breast. Tamoxifen and anastrozole (see above) are undergoing assessment for chemoprevention in women at high risk of breast cancer.

VIRAL IMMUNISATION AND CANCER PREVENTION

In cancers thought to have predominantly viral origins such as cervical cancer (HPV, human papilloma virus) and liver cancer (HCC, hepatocellular cancer) triggered by chronic hepatitis, vaccination against the viruses may have dramatic effects on the incidence of the cancers. The best example of this is HBV vaccination in childhood in Taiwan where the incidence of HCC in children and adolescents fell over 200-fold. More recently HPV vaccinations (such as Gardasil) have been approved, but as HPV is predominantly sexually transmitted, vaccinating pre-pubescent girls and boys (to generate herd immunity) is ethically challenging and may lead to poor uptake and cultural variations of acceptance worldwide.

SUMMARY

Systemic chemotherapy offers prolongation of life and improvements in quality of life for cancer patients. Anti-cancer drugs including cytotoxic agents, hormonal agents, immune stimulants and targeted agents, can be used as curable therapy, adjuvant therapy and palliative therapy according to different strategies. Cytotoxic chemotherapy agents remain the mainstay of systemic anticancer treatment, as an understanding of their pharmacology has enabled clinicians to exploit the benefits of these drugs. Considerations of tumor cell kinetics are of great importance, as cytotoxics treatment alters the behaviour of both malignant and normal cells. Endocrine therapy, such as hormones, or hormone antagonists, of oestrogens, androgens or progestogens and inhibitors of hormone synthesis, can inhibit the growth of some cancers which is hormone dependent. They carries less acute serious consequences for normal tissues than do cytotoxic agents. However, the chronic effects of hormonal therapies are becoming more evident as cancer patients live longer. Non-specific stimulation of active immunity with vaccines along with specific immunization of tumour-specific and tumour-associated antigens are more effectively to kill cancer cells. Also naturally occurring substances are increasingly used to treat cancer. Cytokines are produced in response to various stimuli, such as antigens, e.g. viruses. As anticancer drugs develop, the very real limitations of cytotoxic chemotherapy have forced a concentration of cancer research on trying to understand the carcinogenic process, the aim being to identify specific molecular targets that can be exploited to develop novel therapeutic approaches. So-called targeted therapies are now well-established groups of anticancer drugs. A targeted biological agent may prevent tumour growth or progression and delay recurrence, but may not induce rapid tumour shrinkage, hitherto the key conventional endpoint for evaluating cytotoxic drugs. Targeted antibodies have the advantage of high cancer specificity and relatively low host toxicity. Monoclonal antibodies have been applied in radioimmuno therapy and chemo-immunotherapy. Other approaches are signal transduction inhibition, targeting the cell cycle and protease inhibition. Chemical interventions to reduce cancer risk may be an option for the population as a whole, or for groups at high risk of a specific cancer. In cancers thought to have predominantly viral origins such as cervical cancer (HPV, human papilloma virus) and liver cancer (HCC, hepatocellular cancer) triggered by chronic hepatitis, vaccination against the viruses may have dramatic effects on the incidence of the cancers.

IMPORTANT TERMINOLOGY

adjuvant therapy　辅助性化疗

neoadjuvant therapy　新辅助化疗

palliative therapy　姑息性化疗

cytotoxic chemotherapy　细胞毒化疗

alkylating agents　烷化剂

antimetabolites　抗代谢药

pyrimidine antagonists　嘧啶拮抗剂

purine antagonists　嘌呤拮抗剂

topoisomerase inhibitors　拓扑异构酶抑制剂

spindle poisons　纺锤体抑制剂

synchronisation of cell cycling　细胞周期同步化

multiple drug resistance (MDR)　多药耐药

P-glycoprotein　P糖蛋白

circadian rhythms　生物周期节律

endocrine therapy　内分泌治疗

anti-oestrogen　抗雌激素

aromatase inhibitors　芳香化酶抑制剂

targeted biological therapy　靶向生物治疗

passive immunotherapy　被动免疫治疗

radio immunotherapy　放射免疫治疗

chemo-immunotherapy　化学免疫治疗

signal transduction inhibitors　信号转导治疗

targeting the cell cycle　靶向细胞周期

CHALLENGE YOURSELF

1. As characterised by high proliferative rate, non-Hodgkin's lymphoma is usually treated with 'CHOP' regimen. Please explain why clinicians choose these cytotoxic drugs and design an optimal administration strategy based on different phases of cell growth cycle these drugs attack.

2. Find some methods to avoid the emergence of chemo-resistance.

3. Take some novel molecular targeted drugs of current clinical use for example, what else to concern about except their potential toxicity?

Jianhua Xu

Chapter | 24 |

Anti-inflammatory immunity drugs

INTRODUCTION

The immune system is a complex of interrelated genetic, molecular and cellular components that provides defence against invading microorganisms and aberrant native cells, and repairs tissues once the pathogen is eradicated. The central process by which these are achieved is inflammation: the sequence of events by which a pathogen is detected, cells of the immune system are recruited, the pathogen is eliminated and resulting tissue damage repaired.

Inflammation is appropriate as a response to physical damage, microbial infection or malignancy. A number of illnesses result from abnormal activation or prolongation of the immune response. These include allergy (hay fever, asthma), autoimmunity (rheumatoid arthritis (RA), systemic lupus erythematosus (SLE)), and allograft rejection.

Anti-inflammatory drugs, by acting on and modifying the response of the innate immune system to a challenge, are useful in many settings to damp down an over-exuberant or pathologically prolonged inflammatory response. Immunomodulatory agents, which act on components of the adaptive immune response, are important for the treatment of complex autoimmune diseases and in preventing allograft rejection. Many drugs used in the treatment of these diseases have complex mechanisms of action, working on multiple arms of the immune response, and in some cases the principal way in which they exert their effects is not clear. Partly this is due to the com-

plexity of the immune system itself; many components have overlapping functions, leading to redundancy, and many have several apparently unrelated actions.

Research over the last few decades has vastly improved our appreciation of the complexity of the immune system and of the pathogenesis of many autoimmune diseases. Although there does not appear to be one single factor that leads inexorably to the development or perpetuation of any inflammatory disease, certain mediators that play central roles in specific diseases have been identified. The advent of monoclonal antibodies, fusion proteins and other new drug development technology has allowed the manufacture of a rapidly expanding group of new agents ('biologicals') that target specific components of the immune response thought to be driving particular diseases. These drugs have dramatically changed treatment paradigms, and hopefully will lead to significant improvements in the future outlook for patients suffering rheumatic disease.

INFLAMMATION

The process of acute inflammation is initiated when resident tissue leucocytes (macrophages or mast cells) detect a challenge, for example pathogenic bacteria, or monosodium urate crystals in the case of gout. This sets off a cascade of intracellular signalling that results in activation of the cell, release of soluble cytokines such as tumour necrosis factor-α (TNFα), interleukin-1 (IL-1) and interleukin-6 (IL-6) and other mediators such as histamine and prostaglandins. IL-1, IL-6 and TNFα stimulate endothelial cells at the site of injury to express cellular adhesion molecules, which attract and bind circulating leucocytes, principally neutrophils, and induce them to leave the circulation and migrate into the affected area. They also have systemic effects such as the development of fever and the production of acute phase proteins including C-reactive protein (CRP).

Neutrophils, along with macrophages, phagocytose the injurious stimulus and destroy it. Neutrophils and macrophages may also cause damage to the surrounding host tissue through the release of digesting enzymes such as matrix metalloproteinases and collagenases. The inflammatory process therefore needs to be halted rapidly once the invading organism has been cleared. This occurs partly because neutrophils have a very short lifespan and die quickly once they have left the circulation, and partly through the release of anti-inflammatory mediators.

Several drugs in current use act on the various stages of this inflammatory process. Antagonists of TNFα, IL-1 and IL-6 are available. Colchicine, used in the treatment of gout, interferes with neutrophil chemo-taxis, thus inhibiting their recruitment to the site of inflammation.

Many leucocytes, including mast cells and macrophages, as well as endothelial cells, synthesise pro-inflammatory eicosanoids and platelet-activating factor (PAF) (Fig. 24.1). These are 20-carbon unsaturated fatty acids derived from phospholipid substrates in the plasma membrane by the enzymes phospholipase A_2, cyclo-oxygenase (COX) and lipo-oxygenase (which are induced by IL-1). The prostaglandins, thromboxanes and leukotrienes have diverse pro-inflammatory roles. Leukotrienes promote the activation and accumulation of leucocytes at sites of inflammation. Prostaglandins induce vasodilatation of the microcirculation and are important in pain signalling from locally inflamed tissue. Platelet-activating factor and thromboxane A_2 affect the coagulation and fibrinolytic cascades.

Non-steroidal anti-inflammatory drugs (NSAIDs), including aspirin, inhibit COX and hence prostaglandin and thromboxane synthesis. Glucocorticoids act by inducing the synthesis of lipocortin-1, a polypeptide that inhibits phospholipase A_2, and thereby exert a broad anti-inflammatory effect. The leukotriene receptor antagonists montelukast and zafirlukast cause bronchodilatation and are used to treat asthma.

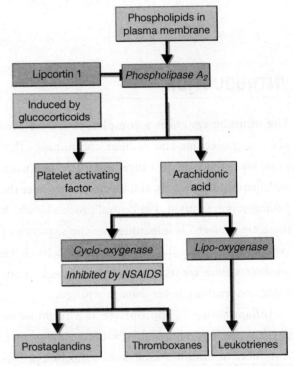

Fig. 24.1 Synthesis of eicosanoids and platelet-activating factor, and drugs acting on this pathway. The enzymes phospholipase A_2, cyclo-oxygenase and lipo-oxygenase are involved in the synthesis of prostaglandins, thromboxanes, leukotrienes and platelet-activating factor, all of which are derived from phospholipid substrates in plasma membranes. Glucocorticoids induce lipocortin 1, which inhibits phospholipase A_2. NSAIDs inhibit cyclo-oxygenases 1 and 2, preventing formation of prostaglandins and thromboxanes.

The adaptive immune response

The adaptive immune response, although integrated into the process of inflammation, becomes active at later stages. Its key properties are ① specificity: each B and T lympho-cyte recognises a single specific peptide sequence; and ② memory: when an invading pathogen has been recognised once, a small number of specific cells remain dormant within the lymph tissue for many years. If that pathogen is detected again, a very rapid response is mounted to eradicate it before the development of clinical symptoms.

An adaptive immune response is initiated when a helper T cell recognises a peptide antigen presented on the surface of an antigen-presenting cell (APC) and is activated (Fig. 24.2). The activated helper T cell is then able to activate other types of T cells and B cells. This results in the proliferation of adaptive cellular effectors, the generation and release of antibodies by plasma cells and the production of a range of cytokines by the participating leucocytes. On occasion, amplification loops may become self-perpetuating, leading to chronic autoimmune disease.

Many immunomodulatory drugs, such as the calcineurin inhibitors, seek to break these loops by inhibiting lymphocyte proliferation. Other newer approaches target specific components of the immune system. For example, rituximab binds CD20, a cell surface molecule found only on B lymphocytes and not memory cells. It is used to treat diseases in which pathogenic autoantibody production is prominent,

such as rheumatoid arthritis and SLE. Abatacept blocks co-stimulatory signals, which are required when a helper T cell is activated, by recognising bound antigen presented by an APC. This is a central process in the pathogenesis of rheumatoid arthritis, and abatacept is licensed to treat this.

Non-steroidal anti-inflammatory drugs (NSAIDs)

NSAIDs are an extremely widely prescribed group of drugs that are mainly used for their analgesic effects. They possess a single common mode of action: inhibition of cyclooxygenase, thereby reducing prostaglandin synthesis. This is also the mode of action of paracetamol (acetaminophen) and aspirin.

Recently concern has arisen over the effect of traditional NSAIDs and COX-2 inhibitors on the cardiovascular system, with analysis of the VIGOR study showing that rofecoxib in particular increases the risk of myocardial infarction (rofecoxib has since been withdrawn from use). While they retain an important role in the treatment of acute gout,

Fig.24.2 Three general mechanisms of action of glucocorticoids and the glucocorticoid receptor in the inhibition of inflammation. TNFα, tumour necrosis factor α; HSP, heat-shock protein; mRNA, messenger RNA; P, phosphate. The three mechanisms are non-genomic activation, DNA-dependent regulation, and protein interference mechanisms (e.g. NF-KB elements). Black arrows denote activation, the red line inhibition, the red dashed arrow repression, and the red X lack of product (i.e. no mRNA).

inflammatory arthritis, ankylosing spondylitis and dysmenorrhea, long-term prescription should only be undertaken following a full discussion with the patient regarding the balance of risks and benefits.

Pharmacokinetics

NSAIDs are absorbed almost completely from the gastrointestinal tract, tend not to undergo first-pass elimination, are highly protein bound and have small volumes of distribution. Their $t_{1/2}$ values in plasma tend to group into short (1–5 h) or long (10–60 h). Differences in $t_{1/2}$ are not necessarily reflected proportionately in duration of effect, as peak and trough drug concentrations at their intended site of action following steady-state dosing are much less than those in plasma. The vast majority of NSAIDs are weak organic acids and localise preferentially in the synovial tissue of inflamed joints.

Mode of action

NSAIDs inhibit cyclo-oxygenase (COX), which catalyses the synthesis of prostaglandins and thromboxane from arachidonic acid (Fig. 24.1). There are two isoforms of COX:

- COX-1 is constitutively expressed in most cell types.
- COX-2 is induced when inflammatory cells (fibroblasts, endothelial cells and macrophages) are activated by cytokines such as IL-1β and TNFα. It is also often upregulated in cancer cells, and is constitutively expressed in the kidney and brain.

Both isoforms generate prostaglandins during an inflammatory response, while COX-1 activity is required for prostaglandin synthesis for tissue homeostasis. Thus, many NSAID adverse effects are due to reductions in beneficial prostaglandin production, for example in the gastric mucosa (PGI_2 and PGE_2) and renal medulla. Recognition of this led to the development of COX-2 selective drugs.

NSAIDs can be categorised according to their COX specificity as:

- COX-2-selective compounds (coxibs), which inhibit COX-2 with at least five times greater potency than COX-1. The group includes celecoxib, etori-

coxib, lumiracoxib, meloxicam and etodolac.
- Non-COX-2-selective compounds, which comprise all other NSAIDs. These drugs inhibit COX-1 as well as COX-2.

Uses

Analgesia. All NSAIDs are analgesics and are particularly effective for disorders with an inflammatory component, as the analgesic action is due to COX inhibition, both in the brain and at the site of inflammation. The non-selective and COX-2-selective agents have generally comparable analgesic efficacies.

Anti-inflammatory action. The majority of NSAIDs are anti-inflammatory because they inhibit COX in the periphery. COX inhibition in most chronic inflammatory conditions, while useful for symptomatic relief, does not modify the course of disease.

Antipyretic action. Paracetamol and all other NSAIDs reduce cytokine-induced prostaglandin synthesis in the hypothalamus, thus reducing fever.

Antiplatelet action. Aspirin irreversibly acetylates a serine residue in COX-1. In platelets the main result is inhibition of thromboxane A_2 (which promotes platelet adhesion, coagulation and vasoconstriction) production for the life of the platelet (7 days). This is the basis for the use of aspirin to prevent and treat arterial thromboses secondary to atherosclerosis and other predisposing illnesses such as the antiphospholipid syndrome.

Other non-selective NSAIDs bind reversibly to COX-1 and produce a variable antiplatelet action. Ibuprofen may block access of aspirin to the active site on platelets and interfere with its cardioprotective effect when taken regularly (but not intermittently, and aspirin taken 2 h before ibuprofen may avoid the problem). Other NSAIDs do not appear to have this interaction.

It has been suggested that inhibition of COX-2 reduces synthesis of endothelial PGI_2 (prostacyclin – which acts to prevent platelet aggregation and causes vasodilatation), while allowing the continued production of COX-1-derived thromboxane A_2. In theory this could alter the balance within the vasculature in favour of thromboxane A_2, and increase the risk of cardiovascular events, although the relative contributions of COX-1 and COX-2 in endothelial prostacyclin synthesis remain to be determined.

Colorectal cancer. Long-term administration of NSAID reduces the incidence of colonic cancer by approximately 50%. This appears to be related to the inhibition of COX-2, which is up-regulated in colon tumours.

Adverse effects

Gastrointestinal. Dyspepsia is one of the commonest side-effects of NSAIDs. The propensity to gastrointestinal (GI) ulceration may result in occult or overt blood loss. Use of NSAIDs is associated with an approximately four-fold increased incidence of severe gastrointestinal haemorrhage, and such complications account for between 700 and 2000 deaths in the UK each year. In addition, ulceration and stricture of the small intestine can result in anaemia, diarrhoea and malabsorption, similar to Crohn's disease. The risk of NSAID-induced GI haemorrhage is associated with high doses and prolonged use, age over 65 years, previous history of peptic ulceration, concomitant use of glucocorticoids, anticoagulants or other NSAIDs, heavy smoking and alcohol use, and the presence of Helicobacter pylori infection.

NSAID-associated gastrointestinal disease appears to result from the inhibition of COX–1–mediated production of cytoprotective mucosal prostaglandins, especially PGI_2 and PGE_2, which inhibit acid secretion in the stomach, promote mucus production and enhance mucosal perfusion. Several large randomised controlled trials have investigated the incidence of gastrointestinal adverse effects in traditional NSAIDs compared with coxibs. The VIGOR (rofecoxib versus naproxen), CLASS[2] (celecoxib versus ibuprofen and diclofenac) and TARGET (lumiracoxib versus ibuprofen and naproxen) studies all indicate that coxib use leads to an approximately 50% reduction of upper gastrointestinal adverse events.

The gastrointestinal toxicity of traditional NSAIDs may be reduced by co-prescription of a proton pump inhibitor, e.g. omeprazole, an H_2-receptor blocker, e.g. ranitidine, or the prostaglandin analogue misoprostol. Proton pump inhibitors are more effective than the other classes of gastro-protective agent and should be considered in all patients with at least one of the above risk factors. In fact, it is now recommended by the UK National Institute for Health and Clinical Effectiveness (NICE) that all patients over 45 years prescribed an NSAID, whether COX-2 selective or not, also receive a proton pump inhibitor.

Cardiovascular. The VIGOR and APPROVE trials reported increased thrombotic cardiovascular events in patients treated with rofecoxib, leading to concerns about a class effect of the coxibs. It was suggested that COX-2 selectivity resulted in an imbalance between prostacyclin and thromboxane production, an effect which would not be seen with traditional NSAIDs which inhibited the synthesis of both equally. Subsequent data from the prospective MEDAL and TARGET trials have not supported a class effect based on COX-2 selectivity. These studies suggest that treatment with either a coxib or an NSAID results in a small increase in cardiovascular risk. The risk is dose-related and rofecoxib, particularly at doses exceeding 50 mg per day, confers the highest cardiovascular risk in the majority of studies. A recent study of more than 1 million patients quantified cardiovascular risk as a composite of coronary death, non-fatal myocardial infarction and fatal and non-fatal stroke, and reported that diclofenac and rofecoxib were associated with the highest cardiovascular risk, while naproxen and perhaps celecoxib at doses 200 mg per day were the least likely to cause a cardiovascular event. NICE guidelines recommend that patients with pro-thrombotic risk, coronary artery or cerebrovascular disease should not be prescribed NSAIDs or a coxib. For other patients, treatment decisions should be made on an individual patient basis taking into account both cardiovascular and gastrointestinal risk factors. The medication should be prescribed for the shortest possible time and regularly reviewed.

Renal. NSAIDs decrease renal perfusion in individuals with congestive cardiac failure, chronic renal disease and cirrhosis with ascites: states in which renal perfusion are dependent upon prostaglandin-mediated vasodilatation. NSAIDs may also promote sodium and water retention, causing oedema and hypertension in some individuals. Papillary necrosis and interstitial nephritis are rare complications, often in the context of chronic and excessive NSAID use.

Worsening of asthma. NSAID intolerance in asthmatics probably reflects diversion of arachidonic acid metabolism towards excessive products of the lipo-oxygenase pathway. It is not immune-mediated but clinically may resemble hypersensitivity, with manifestations including vasomotor rhinitis, urticaria, bronchoconstriction, flushing, hypotension and shock.

Other unwanted effects include headache, confusion, photosensitivity, erythema multiforme, toxic epidermal necrolysis, deranged liver function, cytopenias, haemolytic anaemia and inhibition of ovulation.

Principal interactions

NSAID interactions include:

- Angiotensin-converting enzyme (ACE) inhibitors and angiotensin II receptor blockers: there is a risk of renal impairment and hyperkalaemia.
- Quinolone antimicrobials: convulsions may occur if NSAIDs are co-administered.
- Anticoagulant (warfarin) and antiplatelet agents (dypiridamole, clopidogrel): increase risk of gastrointestinal bleeding with NSAIDs.
- Antihypertensives: their effect is lessened due to sodium retention by inhibition of renal prostaglandin formation.
- Ciclosporin and tacrolimus: nephrotoxic effect is exacerbated by NSAIDs.
- Cytotoxics: renal tubular excretion of methotrexate is reduced by competition with NSAIDs, with risk of methotrexate toxicity (low-dose methotrexate given weekly avoids this hazard).
- Diuretics: NSAIDs cause sodium retention and reduce diuretic efficacy and there is a risk of hyperkalaemia with potassium-sparing diuretics.
- Lithium: NSAIDs delay the excretion of lithium by the kidney and may cause lithium toxicity.

Major NSAID

Aspirin (acetylsalicylic acid)

In the 18th century, the Reverend Edmund Stone wrote about the value of an extract of bark from the willow tree (of the family Salix) for alleviating pain and fever. The active ingredient was salicin, which is metabolised to salicylic acid in vivo. Sodium salicylate manufactured from salicin proved highly successful in the treatment of rheumatic fever and gout, but it was a gastric irritant. In 1897, Felix Hoffman, a chemist at the Bayer Company, whose father developed abdominal pain with sodium salicylate, succeeded in producing acetylsalicylic acid in a form that was chemically stable. The new preparation proved acceptable to his father and paved the way for the production of aspirin.

Pharmacokinetics. Aspirin ($t_{1/2}$ 15 min) is well absorbed from the stomach and upper GI tract. Hydrolysis removes the acetyl group, and the resulting salicylate ion is inactivated largely by conjugation with glycine. At low doses this reaction proceeds by first-order kinetics with a t½ of about 4 h, but at high doses and in overdose the process becomes saturated, i.e. kinetics become zero order, and most of the drug in the body is present as the salicylate. The challenge in overdose is to remove salicylate.

Mode of action. The anti-inflammatory, analgesic and antipyretic actions of aspirin are those of NSAIDs in general. The following additional actions are relevant:

- An antiplatelet effect due to permanent inactivation, by acetylation, of COX-1 in platelets, preventing synthesis of thromboxane A_2. Platelets cannot regenerate the enzyme and the resumption of thromboxane A_2 production is dependent on the entry of new platelets into the circulation (platelet lifespan is 7 days). Thus a continuous antiplatelet effect is achieved with low doses.
- Respiratory stimulation is a characteristic of aspirin intoxication and occurs both directly by stimulation of the respiratory centre and indirectly through increased carbon dioxide production.
- Although aspirin in high dose reduces renal tubular

reabsorption of uric acid so increasing its elimination, other treatments for hyperuricaemia are preferred. Indeed aspirin should be avoided in gout as low doses inhibit uric acid secretion and on balance its effects on uric acid elimination are adverse.

Dose. Doses of 100–200 mg/day are used to prevent thrombotic vascular occlusion; 300 mg as immediate treatment for myocardial infarction; 300–600 mg every 4–6 h for analgesia.

Uses. The main use of aspirin is as an antiplatelet agent to prevent arterial thrombotic events due to atherosclerosis. It has largely been overtaken by NSAIDs and paracetamol as an analgesic. In high doses it is used to treat inflammation in Kawasaki disease, in combination with intravenous immunoglobulin, but in other inflammatory illnesses it has now been superseded by other, more effective agents with fewer side-effects.

Adverse effects. Gastrointestinal effects are those of NSAIDs in general. Effects particularly associated with aspirin are:

- Salicylism (the symptoms of an excessive dose): tinnitus and hearing difficulty, dizziness, headache and confusion.
- Allergy. Aspirin is a common cause of allergic or pseudoallergic symptoms and signs. Patients exhibit severe rhinitis, urticaria, angioedema, asthma or shock. Those who already suffer from recurrent urticaria, nasal polyps or asthma are more susceptible.
- Reye's syndrome. Epidemiological evidence relates aspirin use to the development of the rare Reye's syndrome (encephalopathy, liver injury) in children recovering from febrile viral infections. Consequently, aspirin should not be given to children aged under 15 years.

Acute overdose. A moderate overdose (plasma salicylate acetylation 200–250 mg/L) will cause nausea, vomiting, epigastric discomfort, tinnitus, deafness, sweating, pyrexia, restlessness, tachypnoea and hypokalaemia. A large overdose (plasma salicylate concentration above 250 mg/L) may result in pulmonary oedema, convulsions and coma, with severe dehydration and ketosis. Bleeding is unusual, despite the anti-platelet effect of aspirin.

Adults who have taken a single large quantity usually develop a respiratory alkalosis. Metabolic acidosis suggests severe poisoning but a mixed picture is commonly seen. In children under 4 years, severe metabolic acidosis is more likely than respiratory alkalosis, especially if the drug has been ingested over many hours (e.g. mistaken for sweets).

Serial measurements of plasma salicylate are necessary to monitor the course of the overdose, for the concentration may rise in the early hours after ingestion. The general management of overdose applies, but the following are relevant for salicylate overdose:

- Activated charcoal 50 g by mouth prevents salicylate absorption from the GI tract. Gastric lavage or the use of an emetic is no longer recommended.
- Correction of dehydration, using dextrose 5% i.v. is often indicated.
- Acid–base disturbance. Alkalosis or mixed alkalosis/ acidosis need no specific treatment. Metabolic acidosis is treated with sodium bicarbonate, which alkalinises the urine and accelerates the removal of salicylate in the urine.
- Haemodialysis may be necessary if renal failure develops or the plasma salicylate concentration exceeds 900 mg/L.

Paracetamol (acetaminophen)

Pharmacokinetics. Paracetamol ($t_{1/2}$ 2 h) is well absorbed from the GI tract. It is inactivated in the liver, principally by conjugation as glucuronide and sulphate. Minor metabolites of paracetamol are also formed, of which one oxidation product, N-acetyl-p-benzoquinone imine (NAPQI), is highly reactive chemically. This substance is normally rendered harmless by conjugation with glutathione. The supply of hepatic glutathione is limited and, if the amount of NAPQI formed is greater than the amount of glutathione available, the excess metabolite oxidises thiol (SH-) groups on key enzymes, causing cell death. This is the mechanism of hepatic necrosis in paracetamol overdose.

Mode of action and uses. Paracetamol is an

effective treatment for mild-moderate pain and for relieving fever. It does not affect platelet function or disrupt the GI mucosal barrier. Paracetamol has analgesic efficacy equivalent to aspirin, but in therapeutic doses it has only weak anti-inflammatory effects, a functional separation that reflects its differential inhibition of enzymes responsible for prostaglandin synthesis. For this reason, some would not class paracetamol as an NSAID.

Dose. The oral dose is 0.3–0.6 g every 4–6 h; maximum daily dose 2 g.

Adverse effects. Paracetamol is usually well tolerated. Allergic reactions and rash sometimes occur. Maximal, long-term, daily dosing may predispose to chronic renal disease.

Acute overdose. Severe hepatocellular damage and renal tubular necrosis can result from taking 75 mg/kg body-weight (about 10 or 15 tablets) in one dose. Patients at particular risk include:

- Those whose enzymes are induced as a result of taking drugs or alcohol; their liver and kidneys form more NAPQI.
- Those who are malnourished (chronic alcohol abuse, eating disorders, HIV infection) to the extent that the liver and kidneys are depleted of glutathione to conjugate with NAPQI.

Clinical signs of hepatic damage (jaundice, abdominal pain, hepatic tenderness) and increased liver enzymes do not become apparent for 24–48 h after the overdose. Hepatic failure may ensue 2–7 days later; and is best monitored using prothrombin time.

The general principles for limiting drug absorption apply if the patient is seen within 4 h. Activated charcoal by mouth is effective and should be considered if paracetamol in excess of 75 mg/kg body-weight or 4 g, whichever is the smaller, is thought to have been ingested within the previous hour. The decision to use activated charcoal must take into account its capacity to bind the oral antidote methionine.

Specific therapy involves replenishing stores of liver glutathione, which conjugates NAPQI and so diminishes the amount available to do harm. Glutathione itself cannot be used as it penetrates cells poorly, but N-acetylcysteine (NAC) and methionine are effective as they are precursors for the synthesis of glutathione. NAC is administered intravenously – an advantage if the patient is vomiting. The earlier such therapy is instituted the better, and it should be started if:

- a patient is estimated to have taken more than 150 mg/kg body-weight, without waiting for the measurement of the plasma concentration
- plasma concentration indicates the likelihood of liver damage (above), or
- there is uncertainty about the amount taken, or its timing

Colchicine

Colchicine is derived from the autumn crocus (Colchicum autumnale). Its anti-inflammatory properties have long been recognised: Alexander of Tralles recommended colchicum for gout in the 6th century AD. Nowadays, in addition to relieving inflammation in acute gout attacks, it is used to treat other inflammatory disorders including Behcet's syndrome and the hereditary fever syndrome familial Mediterranean fever. The precise way in which colchicine reduces inflammation is not completely understood but relates to its effects on neutrophils (which play a prominent role in the pathology of these conditions). It inhibits the assembly of microtubules, thus interfering with mitotic spindle formation and arresting cell division as well as inhibiting cell migration.

The most common adverse effect of colchicine is diarrhoea, due to its effects on rapidly proliferating gastrointestinal epithelial cells. If this is ignored, severe neutropenia may follow and it is therefore a sign to stop the drug and restart at a lower dose. Agranulocytosis and aplastic anaemia may complicate chronic use.

Steroidal anti-inflammatory-immunity drugs (SAIIDs)

Glucocorticoids (GCs) are among the most widely prescribed anti-inflammatory drugs, due to their profound efficacy, long history of use and familiarity. Besides their anti-inflammatory actions they exert effects on carbohydrate, protein and lipid metabolism, some of which contribute to their substantial adverse effect profile.

GCs are used in acute and chronic settings to treat inflammatory conditions ranging from asthma and allergy, to prevention of allograft rejection, to rheumatoid arthritis and systemic vasculitis. Because of their rapid onset of action (less than 24 h) and potency, they remain the preferred acute treatment for severe inflammatory disease in a wide variety of settings despite their adverse effects. In chronic disease the aim now is to minimise cumulative exposure by using other immunomodulatory 'steroid-sparing' drugs, and proactively to manage potential long-term side-effects such as osteoporosis.

Mode of action

GCs, being lipophilic, diffuse across the cell membrane and bind the cytosolic glucocorticoid receptor (GR) (Fig. 24.3). Receptor polymorphisms influence the strength of the receptor interaction, and represent one source of variation in sensitivity to exogenous steroids. Once bound, the GC-GR complex translocates to the nucleus where it acts in at least two ways to alter gene transcription:

1. The GC-GR complex binds to the glucocorticoid response element within target gene promoters, increasing transcription of various anti-inflammatory genes. These include I-κB, which inhibits the activation of nuclear factor (NF)-κB, and the cytokines IL-4, IL-10, IL-13 and transforming growth factor (TGF) β, which have immunosuppressive and anti-inflammatory activity.

2. The GC-GR complex interferes with the binding of the transcription factors activating protein (AP)-1 and NF-κB to their response elements. This action decreases the transcription of a range of pro-inflammatory mediators. These include IL-1b and TNFα; IL-2, which stimulates T-cell proliferation; a range of chemokines and cellular adhesion molecules; metalloproteinases; COX-2; and inducible nitric oxide synthase.

3. GCs increase synthesis of the polypeptide lipocortin-1 which inhibits phospholipase A_2 and thereby the synthesis of prostaglandins, thromboxane A_2 and PAF. (Fig. 24.1)

At the cellular level, GCs reduce the numbers of circulating lymphocytes, eosinophils and monocytes. This is maximal 4–6 hours after administration and is achieved by a combination of apoptosis induction

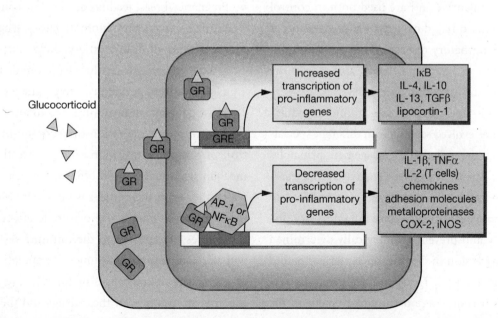

Fig.24.3 Mechanisms of glucocorticoid anti-inflammatory effects. Glucocorticoids exert pleiotropic effects on cellular metabolism. They increase transcription of a number of genes encoding anti-inflammatory proteins and decrease transcription of proinflammatory genes. AP-1, activating protein-1; COX, cyclo-oxygenase; GR, glucocorticoid receptor; GRE, glucocorticoid response element; IL, interleukin; iNOS, inducible nitric oxide synthase; NF, nuclear factor; TGF, transforming growth factor.

and inhibition of proliferation. Chronic administration of GC is associated with a neutrophilia caused by release of neutrophils from the bone marrow and reduced adherence to vascular walls.

In inflammatory disease, the choice of GC preparation will reflect the site and the extent of inflamed tissue, e.g. oral or parenteral for systemic disease, inhaled in asthma, topical in cutaneous, ocular, oral or rectal disease. Different corticosteroid preparations, their pharmacokinetics, modes of delivery and adverse effects are discussed elsewhere, except for the management of steroid-induced osteoporosis, which is found in the section on management of rheumatoid arthritis at the end of this chapter.

Disease-modifying drugs (DMDs)

Disease modifying drugs (DMD) are including immunomodulatory drugs and biologic agents, widely used in inflammatory immune disease, tumor, and treatment of transplantation rejection. Although their chemical structures are different, they all have anti-inflammatory and immune regulation effect.

IMMUNOMODULATORY DRUGS

Immunomodulaory drugs are used both to control symptoms and to retard or arrest the progression of chronic inflammatory diseases. They act to inhibit inflammation in a variety of ways, and reduce the proliferation and activation of lymphocytes.

The terminology surrounding immunomodulatory drugs has evolved separately in different specialties, although the underlying management principles are similar. Rheumatologists use the term 'disease-modifying anti-rheumatic drugs' (DMARDs) to describe those agents that reduce inflammatory disease activity and prevent radiologically determined disease progression in illnesses such as rheumatoid or psoriatic arthritis. Treatment regimens for systemic vasculitis or severe organ involvement in the connective tissue diseases make use of terminology drawn from oncology, with 'remission induction' followed by 'maintenance' phases. Many of these drugs are described as 'steroid-sparing' as their concomi-

tant use with glucocorticoids substantially reduces the total cumulative dose of steroid required for disease suppression. Many can be used in combination: with steroids, with each other or with biologic agents. This is discussed in the section on specific disease management at the end of the chapter.

The choice and combination of immunomodulatory agent in an individual patient depends on the following considerations:

- Severity of disease: this determines the risk: benefit ratio. For example, cerebral or renal lupus is more hazardous than rash or arthritis and therefore a more potent but potentially more toxic drug regimen is justified.
- Adverse-effect profile: both the probability and severity of potential adverse effects need to be considered.
- Evidence base: this, disappointingly, is often patchy but where it exists affords greater confidence for the prescribing physician.
- Age: the risk of future malignancy is less significant in elderly patients.
- Co-morbidity: drugs causing hypertension or adverse lipid profiles may be avoided in patients with high cardiovascular risk.
- Pregnancy/breast feeding: an absolute contraindication for many immunomodulatory drugs.
- Importance of future fertility: cyclophosphamide is likely to decrease fertility; leflunomide requires a long washout period prior to pregnancy.

Most conventional immunomodulatory agents act by inhibiting activation or reducing proliferation of lymphocytes. Many have more than one mechanism of action and often the precise way in which they exert their effects is unknown. Moreover, their antiproliferative and cytotoxic effects are in most cases not specific to the immune system but will affect any rapidly dividing cell population. This is one of the major causes of toxicity. Figure 24.4 presents an overview of these drugs and the known mechanisms of action that are relevant to the following discussion.

Methotrexate, azathioprine, mycophenolate mofetil and leflunomide are antimetabolites, interfering with

Fig.24.4 Overview of action of immunomodulatory drugs. Many conventional immunomodulatory drugs used in rheumatology practice are anti-metabolites, inhibiting de novo synthesis of purines or pyrimidines; pathways upon which activated lymphocytes are particularly dependent. The mechanisms of action of sulfasalazine, hydroxychloroquine and thalidomide appear to involve inhibition of expression of pro-inflammatory cytokines. The calcineurin inhibitors and sirolimus interfere with either the expression of IL-2 or signalling downstream of the IL-2 receptor; these effects target activated T cells. Cyclophosphamide is a cytotoxic agent that indiscriminately targets proliferating cells. Several biological agents block specific pro-inflammatory cytokines. Agents in current use include those targeting TNFα, IL-1 and IL-6.

the de novo synthesis of purines and pyrimidines, on which proliferating (but not resting) lymphocytes depend. Methotrexate is thought to have additional anti-inflammatory effects. The calcineurin antagonists (ciclosporin and tacrolimus) and sirolimus selectively inhibit T-cell activation and proliferation, by inhibiting cytokine expression and cytokine-driven proliferation, respectively. Cyclophosphamide is an alkylating agent that is cytotoxic in dividing cells and, in an autoimmune response, is particularly toxic to rapidly proliferating lymphocytes. Intravenous immunoglobulin has immunomodulatory effects through interference with Fcγ receptor signalling, among other mechanisms. The precise mechanisms of action of sulfasalazine, hydroxychloroquine, thalidomide, dapsone and gold are less clear, but they have been shown to influence the expression of a range of pro-inflammatory cytokines.

Immunomodulatory drugs have well recognised and occasionally very serious toxic side-effects but these only occur in a proportion of patients and/or are reversible on cessation of drug. They also often have less impact on quality of life than the inevitable effects of chronic high-dose glucocorticoid.

The complexity of prescribing and monitoring of toxicity with most immunomodulatory drugs demands collaboration between specialists, general practitioners and a well-informed patient. All should only be initiated under specialist supervision and all call for close monitoring, for example of bone marrow, liver, kidney or other organs, as known toxicity dictates. Live vaccines in general should not be given to immunosuppressed patients as there is a risk of disseminated infection.

Methotrexate

Methotrexate was first developed as an anticancer drug 50 years ago. Studies in the 1980s demonstrated its efficacy in rheumatoid arthritis and it is now the principal DMARD used in this disease. It is also used to treat many other chronic inflammatory illnesses, particularly psoriatic arthritis, and in the maintenance phase of therapy for systemic vasculitis.

Mechanism of action. As a folate analogue, methotrexate inhibits folate-dependent enzymes involved in purine biosynthesis, thus reducing lymphocyte proliferation, and this was originally thought to be its principal mechanism of action (and is likely to be the source of many of its toxic effects). In recent years, however, it has become clear that methotrexate has a number of other anti-inflammatory effects, and inhibition of 5-aminoimidazole-4-carboxamide ribonucleotide (AICAR) transformylase, another folate dependent enzyme, is now thought to be the likely pathway responsible for its efficacy in chronic inflammatory conditions. This results in a rise in intracellular levels of AICAR, which then inhibits adenosine deaminase and prevents the degradation of adenosine. Increased plasma concentrations of adenosine are thought to mediate many anti-inflammatory effects such as decreased TNFα and IFNγ production.

Prescription. Methotrexate is usually prescribed orally, starting at 5–10 mg once weekly and increasing as bone marrow and liver function allows, up to 20 mg. Parenteral administration is also possible, but is principally used in paediatric practice. Folic acid is usually prescribed (variably 5 mg weekly, three times weekly or on all days apart from on the methotrexate dosing day), in order to mitigate the adverse effects. This appears to have little effect on the blockade of de novo purine synthesis, unlike folinic acid (tetrahydrofolic acid).

Adverse effects. The most serious adverse effects of methotrexate are bone marrow toxicity, hepatic toxicity and pneumonitis; regular (at least monthly) monitoring of full blood count and liver function testing are recommended and a baseline chest X-ray is performed prior to first prescription. Methotrexate is also embryotoxic. Mouth ulcers and nausea occur commonly but may be improved by co-prescription of folic acid.

Interactions. Methotrexate used with trimethoprim, cotrimoxazole or sulphonamides creates a risk of megaloblastic anaemia and pancytopenia due to the additive antifolate effect. Folinic acid rescue may be effective should this occur.

Contraindications. Methotrexate should not be prescribed to patients with moderate to severe renal impairment, liver disease or an active infection. Because of its teratogenicity it must not be prescribed for women who are or may become pregnant or who are breast feeding. Both men and women should be counselled to use effective contraception while taking methotrexate and for 6 months afterwards.

Azathioprine

Azathioprine is another antimetabolite which acts by inhibiting purine biosynthesis, thus preferentially acting on proliferating lymphocytes. Besides its use to prevent rejection in organ transplant recipients, it has a well-established role as a disease-modifying or steroid-sparing agent in the maintenance phase of treatment of chronic inflammatory diseases, such as SLE, ANCA-associated and large vessel vasculitis, and interstitial lung disease.

Mechanism of action. Azathioprine undergoes reduction in the presence of glutathione to 6-mercaptopurine and then to 6-thioguanine. This forms a false purine nucleotide that is then incorporated into DNA, thus inhibiting DNA replication and cell proliferation. It may also trigger apoptosis. These actions result in a reduction in circulating B and T lymphocytes, reduced IL-2 secretion and reduced IgM and IgG synthesis.

Azathioprine and 6-mercaptopurine are metabolised predominantly by methylation and oxidation in the liver and/or erythrocytes, via thiopurine methyltransferase (TPMT).

Prescription. Azathioprine is taken orally, starting at 5 mg/kg and rising over the course of several weeks to a daily dose of 1–3 mg/kg. Polymorphisms in the gene encoding TPMT are associated with variable catabolism and hence toxicity and in most centres erythrocyte TPMT activity is assessed prior to its prescription, to guide use, dose and escalation.

Adverse effects. The major serious reactions are bone marrow suppression resulting in leucopenia, anaemia and thrombocytopenia; hepatotoxicity; increased susceptibility to infection; and in the long term an increased risk of neoplasia. As with methotrexate, regular monitoring of full blood count and liver function is mandatory. Other side-effects include nausea, alopecia and, rarely, allergy.

Interactions. Xanthine oxidase, the enzyme inhibited by allopurinol and febuxostat to therapeutic effect in the management of gout, is involved in the catabolism of azathioprine. Concomitant use of xanthine oxidase inhibitors and azathioprine may result in profound myelosuppression and should be avoided. If the combination is unavoidable, azathioprine must be decreased to 25%–33% of the usual dose. Sulfasalazine and NSAIDs inhibit TPMT and thereby the metabolism of azathioprine, also increasing the risk of myelotoxicity. Lastly, co-prescription of angiotensin-converting enzyme inhibitors and azathioprine increases the risk of myelosuppression; the mechanism is incompletely understood but has assumed greater importance with the recent appreciation that patients with SLE and other chronic inflammatory disorders have an increased risk of cardiovascular disease and are thus more likely to be prescribed both.

Contraindications. Experience with azathioprine in pregnant women with renal transplants indicates that it is relatively safe, probably because the fetus cannot metabolise 6-mercaptopurine. Although a teratogenic metabolite is present in breast milk, its concentration is low and no evidence for harm exists; nevertheless, breast feeding while taking azathioprine is best regarded as unsafe.

Mycophenolate mofetil

Mycophenolate mofetil (MMF) is also an antimetabolite that inhibits purine synthesis. It is licensed for the prophylaxis of acute rejection following organ transplantation and is also used (unlicensed in the UK) as a treatment for SLE nephritis, other connective tissue diseases with severe major organ involvement and systemic vasculitis.

Mechanism of action. MMF is metabolised to mycophenolic acid, which inhibits inosine monophosphate dehydrogenase, an enzyme in the guanine nucleotide synthesis pathway used by lymphocytes. As other cells have salvage pathways, MMF selectively inhibits lymphocyte proliferation.

Adverse effects. These are similar to azathioprine and include gastrointestinal disturbances (diarrhoea is particularly common), myelosuppression, hepatotoxicity, electrolyte disturbances, adverse lipid profile, increased risk of malignancy and pancreatitis. MMF is teratogenic and thus is contraindicated during pregnancy.

Leflunomide

The active metabolite of leflunomide (A771726) inhibits dihydroorotate dehydrogenase, a mitochondrial enzyme required for the synthesis of pyrimidines. It arrests the proliferation of activated lymphocytes and is licensed for the treatment of rheumatoid arthritis and psoriatic arthritis.

Adverse effects. Diarrhoea is the commonest; other gastrointestinal disturbances, hepatitis, leucopenia, alopecia, hypertension and allergy also occur. In the event of a serious adverse event, the elimination of leflunomide can be accelerated by colestyramine (4–6 g three times daily).

Contraindications. Leflunomide is contraindicated in liver disease, severe hypoproteinaemia, immunodeficiency, pregnancy, breast feeding or if there is a possibility of future pregnancy. A gap of at least 2 years is recommended between cessation of leflunomide treatment and conception.

Calcineurin inhibitors

The calcineurin inhibitors ciclosporin and tacrolimus inhibit cytokine-driven activation and proliferation of activated T cells by interfering with synthesis of IL-2. Both bind cytosol receptors called immunophilins (ciclophilin and FKBP-12 respectively) and form complexes that inhibit IL-2 production via the calcineurin pathway. They are used orally to prevent rejection after solid organ transplantation and in chronic inflammatory disorders including cutaneous psoriasis, Behcet's syndrome, systemic vasculitis and, occasionally, rheumatoid arthritis. However, other preparations are also becoming accepted: topical tacrolimus is used in cutaneous SLE and severe atopic dermatitis.

Adverse effects. The use of ciclosporin has in recent years been curtailed a little by the substantial incidence of hypertension and nephrotoxicity associated with long-term use, and the development of more effective, less toxic competitors. Both ciclospoin and tacrolimus can cause myelosuppression and hepatotoxicity and regular blood monitoring is required; gastrointestinal problems are also common, particularly diarrhoea with tacrolimus.

Sirolimus

Sirolimus (rapamycin) is a macrolide antibiotic, structurally very similar to tacrolimus, that is licensed for use in pre-venting rejection after solid organ transplantation, and is occasionally used (unlicensed) to treat autoimmune inflammatory disorders such as SLE and Behcet's syndrome. Sirolimus-coated stents are also commonly used in percutaneous coronary artery intervention, as the presence of sirolimus reduces neo-intimal proliferation. It acts by binding FKBP-12, like tacrolimus, but the complex in this case has no effect on the calcineurin pathway and instead binds to and inhibits activation of mTOR (mammalian target of rapamycin), an important signalling kinase. This in turn suppresses cytokine-driven T-cell and B-cell proliferation and antibody production. Adverse effects are similar to those of tacrolimus.

Cyclophosphamide

Cyclophosphamide, an alkylating cytotoxic agent, dam-ages DNA by forming cross-links which trigger apoptosis in dividing cells. In autoimmunity it is particularly toxic to rapidly proliferating lymphocytes and has also been used as a cancer chemotherapy drug. It is used to induce remission in severe inflammatory conditions with life-threatening organ involvement such as SLE nephritis, ANCA-associated vasculitis causing nephritis or pulmonary haemorrhage, or rapidly progressive interstitial lung disease.

Prescription and adverse effects. In rheumatological practice, cyclophosphamide is most commonly given as an intravenous pulse, repeated at 3–4 week intervals, for six pulses. Oral cyclophosphamide is less frequently used due to the larger cumulative dose and thus increased risk of long-term toxicities. A serious consequence is haemorrhagic cystitis, due to the action of acrolein (a drug metabolite) on the urinary tract epithelium. This is minimised by intravenous pre-hydration and oral administration of 2-mercaptoethane sulphonate (mesna), which reacts with and inactivates acrolein. Other adverse effects are highly significant and include bone marrow toxicity and consequent increased risk of opportunistic infection, infertility, teratogenicity, severe nausea and increased incidence of malignancy, especially of the bladder. In male patients, sperm may be stored prior to cyclophosphamide treatment.

Hydroxychloroquine

Hydroxychloroquine, an antimalarial drug, is used commonly for mild manifestations of SLE and other connective tissue diseases, particularly rashes and arthralgia, at doses of 200–400 mg daily. In rheumatoid arthritis, it is used as an adjunct to other disease-modifying agents.

Mechanism of action. It is not well understood how hydroxychloroquine exerts its disease-modifying effects. In vitro studies suggest that chloroquine and hydroxychloroquine can reduce the production of pro-inflammatory cytokines including TNFα and IL-1β, and both are known to be concentrated in lysosomes, inhibiting the metabolism of deoxyribonucleotides.

Adverse effects. Hydroxychloroquine is normally very well tolerated and has a low incidence of side-effects. GI disturbances, rashes, and, rarely, blood dyscrasias may occur. Retinal toxicity may rarely occur with long-term use; measurement of visual acuity initially and at annual intervals is recommended.

Contraindications. Hydroxychloroquine should be used with caution in hepatic or renal impairment, in neurological disorders, in glucose 6-phosphate dehydrogenase deficiency and in porphyria. The manufacturer's instructions advise against use in pregnancy and breast feeding, but data on over 250 pregnancies in women with connective tissue disease who were taking hydroxychloroquine provide evidence that the treatment is safe in pregnancy, and probably also during breast feeding.

Sulfasalazine

Sulfasalazine (SSZ) is a conjugate of mesalazine (5-aminosalicylic acid, 5-ASA) coupled to sulfapyridine. It is used to treat rheumatoid arthritis, either alone or in combination with methotrexate, and peripheral joint involvement in the spondyloarthropathies, including ankylosing spondylitis and reactive arthritis.

Mechanism of action. SSZ is cleaved by bacterial azoreductases in the colon to release 5-ASA and sulfapyridine (Fig. 24.5). 5-ASA is retained mostly in the colon and excreted, but 30% of intact SSZ and all sulfapyridine are absorbed. Anti-inflammatory effects of mesalazine, both in the colonic epithelial cell and in peripheral blood mononuclear cells, include inhibition of cyclooxygenase and lipooxygenase, scavenging of free radicals, and inhibition of the production of pro-inflammatory cytokines and immunoglobulins. In the treatment of inflammatory bowel disease, preparations containing 5-ASA alone have efficacy comparable to that of SSZ, but with fewer side-effects. In contrast, the sulfapyridine component appears to be the active moiety in rheumatoid arthritis. SSZ has been shown to reduce rheumatoid factor titres, inhibit IL-2-induced T-cell proliferation and inhibit macrophage IL-1 and IL-12 production, but the relative importance of these effects on its anti-inflammatory activity remains unclear.

Adverse effects. Sulfasalazine is associated with a number of adverse effects including cytopenias and hepatitis, which appear to be caused by the sulfapyridine moiety. A lupus-like syndrome may occur; the risk of this is higher in rheumatoid patients who are antinuclear antibody-positive.

Intravenous immunoglobulin

Intravenous immunoglobulin (IvIg) was first used in 1952 to treat primary immune deficiencies. It is composed of pooled IgG extracted from the plasma of 3 000–10 000 blood donors, and contains the entire repertoire of naturally occurring antibodies. Besides its uses as a treatment for primary immune deficiencies and hypogammaglobulinaemia, it has immuno-modulatory properties, making it an effective therapy for a number of autoimmune conditions. However, it has also been used in scenarios where there is no evidence of efficacy and little theoretical basis to suggest benefit. As there is a national shortage, the UK NHS

Fig. 24.5 Metabolism and activity of sulfasalazine. Sulfasalazine is reduced to sulfapyridine and mesalazine in the colon by bacterial azoreductases. The two components have distinct anti-inflammatory activities.

has recently introduced guidelines to restrict its use only to those conditions in which there is a known benefit.

Diseases in which IvIg is known to be of benefit include: Kawasaki disease, immune thrombocytopenic purpura (ITP), dermatomyositis, Guillain–Barre' syndrome and chronic inflammatory demyelinating polyneuropathy. There are many others in which it may be used as part of a range of treatments.

Mechanism of action. The immunomodulatory mecha-nism of action of IvIg is thought primarily to be through the Fc region of the IgG molecule. Binding to Fc receptors and altering Fc receptor signalling in macrophages, other phagocytes and B cells has been shown to be an important effect in ITP and other autoimmune cytopenias. In dermatomysitis and Kawasaki disease, modulation of complement cascade activation is important. IvIg binds C3b and C4b, thus inhibiting formation of the membrane attack complex. Other functions of IvIg such as suppression of autoantibodies and of cytokines and chemokines have also been demonstrated.

Adverse effects. These include infusion reactions during or shortly after treatment, acute renal failure and rarely thrombosis, hyperproteinaemia and disseminated intravascular coagulation. As IvIg contains trace amounts of IgA, IgA-deficient patients may develop a hypersensitivity reaction following repeated infusions, which may progress to anaphylaxis.

BIOLOGIC AGENTS

The biggest change in treatment of inflammatory disease over the last 10 years has been the development of monoclonal antibodies and fusion proteins that target a specific component of the inflammatory response. This allows selective modification of the abnormal immune response underlying many chronic inflammatory diseases, resulting in greater efficacy and potentially fewer side-effects than conventional 'dirtier' immunosuppressants. The first drugs of this sort to enter widespread clinical use were TNFα antagonists, which now have an established role in the treatment of rheumatoid arthritis,

juvenile idiopathic arthritis, ankylosing spondylitis, psoriasis and Crohn's disease.

In recent years there has been a dramatic increase in the variety of different biological drugs, and their indications. Their major drawbacks, shared by all, are an increased susceptibility to infection, and price, which in the UK at least severely curtails their use. A brief overview only is given here.

Anti-TNFα therapies

TNFα, a pro-inflammatory cytokine, is produced predominantly by macrophages and in smaller amounts by CD4+Th1 lymphocytes. It plays an important role in macrophage activation and the eradication of intracellular bacterial and fungal infections. TNFα is also a key mediator of the inflammatory response seen in chronic granulomatous conditions such as rheumatoid arthritis and Crohn's disease. TNFα blockade by biological agents has proved highly effective for many chronic inflammatory diseases, and there are now several different agents selectively targeting TNFα available, with more in development.

Infliximab is a chimeric monoclonal IgG1 antibody (Fig. 24.6). In rheumatoid arthritis it is administered by in-travenous infusion at 3–5 mg/kg, repeated 2 and 6 weeks after the initial infusion and then at 6–8 week intervals. In ankylosing spondylitis, psoriasis and Crohn's disease, it is used at doses of 5 mg/kg. Methotrexate is co-prescribed to limit the development of neutralising antibodies.

Adalimumab is a fully human monoclonal IgG1 antibody (Fig. 24.6). The recommended dose is 40 mg by subcutane-ous injection fortnightly, in combination with methotrexate. It is licensed for use in rheumatoid arthritis, ankylosing spondylitis and psoriatic arthritis.

Etanercept is a fusion protein consisting of two human p75 TNFα receptors coupled to an Fc component of human IgG1 (Fig. 24.6). It is licensed for weekly subcutaneous injection in adult patients with rheumatoid arthritis (50 mg).

- does not fix complement and therefore does not cause lysis of cells that express TNFα on their surface

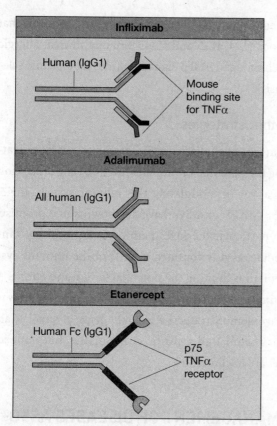

Fig. 24.6 Structure of anti-TNFα biologicals. Infliximab and adalimumab are monoclonal antibodies. Etanercept is a fusion molecule composed of two p75 TNFα receptors coupled to a human immunoglobulin Fc component.

- binds trimeric (active) TNFα only, in contrast with infliximab, which binds both monomeric (inactive) and trimeric (active) TNFα
- also binds lymphotoxin (TNFβ)

There are two further anti-TNFα antibodies that have recently entered clinical practice in the UK. Golimumab is a fully human monoclonal antibody to TNFα which is taken monthly; and certolizumab pegol is a pegylated humanised Fab fragment directed against TNFα.

Adverse effects

The major risk with anti-TNF therapy is increased susceptibility to infection, particularly with intracellular pathogens such as Mycobacteria tuberculosis (M.Tb). In the case of M.Tb this may be reactivation of latent disease, but there is also a risk of new infection with M.Tb, other mycobacteria or intracellular pathogens such as histoplasmosis, coccidiomycosis or nocardiosis. Guidelines for assessing risk and for managing infection with Mycobacterium tuberculosis in the context of anti-TNFα agents are available. Chemoprophylaxis must be started prior to treatment in patients with latent infection.

Antinuclear antibodies develop twice as commonly in rheumatoid arthritis patients taking anti-TNFα agents. The risk of developing anti-double-stranded DNA antibodies is also increased but, in the majority of cases, the clinical significance of these autoantibodies is unclear. Anti-TNFα-induced lupus is a rare complication.

Infusion reactions may occur with infliximab adminis-tration, e.g. fever, pruritus, urticaria, chest pain, hypotension and dyspnoea. These usually resolve if the infusion rate is slowed or suspended temporarily and then restarted at a slower rate.

Symptoms and/or radiological evidence of demyelination may be exacerbated, as may severe cardiac failure.

TNFα blockade presents a theoretical risk of increasing the incidence of malignancy. In patients with rheumatoid arthritis, current data do not suggest an overall augmented tumour risk but the chance of developing lymphoma may be increased.

B-cell depletion

Rituximab is a chimeric monoclonal IgG1 antibody specific for CD20, which is expressed on B cells but not plasma cells. Initially used for B-cell lymphomas, it is now prescribed for a variety of autoimmune disorders, including rheumatoid arthritis and SLE, in which autoantibody production is a significant disease-causing mechanism. Targeting CD20 removes the pathogenic anti-body-producing cells, leaving the memory plasma cells needed to mount a response to infection intact. It is administered by intravenous infusion in doses of 1 g 2 weeks apart. The B-cell count is then monitored to check for depletion. Patients can be retreated if their B-cell count recovers and the disease recurs. The major adverse effects are in-creased susceptibility to infection, and infusion reactions.

Belimumab is a monoclonal antibody that blocks B-lymphocyte stimulator (BLyS), preventing the proliferation of B cells. It recently received FDA approval as a treat-ment for SLE.

Inhibition of T-cell activation

Abatacept is a fusion protein formed from the extracellular domain of human CTLA4 (cytotoxic T lymphocyte an-tigen-4) linked to the Fc portion of human IgG1. Normally, CTLA4 on the T-cell membrane binds CD80 and CD86 on antigen presenting cells to provide the co-stimulation signal required for full T-cell activation when it recognises a Class II MHC-antigen complex. Abatacept competes with T-cell-bound CTLA4 and binds CD80 or CD86 itself, thus preventing co-stimulation, and this leads to a reduction in T-cell proliferation and cytokine production. It has been shown to be effective in reducing rheumatoid arthritis activity and is given as an intravenous infusion.

Other biologic anticytokine agents

Interleukin-1 (IL-1) is a pro-inflammatory cytokine with a central role in the activation of an inflammatory re-sponse. Anakinra is recombinant IL-1Ra, an endogenous antagonist of the IL-1 receptor. Clinical trials in rheumatoid arthritis, SLE and psoriasis have had disappointing results, but anakinra is dramatically effective in treating rare hereditary fever syndromes characterised by excess IL-1 signalling. These include cryopyrin-associated periodic syndromes (CAPS) such as Muckle–Wells syndrome, and hyper-IgD syndrome. Anakinra is also effective in treating systemic onset juvenile inflammatory arthritis and adult-onset Still's disease, and may be effective in severe gout.

Interleukin-6 (IL-6) is another pro-inflammatory cytokine that is of critical importance to the mounting of an immune response, and is the most abundant cytokine found in the synovium of rheumatoid arthritis patients. Tocilizumab is a monocloncal antibody that binds IL-6 receptors and inhibits their intracellular signalling. It has been shown to be effective in controlling disease activity in rheumatoid arthritis, and is licensed for use in this condition in the UK. It is given by intravenous infusion on a monthly basis.

Other anticytokine biological agents in development or undergoing clinical trials include agents that block IL-4, IL-5 and IL-13 (mainly to treat allergic asthma), and TGFβ signalling (to treat systemic sclerosis).

Other strategies

Current drug discovery programmes are investigating the potential of protein kinase cascade disruption as a way of modulating the immune system. JAK3, p38 MAPK and Syk have all shown some promise. In particular the JAK3 pathway is a promising candidate, as it is confined to cells of the immune system, thus limiting the potential for adverse effects. A number of small molecule inhibitors of this pathway have demonstrated beneficial effects in small trials for rheumatoid arthritis and psoriasis, but none as yet are in clinical use.

MANAGEMENT OF DISEASES ASSOCIATED WITH INFLAMMATION

Osteoarthritis

Osteoarthritis (OA) is the most common form of arthritis, with radiographic evidence of knee OA in up to 15% of people aged over 55 years. It reflects a dynamic bone and cartilage response to joint trauma and ageing. OA is a common cause of disability, particularly in the elderly, and is the major indication for joint replacement.

The aims of management of OA are to control pain, reduce progression of joint damage and minimise disability. The major strategies employed are non-pharmacological; there are no disease-modifying drugs in clinical use. Patient education in pain management is important to minimise the adverse effects of analgesics. NSAIDs have been shown to be marginally more effective but are associated with more adverse effects than paracetamol. Regular paracetamol or codydramol should therefore be tried before introducing a NSAID. Other options include topical NSAID gel, which may provide a modest improvement in symptoms at least in the short term. For patients with large-joint OA, occasional intra-articular injection of corticosteroid and local anaesthetic can provide some respite for up to 6 weeks.

Gout

Gout is a recurrent acute inflammatory arthritis caused by monosodium urate (MSU) crystals within synovial joints, affecting 1.4% of the UK population. Hyperuricaemia is due to over-production or under-excretion of uric acid. Both mechanisms may operate in the same patient, but reduced renal clearance is the main cause of hyperuricaemia in most cases. Drugs may influence these processes as follows:

- Over-production of uric acid occurs if there is excessive cell destruction releasing nucleic acids. This may occur when myeloproliferative and lymphoproliferative disorders are first treated.
- Under-excretion of uric acid is caused by thiazide and loop diuretics, low dose aspirin, ethambutol, pyrazinamide, nicotinic acid, ciclosporin and alcohol (which increases uric acid synthesis and also causes a rise in serum lactic acid that inhibits tubular secretion of uric acid). Conversely, a small number of drugs have a mild uricosuric effect and increase renal clearance of urate. Losartan and fenofibrate are examples of this.

Patients with gout but no visible tophi have a uric acid pool that is two to three times normal. This exceeds the amount that can be carried in solution in extracellular fluid, so MSU crystals precipitate and form deposits in tissues, including the joints and occasionally in subcutaneous tissues (tophi). These crystals then trigger acute attacks of inflammatory arthritis.

The priority in an acute attack is to relieve the intense pain by reducing the inflammatory response. NSAIDs are most commonly prescribed, but if contraindicated, colchicine (EULAR guidelines suggest 0.5 mg three times daily) is an alternative. A short course of oral prednisolone or intra-articular corticosteroid is also effective, although the severity of joint pain may preclude intra-articular injection during an acute attack.

Management of chronic gout should include a review of modifiable risk factors for hyperuricaemia, including obesity, hypertension, excessive alcohol consumption, high dietary intake of purines (red meat, game, seafood, legumes) and drugs. If these measures are insufficient, plasma uric acid levels may be reduced by inhibiting the formation of uric acid (allopurinol, febuxostat), or increasing renal excretion (sulfinpyrazone, probenecid or benzbromarone). In treatment-resistant cases, 'biologic' therapy with recombinant uricase, which metabolises urate further, can be considered. Rapid lowering of plasma uric acid by any means can precipitate an acute flare, probably by causing the dissolution of crystal deposits. Colchicine prescribed concomitantly for up to 6 months or an NSAID for 6 weeks protect against this.

Allopurinol inhibits xanthine oxidase, the enzyme that converts xanthine and hypoxanthine to uric acid. Patients taking allopurinol excrete less uric acid and more xanthine and hypoxanthine in the urine. It is readily absorbed from the GI tract, metabolised in the liver to oxypurinol, which is also a xanthine oxidase inhibitor, and excreted unchanged by the kidney. Allopurinol is indicated in recurrent gout and during treatment of myeloproliferative disorders where cell destruction creates a high uric acid load. It pre-vents the hyperuricaemia due to diuretics and may be combined with a uricosuric agent.

Adverse effects of allopurinol include precipitation of an acute gout attack and the allopurinol hypersensitivity syndrome (AHS) which is rare but can be severe. Features include hepatitis, desquamating erythematous rash, eosinophilia and worsening renal function. For this reason, allopurinol should not be commenced unless the diagnosis is certain, and attacks of gout are frequent despite lifestyle changes. It also interferes with the metabolism of azathioprine and co-prescription may cause severe myelosuppression.

Febuxostat is a newly licensed non-purine selective xanthine oxidase inhibitor. Although it is at least as effective, if not more, than allopurinol at lowering serum urate levels, its safety in patients who are allergic to allopurinol has not been fully established. Diarrhoea, liver function disturbance and other GI symptoms are the commonest adverse effects. Febuxostat also interferes with azathioprine metabolism.

Sulfinpyrazone competitively inhibits the active transport of organic anions across the kidney tubule, both from the plasma to the tubular fluid and vice versa. The effect is dose-dependent: at low dose sulfinpyrazone prevents secretion of uric acid into tubular fluid, and at high dose, and more powerfully, it prevents reabsorption, increasing its excretion in the urine. A net beneficial uricosuric action is obtained with an initial dose of 100–200 mg/day by mouth with food, increasing over 2–3 weeks to 200–400 mg/day, which should be continued until the plasma uric acid level is normal. The dose may then be reduced for maintenance, to as little as 100 mg daily. During initial therapy ensure that fluid intake is at least 2 L/day to prevent uric acid crystalluria. Other adverse effects are mainly gastro-intestinal; sulfinpyrazone is contraindicated in peptic ulcer.

Rasburicase is a recombinant uricase which converts urate into allantoin, a more soluble metabolite which is readily excreted renally. It rapidly and profoundly lowers serum uric acid concentration and is licensed for use in tumour lysis syndrome. It has also been used in small numbers of patients with gout, but antibody development limits its effectiveness with repeated infusions, as would be needed to treat chronic tophaceous gout. A pegylated uricase (pegloticase), which has a longer half-life and is less immunogenic, has shown promise in recent trials.

Rheumatoid arthritis

Rheumatoid arthritis (RA) is a chronic symmetrical polyarthritis affecting approximately 1% of the UK population. The principal pathology is inflammation within synovial joints, causing pain, swelling and stiffness and progressing to erosion and eventually joint destruction. RA is a systemic autoimmune inflammatory disorder and may cause extra-articular manifestations affecting blood vessels, bone marrow, GI tract, skin, lungs and eyes. Further sources of morbidity reflect the interaction of the disease process with adverse effects of medication and include osteoporosis, gastrointestinal haemorrhage and accelerated atherosclerosis. Mortality in patients with RA is increased up to three-fold compared with the general population; most of the excess is due to cardiovascular disease.

The initial management of a patient presenting with new inflammatory polyarthritis consists of reducing systemic inflammation, joint pain and stiffness while the diagnosis is confirmed. This may be achieved by short-term glucocorticoids such as Depo-Medrone 250–500 mg daily i.m., com-bined with analgesia and an NSAID (e.g. diclofenac 25–50 mg three times daily).

Once a diagnosis of RA is made, a DMARD should be initiated. As these reduce the progression of joint damage, it is imperative to start treatment in early disease; it is not acceptable to attempt to treat patients with early RA solely symptomatically. Methotrexate is the most common first-line DMARD. Careful education and counselling of the patient is important to ensure regular monitoring (of bone marrow, liver and lung function) and early detection of adverse effects. Folic acid 5 mg (up to 6 days weekly) is co-prescribed to reduce side-effects such as mouth ulcers.

Hydroxychloroquine is often used as an adjunct DMARD with methotrexate, and combination therapy of methotrexate, sulfasalazine and hydroxychloroquine can have added benefits beyond that of the individual drugs. Where methotrexate is contraindicated, ineffective or toxic, sulfasalazine alone, leflunomide or gold are alternatives. At any point in the disease course, glucocorticoids can be used as an adjunct to control flares, administered orally, intra-articularly or intra-muscularly.

If adequate disease control is not achieved after use of two DMARDs, UK guidelines recommend starting anti-TNFα agents: infliximab, etanercept or adalimumab. If this is not effective, current practice involves switching to an alternative anti-TNFα agent with a different mechanism of action, or to the anti-CD20 mAb, rituximab. In 2010, tocilizumab (anti IL-6R) and abatacept (T-cell co-stimulation blockade) were approved for those patients who have not responded to other biologics. Many other biologic agents targeting cytokine expression, immune cell subtypes and intracellular signalling are currently in development.

It is particularly important to address cardiovascular risk reduction in patients with RA, given the increased risk of cardiovascular disease associated with chronic inflammation. Aggressive management of RA with DMARDs may reduce cardiovascular disease incidence at the same time as controlling inflammation. Moreover, atorvastatin has been reported to improve disease activity scores in RA.

Protection against osteoporosis is particularly important for patients who receive long-term glucocorticoids; The UK guideline for the prevention and treatment of glucocorticoid-induced osteoporosis is summarised in Figure 24.7. Bone loss is most rapid in the first few months of treatment, therefore protection must be considered at the onset of treatment, whenever the intention is to continue for more than 3 months, at any dose. Strategies include minimising the dose of corticosteroid, concomitant prescription of vitamin D 800 IU and calcium 1 g daily and advice on smoking cessation, alcohol intake, nutrition and exercise. Bisphosphonates should be prescribed for all patients aged over 65 years, or those with a history of a fragility fracture. Other patients should undergo bone densitometry and should be prescribed a bisphosphonate if the T score is 1.5 or less[16] at either lumbar spine or hip.

Patients with RA have a five-fold increased risk of gastrointestinal haemorrhage compared with the general population, mainly due to NSAID use, alone or in combination with corticosteroids. Any patient with RA taking regular NSAIDs should also be prescribed a proton pump inhibitor or other gastroprotective agent.

Systemic lupus erythematosus

Systemic lupus erythematosus (SLE) is a chronic multi-organ autoimmune condition affecting primarily young women, those may have life-threatening manifestations. Management depends on the degree and severity of organ involvement, which may range from mild rashes and arthralgia to pancytopenia or renal and cerebral vasculitis.

Mild lupus may be treated with hydroxychloroquine and lifestyle advice, such as avoidance of sun exposure or extreme stress, but many require a more potent immunomodulator, such as azathioprine or mycophenolate mofetil (MMF). Flares may be controlled by pulses of glucocorticoid i.v. or i.m. or a progressively reduced oral course, although some patients require long-term low-dose GC. Topical or intra-articular steroids are used if appropriate. Severe manifestations such as lupus nephritis are traditionally managed with i.v. pulses of methylprednisolone and cyclophosphamide. MMF is now increasingly used, in light of the risk of infertility associated with cyclophosphamide. B-cell depletion with rituximab may also be effective.

Co-morbidities result from both the disease and its treatment; in addition to excess cardiovascular mortality there is a risk long term of developing other autoimmune diseases or malignancy as well as osteoporosis or opportunistic infection. Patients with SLE should be screened for anti-phospholipid antibodies, and antiplatelet therapy should be considered in those who are positive.

Poly myalgia rheumatic and giant cell arteritis

These are chronic inflammatory conditions that occur mainly in patients over 60 years and present with proximal pain and stiffness, fever and night sweats or headache. The most feared complication is sudden visual loss due to involvement of the ophthalmic artery. They respond exquisitely to corticosteroids. If

Fig. 24.7 Prevention and treatment of glucocorticoid-induced osteoporosis. UK guidelines for osteoprotection in patients treated with glucocorticoids.

giant cell arteritis is suspected or diagnosed, high dose prednisolone (30–60 mg daily) is used. Other immunomodulators such as azathioprine or methotrexate do not have proven efficacy but are sometimes used in patients whose disease requires unacceptably high doses of glucocorticoid for suppression. As treatment is normally required for at least 2 years, osteoprotection and gastroprotection must be used.

SUMMARY

A vast burden of human disease involves the process of inflammation and the engagement of an immune response, often entirely appropriately as in the case of defence against infection. By contrast, a number of organ-specific and multisystem rheumatic diseases are characterised by a primary abnormality within the immune response, requiring treatments that modify or suppress it. Anti-inflammatory -immunity drugs make up about half of analgesics, remedying pain by reducing inflammation as opposed to opioids, which affect the central nervous system. Anti-inflammatory-immunity drugs involves three classes: non-steroidal anti-inflammatory-immunity drugs (NSAIIDs), steroidal anti-infalmmatory-immunity drugs (SAIIDs) and disease-modifying drugs (DMDs). This chapter reviews some development of these drugs in clinical research: some new NSAIIDs have little side-effects because of their selective inhibiting cyclooxygenase; Low doses of SAIIDs are effective and of little side-effects in the treatment of rheumatoid arthritis; SAIIDs might have immune-regulatory effect when their doses are low; Some new DMDs have been developed in these years; Biologic interventions in inflammatory-immune disease have been paid great attention. Even though, much effort should be made to develop new anti-inflammatory-immunity drugs with effectiveness and little side-effects in future.

IMPORTANT TERMONOLOGY

non-steroidal anti-inflammatory drugs (NSAIDs) 非甾体抗炎药

tumour necrosis factor-α (TNFα) 肿瘤坏死因子 α

C-reactive protein (CRP) C- 反应蛋白

cyclo-oxygenase (COX) 环加氧酶

antigen-presenting cell (APC) 抗原呈递细胞

glucocorticoid receptor (GR) 糖皮质激素受体

transforming growth factor (TGF) 转化生长因子

angiotensin-converting enzyme (ACE) 血管紧张素转化酶

N-acetyl-p-benzoquinone imine (NAPQI) N- 乙酰基 - 对苯醌亚胺

disease-modifying anti-rheumatic drugs (DMARDs) 改善病情抗风湿药

thiopurine methyltransferase (TPMT) 硫代嘌呤甲基转移酶

5-aminosalicylic acid (5-ASA) 5- 氨基水杨酸

intravenous immunoglobulin (Ivlg) 静脉注射免疫球蛋白

mammalian target of rapamycin (mTOR) 哺乳动物雷帕霉素靶向基因

B-lymphocyte stimulator (BLyS) B 淋巴细胞刺激因子

cryopyrin-associated periodic syndromes (CAPS) 蛋白相关周期性综合征

the allopurinol hypersensitivity syndrome (AHS) 别嘌醇过敏综合征

psoriatic arthritis (PsA) 银屑病关节炎

rheumatoid arthritis (RA) 类风湿性关节炎

systemic lupus erythematosus (SLE) 系统性红斑狼疮

platelet-activating factor (PAF) 血小板活化因子

CHALLENGE YOURSELF

1. What are the pharmacologic characteristics of non steroidal anti-inflammatory drugs?
2. What are the adverse effects of non steroidal anti-inflammatory drugs?
3. What is the pharmacological action and clinical application of aspirin?
4. Please descript the pharmacological action, mechanism of action and the main adverse effects of glucocorticoid?

Shuwen Liu

Chapter | 25 |

Vitamins, calcium, bone

VITAMIN A: RETINOL

Vitamin A is a generic term embracing substances having the biological actions of retinol and related substances (called *retinoids*). The principal functions of retinol are to:

- sustain normal epithelia
- promote corneal and conjunctival development
- form retinal photochemicals
- enhance immune functions
- protect against infections and probably some cancers

Deficiency of retinol leads to xerophthalmia, squamous metaplasia, hyperkeratosis and impairment of the immune system.

Therapeutic uses

Retinol and derivatives provide therapeutic benefit in a number of clinical areas.

Psoriasis

Tazorotene, a topical retinoid, is effective in the treatment of chronic stable plaque psoriasis. Skin irritation is common, making it unsuitable for the treatment of inflammatory forms of psoriasis. The 0.05% cream is better tolerated than 0.1% although less effective. *Acitretin* is a retinoic acid derivative ($t_{1/2}$ 48 h) that is used orally for severe psoriasis. Dose range 25 mg alternate days – 50 mg daily.

Acne

Tretinoin is retinoic acid and is used in acne by topi-cal application. *Isotretinoin* is a retinoic acid isomer ($t_{1/2}$ 20 h) given orally for acne. It is also effective for preventing second tumours in patients following treatment for primary squamous cell carcinoma of the head and neck.

Acute promyelocytic leukaemia

Tretinoin can be used to induce remission in conjunction with chemotherapy in acute promyelocytic leukaemia, a subgroup of acute myeloid leukaemia (AML) involving chromosomal translocation of the retinoic acid receptor-alpha gene. Initially, it proved remarkably successful, but the high doses given caused the fatal 'differentiation syndrome' (previously called 'retinoic acid syndrome'; respiratory distress, fever and hypotension) and the duration of treatment is now shorter.

Vitamin A deficiency

Primary deficiency is common in developing countries. *Retinol* is used to prevent and treat deficiency; 1 microgram = 3.3 IU ($t_{1/2}$ 7–14 days). For prevention of deficiency in susceptible individuals, supplements are given at 4–6-monthly intervals. Dosing is according to age. More frequent doses are required for treatment of xerophthalmia. Secondary deficiency resulting from fat malabsorption is seen with pancreatic insufficiency and disorders of the gastrointestinal tract. Vitamin A supplementation at pharmacological doses is standard for patients with cystic fibrosis. This can result in chronic toxicity and serum retinol levels should be monitored.

Adverse effects

Acute toxicity occurs in adults with a single dose of more than 600 000 IU/day. Symptoms include headache, nausea, vomiting and drowsiness. Travellers have become ill by eating the livers of Arctic carnivores.

Chronic toxicity occurs with prolonged high intake (in children 25 000–50 000 IU/day, 10 times the recommended daily allowance, RDA). A diagnostic sign is the presence of painful tender swellings on long bones. Anorexia, skin lesions, hair loss, hepatosplenomegaly, papilloedema, bleeding and general malaise also occur. Vitamin A accumulates in liver and fat, and effects take weeks to wear off. Chronic overdose also makes the biological membranes and the outer layer of the skin more liable to peel.

Teratogenicity. Vitamin A and its derivatives are teratogenic at pharmacological doses. Supplements should not exceed 8 000 IU (2 400 micrograms) per day.

VITAMIN B: COMPLEX

A number of widely differing substances are now, for convenience, classed as the 'vitamin B complex'. Those used for pharmacotherapy include the following:

Thiamine (B_1). Deficiency is associated with three distinct conditions: Wernicke–Korsakoff syndrome, beriberi, and Leigh's syndrome. The UK RDA of thiamine is 1 mg for men and 0.8 mg for women. It is given orally for nutritional purposes, but intravenously in serious emergencies, e.g. Wernicke–Korsakoff syndrome. Give the injection over 10 min (intramuscularly); note that it can cause anaphylactic shock.

Pyridoxine (B_6) is a coenzyme in the metabolic transformation of many amino acids, including decarboxylation and transamination. The UK RDA of vitamin B_6 is 1.4 mg for men and 1.2 mg for women. As pharmacotherapy, pyridoxine is given to treat certain pyridoxine-dependent inborn errors of metabolism, e.g. homocystinuria, hereditary sidero-

blastic anaemia and primary hyperoxaluria. Deficiency may be induced by drugs such as isoniazid, hydralazine and penicillamine; pyridoxine 10 mg/day prevents the development of peripheral neuritis without interfering with therapeutic action.

Pyridoxine, in doses sometimes exceeding 100 mg/day, has found use for a variety of conditions including premenstrual syndrome and nausea in pregnancy.

Niacin (nicotinic acid, B_3) is converted to nicotinamide, and subsequently to nicotinamide adenine dinucleotide (NAD) and nicotinamide adenine dinucleotide phosphate (NADPH), the cofactors that are essential for the oxidation–reduction reactions that comprise tissue respiration. Nicotinamide is used for nutritional purposes. Pellagra resulting from dietary deficiency of niacin is rarely seen in developed countries. Causes other than dietary include alcoholism, carcinoid syndrome and Hartnup disease. Nicotinic acid at pharmacological doses is used for the treatment of some hyperlipidaemias. Adverse effects include peripheral vasodilatation, unpleasant flushing, itching and fainting.

VITAMIN C: ASCORBIC ACID

Vitamin C is a powerful *reducing agent* (antioxidant) and is an essential cofactor and substrate in a number of enzymatic reactions, including collagen synthesis and noradrenaline synthesis. It also functions as an antioxidant, mopping up free radicals produced endogenously or in the environment, e.g. cigarette smoke. There has been considerable interest in using vitamin C as an antioxidative agent to reduce oxidation of low-density lipoproteins (LDL) in atherosclerosis and prevent formation of carcinogens to reduce risk of cancer. However, randomised trials have not shown any beneficial effect thus far of vitamin C on either cancer incidence or primary or secondary prevention of coronary heart disease.

Indications

- The prevention and cure of scurvy.
- Methaemoglobinaemia.

Scurvy

Deficiency of ascorbic acid leads to *scurvy*, which is characterised by petechial haemorrhages, haematomas, bleeding gums (if teeth are present) and anaemia.

Methaemoglobinaemia

A reducing substance is needed to convert the methaemoglobin (ferric iron) back to oxyhaemoglobin (ferrous iron) whenever enough has formed seriously to impair the oxygen-carrying capacity of the blood. Ascorbic acid is non-toxic (it acts by direct reduction) but is less effective than *methylene blue* (methylthioninium chloride). Both can be given orally, intravenously or intramuscularly. Excessive doses of methylene blue can cause methaemoglobinaemia (by stimulating NADPH-dependent enzymes).

Methaemoglobinaemia may be induced by oxidising drugs: sulphonamides, nitrites, nitrates (may also occur in drinking water), primaquine, -caine local anaesthetics, dapsone, nitrofurantoin, nitroprusside, vitamin K analogues, chlorates, aniline and nitrobenzene. Where symptoms are severe enough to warrant urgent treatment, methylene blue given intravenously at 1–2 mg/kg gives response within 30 min. Patients should be monitored for rebound methaemoglobinaemia. Methylene blue turns the urine blue and high concentrations can irritate the urinary tract, so that fluid intake should be high when large doses are used. Methlyene blue should not be administered to patients with glucose-6-phosphate dehydrogenase (G6PD) deficiency since its action is dependent on NADPH produced by G6PD. In addition to being ineffective in this circumstance it may induce haemolysis. Ascorbic acid is inadequate for the treatment of acute methaemoglobinaemia requiring treatment.

Congenital methaemogobinaemia can be treated long term with either oral methylene blue or ascorbic acid with partial effect.

Adverse effects

High doses may cause sleep disturbances, headaches and gut upsets. Ascorbic acid is eliminated partly in the urine unchanged and partly metabolised to oxalate. Doses above 4 g/day increase urinary oxalate concentration and there is a potential risk of renal oxalate stones with chronic ascorbic acid administration. Intravenous ascorbic acid may precipitate a haemolytic attack in subjects with G6PD deficiency.

VITAMIN D, CALCIUM, PARATHYROID HORMONE, CALCITONIN, BISPHOSPHONATES, BONE

Vitmain D is closely interrelated with calcium homeostasis and bone metabolism and these topics are therefore discussed together.

Vitamin D

Vitamin D comprises a number of structurally related sterol compounds having similar biological properties (but different potencies) in that they prevent or cure the vitamin D-deficiency diseases, rickets and osteomalacia. The most relevant form of vitamin D is vitamin D_3 (colecaciferol). This is made by ultraviolet irradiation of 7-dehydrocholesterol in the skin. It is also absorbed in the intestinal tract; however, few foods contain significant levels of vitamin D (Fig. 25.1). Vitamin D_2 (*ergocalciferol*) is made by ultraviolet irradiation of ergosterol in plants. This is not the naturally occurring form.

Vitamin D_3 (and D_2) undergo two successive hydroxylations: first in the liver to form 25-hydroxyvitamin D and second in the proximal tubules of the kidney (under the control of parathyroid hormone, PTH) to form $1\alpha,25$-dihydroxyvitamin D_3 (*calcitriol*), the most *physiologically active* form of vitamin D.

There exist also a variety of synthetic vitamin D analogues, developed to treat vitamin D deficiency and hypoparathyroidism. The vitamin D derivative 1α-hydroxycolecalciferol (*alfacalcidol*) requires only hepatic hydroxylation to become calcitriol. The usual adult maintenance dose, 0.25–1 micrograms/day, indicates its potency.

Other 1α-hydroxylated vitamin D analogues include *paricalcitol*. In addition, a structural variant

Fig. 25.1 Metabolism of vitamin D. D₃, Vitamin D₃ (cholecalciferol); pre-D₃, pre-vitamin D₃; DBP, vitamin D-binding protein; 25-OHase, liver 25-hydroxylase; 25(OH)D₃, 25-hydroxycholecalciferol 25(OH)D₃; 1-OHase, 25-hydroxyvitamin D3-1-hydroxylase; 1,25(OH)₂D₃, calcitriol; PTH, parathyroid hormone.

of vitamins D₂ and D₃, dihydrotachysterol (ATIO, Tachyrol), is also biologically activated by hepatic 25-hydroxylation. All are effective in renal failure as they bypass the defective renal hydroxylation stage.

Pharmacokinetics

Alfacalcidol and *dihydrotachysterol* have a fast onset and short duration of clinical effect (days) which renders them suitable for rapid adjustment of plasma calcium, e.g. in hypoparathyroidism. Such factors are not relevant to the slower adjustment of plasma

calcium (weeks) with vitamins D₂ and D₃ in the ordinary management of vitamin D deficiency.

Actions are complex. Vitamin D promotes the active transport of calcium and phosphate in the gut (increased absorption) and renal tubule (reduced excretion), and thus controls, with PTH, the plasma calcium concentration and the mineralisation of bone (Fig. 25.1). After a dose of D₂ or D₃ there is a lag of about 21 h before the intestinal effect begins; this is probably due to the time needed for its metabolic conversion to the more active forms. With the biologically more active calcitriol, the lag is only 2 h.

A large single dose of vitamin D has biological effects for as long as 6 months (because of metabolism and storage). Thus, the agent is cumulative.

Indications

- The prevention and cure of rickets of all kinds and osteomalacia (vitamin D deficiency).
- Osteoporosis.
- Hypoparathyroidism.
- Psoriasis.
- CKD-MBD (renal osteodystrophy).

Vitamin D deficiency

This can be treated with a variety of vitamin D analogues. Selecting the appropriate preparation requires a knowledge of the underlying aetiology. There are no absolute criteria for vitamin D deficiency; however, serum 25(OH)VitD$_3$ levels are used as a guide to vitamin D levels and there is a general consensus that a 25(OH)D concentration of 50 –75–nmol/L reflects insufficiency, and concentrations of less than 50–nmol/L indicate deficiency.

Although rickets due to *primary* vitamin D deficiency is rare in developed countries, subclinical vitamin D *deficiency* and vitamin D *insufficiency* are now recognised to be extremely common in the UK and in other populations with limited exposure to sunlight, particularly in individuals with increased skin pigmentation, in whom greater amounts of sun exposure are required for adequate synthesis, or in those with excessive body cover. There is accumulating evidence that subclinical vitamin D deficiency has adverse effects on health. Vitamin D deficiency in pregnancy is a significant public health issue: babies born to mothers with low vitamin D levels are at increased risk of neonatal hypocalcaemia and other vitamin D deficiency-related symptoms. Vitamin D deficiency can be prevented in susceptible individuals by taking an oral supplement of *ergocalciferol* 20 micrograms (800 units) daily. All pregnant and lactating women should receive vitamin D supplementation. Breast milk contains negligible amounts of vitamin D thus breast-fed infants receiving less

than 500 mL of formula should be supplemented with vitamin D: *Abidec* and *Dalivit* are two paediatric multivitamin preparations, both containing colecalciferol 400 IU.

For the treatment of simple nutritional vitamin D *deficiency* oral doses of either *colecalciferol* or *ergocalciferol*, 10 000 units daily or 60 000 units weekly, should be given for 12 weeks. Infants and children should receive between 1 000 and 5 000 units of vitamin D$_3$ daily, depending on age (usually *ergocalciferol*), for 12 weeks. Where there are concerns with regards to compliance, 'Stoss' therapy – a single dose of intramuscular *ergocalciferol* 500–000 units – can be given. Nutritional vitamin D *insufficiency* can be treated with 800–1000 units daily for 12 weeks. 25(OH)-vitamin D$_3$ levels should be measured after 12 weeks of treatment. *Alfacalcidol* should not be given for the treatment of vitamin D deficiency as it does not replete vitamin D stores.

Vitamin D deficiency resulting from *intestinal malabsorption or chronic liver disease* usually requires vitamin D in pharmacological doses, e.g. *ergocalciferol* tablets up to 50 000 units daily. The maximum antirachitic effect of vitamin D occurs after 1–2 months, and the plasma calcium concentration reflects the dosage given days or weeks before. Frequent changes of dose are therefore not required. Vitamin D deficiency resulting from *chronic renal failure* is discussed below.

Epileptic patients taking enzyme-inducing drugs long term can develop osteomalacia (adults) or rickets (children). This may arise from the accelerated metabolism, increasing vitamin D breakdown and causing deficiency, or from inhibition of one of the hydroxylations that increase biological activity.

Osteoporosis

Calcitriol is licensed for the management of postmenopausal osteoporosis.

Hypoparathyroidism

The hypocalcaemia of hypoparathyroidism requires 1 000–1 500 mg of elemental calcium daily in divided doses as well as vitamin D. Ergocalciferol may be required in doses up to 100 000 units daily to achieve normocalcaemia, but the dose is difficult to titrate and hypercalcaemia from overdose may take weeks to resolve. *Alfacalcidol* (0.5–2.0 micrograms daily) or *calcitriol* (0.5–1.0 micrograms daily) are therefore preferred, as their rapid onset and offset of action makes for easier control of plasma calcium levels.

Psoriasis

Calcipotriol and *tacalcitol* are vitamin D analogues available as creams or ointments for the treatment of psoriasis.

Renal osteodystrophy

Adverse effects

Vitamin D *toxicity* has been reported in children accidentally overdosed on vitamin D supplements. Symptoms of overdosage are due mainly to an excessive increase in plasma calcium concentration and include anorexia, nausea and vomiting, diarrhoea, constipation, weight loss, polyuria and thirst. Other long-term effects include ectopic calcification almost anywhere in the body, renal damage and an increased calcium output in the urine; renal calculi may form. Recent research has suggested that the safe upper limit of vitamin D therapy be revised. It was previously considered dangerous to exceed 10 000 units daily of vitamin D in an adult for more than about 12 weeks; however, it has now become apparent that such doses are required to render a vitamin D-deficient individual replete. In general, use of vitamin D at pharmacological doses requires monitoring of plasma calcium.

TREATMENT OF CALCIUM AND BONE DISORDERS

Hypocalcaemia

In *acute hypocalcaemia* requiring systemic therapy, give a slow intavenous infusion of 10 mL of 10% *calcium gluconate injection* over 10 min. This should not be given at a faster rate because of the risk of cardiac arrhythmias and arrest. Correction of hypo-

calcaemia is temporary and this should be followed by a continuous intravenous infusion containing ten 10 mL ampoules of 10% calcium gluconate in 1 L of 0.9% saline given at an initial infusion rate of 50 mL/h. Plasma calcium should be monitored and the rate adjusted accordingly. Oral calcium therapy should be initiated meanwhile and the intravenous infusion stopped once the oral agents take effect. Avoid infusing with solutions containing bicarbonate or phosphate, which cause calcium to precipitate. Intramuscular injection is contraindicated as it is painful and causes tissue necrosis. Calcium glubionate (Calcium Sandoz) can be given by deep intramuscular injection in adults. Concurrent hypomagnesaemia should be corrected as hypocalcaemia is resistant to treatment without normal serum magnesium levels.

Treatment of *chronic hypocalcaemia* is with 1 500–2 000 mg of oral elemental calcium daily in divided doses, as either *calcium carbonate* or *calcium citrate*. Additional treatment depends on the cause. Hypocalcaemia secondary to vitamin D deficiency should be treated with vitamin D as described above and there are preparations which combine calcium tablets with colecalciferol. Hypocalcaemia secondary to hypoparathyroidism requires alfacalcidol or calcitriol as PTH is required for hydroxylation of 25-hydroxy-vitamin D_3, thus ergocalciferol or colecalciferol have reduced efficacy.

Adverse effects of intravenous calcium may be very dangerous. An early sign is a tingling feeling in the mouth and of warmth spreading over the body. Serious effects are those on the heart, which mimic and synergise with digitalis, and it is advisable to avoid intravenous calcium administration in any patient taking a digitalis glycoside (except in severe symptomatic hypocalcaemia). The effect of calcium on the heart is antagonised by potassium, and similarly the toxic effects of hyperkalaemia in acute renal failure may be to an extent counteracted by calcium.

Hypercalcaemia

Treatment of severe acute hypercalcaemia causing symptoms is needed whether or not the cause can be removed; generally a plasma concentration of

3.0 mmol/L (12 mg/100 mL) needs urgent treatment if there is also clinical evidence of toxicity (individual tolerance varies greatly).

Temporary measures

After taking account of the patient's cardiac and renal function, the following measures may be employed selectively:

- *Physiological saline solution* is important, firstly to correct sodium and water deficit, and secondly to promote sodium-linked calcium diuresis in the proximal renal tubule. Initially, 500 mL 0.9% saline should be given intravenously over 4 h and then adjusted to maintain urine output at 100-150 mls/hour until the plasma Ca^{2+} level falls below 3.0 mmol/L and the oral intake is adequate. The regimen requires careful attention to fluid and electrolyte balance, particularly in patients with renal insufficiency secondary to hypercalcaemia or heart failure who are unable to excrete excess sodium. The use of furosemide to enhance renal Ca^{2+} excretion has been largely abandoned owing to the exacerbation of electrolyte disturbances and the increased availability of newer agents.

- *Bisphosphonates* are the agents of choice in moderate to severe hypercalcaemia, There are a number of bisphosphonates licensed for this indication but *pamidronate* and *zoledronic acid* are the most widely used agents. *Pamidronate* is active in a wide variety of hypercalcaemic disorders. A fall in the serum calcium concentration begins within the first day, reaches a nadir in 5–6 days and lasts for 20–30 days. *Zoledronic acid* has the advantage of being more potent and it can be administered over a shorter time (4 mg over 15 min versus 2 h). It is a convenient regimen for patients with hypercalcaemia of malignancy where repeat courses may be required every 3–4 weeks.

- *Calcitonin.* When the hypercalcaemia is at least partly due to mobilisation from bone, calcitonin (4 units/kg) can be used to inhibit bone resorption, and may enhance urinary excretion of calcium. The effect develops in a few hours but responsiveness is lost over a few days owing to tachyphylaxis. Calcitonin is not as effective as the bisphosphonates; however, its shorter onset of action makes it a valuable agent for initial management of hypercalcaemia until the peak onset of action of the bisphosphonate at 2–4 days.

- An *adrenocortical steroid*, e.g. prednisolone 20–40 mg/day orally, is effective in particular situations; it reduces the hypercalcaemia of hypervitaminosis D (which is due to excessive intestinal absorption of calcium either secondary to intoxication or granulomatous disease, e.g. sarcoidosis). Corticosteroid may be effective in the hypercalcaemia of malignancy where the disease itself is responsive, e.g. myeloma of lymphoma. Patients with hyperparathyroidism do not respond.

- *Dialysis* is quick and effective and is likely to be needed in severe cases or in those with renal failure.

Longer-term treatment

Sodium cellulose phosphate (Calcisorb) is an oral ion exchange substance with a particular affinity for calcium which is bound in the gut, and the complex eliminated in the faeces. It is effective for patients who over-absorb dietary calcium and develop hypercalciuria and renal stones.

Inorganic phosphate e.g. sodium acid phosphate (Phosphate Sandoz), taken orally, also binds calcium in the gut. It is of particular use for hypercalcaemia resulting from increased intestinal absorption of calcium, e.g. vitamin D intoxication, or increased calcitriol production (as seen with chronic granulomatous disease).

Hypercalciuria

In renal stone formers, in addition to general measures (low calcium diet, high fluid intake), urinary calcium may be diminished by a *thiazide* diuretic (with or without citrate to bind calcium) and oral *phosphate.*

Parathyroid hormone

Parathyroid hormone (PTH) acts chiefly on the kidney, increasing renal tubular reabsorption of calcium and excretion of phosphate; it increases calcium absorption from the gut, indirectly, by stimulating the renal synthesis of 1α,25-vitamin D (Fig. 25.1). PTH increases the rate of bone remodelling (mineral and collagen) and osteocyte activity with, at *high* doses, an overall balance in favour of resorption (*osteoclast activity*) with a rise in plasma calcium concentration (and fall in phosphate); but, at *low* doses, the balance favours bone formation (*osteoblast activity*).

Calcitonin

Calcitonin is a peptide hormone produced by the C cells of the thyroid gland (in mammals). It acts on bone (inhibiting osteoclasts) to reduce the rate of bone turnover, and on the kidney to reduce reabsorption of calcium and phosphate. It is obtained from natural sources (pork, salmon, eel) or synthesised. The $t_{1/2}$ varies according to source; the human $t_{1/2}$ is 10 min. Antibodies develop particularly to pork calcitonin and neutralise its effect; synthetic salmon calcitonin (salcatonin) is therefore preferred for prolonged use; loss of effect may also be due to downregulation of receptors.

Calcitonin is used (subcutaneously, intramuscularly or intranasally) for Paget's disease of bone (relief of pain, and compression of nerves, e.g. auditory cranial), metastatic bone cancer pain, post-menopausal osteoporosis, and for initial control of hypercalcaemia.

Adverse effects include allergy, nausea, flushing and tingling of the face and hands.

Bisphosphonates

Bisphosphonates are synthetic, non-hydrolysable analogues of pyrophosphate (an inhibitor of bone mineralisation) in which the central oxygen atom of the -P-O-P- structure is replaced with a carbon atom to give the -P-C-P- group. There are two classes of bisphosphonates: nitrogen containing (*alendronate, risedronate, ibandronate, pamidronate* and *zoledronate*) and non-nitrogen containing (*clodronate, etidronate* and *tiludronate*).

Actions. These compounds are effective calcium chelators that rapidly target exposed bone mineral surfaces, are imbibed by bone-resorbing osteoclasts, inhibit their function and cause osteoclast apoptosis. An additional action may be to stimulate bone formation by osteoblasts, but the therapeutic utility of bisphosphonates rests on their capacity to inhibit bone resorption.

Bisphosphonate binding to hydroxyapatite crystals can, in high doses, *inhibit* bone mineralisation (potentially causing osteomalacia), an effect that is unrelated to their anti-resorptive efficacy. This disadvantageous effect, prominent with non-nitrogen containing bisphosphonates, is less with newer nitrogen containing members.

Pharmacokinetics

Bisphosphonates are poorly absorbed after ingestion. Absorption is further impaired by food, drinks, and drugs containing calcium, magnesium, iron or aluminium salts. A proportion of bisphosphonate that is absorbed is rapidly incorporated into bone; the remaining fraction is excreted unchanged by the kidneys. Once incorporated into the skeleton, bisphosphonates are released only when the bone is resorbed during turnover. They may be given orally or intravenously. One trial has shown that bioavailability of oral bisphosphonates are greatest if the drug is administered in the early morning, before the first meal of the day.

Indications

- Osteoporosis.
- Paget's disease of bone.
- Hypercalcaemia due to malignancy and metastatic bone disease Bisphosphonates reduce skeletal fractures and loss of skeletal integrity associated with metastatic bone disease. The best evidence for such a benefit comes from use of intravenous *zoledronic acid* in patients with metastatic lung cancer, prostate cancer or breast cancer. There is no evidence that bisphosphonates can prevent bone metastases in these cancers.

Adverse effects of orally administered bisphosphonates include gastrointestinal disturbances, and oesophageal irritation – a particular problem with alendronate. This drug should be taken at least 30 min before food, with the patient remaining erect during this period. Oral bisphosphonates should not be used in patients with Barrett's oesophagus. Disturbances of calcium and mineral metabolism (e.g. vitamin D deficiency, PTH dysfunction) should be corrected before starting a bisphosphonate. Increased bone pain (as well as relief) and fractures (high dose, prolonged use only) can occur due to bone demineralisation. Potential nephrotoxicity is a concern with bisphosphonate therapy although zoledronic acid has been used in patients with severe renal impairment. Intravenous administration can cause acute 'flu-like symptoms (fever, myalgia, malaise). Repeated courses of intravenous bisphosphonates for treatment of hypercalcaemia of malignancy are associated with increased risk of osteonecrosis of the jaw in patients with metastatic bone disease or multiple myeloma. The risk may be slightly greater with zoledronic acid compared with pamidronate.

Osteoporosis

Osteoporosis is a disease characterised by increased skeletal fragility, low bone mineral density (less than 2.5 standard deviations below the mean for young people; Fig. 25.2) and deterioration of bone microarchitecture. It occurs most commonly in postmenopausal women and patients taking long-term corticosteroid. Exclude underlying causes such as hyperthyroidism, hyperparathyroidism and hypogonadism (in both sexes) before treatment is initiated.

Post-menopausal osteoporosis is due to gonadal deficiency; it can be *prevented*. In the UK, one in four women in their sixties and one in two in their seventies experience an osteoporotic fracture. Prevention with combined oestrogen–progestogen therapy was widespread until data from the UK Women's Health Initiative showed an increased risk of breast cancer, stroke and venous thromboembolic disease.

Now, patients at risk of osteoporosis are advised to increase daily exercise, stop smoking and optimise diet to ensure sufficient calories and an adequate intake of calcium and vitamin D. The recommended daily calcium intake of 1 500 mg can be achieved with calcium supplementation (500–1 000 mg in divided doses daily). Vitamin D supplementation with ergocalciferol can be given to ensure a daily intake of 800 IU.

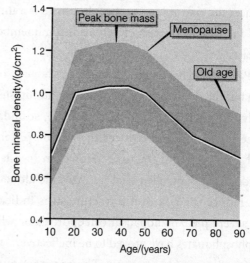

Fig. 25.2 Bone mineral density of the lumbar spine in women. The shaded area represents two standard deviations above and below the mean for bone mineral density.

Pharmacotherapy

Bisphosphonates are the first-line treatment for postmenopausal osteoporosis. Four bisphosphonates (alendronate, etidronate, risedronate, ibandronate) are currently licensed in the UK for the treatment of osteoporosis (zoledronate is also effective). Alendronate (10 mg once daily or 70 mg once weekly) and risedronate (5 mg daily or 35 mg once weekly) are effective both at preventing post-menopausal osteoporosis and at reducing hip and vertebral fracture incidence. Ibandronate is effective as a once-monthly preparation, or intravenously every 3 months for those unable to tolerate oral bisphosphonates. Ibandronate has been shown to have efficacy in reducing the risk of new vertebral fractures; however, randomised controlled trials conducted with ibandronate did not have sufficient power to demonstrate efficacy in hip fractures All post-menopausal women with a history of hip or verterbral fracture, or with osteoporosis based on bone mineral density measurement should receive bisphosphonate therapy.

Selective oestrogen receptor modulator. Raloxifene is effective for both the prevention and treatment of osteoporosis; it reduces the incidence of vertebral but not of non-vertebral fractures. It is probably less effective than bisphosphonates but no direct comparisons have been made. Raloxifene reduces the risk of breast cancer but there is a three-fold increase in the risk of venous thromboembolic disease.

Parathyroid hormone. PTH increases bone resorption but the synthetic PTH, teriparatide, administered daily (20 micrograms, subcutaneously), stimulates bone formation and reduces the risk of vertebral and non-vertebral fractures. However, in a large randomised controlled trial, teriparatide alone did not reduce the risk of hip fracture. It is indicated for severe post-menopausal osteoporosis or where bisphosphonates have proved to be ineffective.

Oestrogen–progestogen. Though now out of favour, oestrogen–progestogen therapy may yet be indicated in a small proportion of post-menopausal women with documented osteoporosis or osteopenia, or those at increased risk of osteoporosis, who do not have a personal or family history of breast cancer or cardiovascular disease and are unable to tolerate alternative anti-resorptive agents.

Calcitonin. The mode of administration (subcutaneous, intramuscular or nasal) and possible tachyphylaxis make calcitonin a less suitable choice for treatment of osteoporosis. Additionally, the increase in bone mineral density and reduction in fracture risk is small compared with alternative agents.

Fracture (usually assessed by vertebral and hip fractures) is the only important outcome of osteoporosis.

Corticosteroid-induced osteoporosis. Most bone loss occurs during the first 6–12 months of use. Patients taking the equivalent of prednisolone 7.5 mg or more each day for more than 3 months should be considered for prophylactic treatment, and it is mandatory in those aged over 65 years. All patients should receive vitamin D and calcium supplements. Bisphosphonates are first line for both prophylaxis and treatment; calcitonin may be considered where bisphosphonates are contraindicated or not tolerated.

Chronic kidney disease – mineral bone disorder (CKD-MBD)

The pathogenesis of CKD-MBD is complex reflecting the combined contribution of hyperphosphataemia, vitamin D deficiency and secondary hyperparathyroidism. Vitamin D deficiency in chronic renal failure results from reduced synthesis of *calcitriol*. High serum phosphate and high levels of the phosphaturic hormone fibroblast growth factor-23 (FGF-23) both suppress 1α-hydroxylase activity and this, combined with reduced levels of renal 1α-hydroxylase, results in reduced $1\alpha,25$-dihydroxyvitamin D_3 synthesis. Failure of $1\alpha,25$-dihydroxyvitamin D_3 to occupy receptors on the parathyroid glands leads to increased release of PTH. In addition, reduced calcitriol results in decreased intestinal absorption of calcium and the subsequent hypocalcaemia further stimulates PTH release. The aim of treatment is to maintain normal serum phosphate and calcium levels and suppress secondary hyperparathyroidism in order to prevent disordered bone metabolism. An elevated PTH is the earliest sign of disordered bone and mineral metabolism and is usually apparent once the glomerular filtration rate (GFR) falls below 60 mL/min/1.73 m^2 (CKD Stage 3).

Phosphate binders are the first step in the management of hyperphosphataemia and prevention of renal osteodystrophy. The aim of treatment has been to prevent secondary hyperparathyroidism; however, recent observational studies have suggested a link between hyperphosphataemia and adverse clinical outcomes, possible secondary to accelerated vascular calcification, providing aditional rationale for normalising serum phosphate levels. Calcium-based phosphate binders, such as *calcium carbonate* and *calcium acetate*, are the most commonly used agents with similar efficacy. Newer non calcium-based phosphate binders include the anion exchange resins *sevelamer hydrocholoride* and *sevelamer carbonate*. These have a similar phosphate lowering effect compared to calcium based agents but are associated with reduced risk of hypercalcaemia. Sevelamer hydrochloride may worsen metabolic acidosis thus sevelamer carbonate is the preferred agent. *Lanthanum carbonate* is a non-aluminium, non-calcium-based phosphate binder with similar efficacy to calcium-based phosphate binders. There are fewer data from good quality, large clinical trials evaluating lanthanum; short-term trials suggest increased adverse effects compared with other binders.

Phosphate binders alone may not be sufficient to control phosphate levels and prevent secondary hyperparathyroidism. Vitamin D analogues or the calcimimetic *cinacalcet* are instituted once PTH levels rise. There is a lack of evidence and thus consensus with regards to the 'optimum' PTH levels in CKD. US National Kidney Foundation Kidney Disease Outcomes Quality Initiative (K/DOQI) guidelines recommend instituting therapy when PTH levels rise above 75, 110 and 300 picograms/mL for CKD 3, 4, and 5 respectively, despite optimal phosphate binder therapy, i.e. to achieve the aim of preventing hyperparathyroidism, rather than treating established osteodystrophy. However, the target PTH remains uncertain as there is currently no good evidence that normalisation of PTH levels in adults results in reduced morbidity and mortality. Recent Kidney Disease: Improving Global Outcomes (KDIGO) guidelines reflect this uncertainty and do not set target PTH levels for pre-dialysis patients.

Calcitriol and vitamin D analogues (e.g. *alfacalcidol*, above) inhibit PTH gene transcription by the vitamin D receptor and will also increase the serum concentration of Ca^{2+}, which acts on the parathyroid Ca^{2+} receptor further to inhibit PTH secretion. Note that vitamin D analogues, by increasing intestinal phosphate absorption, can worsen hyperphosphataemia. Because of the increase in serum calcium and phosphate that can occur with vitamin D therapy, *cinacalcet* is preferred in patients with serum phosphate or calcium levels at the upper limit of normal. *Cinacalcet* is a calcium analogue that binds to the calcium sensing receptor (CaSR) in the parathyroids and increases the sensitivity of the receptor to Ca (it is the only example of an allosteric agonist in clinical use). Calcium signalling through the CaSR is the main determinant of PTH secretion. It is indicated for patients with end-stage renal disease with secondary hyperparathyroidism refractory to standard treatment.

Osteomalacia

Osteomalacia is due to *primary* or *secondary* vitamin D deficiency (see above).

Paget's disease of bone

This disease is characterised by increased bone turnover (resorption and formation) – as much as 50 times normal. The result is large, vascular, deformed and painful bones that fracture.

Bisphosphonates

The newer nitrogen-containing bisphosphonates (*pamidronate, zoledronic acid, risedronate, alendronate*) are the agents of choice. These bisphosphonates suppress bone turnover without impairing bone mineralisation. *Alendronate* and *risedronate* are administered orally whereas *pamidronate* and *zoledronic acid* are given intravenously. Their response is dose related and biochemical remission (normalisation of alkaline phosphatase) after a course may last for up to 2 years. Supplementation with calcium and vitamin D is required to prevent hypocalcaemia.

Calcitonin (which also inhibits bone resorption) has been largely superseded by the bisphosphonates but retains usefulness because it reduces bone blood flow before surgery.

VITAMIN E: TOCOPHEROL

The functions of vitamin E may be to take up (scavenge) the free radicals generated by normal metabolic processes and by substances in the environment, e.g. hydrocarbons. This prevents free radicals from attacking polyunsaturated fats in cell membranes with resultant cellular injury.

A deficiency syndrome is recognised, including peripheral neuropathy with spinocerebellar degeneration, and a haemolytic anaemia in premature infants.

α-*Tocopheryl acetate* (Ephynal) pharmacotherapy may benefit the neuromuscular complications of congenital cholestasis and abetalipoproteinaemia.

SUMMARY

Vitamins, nutrients indispensable to normal functions of the body, are comprised a class of low molecular organic compounds closely related to metabolism. Despite the trace amount as needed by the body, the role of vitamins cannot be neglected. At present, vitamins are an important treatment of clinical malnutrition. Rational usage of vitamins is an important management for recovery of disease and prevention regression.

Vitamins are classified as either water-soluble or fat-soluble. In humans, among 13 vitamins, 4 of them are fat-soluble (A, B, E and K), and 9 of them are water-soluble (8 B vitamins and vitamin C).

Vitamins have diverse biochemical functions. The B complex vitamins, which are the largest group of vitamins, function as enzyme cofactors or the precursors for them; For example, vitamin D has hormone-like functions that regulates mineral metabolism, or regulates cell and tissue growth and differentiation. Others function as antioxidants, e.g., vitamin E and vitamin C.

Our body cannot synthesize vitamins except some vitamin D, which are made from nicotinamide from tryptophan. Lack of a particular vitamin may lead to a specific deficient syndrome. Well-known vitamin deficiencies involve thiamine (beriberi), niacin (pellagra), and vitamin C (scurvy) and vitamin D (rickets). Vitamin deficiencies may be primary (inadequate diet) or secondary, due to failure of absorption (intestinal abnormality or chronic diarrhoea) or to increased metabolic need (growth, pregnancy, lactation, hyperthyroidism). Vitamin deficiencies are commonly multiple and complex clinical pictures occur. There are numerous single and multivitamin preparations available to provide prophylaxis and therapy.

In most cases, vitamins are used only as adjunctive medications. Exaggerate the role of vitamins, blindly supplement vitamins or taking large doses of vitamins can only be more harm than good.

IMPORTANT TERMINOLOGY

acute promyelocytic leukaemi 急性早幼粒细胞白血病

scurvy 坏血病

methaemoglobinaemia 高铁血红蛋白血症

hypocalcaemia 低钙血症

hypercalcaemia 高钙血症

osteoporosis 骨质疏松症

CHALLENGE YOURSELF

1. Which are commonly used water-soluble and fat-soluble vitamins, respectively?
2. What are their physiological and pharmacological functions?
3. What is the clinical manifestation of each vitamin deficiency? How to prevent or treat vitamin deficiency?
4. What are the clinical applications of various vitamins? What are the side effects of excessive usage of vitamins?

Jinhan He

INDEX